Quantification
of Brain Function
Using PET

Quantification of Brain Function Using PET

Edited by

Ralph Myers
Vin Cunningham
Dale Bailey
Terry Jones

PET Methodology Group, Cyclotron Unit
MRC Clinical Sciences Centre
Royal Postgraduate Medical School
Hammersmith Hospital
London, United Kingdom

Academic Press

San Diego   New York   Boston   London   Sydney   Tokyo   Toronto

Find Us on the Web! http://www.apnet.com

Academic Press, Inc.
A Division of Harcourt Brace & Company
525 B Street, Suite 1900, San Diego, California 92101-4495

United Kingdom Edition published by
Academic Press Limited
24-28 Oval Road, London NW1 7DX

Library of Congress Cataloging-in-Publication Data

Quantification of brain function using PET / edited by Ralph Myers,
    ... [et al.].
        p.   cm.
    Includes index.
    ISBN 0-12-389760-2 (alk. paper)
    1. Brain--Tomography.   2. Brain-Radionuclide imaging.   3. Brain-
-Metabolism.   I. Myers, Ralph, date.
    QP376.Q363   1996
    612.8'2--dc20   96-10926
                                                 CIP

PRINTED IN THE UNITED STATES OF AMERICA
96 97 98 99 00 01 EB 9 8 7 6 5 4 3 2 1

Contents

6. Autoradiography as a Tool for PET/SPECT Tracer Selection and Assessment

A. BIEGON, C. MATHIS, AND W. JAGUST

7. Radioactive Metabolites of the 5-HT$_{1A}$ Receptor Radioligand, [O-methyl-^{11}C]WAY-100635, in Humans

S. OSMAN, J. A. MCCARRON, S. P. HUME, S. ASHWORTH, V. W. PIKE, S. K. LUTHRA, A. A. LAMMERTSMA, C. BENCH, P. GRASBY, I. A. CLIFFE, AND A. FLETCHER

8. [^{11}C]Nefopam as a Potential PET Tracer of Serotonin Reuptake Sites: Initial Findings in Living Pig Brain

DONALD F. SMITH, ROBERT GLASER, ANTHONY GEE, AND ALBERT GJEDDE

9. The Effect of Amine pK_a on the Transport and Binding of Amphetamine Analogs in the Pig Brain: An in Vivo Comparison of β,β-Difluoro[N-methyl-^{11}C]methamphetamine and [N-methyl-^{11}C]Methamphetamine Using PET

A. D. GEE, N. GILLINGS, D. SMITH, O. INOUE, K. KOBAYASHI, AND A. GJEDDE

10. Tracer Selection Summary 47

MICHAEL R. KILBOURN

PART

II

DATA ACQUISITION

11. Application of Simultaneous Emission and Transmission Scanning to Quantitative Cerebral PET

STEVEN R. MEIKLE, STEFAN EBERL, BRIAN F. HUTTON, PATRICK K. HOOPER, AND MICHAEL J. FULHAM

12. A New PET Camera for Noninvasive Quantitation of Physiological Functional Parametric Images: Headtome-V-Dual

HIDEHIRO IIDA, SHUICHI MIURA, IWAO KANNO, TOSHIHIDE OGAWA, AND KAZUO UEMURA

P A R T

V

STATISTICAL ANALYSIS

Contributors

Numbers in parentheses indicate the pages on which the authors' contributions begin.

M. Adam (227) Neurodegenerative Disorders Centre and TRIUMF, University of British Columbia, Vancouver, British Columbia, Canada

Nathaniel M. Alpert (141, 249, 425) PET Imaging Laboratory and Radiology Department, Massachusetts General Hospital, and Harvard Medical School, Boston, Massachusetts 02114

J. R. Anderson (378) PET Imaging Section, VA Medical Center, Minneapolis, Minnesota 55417

Nancy C. Andreasen (365, 389) The Mental Health Clinical Research Center, Department of Psychiatry, University of Iowa Hospitals and Clinics, Iowa City, Iowa 52242

A. Antonini (224) PET Department, Paul Scherrer Institute, CH-5232 Villigen, Switzerland

Babak A. Ardekani (113) Department of Applied Physics, University of Technology, Sydney, New South Wales 2007, Australia

Stephan Arndt (365, 389) The Mental Health Clinical Research Center, Department of Psychiatry, and Department of Preventive Medicine and Environmental Health, The University of Iowa Hospitals and Clinics, Iowa City, Iowa 52242

John Ashburner (301, 317) Cyclotron Unit, MRC Clinical Sciences Centre, Hammersmith Hospital, London W12 0NN, United Kingdom

Sharon Ashworth (12, 34, 62) PET Methodology Group, Cyclotron Unit, MRC Clinical Sciences Centre, Royal Postgraduate Medical School, Hammersmith Hospital, London W12 0NN, United Kingdom

Dale L. Bailey (82) MRC Cyclotron Unit, Hammersmith Hospital, London W12 0NN, United Kingdom

E. Baker (9) Department of Medical Physics, University of Wisconsin Medical School, Madison, Wisconsin 53706

D. G. Barnes (415) Centre for Positron Emission Tomography, Austin Repatriation Medical Centre, Melbourne 3084, Australia

C. Bench (34) PET Neuroscience Group, MRC Clinical Sciences Centre, Royal Postgraduate Medical School, Hammersmith Hospital, London W12 0NN, United Kingdom; and Charing Cross and Westminster Medical School, London W6 8RF, United Kingdom

B. Bendriem (88, 243) CEA, Service Hospitalier Frédéric Joliot, Orsay 91406, France

D. Berdichevsky (141) PET Imaging Laboratory, Massachusetts General Hospital, Boston, Massachusetts 02114

A. Biegon (26) Pharmos Ltd., Kiryat Weizmann Science Park, Rehovot, Israel

R. C. Blair (334) Department of Epidemiology and Biostatistics, College of Public Health, University of South Florida, Tampa, Florida

G. Blomqvist (170) Department of Clinical Neuroscience, Experimental Alcohol and Drug Addiction Research Section, and Section of Clinical Neurophysiology, Karolinska Hospital, S-17176 Stockholm, Sweden

Peter M. Bloomfield (12, 62, 191) PET Methodology Group, Cyclotron Unit, MRC Clinical Sciences Centre, Royal Postgraduate Medical School, Hammersmith Hospital, London W12 0NN, United Kingdom

Laura L. Boles Ponto (365, 384, 389) Positron Emission Tomography Imaging Center, Department of Radiology, University of Iowa Hospitals and Clinics, Iowa City, Iowa 52242

Paul Brakeman (152) Department of Neuroscience, The Johns Hopkins Medical Institutions, Baltimore, Maryland 21205

Michael Braun (113) Department of Applied Physics, University of Technology, Sydney, New South Wales 2007, Australia

David J. Brooks (82) MRC Cyclotron Unit, Hammersmith Hospital, London W12 0NN, United Kingdom; and Institute of Neurology, London W12 0NN, United Kingdom

C. K. Brown (384) Department of Preventive Medicine and Environmental Health, University of Iowa, Iowa City, Iowa 52242

W. D. Brown (9, 138) Department of Radiology, University of Wisconsin Medical School, Madison, Wisconsin 53792

T. Bruckbauer (410) Max Planck Institute for Neurological Research, 50931 Cologne, Germany

K. R. Buckley (227) Neurodegenerative Disorders Centre and TRIUMF, University of British Columbia, Vancouver, British Columbia, Canada

C. Calonder (307) Paul Scherrer Institute, CH 5232 Villigen PSI, Switzerland

Gregory Campbell (98) Biometry and Field Studies Branch, National Institute of Neurological Disorders and Stroke, National Institutes of Health, Bethesda, Maryland 20892

Richard E. Carson (98, 185, 321) PET Department, Clinical Center, National Institutes of Health, Bethesda, Maryland 20892

Thomas Chaly (219, 232) Departments of Neurology, Research, Medicine, and Biostatistics, North Shore University Hospital, Cornell University Medical College, Manhasset, New York 11030

G. L-Y. Chan (227) Neurodegenerative Disorders Centre and TRIUMF, University of British Columbia, Vancouver, British Columbia, Canada

Chin-Tu Chen (109, 292) Franklin McLean Memorial Research Institute, Department of Radiology, The University of Chicago, Chicago, Illinois 60637

Ted Cizadlo (365, 389) The Mental Health Clinical Research Center, Department of Psychiatry, University of Iowa Hospitals and Clinics, Iowa City, Iowa 52242

I. A. Cliffe (34) Wyeth Research (U.K.) Ltd., Taplow, Maidenhead, Berkshire SL6 0PH, United Kingdom

D. L. Collins (123) Montreal Neurological Institute, McGill University, McConnell Brain Imaging Centre, Montreal, Quebec H3A 2B4, Canada

Malcolm Cooper (109, 292) Franklin McLean Memorial Research Institute, Department of Radiology, The University of Chicago, Chicago, Illinois 60637

F. Crivello (342) Groupe d'Imagerie Neurofonctionnelle, Service Hospitalier Frédéric Joliot, CEA-DRM, 91401 Orsay, France; and EA 1555, Université Paris 7, Paris, France

M. Crossnoe (138) Department of Radiology, University of Wisconsin Medical School, Madison, Wisconsin 53792

Paul Cumming (237) McConnell Brain Imaging Center, Montreal Neurological Institute and Department of Neurology and Neurosurgery, McGill University, Montreal, Quebec H3A 2B4, Canada

Vincent J. Cunningham (191, 266, 292, 301, 317) Cyclotron Unit, MRC Clinical Sciences Centre, Hammersmith Hospital, London W12 0NN, United Kingdom

J. Czernin (147) Division of Nuclear Medicine and Biophysics, Department of Molecular and Medical Pharmacology, UCLA School of Medicine, Los Angeles, California 90095

M. Dahlbom (147) Division of Nuclear Medicine and Biophysics, Department of Molecular and Medical Pharmacology, UCLA School of Medicine, Los Angeles, California 90095

H. Damasio (384) Department of Neurology, Division of Behavioral Neurology and Cognitive Neuroscience, University of Iowa, Iowa City, Iowa 52242

J. DaSilva (262) PET Centre, Clarke Institute of Psychiatry, University of Toronto, Toronto M5T 1R8, Canada

Margaret E. Daube-Witherspoon (98) PET Department, Clinical Center, National Institutes of Health, Bethesda, Maryland 20892

O. T. DeJesus (9) Department of Medical Physics, University of Wisconsin Medical School, Madison, Wisconsin 53792

J. Delforge (243) C. E. A. Service Hospitalier F. Joliot, 91400 Orsay, France

Vijay Dhawan (219, 232) Departments of Neurology, Research, Medicine, and Biostatistics, North Shore University Hospital, Cornell University Medical College, Manhasset, New York 11030

S. Dickhoven (175) Max Planck Institute for Neurological Research and University Hospital, Department of Neurology, D-50931 Cologne, Germany

Mirko Diksic (237) McConnell Brain Imaging Center, Montreal Neurological Institute and Department of Neurology and Neurosurgery, McGill University Faculty of Medicine, Montreal, Quebec H3A 2B4, Canada

Stefan Eberl (51) The PET Department, Division of Medical Imaging Services, Royal Prince Alfred Hospital, Sydney, Australia

G. F. Egan (415) Centre for Positron Emission Tomography, Austin Repatriation Medical Centre, Melbourne 3084, Australia

David Eidelberg (219, 232) Departments of Neurology, Research, Medicine, and Biostatistics, North Shore University Hospital, Cornell University Medical College, Manhasset, New York 11030

Lars Eriksson (102, 170) Department of Clinical Neurophysiology and Department of Clinical Neuroscience, Experimental Alcohol and Drug Addiction Research Section, Section of Clinical Neurophysiology, Karolinska Hospital Institute, S-17176 Stockholm, Sweden

Alan C. Evans (123, 158, 201, 327, 421, 434) Positron Imaging Laboratories, McConnell Brain Imaging Centre, Montreal Neurological Institute, McGill University, Montreal, Quebec H3A 2B4, Canada

G. R. Fink (410) Max Planck Institute for Neurological Research, Cologne, Germany; and Neurology Clinic of the University of Cologne, 50931 Cologne, Germany

Alan J. Fischman (249, 425) Radiology Department, Massachusetts General Hospital and Harvard Medical School, Boston, Massachusetts 02114

Ronald E. Fisher (425) Radiology Department, Massachusetts General Hospital and Harvard Medical School, Boston, Massachusetts 02114

A. Fletcher (34) Wyeth Research (U.K.) Ltd., Taplow, Maidenhead, Berkshire SL6 0PH, United Kingdom

A. Fontaine (88) CEA, Service Hospitalier Frédéric Joliot, Orsay 91406, France

I. Ford (334) Department of Statistics, University of Glasgow, Glasgow, Scotland, United Kingdom

G. Forse (20) PET Methodology Group, Clinical Sciences Centre, Royal Postgraduate Medical School, Hammersmith Hospital, London W12 0NN, United Kingdom

R. S. J. Frackowiak (359) The Wellcome Department of Cognitive Neurology, Institute of Neurology, Queen Square, London WC1N 3BG, United Kingdom

R. J. Frank (384) Department of Preventative Medicine and Environmental Health, University of Iowa, Iowa City, Iowa 52242

K. J. Friston (266, 359) MRC Cyclotron Unit, Hammersmith Hospital, London W12 0HS, United Kingdom; and Wellcome Cognitive Neurology Department, London WC1 3BG, United Kingdom

J. James Frost (152) Departments of Environmental Health Sciences and Neuroscience, Division of Nuclear Medicine, The Johns Hopkins Medical Institutions, Baltimore, Maryland 21205

V. Frouin (88) CEA, Service Hospitalier Frédéric Joliot, Orsay 91406, France

Hideaki Fujita (362) Department of Radiology and Nuclear Medicine, Akita Research Institute of Brain and Blood Vessels, Akita 010, Japan

Takehiko Fujiwara (67, 191, 206, 317) Division of Nuclear Medicine, Cyclotron and Radioisotope Center, Tohoku University, Sendai 980-77, Japan

H. Fukuda (317) Department of Radiology and Nuclear Medicine, Institute of Development, Aging and Cancer, Tohoku University, Sendai 980-77, Japan

Michael J. Fulham (51) The PET Department, Division of Medical Imaging Services, Royal Prince Alfred Hospital, Sydney, Australia

Anthony D. Gee (38, 42) PET Center, Aarhus University Hospitals, 8000 Aarhus C, Denmark

N. Gillings (42) PET Centre, Aarhus University Hospital, 8000 Aarhus C, Denmark

Albert Gjedde (38, 42, 72, 201, 237, 421) PET Centre, Aarhus University Hospital, 8000 Aarhus C, Denmark; and Positron Imaging Laboratories, McConnell Brain Imaging Centre and Montreal Neurological Institute, McGill University, Montreal, Quebec H3A 2B4, Canada

Robert Glaser (38) Department of Chemistry, Ben-Gurion University of the Negev, Beersheva 84105, Israel

T. J. Grabowski (384) Department of Neurology, Division of Behavioral Neurology and Cognitive Neuroscience, University of Iowa, Iowa City, Iowa 52242

R. Graf (16) Max Planck Institute for Neurological Research and University of Cologne Neurology Clinic, D-50931 Cologne, Germany

S. T. Grafton (353) Departments of Neurology and Nuclear Medicine, University of Southern California, Los Angeles, California

Michael M. Graham (277, 297, 312) Department of Radiology (Nuclear Medicine) and Division of Nuclear Medicine, University of Washington Medical Center, Seattle, Washington 98195

P. Grasby (34) PET Neuroscience Group, MRC Clinical Sciences Centre, Royal Postgraduate Medical School, Hammersmith Hospital, London W12 0NN, United Kingdom

R. N. Gunn (20, 266) PET Neuroscience and Methodology Groups, Clinical Sciences Centre, Royal Postgraduate Medical School, Hammersmith Hospital, London W12 0NN, United Kingdom

I. Günther (224) PET Department, Paul Scherrer Institute, CH 5232 Villigen, Switzerland

S. Hagisawa (67) Division of Nuclear Medicine, Cyclotron Radioisotope Center, Tohoku University, Sendai 980-77, Japan

A. Haida (20) PET Methodology Group, Clinical Sciences Centre, Royal Postgraduate Medical School, Hammersmith Hospital, London W12 0NN, United Kingdom

M. Halber (175, 209, 410) Max Planck Institute for Neurological Research and University Hospital, Department of Neurology, D-50931 Cologne, Germany

Mark Hallett (98) Human Motor Control Section, Medical Neurology Branch, National Institutes of Health, Bethesda, Maryland 20892

Lars K. Hansen (271, 378) CONNECT, Electronics Institute, Technical University of Denmark, DK-2800 Lyngby, Denmark

Greg Harris (389) The Mental Health Clinical Research Center, Department of Psychiatry, The University of Iowa Hospitals and Clinics, Iowa City, Iowa 52242

Jane Haslam (301) Medical Biophysics, Medical School, Manchester, United Kingdom

Steen Hasselbalch (271) Department of Neurology, National University Hospital, Rigshospitalet, DK-2100 Copenhagen, Denmark

Jun Hatazawa (362) Department of Radiology and Nuclear Medicine, Akita Research Institute of Brain and Blood Vessels, Akita 010, Japan

W.-D. Heiss (16, 175, 209, 410) Max Planck Institute for Neurological Research and University of Cologne Neurology Clinic, D-50931 Cologne, Germany

K. Herholz (175, 209, 410) Max Planck Institute for Neurological Research and University Hospital, Department of Neurology, D-50931 Cologne, Germany

Peter Herscovitch (98) PET Department, Clinical Center, National Institutes of Health, Bethesda, Maryland 20892

H. Herzog (118, 393) Institute of Medicine, Research Centre, Jülich 52425, Germany

Richard D. Hichwa (365, 384, 389) Positron Emission Tomography Imaging Center, Department of Radiology, University of Iowa Hospitals and Clinics, Iowa City, Iowa 52242

C. Hoh (147) Division of Nuclear Medicine and Biophysics, Department of Molecular and Medical Pharmacology, UCLA School of Medicine, Los Angeles, California 90095

J. E. Holden (9, 138, 227) Department of Medical Physics, University of Wisconsin Medical School, Madison, Wisconsin 53792

Søren Holm (93, 271) Departments of Neurology and Nuclear Medicine, The National University Hospital, Rigshospitalet, DK-2100 Copenhagen, Denmark

A. P. Holmes (334, 359) Department of Statistics, University of Glasgow, Glasgow, United Kingdom; and Wellcome Department of Cognitive Neurology, Institute of Neurology, London W12 0NN, United Kingdom

C. J. Holmes (123) Montreal Neurological Institute, McGill University, McConnell Brain Imaging Centre, Montreal, Quebec H3A 2B4, Canada

Patrick K. Hooper (51) The PET Department, Division of Medical Imaging Services, Royal Prince Alfred Hospital, Sydney, Australia

S. Houle (262) PET Centre, Clarke Institute of Psychiatry, University of Toronto, Toronto, Ontario M5T 1R8, Canada

D. Houser (9) Primate Research Center, University of Wisconsin, Madison, Wisconsin 53792

Sung-Cheng Huang (147, 404) Division of Nuclear Medicine and Biophysics, Department of Molecular and Medical Pharmacology, UCLA School of Medicine, Los Angeles, California 90095

S. P. Hume (12, 34) PET Methodology Group, MRC Clinical Sciences Centre, Royal Postgraduate Medical School, Hammersmith Hospital, London W12 0NN, United Kingdom

Richard R. Hurtig (365) Department of Speech, Pathology and Audiology, University of Iowa Hospitals and Clinics, Iowa City, Iowa 52242

D. Hussey (262) PET Centre, Clarke Institute of Psychiatry, University of Toronto, Toronto, Ontario M5T 1R8, Canada

Brian F. Hutton (51, 113) The PET Department, Division of Medical Imaging Services, Royal Prince Alfred Hospital, Sydney, Australia; and Department of Medical Physics, Westmead Hospital, Westmead, New South Wales, Australia

M. Iacoboni (353) Department of Neurology and Division of Brain Mapping, UCLA School of Medicine, Los Angeles, California 90095

T. Ido (67, 317) Division of Radiopharmaceutical Chemistry, Cyclotron Radioisotope Center, Tohoku University, Sendai 980-77, Japan

Hidehiro Iida (57, 404) Akita Research Institute of Brain and Blood Vessels, Akita City 010, Japan

O. Inoue (42) National Institute of Radiological Sciences, Chiba-shi 260, Japan

Kazunari Ishii (362) Department of Radiology and Nuclear Medicine, Akita Research Institute of Brain and Blood Vessels, Akita 010, Japan

Tatsuya Ishikawa (219, 232) Departments of Neurology, Research, Medicine, and Biostatistics, North Shore University Hospital, Cornell University Medical College, Manhasset, New York 11030

H. Itoh (317) Department of Radiology and Nuclear Medicine, Institute of Development, Aging and Cancer, Tohoku University, Sendai 980-77, Japan

Masatoshi Itoh (67, 191, 206, 317) Division of Nuclear Medicine, Cyclotron and Radioisotope Center, Tohoku University, Sendai 980-77, Japan

R. Iwata (67, 317) Division of Radiopharmaceutical Chemistry, Cyclotron and Radioisotope Center, Tohoku University, Sendai 980-77, Japan

F. Jadali (76) PET Facility, Department of Radiology, University of Pittsburgh Medical Center, Pittsburgh, Pennsylvania 15213

W. Jagust (26) Lawrence Berkeley Laboratory Center for Functional Imaging, Berkeley, California 94720

S. Jivan (227) Neurodegenerative Disorders Centre and TRIUMF, University of British Columbia, Vancouver, British Columbia, Canada

M. Joliot (342) Groupe d'Imagerie Neurofonctionnelle, Service Hospitalier Frédéric Joliot, CEA-DRM, 91401 Orsay, France; and EA 1555, Université Paris 7, Paris, France

A. K. P. Jones (191) Rheumatic Diseases Centre, Hope Hospital, Manchester, United Kingdom

C. Jones (262) PET Centre, Clarke Institute of Psychiatry, University of Toronto, Toronto, Ontario M5T 1R8, Canada

Terry Jones (12, 20, 62, 191, 266, 301, 317) PET Methodology Group, Cyclotron Unit, MRC Clinical Sciences Centre, Royal Postgraduate Medical School, Hammersmith Hospital, London W12 0NN, United Kingdom

Iwao Kanno (57, 113, 362, 404) Department of Radiology and Nuclear Medicine, Akita Research Insitute for Brain and Blood Vessels, Akita City 010, Japan

Chien-Min Kao (109) Franklin McLean Memorial Research Institute, Department of Radiology, The University of Chicago, Chicago, Illinois 60637

S. Kapur (262) PET Centre, Clarke Institute of Psychiatry, University of Toronto, Toronto, Ontario M5T 1R8, Canada

H. Karbe (175) Max Planck Institute for Neurological Research and University Hospital, Department of Neurology, D-50931 Cologne, Germany

J. Kessler (410) Max Planck Institute for Neurological Research, D-50931 Cologne, Germany

Michael R. Kilbourn (3, 47) Division of Nuclear Medicine, Department of Internal Medicine, University of Michigan Medical School, Ann Arbor, Michigan 48109

Yuichi Kimura (282, 287) Division of Instrumentation Engineering, Tokyo Medical and Dental University, Tokyo 113, Japan

P. E. Kinahan (76) PET Facility, Department of Radiology, University of Pittsburgh Medical Center, Pittsburgh, Pennsylvania 15213

U. Knorr (393) Department of Neurology, University of Düsseldorf, Düsseldorf, Germany

K. Kobayashi (42) National Institute of Radiological Sciences, Chiba-shi 260, Japan

E. Rota Kops (118) Institute of Medicine, Research Centre, Jülich 52425, Germany

Yukio Kosugi (166) Tokyo Institute of Technology, Yokohama 226, Japan

Mark Kruger (152) Department of Radiology, Division of Nuclear Medicine, The Johns Hopkins Medical Institutions, Baltimore, Maryland 21205

Hiroto Kuwabara (201, 214, 237, 421) Positron Imaging Laboratories, McConnell Brain Imaging Centre, Montreal Neurological Institute and Department of Neurology and Neurosurgery, McGill University Faculty of Medicine, Montreal, Quebec H3A 2B4, Canada

Adriaan A. Lammertsma (12, 34, 62, 191) PET Methodology Group, MRC Clinical Sciences Centre, Cyclotron Unit, Royal Postgraduate Medical School, Hammersmith Hospital, London W12 0NN, United Kingdom

L. Laurier (342) Groupe d'Imagerie Neurofonctionnelle, Service Hospitalier Frédéric Joliot, CEA-DRM, 91401 Orsay, France; and EA 1555, Université Paris 7, Paris, France

Ian Law (93, 271) Department of Neurology, National University Hospital, Rigshospitalet, DK-2100 Copenhagen, Denmark

K. L. Leenders (224, 307, 393) PET Department, Paul Scherrer Institute, CH 5232 Villigen PSI, Switzerland

B. Legg (227) Neurodegenerative Disorders Centre and TRIUMF, University of British Columbia, Vancouver, British Columbia, Canada

Z. Levin (141) PET Imaging Laboratory, Massachusetts General Hospital, Boston, Massachusetts, 02114

Kang-Ping Lin (404) Department of Electrical Engineering, Chung-Yuan University, Taiwan

Jonathan M. Links (152) Departments of Radiology and Environmental Health Sciences, Division of Nuclear Medicine, The Johns Hopkins Medical Institutions, Baltimore, Maryland 21205

B. Lipinski (118) Institute of Medicine, Research Centre, Jülich 52425, Germany

B. J. Lopresti (76) PET Facility, Department of Radiology, University of Pittsburgh Medical Center, Pittsburgh, Pennsylvania 15213

J. Löttgen (16) Max Planck Institute for Neurological Research, University of Cologne Neurology Clinic, D-50931 Cologne, Germany

S. K. Luthra (34) PET Methodology Group, MRC Clinical Sciences Centre, Royal Postgraduate Medical School, Hammersmith Hospital, London W12 0NN, United Kingdom

Yilong Ma (158) Positron Imaging Laboratories, McConnell Brain Imaging Centre, Montreal Neurological Institute, McGill University, Montreal, Quebec H3A 2B4, Canada

R. P. Maguire (307, 393) PET Program, Paul Scherrer Institute, CH 5232 Villigen, Switzerland

K. Mahmood (257) PET Facility, Department of Radiology, University of Pittsburgh, Pittsburgh, Pennsylvania,15213

Andrea L. Malizia (20, 266) PET Neuroscience Group, MRC Cyclotron Unit, Clinical Sciences Centre, Royal Postgraduate Medical School, Hammersmith Hospital, London W12 0NN, United Kingdom; and Psychopharmacology Unit, University of Bristol, Bristol BS8 1TD, United Kingdom

David A. Mankoff (312) Division of Nuclear Medicine, University of Washington, Seattle, Washington 98195

Stefano Marenco (158) Department of Radiology, Johns Hopkins Medical Institution, Baltimore, Maryland 21205

S. Marrett (327) McConnell Brain Imaging Centre, Montreal Neurological Institute, Montreal, Quebec H3A 2B4, Canada

C. A. Mathis (26, 76, 257) PET Facility, Department of Radiology, University of Pittsburgh, Pittsburgh, Pennsylvania 15213

Y. Matsumura (287) School of Science and Engineering, Waseda University, Tokyo 169, Japan

B. Mazoyer (342) Groupe d'Imagerie Neurofonctionnelle, Service Hospitalier Frédéric Joliot, CEA-DRM, 91401 Orsay, France; and EA 1555, Université Paris 7, Paris, France

John C. Mazziotta (353, 398) Department of Neurology and Division of Brain Mapping, Department of Pharmacology, and Department of Radiological Sciences, UCLA School of Medicine, Los Angeles, California 90095

J. A. McCarron (34) PET Methodology Group, MRC Clinical Sciences Centre, Royal Postgraduate Medical School, Hammersmith Hospital, London W12 0NN, United Kingdom

K. Meguro (317) Department of Geriatric Medicine, Tohoku University School of Medicine, Sendai 980-77, Japan

Steven R. Meikle (51, 415) The PET Department and Department of Nuclear Medicine, Division of Medical Imaging Services, Royal Prince Alfred Hospital, Sydney 2050, Australia

Marco A. Mejia (191, 206, 317) Department of Nuclear Medicine, Cyclotron and Radioisotope Center, Tohoku University, Sendai 980-77, Japan

E. Mellet (342) Groupe d'Imagerie Neurofonctionnelle, Service Hospitalier Frédéric Joliot, CEA-DRM, 91401 Orsay, France; and EA 1555, Université Paris, Paris, France

Carolyn Cidis Meltzer (152) Department of Radiology, Divisions of Neuroradiology and Nuclear Medicine, The Johns Hopkins Medical Institutions, Baltimore, Maryland 21205

Ernst Meyer (72, 196, 201, 214, 421) Positron Imaging Laboratories, McConnell Brain Imaging Centre and Montreal Neurological Institute, McGill University, Montreal, Quebec H3A 2B4, Canada

P. Millet (243) CERMEP, Lyon, France

S. Minoshima (209) University of Michigan Medical School, Cyclotron/PET Facility, Ann Arbor, Michigan 48109

M. A. Mintun (76, 257) PET Facility, Department of Radiology, University of Pittsburgh Medical Center, Pittsburgh, Pennsylvania 15213

J. Missimer (393) PET Program, Paul Scherrer Institute, Villigen, Switzerland

Shuichi Miura (57) Research Institute for Brain and Blood Vessels, Akita City 010, Japan

M. Miyake (67) Division of Radioprotection, Cyclotron Radioisotope Center, Tohoku University, Sendai 980-77, Japan

Toshimitsu Momose (166) University of Tokyo, School of Medicine, Bunkyoku, Tokyo 113, Japan

Niels Mørch, (271) Department of Neurology, National University Hospital, Rigshospitalet, DK-2100 Copenhagen, Denmark; and CONNECT, Electronics Institute, Technical University of Denmark, DK-2800 Lyngby, Denmark

Evan D. Morris (141, 249, 425) Radiology Department, PET Imaging Laboratory, Massachusetts General Hospital and Harvard Medical School, Boston, Massachusetts 02114

Paul K. Morrish (82) MRC Cyclotron Unit, Hammersmith Hospital, London W12 0NN, United Kingdom

S. Morrison (227) Neurodegenerative Disorders Centre and TRIUMF, University of British Columbia, Vancouver, British Columbia, Canada

H. W. Müller-Gärtner (118) Institute of Medicine, Research Centre, Jülich 52425, Germany

Kenya Murase (72, 201, 421) Positron Imaging Laboratories, McConnell Brain Imaging Centre and Montreal Neurological Institute, McGill University, Montreal, Quebec H3A 2B4, Canada

Mark Muzi (297) University of Washington Medical Center, Seattle, Washington 98195

R. Myers (12) PET Methodology Group, MRC Clinical Sciences Centre, Royal Postgraduate Medical School, Hammersmith Hospital, London W12 0NN, United Kingdom

Takashi Nakamura (67, 191, 206) Division of Radioprotection, Cyclotron and Radioisotope Center, Tohoku University, Sendai 980-77, Japan

Tadashi Nariai (282) Tokyo Medical and Dental University, Tokyo 101, Japan

P. Neelin (327) McConnell Brain Imaging Centre, Montreal Neurological Institute, Montreal, Quebec H3A 2B4, Canada

R. J. Nickles (9) Department of Medical Physics, University of Wisconsin Medical School, Madison, Wisconsin 53792

Junichi Nishikawa (166) University of Tokyo, School of Medicine, Bunkyoku, Tokyo 113, Japan

Sadahiko Nishizawa (214) Positron Imaging Laboratories, McConnell Brain Imaging Centre, Montreal Neurological Institute and McGill University, Montreal, Quebec H3A 2B4, Canada

D. J. Nutt (20, 266) Psychopharmacology Unit, University of Bristol, Bristol BS8 1TD, United Kingdom

G. J. O'Keefe (415) Centre for Positron Emission Tomography, Austin Repatriation Medical Centre, Melbourne 3084, Australia

Daniel S. O'Leary (365, 389) Department of Psychiatry, The Mental Health Clinical Research Center, University of Iowa Hospitals and Clinics, Iowa City, Iowa 52242

B. T. O'Sullivan (415) Department of Psychiatry, Royal Prince Alfred Hospital, Sydney 2050, Australia

Finbarr O'Sullivan (277, 297) Department of Statistics, University of Washington Medical Center, Seattle, Washington 98195

W. Oberschelp (118) Institute of Applied Mathematics, Aachen 52054, Germany

Toshihide Ogawa (57) Research Institute for Brain and Blood Vessels, Akita City 010, Japan

S. Ono (317) Department of Radiology and Nuclear Medicine, Institute of Development, Aging and Cancer, Tohoku University, Sendai 980-77, Japan

S. Osman (34) PET Methodology Group, MRC Clinical Sciences Centre, Royal Postgraduate Medical School, Hammersmith Hospital, London W12 0NN, United Kingdom

Clifford Patlak (219, 232) State University of New York at Stony Brook, Stony Brook, New York 11794

Olaf B. Paulson (93, 271) Department of Neurology, The National University Hospital, Rigshospitalet, DK-2100 Copenhagen Ø, Denmark

Gunter Pawlik (349) Max Planck Institute for Neurological Research and Neurology Clinic of the University of Cologne, D-50931 Cologne, Germany

L. Petit (342) Groupe d'Imagerie Neurofonctionnelle, Service Hospitalier Frédéric Joliot, CEA-DRM, 91401 Orsay, France; and EA 1555, Université Paris 7, Paris, France

U. Pietrzyk (16, 175, 410) Max Planck Institute for Neurological Research and Department of Neurology, University Hospital, and University of Cologne Neurology Clinic, D-50931 Cologne, Germany

V. W. Pike (34) PET Methodology Group, MRC Clinical Sciences Centre, Royal Postgraduate Medical School, Hammersmith Hospital, London W12 0NN, United Kingdom

J.-B. Poline (342, 359, 372) The Wellcome Department of Cognitive Neurology, Institute of Neurology, Queen Square, London WC1N 3BG, United Kingdom

K. Poole (20) PET Methodology Group, Clinical Sciences Centre, Royal Postgraduate Medical School, Hammersmith Hospital, London W12 0NN, United Kingdom

J. C. Price (76, 257) PET Facility, Department of Radiology, University of Pittsburgh Medical Center, Pittsburgh, Pennsylvania 15213

M. Psylla (224) PET Department, Paul Scherrer Institute, CH 5232 Villigen, Switzerland

Robert Pyzalski (138) Department of Radiology, University of Wisconsin Medical School, Madison, Wisconsin 53792

S. Rajeswaran (12, 20) PET Methodology Group, MRC Clinical Sciences Centre, Royal Postgraduate Medical School, Hammersmith Hospital, London W12 0NN, United Kingdom

James S. Rakshi (82) MRC Cyclotron Unit, Hammersmith Hospital, London W12 0NN, United Kingdom

Alex Ranicar (62) PET Methodology Group, Cyclotron Unit, MRC Clinical Sciences Centre, Royal Postgraduate Medical School, Hammersmith Hospital, London W12 0NN, United Kingdom

Scott L. Rauch (425) Psychiatry Department, Massachusetts General Hospital and Harvard Medical School, Boston, Massachusetts 02114

P. Remy (88) CEA, Service Hospitalier Frédéric Joliot, Orsay 91406, France

David C. Reutens (214) Positron Imaging Laboratories, McConnell Brain Imaging Centre, Montreal Neurological Institute and McGill University, Montreal, Quebec H3A 2B4, Canada

Andy Roberts (9) Department of Medical Physics, University of Wisconsin Medical School, Madison, Wisconsin 53792

G. Rosenqvist (170) Department of Clinical Neuroscience, Experimental Alcohol and Drug Addiction Research Section, and Section of Clinical Neurophysiology, Karolinska Hospital, S-17176 Stockholm, Sweden

D. A. Rottenberg (378) PET Imaging Section, VA Medical Center, Minneapolis, Minnesota 55417; and Neurology and Radiology Departments, University of Minnesota, Minneapolis, Minnesota 55455

Olivier G. Rousset (158) Positron Imaging Laboratories, McConnell Brain Imaging Centre, Montreal Neurological Institute, McGill University, Montreal, Quebec H3A 2B4, Canada

T. J. Ruth (227) Neurodegenerative Disorders Centre and TRIUMF, University of British Columbia, Vancouver, British Columbia, Canada

Norihiro Sadato (98) Human Motor Control Section, Medical Neurology Branch, National Institutes of Health, Bethesda, Maryland 20892

Y. Samson (243) C. E. A. Service Hospitalier F. Joliot, 91400 Orsay, France

H. Sasaki (317) Department of Geriatric Medicine, Tohoku University School of Medicine, Sendai 980-77, Japan

Mikiya Sase (166) University of Tokyo, School of Medicine, Bunkyoku, Tokyo 113, Japan

D. Sashin (76) PET Facility, Department of Radiology, University of Pittsburgh Medical Center, Pittsburgh, Pennsylvania 15213

K. Schaper (378) PET Imaging Section, VA Medical Center, Minneapolis, Minnesota 55417

G. Schlaug (393) Department of Neurology, University of Düsseldorf, Düsseldorf, Germany

L. Schnorr (20) PET Methodology Group, Clinical Sciences Centre, Royal Postgraduate Medical School, Hammersmith Hospital, London W12 0NN, United Kingdom

R. J. Seitz (393) Department of Neurology, University of Düsseldorf, Düsseldorf, Germany

Michio Senda (282, 287) Positron Medical Center and PET Center, Tokyo Metropolitan Institute of Gerontology, Tokyo 173, Japan

S. E. Shelton (9) Primate Center, University of Wisconsin, Madison, Wisconsin 53792

Anthony F. Shields (312) Department of Medicine and Veterans Affairs Medical Center and University of Washington, Seattle, Washington

Eku Shimosegawa (362) Department of Radiology and Nuclear Medicine, Akita Research Institute of Brain and Blood Vessels, Akita 010, Japan

Masahiro Shiraishi (237) McConnell Brain Imaging Center, Montreal Neurological Institute and Department of Neurology and Neurosurgery, McGill University, Montreal, Quebec H3A 2B4, Canada

Richard Shrager (185) Division of Computer Research and Technology, National Institutes of Health, Bethesda, Maryland 20892

J. J. Sidtis (378) Neurology Department, University of Minnesota, Minneapolis, Minnesota 55455

N. R. Simpson (76, 257) PET Facility, Department of Radiology, University of Pittsburgh Medical Center, Pittsburgh, Pennsylvania 15213

D. Smith (42) PET Center, Aarhus University Hospital, 8000 Aarhus C, Denmark; and Department of Biological Psychiatry, Psychiatric Hospital of Aarhus University, 8240 Risskov, Denmark

Donald F. Smith (38) Department of Biological Psychiatry, Psychiatric Hospital of Aarhus University, 8240 Risskov, Denmark

B. J. Snow (227) Neurodegenerative Disorders Centre and TRIUMF, University of British Columbia, Vancouver, British Columbia, Canada

Abraham Z. Snyder (131) Department of Neurology and Neurosurgery, Washington University School of Medicine, St. Louis, Missouri 63110

V. Sossi (227) Neurodegenerative Disorders Centre and TRIUMF, University of British Columbia, Vancouver, British Columbia, Canada

L. Spelle (243) C. E. A. Service Hospitalier F. Joliot, 91400 Orsay, France

Alexander Spence (297) University of Washington Medical Center, Seattle, Washington 98195

S. C. Strother (181, 378) PET Imaging Section, VA Medical Center, Minneapolis, Minnesota 55417; and Radiology Department, University of Minnesota, Minneapolis, Minnesota 55455

Martin J. Stumpf (152) Department of Radiology, Division of Nuclear Medicine, The Johns Hopkins Medical Institutions, Baltimore, Maryland 21205

Yusuke Suganami (166) Tokyo Institute of Technology, Yokohama 226, Japan

Claus Svarer (271) Department of Neurology, National University Hospital, Rigshospitalet, DK-2100 Copenhagen, Denmark

S. J. Swerdloff (9, 138) Department of Medical Physics, University of Wisconsin Medical School, Madison, Wisconsin 53792

A. Syrota (243) C. E. A. Service Hospitalier F. Joliot, 91400 Orsay, France

A. Taguchi (287) School of Science and Engineering, Waseda University, Tokyo 169, Japan

E. Talarico (342) Groupe d'Imagerie Neurofonctionnelle, Service Hospitalier Frédéric Joliot, CEA-DRM, 91401 Orsay, France; and EA 1555, Université Paris 7, Paris, France

Chris Taylor (301) Medical Biophysics, Medical School, Manchester, United Kingdom

L. Tellman (393) Institute of Medicine Research Center, Jülich, Germany

A. Thiel (349) Max Planck Institute for Neurological Research and Neurology Clinic of the University of Cologne, D-50931 Cologne, Germany

H. J. Tochon-Danguy (415) Centre for Positron Emission Tomography, Austin Repatriation Medical Centre, Melbourne 3084, Australia

Arthur W. Toga (398) Department of Neurology, Division of Brain Mapping, UCLA School of Medicine, Los Angeles, California 90095

P.-J. Toussaint (196, 201) Positron Imaging Laboratories, McConnell Brain Imaging Centre and Montreal Neurological Institute, McGill University, Montreal, Quebec H3A 2B4, Canada

D. W. Townsend (76) PET Facility, Department of Radiology, University of Pittsburgh Medical Center, Pittsburgh, Pennsylvania 15213

Hinako Toyama (282) PET Center, Tokyo Metropolitan Institute of Gerontology, Tokyo 173, Japan

R. Trébossen (88) CEA, Service Hospitalier Frédéric Joliot, Orsay 91406, France

N. Tzourio (342) Groupe d'Imagerie Neurofonctionnelle, Service Hospitalier Frédéric Joliot, CEA-DRM, 91401 Orsay, France; and EA 1555, Université Paris 7, Paris, France

A. Uchiyama (287) School of Science and Engineering, Waseda University, Tokyo 169, Japan

Kazuo Uemura (57) Research Institute for Brain and Blood Vessels, Akita City 010, Japan

H. Uno (9) Primate Research Center, University of Wisconsin, Madison, Wisconsin 53792

M. Vafaee (72, 201) Positron Imaging Laboratories, McConnell Brain Imaging Centre and Montreal Neurological Institute, McGill University, Montreal, Quebec H3A 2B4, Canada

F. J. G. Vingerhoets (227) Neurodegenerative Disorders Centre and TRIUMF, University of British Columbia, Vancouver, British Columbia, Canada

P. Vontobel (224) PET Department, Paul Scherrer Institute, CH 5232 Villigen, Switzerland

R. Wagner (16) Max Planck Institute for Neurological Research, University of Cologne Neurology Clinic, D-50931 Cologne, Germany

Hiroshi Watabe (67, 191, 206, 317) Department of Investigative Radiology, National Cardiovascular Center Research Institute, Suita 565, Japan; Department of Radiation Protection, Division of Radioprotection, Cyclotron and Radioisotope Center, Tohoku University, Sendai 980-77, Japan; and National Cardiovascular Center Research Institute, Osaka, Japan

G. Leonard Watkins (365, 384, 389) PET Imaging Center, Department of Radiology, The University of Iowa Hospitals and Clinics, Iowa City, Iowa 52242

J. D. G. Watson (334, 415) Medical Research Council Cyclotron Unit, Hammersmith Hospital, London W12 0NN, United Kingdom; and Department of Anatomy, University College, London, United Kingdom

Miles Wernick (109) Department of Electrical and Computer Engineering, Illinois Institute of Technology, Chicago, Illinois

K. Wienhard (16, 410) Max Planck Institute for Neurological Research, University of Cologne Neurology Clinic, D-50931 Cologne, Germany

A. A. Wilson (262) PET Centre, Clarke Institute of Psychiatry and University of Toronto, Toronto, Ontario M5T 1R8, Canada

S. Wilson (266) Psychopharmacology Unit, University of Bristol, Bristol BS8 1TD, United Kingdom

Scott D. Wollenweber (365) PET Imaging Center, Department of Radiology, University of Iowa Hospitals and Clinics, Iowa City, Iowa 52242

Dean F. Wong, (158) Department of Radiology, Johns Hopkins Medical Institution, Baltimore, Maryland 21205

Roger P. Woods (353, 398) Department of Neurology, Division of Brain Mapping, UCLA School of Medicine, Los Angeles, California 90095

K. J. Worsley (327, 359) Department of Mathematics and Statistics, McGill University, Montreal, Quebec H3A 2K6, Canada

Yuchen Yan (185) PET Department, National Institutes of Health, Bethesda, Maryland 20892

K. Yanai (317) Department of Pharmacology I, Tohoku University School of Medicine, Sendai 980-77, Japan

J. Yang (147) Division of Nuclear Medicine and Biophysics, Department of Molecular and Medical Pharmacology, UCLA School of Medicine, Los Angeles, California 90095

Jeffrey T. Yap (109, 292) Franklin McLean Memorial Research Institute, Department of Radiology, The University of Chicago, Chicago, Illinois 60637

D. C. Yu (147) Division of Nuclear Medicine and Biophysics, Department of Molecular and Medical Pharmacology, UCLA School of Medicine, Los Angeles, California 90095

Gene Zeien (389) The Mental Health Clinical Research Center, Department of Psychiatry, The University of Iowa Hospitals and Clinics, Iowa City, Iowa 52242

Y. Zhou (147) Division of Nuclear Medicine and Biophysics, Department of Molecular and Medical Pharmacology, UCLA School of Medicine, Los Angeles, California 90095

Jon Kar Zubieta (152) Division of Nuclear Medicine, The Johns Hopkins Medical Institutions, Baltimore, Maryland 21205

Foreword

The basis for this book was an international symposium held in Oxford, United Kingdom in July 1995, on the quantification of brain function with PET. The focus of the book is on advances in quantification and the integration of methods to provide accurate parametric images with PET. The symposium was held as a satellite meeting to the XVII International Symposium on Cerebral Blood Flow and Metabolism held in Cologne, Germany.

PET stands for Positron Emitting Tracers and Positron Emission Tomography. As a result of the specificity of the tracers and sensitivity of the tomographs, it is one of the most specific and sensitive means for studying molecular pathways and molecular interactions in the living human body. In exploiting these advantages, there clearly needs to be an emphasis on achieving maximum accuracy and formulating strategies for addressing research and diagnostic questions. Other books cover many components that contribute to these strategies but few are also structured to comprehensively address these central themes. Figure 1 depicts the methodological flow from the research and diagnostic questions to the formation of functional images. This scheme was used as the structure for the symposium which systematically addressed tracer selection, data acquisition, processing, kinetic analysis, parametric imaging, and statistical analysis. The meeting, which aimed at identifying strengths and weaknesses in the strategy, was attended by representatives of many of the leading groups concerned with the development and application of PET. Here the motivation was to create a critical mass of like-minded enthusiasts for a comparatively small methodological field. The full development and exploitation of PET is expensive and requires an institutional approach to ensure all relevant facets are advanced. At a time of recession in the science economy, accountability in the healthcare area, and the large scientific vote in molecular biology, such

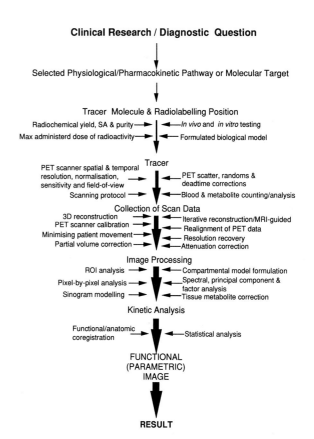

FIGURE 1   The scientific and technical strategy for addressing clinical research and diagnostic questions and for recording accurate functional images with PET.

institutional approaches are being threatened, especially when they are still in their infancy, as far as realizing their potential and exploitation is concerned. It is hoped that this book will help to illustrate the interrelated components of this field and the need for a multidisciplinary approach.

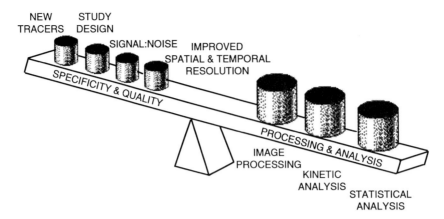

FIGURE 2   The balance in PET methodology between the specificity and quality of PET data and its processing and analysis.

As an overview of the field, it appears that the ability to process and analyze data both kinetically and statistically is outbalancing the specificity and quality of the data, especially with respect to tracer strategies, temporal resolution, and the statistical accuracies provided by the scanners themselves (Fig. 2). The inference is not that there are insufficient tracers but that paradigms for their use need broader consideration, e.g., multiple tracers and challenge studies. Although high sensitivity tomographs are commonly installed, few centers have invested in exploiting this enhanced accuracy in a systematic fashion. New detector materials are on the horizon with the promise of improved spatial and kinetic resolutions and signal : noise, yet currently there is little emphasis on seeking to record cleaner data at the time of its collection.

Data processing is seen to be healthy with ingenious reconstructions and considerations for reducing noise. Little movement is seen in advancing the applications of clearly defined compartmental models for kinetic analysis. This seems to arise from the fact that they are not in the first instance statistically conducive to a voxel by voxel analysis to provide parametric images. A more pragmatic approach for kinetic analysis is in evidence with an aim of producing "functional" images. The maturity of the use of statistics to detect and characterize change in images is a refreshing advance and bodes well for exploitation in other imaging areas. This is clearly highly desirable since objective, common endpoints for assessing data quality, significance of change, and reproducibility are germane to the advancement of this field.

Terry Jones

Acknowledgments

The editors gratefully acknowledge the assistance of Andrew Holmes, Vic Pike, and Susan Hume in the preparation of these Proceedings.

The generous support from GE Medical Systems, CTI PET Systems (Knoxville, Tennessee), and Academic Press (San Diego, California) is also gratefully acknowledged.

The Scientific and Organizing Committees are recognized for their efforts in organizing and coordinating the meeting that inspired the papers presented here.

International Scientific Committee

N. M. Alpert Boston
J. C. Baron Caen
R. G. Blasberg New York
R. E. Carson Bethesda
S. Cherry Los Angeles
J. Delforge Orsay
S. Derenzo Berkeley
L. Eriksson Stockholm
A. C. Evans Montreal
I. Ford Glasgow
J. Fowler Brookhaven
A. Gjedde Aarhus
M. Graham Seattle

W. D. Heiss Cologne
C. Halldin Stockholm
J. E. Holden Madison
S. C. Huang Los Angeles
I. Kanno Akita
M. R. Kilbourn Ann Arbor
R. A. Koeppe Ann Arbor
B. Langström Uppsala
N. A. Lassen Copenhagen
B. Maziere Orsay
B. M. Mazoyer Orsay
M. A. Mintun Pittsburgh
C. Patlak New York
M. Phelps Los Angeles
S. C. Strother Minneapolis
D. Townsend Pittsburgh
K. Wienhard Cologne

Local Organizing and Scientific Committee

Dale Bailey, David Brooks, Vin Cunningham, Richard Frackowiak, Karl Friston, Sylke Grootoonk, Roger Gunn, Andrew Holmes, Susan Hume, Terry Jones (convenor), Adriaan Lammertsma, Jindy Luthra, Jean-Baptiste Poline, Ralph Myers, Vic Pike, Jimmy Seaward, Greg Stachowski, and Terry Spinks.

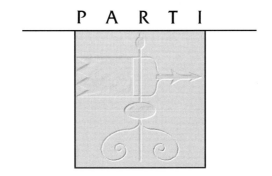

PART I

TRACER SELECTION

In Vivo–in Vitro Correlations:
An Example from Vesicular Monoamine Transporters

MICHAEL R. KILBOURN

Division of Nuclear Medicine
Department of Internal Medicine
University of Michigan Medical School
Ann Arbor, Michigan 48109

In the development and evaluation of new radiotracers for in vivo imaging using PET (positron emission tomography), researchers often make use of correlations between in vitro and in vivo measures of binding affinities and regional organ distributions of radioligand binding in animals. Using examples drawn from a series of radioligands for the vesicular monoamine transporter, the value of such correlations in choosing candidate radioligands is discussed. In vitro binding affinities are useful in initial selection of candidate radioligands, but other factors such as nonspecific binding and metabolism may be of equivalent importance. Correlations between in vitro and in vivo distributions of radioligand binding sites, if correctly drawn, can provide useful insights into radiotracer selection. Such comparisons of in vitro and in vivo properties of new compounds are thus important components of an overall program to design, synthesize, and validate a new radiotracer for in vivo imaging applications.

I. INTRODUCTION

Positron emission tomography (PET) holds great promise as a noninvasive means to examine the biochemistry of the human body. As the field has matured, more complex physiological systems are being studied, using increasingly complicated imaging instrumentation and increasingly sophisticated pharmacokinetic models. All this has the goal of developing new, valuable imaging protocols for the study of normal and pathophysiological functions of the human body. One crucial component of every imaging study is the radiopharmaceutical. As considerable time, effort, and cost is associated with bringing a new radiopharmaceutical to human use, timely and efficient selection of candidate radiotracers is of paramount importance. The requirements for successful radiotracers vary with the intended use, and the "optimum" characteristics have been repeatedly discussed, rarely with consensus.

As part of the preclinical evaluation process of radiotracers for specific, saturable high-affinity binding sites (e.g., receptors, transporters, ion channels of enzymes), the *in vivo* properties of new or potential radiotracers are often compared with independent, *in vitro* measures of binding affinities or *in vitro* distributions of high-affinity radioligand binding sites within an organ such as the brain. Such correlations can be extremely helpful in identifying valuable new radiotracers and, perhaps just as important, indicate compounds that in all likelihood would be rather poor choices for further development into PET imaging radiopharmaceuticals. In this chapter, we draw upon our experiences with radioligands for the brain synaptic vesicle monoamine transporter (VMAT2) to provide examples of how *in vivo–in vitro* correlations can be used to identify good candidate radioligands for human imaging with PET.

II. MATERIALS AND METHODS

Syntheses of $(\pm)$-α-dihydrotetrabenazine $((\pm)$-α-DTBZ), $(+)$-α-dihydrotetrabenazine $((+)$-α-DTBZ) and a series of 2-alkyl-($\pm$)-α-dihydrotetrabenazine derivatives have been described previously (DaSilva et al., 1993; Lee et al., 1994; Kilbourn et al., 1995b). Radiochemical syntheses of ($\pm$)-[^{11}C]tetrabenazine (($\pm$)-[^{11}C]TBZ), ($\pm$)-α-[^{11}C]methoxytetrabenazine (($\pm$)-α-[^{11}C]MTBZ), ($\pm$)-α-[^{11}C]dihydrotetrabenazine (($\pm$)-α-[^{11}C]DTBZ), and (+)-α-[^{11}C]dihydrotetrabenazine ((+)-α-[^{11}C]DTBZ) were done using [^{11}C]methylation of the appropriate desmethyl precursors, by methods previously described (DaSilva et al., 1993; DaSilva et al., 1993b; Kilbourn et al., 1995b). The ($\pm$)-α-[^{3}H]methoxytetrabenazine ([^{3}H]MTBZ) was prepared by custom tritiation (Amersham) of the desmethyl precursor. In vivo regional brain distributions in mice were done using iv injections of radiotracer, sacrifice 15 min after injection, and rapid dissection, counting and weighing of tissue samples (DaSilva and Kilbourn, 1992; DaSilva et al., 1994). K_i values for unlabeled ligands were determined using an autoradiographic method, with [^{3}H]MTBZ as the radioligand (Vander Borght et al., 1995b). Regional distribution of in vitro binding of [^{3}H]MTBZ in rat brain was determined using quantitative autoradiography, as previously reported (Vander Borght et al., 1995b).

III. RESULTS AND DISCUSSION

Using the data we have obtained from our series of in vitro and in vivo experiments, as well as the extensive literature data regarding the in vitro properties of ($\pm$)-α-[^{3}H]dihydrotetrabenazine (($\pm$)-α-[^{3}H]DTBZ) (Masuo et al., 1990; Scherman, 1986; Scherman et al., 1986, 1988), we can examine whether in vitro–in vivo correlations can be utilized to properly identify the most appropriate radioligand for in vivo PET imaging of the brain synaptic vesicle monoamine transporter in humans. The vesicular monoamine transporter (VMAT2) is a specific protein located in small synaptic vesicles of the monoaminergic neurons of the brain (Schuldiner, 1994). Its function in dopaminergic, noradrenergic, and serotonergic neurons is to transport monoamines (dopamine, norepinephrine, and serotonin) from the cytoplasm into the lumen of the vesicle, protecting the neurotransmitters from degradative enzymes as well as packaging them for exocytotic release. Monoaminergic neurons are found in many regions of the mammalian brain, providing a wide range of in vitro values with which to correlate in vivo radiotracer binding.

A. In Vivo–in Vitro Correlations: Binding Affinities vs. Regional Brain Distribution

By the application of in vitro radioligand binding assays, it is now relatively straightforward to determine

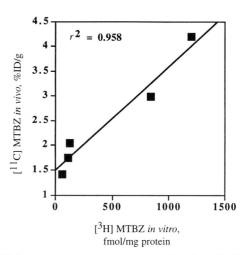

FIGURE 1 Correlation between in vitro binding affinities and in vivo ability to block radioligand localization in mouse brain striatum. In vitro binding affinities are for competition with [^{3}H]MTBZ binding to rat brain striatal slices. In vivo values are for inhibition of [^{11}C]MTBZ localization in mouse brain striatum following 10 mg/kg. iv coinjections of competing compounds, expressed as a percentage of control values (saline injection). Compounds: **1**, 2-β-methyl-α-dihydrotetrabenazine; **2**, tetrabenazine; **3**, 2-α-methyl-β-dihydrotetrabenazine; **4**, 2-α-ethyl-β-dihydrotetrabenazine; **5**, 2-α-n-propyl-β-dihydrotetrabenazine; **6**, 2-α-isopropyl-β-dihydrotetrabenazine; **7**, 2-α-isobutyl-β-dihydrotetrabenazine. The correlation ($r^2 = 0.994$) is shown for compounds **1–6**.

the in vitro relative binding affinities of a series of compounds, and this is often a first step in the development of new drugs or radiopharmaceuticals. Do such in vitro assays, which determine the ability of test compounds to compete for binding of a well-characterized, high-affinity radioligand to a specific site, necessarily predict eventual in vivo binding to the same site? Can they be used to predict the best compound, or are they more suited to separate a larger series of compounds into good lead candidates (which can then be followed up) and likely failures?

Our data using the benzoisoquinoline derivatives suggest that the latter option is more appropriate. As shown in Figure 1, there is a reasonable correlation between the in vitro binding affinities of these compounds and the ability of to occupy brain VMAT2 binding sites in vivo when all are administered (via peripheral injection) at the same dose. This type of in vivo assay provides an indirect measure of the efficacy of a new drug to bind to the target site, but of course, provides no other information regarding what would be the eventual biodistribution of these compounds if each were independently radiolabeled. Nevertheless, such correlations can provide important information, useful for the selection of candidate radioligands. It is apparent that the derivatives with higher in vitro binding affinities (lower n*M* values) are, by and large, more effective at blocking radioligand binding in the rat striatum *in vivo*, with the exception of the isobutyl derivative **7**, which has a reasonably good *in vitro* affinity (K*i* of 33 n*M*) but is ineffective *in vivo*. The reasons for the poor *in vivo* effectiveness of the isobutyl derivative are likely pharmacokinetic (poor brain permeability or high serum protein binding or both), but in any case the isobutyl derivative could easily be ruled out as a potential radioligand, and furthermore the smaller chain alkyl derivatives—such as the methyl compounds—would be most attractive.

Can *in vitro* affinities be used to identify the best candidate? For numerous benzoisoquinolines, the *in vitro* binding affinities have now been measured, and several of these ((±)-TBZ, (±)-MTBZ, (±)-DTBZ, (+)-DTBZ, (±)-β-methyl-α-DTBZ) have *in vitro* binding affinities between 1 and 10 n*M*. As there has never been a firm description of what *in vitro* binding affinity is best (or even required) for successful, quantitative *in vivo* PET imaging, we are left with the question; which one to choose? Fortunately for this discussion, four of these candidate compounds have been carbon-11 labeled and examined in both animals and humans, and we can now take a retrospective look at whether *in vitro* measures might have predicted a "best" radioligand.

B. *In Vivo–in Vitro* Correlations: Regional Brain Distributions

The determination of *in vitro* radioligand binding to various brain regions is easily accomplished, using either tissue homogenate binding or quantitative autoradiography. Both methods are capable of providing good measures of the numbers of specific binding sites for a radioligand: autoradiography can provide regional radioligand binding measures with impressive spatial resolution.

For *in vivo* radiotracer distributions, both cut-and-count dissection techniques as well as *ex vivo* autoradiography can be used. In general, these methods provide accurate measures of radiotracer distribution into tissues; the proportion of the total radiotracer concentration that is specifically bound to the site of interest, as compared to radioligand in other pools (free, nonspecifically bound, or bound to other sites), is generally determined in separate studies employing pharmacological blocking of the target binding site. Most often, the relatively simple single time point determinations of radiotracer distributions are utilized as estimates of *in vivo* specific binding; whether more complicated pharmacokinetic modeling of rodent distribution data (entailing many more animals and probably a metabolite-corrected blood curve) would be more appropriate

is an interesting question, which will not be addressed here. Certainly, single time point determinations introduce bias into the estimates of *in vivo* binding parameters, but the magnitudes of these biases will vary with the characteristics of the radiotracer, and therefore need to be considered for each radiotracer.

Do (or should?) *in vitro* measures of binding sites correlate with such *in vivo* estimates of specific binding? If it is assumed that all binding sites measured *in vitro* are similarly accessible *in vivo*, then the answer to this question is yes; however, if *in vivo* some binding sites are effectively masked (perhaps through physiochemical changes in the tissue or occupation by endogenous ligands), then a direct correlation might not be expected. In the latter case, *in vitro* does not equal *in vivo*, and attempting to correlate such data would prove useless. In most instances, researchers interested in developing *in vivo* radioligands have assumed that the *in vivo* numbers of binding sites do correlate with *in vitro* measures and have determined the appropriate correlation coefficients. However, as demonstrated in the following examples, there is a correct and incorrect way to present such correlations; and if done correctly they are quite useful in identifying a "better" radioligand for *in vivo* imaging.

Using *in vitro* autoradiography, we have recently determined the regional rat brain distribution of binding sites for [³H]MTBZ (Vander Borght *et al.*, 1995b). The pattern of binding sites is essentially identical to that of [³H]DTBZ binding determined some years earlier (Masuo *et al.*, 1990), and both are very similar to the pattern of [³H]DTBZ binding measured in mouse brain (Scherman, 1986; Scherman *et al.*, 1986). These would therefore be representative of the *in vitro* levels of VMAT2 in the rodent brain. For *in vivo* data, we have determined the regional brain distributions of all four carbon-11 labeled benzoisoquinolines in mouse or rat brain (DaSilva and Kilbourn, 1992; DaSilva *et al.*, 1994; Vander Borght *et al.*, 1995a; Kilbourn *et al.*, 1995b). The *in vitro* and *in vivo* data (in this case, for MTBZ binding in the mouse brain) can be plotted against one another, and a very typical correlation graph (similar to that found in many papers dealing with evaluation of *in vivo* radiotracers) is shown in Figure 2. The general assumption is then made that the *in vitro* and *in vivo* data are highly correlated, and thus this would be a "validated" radioligand.

But is this an appropriate correlation graph? Note that the dimensions of the axis are significantly different; replotting the same data with identical axes gives a plot (not shown) with a very flat line that would suggest little sensitivity of the *in vivo* radiotracer measure to rather large changes in the *in vitro* values. But again, this is not an appropriate method to examine

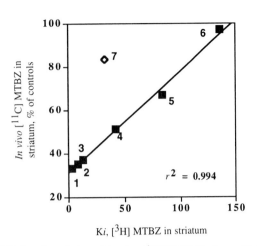

FIGURE 2   Correlation of *in vitro* [³H]MTBZ binding with *in vivo* [¹¹C]MTBZ regional brain localization at a single time point after iv injection, for radioligand binding to VMAT2 of the rodent brain.

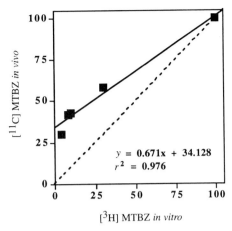

FIGURE 3   Correlation of *in vitro* and *in vivo* binding of MTBZ to the VMAT2 of the rodent brain. Values have been expressed as a percentage of the maximal value, with the striatum assigned as 100%. The dotted line indicates an ideal radiotracer that has no nonspecific binding, a linear relationship between *in vitro* and *in vivo* values, and a slope of 1 for the correlation line.

the characteristics of a radioligand, and certainly not suitable for comparing radioligands as the difference between two very flat lines might well be indistinguishable.

Is there a better way to plot the data? We suggest that both the *in vitro* and *in vivo* data should be normalized to the respective maximum values, such that the brain region with the highest concentrations of binding sites would be 100, and a value of 0 would represent no measurable binding sites. An ideal ligand, with no nonspecific binding, no unbound ligand distribution, and a linear sensitivity to the numbers of sites present, would thus have a slope of 1 and pass through the origin (as depicted by the dotted line in Figure 3). No "ideal" *in vivo* radioligand has yet been made, so the actual correlation line will deviate from the ideal case. As shown in Figure 3 for regional [¹¹C]MTBZ distribution in the mouse brain, the slope may well be less than 1, and the *y*-intercept greater than 0, which represents a nonspecific distribution (free radioligand and nonspecific binding).

Are such normalized plots better suited to discern differences between radioligands? Figure 4 shows such correlation lines for two radioligands, (±)-α-[¹¹C]-DTBZ and (+)-α-[¹¹C]DTBZ. For both radioligands, the *in vitro*–*in vivo* correlation coefficients are very high ($r^2 = 0.976$ and 0.978, respectively). The differences between the radiotracers can now be clearly appreciated, as the single, biologically resolved isomer (+)-DTBZ shows both a larger slope (0.74, but still not 1) and a lower *y*-intercept. This is, of course, consistent with using a resolved isomer rather than a racemic mixture, as the inactive radiolabeled isomer contri-

butes to tissue radioactivity levels in a nonspecific fashion. But this type of graphical comparison would be just as useful in distinguishing between any two radioligands that might differ in the percentage of nonspecific binding but that, independently, show *in vivo* distributions highly correlated with *in vitro* measures of regional binding distributions.

Thus, rather simple correlations between single time point measurements of radiotracer distributions and *in vitro* binding levels can provide meaningful insights into radiotracer selection. But, do they really translate

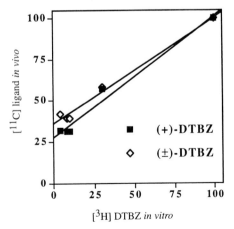

FIGURE 4   Correlation of *in vitro* and *in vivo* binding of (+)- and (±)-DTBZ in the rodent brain. Regional values are expressed as a percentage of the maximal binding in the striatum. Correlation coefficients are (+)-DTBZ, $r^2 = 0.978$; (±)-DTBZ, $r^2 = 0.986$.

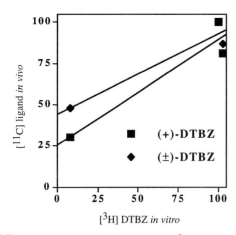

FIGURE 5 Correlation of *in vitro* binding of [³H]DTBZ and *in vivo* binding of (+)- and (±)-[¹¹C]DTBZ in the human brain. *In vivo* values represent the percentage of maximal binding in the putamen, using distribution volumes (DV) calculated through pharmacokinetic modeling.

into significant differences in human PET imaging results? We have had a chance to obtain quantitative PET imaging studies with each of the carbon-11 labeled benzoisoquinolines (Kilbourn *et al.*, 1993; Vander Borght *et al.*, 1995a; Koeppe *et al.*, 1995; Frey *et al.*, 1995; Kilbourn *et al.*, 1995a), as for various reasons they were developed sequentially rather than all at the same time. We can thus, in retrospect, compare the *in vivo* PET imaging results with the *in vitro* determined densities of [³H]DTBZ binding sites in the postmortem human brain (Scherman *et al.*, 1989). These correlations are somewhat limited due to the paucity of regions sampled in the postmortem assay of the human brain but, nevertheless, provide interesting results as shown in Figure 5. Whereas little significant difference was found between (±)-α-[¹¹C]MTBZ and (±)-α-[¹¹C]-DTBZ (data not shown; (±)-α-[¹¹C]MTBZ seemed, by visual inspection of images, to demonstrate slightly higher nonspecific binding), it is very clear that movement to the resolved isomer (+)-α-[¹¹C]DTBZ has significantly improved the *in vivo* PET results. Of course, this is also visually evident on the parametric images of radioligand distribution volumes, due to the lower nonspecific and free distribution for (+)-α-[¹¹C]DTBZ. It is encouraging, however, to see that the animal and human results were so consistent; the simplified animal approach of determining a single time point for radiotracer distribution may have in fact underestimated the actual differences between the radioligands, which was better brought out by the pharmacokinetic modeling.

The correlations shown here and the differences between the different radiotracers are actually not surprising, and certainly do not exemplify all of the radio-

tracers that have been or are being developed for *in vivo* PET imaging. The data we have presented is, however, the only complete set of animal plus human data obtained for four closely related carbon-11 labeled radioligands, with all studies done in the same institution and using the same animals, equipment, analytical methods, and personnel. Our results do indicate that *in vitro* data has a place in the preclinical evaluation of new radiotracers, but other information—such as radiotracer metabolism, toxicity, and serum protein binding—will also play a role in ultimate tracer selection. In our case, (+)-α-[¹¹C]DTBZ is the radioligand of choice, having the best dynamic range *in vivo* (i.e., the slope of the correlation line (Fig. 4) closest to 1), lower serum protein binding, and no *in vivo* metabolites that pass the blood–brain barrier.

Acknowledgments

This work was supported by grants from the National Institutes of Health (MH 47611, NS 15655, AG08671, and T-32-CA09015) and the Department of Energy (DOE-DE-FG021–87ER60561). The author thanks J. N. DaSilva, D. M. Jewett, L. C. Lee, R. A. Koeppe, K. A. Frey, T. M. Vander Borght, P. Sherman, and T. Desmond for all of their hard work in obtaining the data used in this manuscript.

References

DaSilva, J. N., and Kilbourn, M. R. (1992). *In vivo* binding of [¹¹C] tetrabenazine to vesicular monoamine transporters in mouse brain. *Life Sci.* **51:** 593–600.

DaSilva, J. N., Kilbourn, M. R., and Mangner, T.J. (1993a). Synthesis of a [¹¹C]methoxy derivative of α-dihydrotetrabenazine: A radioligand for studying the vesicular monoamine transporter. *Appl. Radiat. Isot.* **44:** 1487–1489.

DaSilva, J. N., Kilbourn, M. R., and Mangner, T. J. (1993b). Synthesis of [¹¹C]tetrabenazine: A vesicular monoamine uptake inhibitor, for PET imaging studies. *Appl. Radiat. Isot.* **44:** 673–676.

DaSilva, J. N., Kilbourn, M. R., Carey, J. E., Sherman, P., and Pisani, T. (1994). Characterization of [¹¹C]tetrabenazine as an *in vivo* radioligand for the vesicular monoamine transporter. *Nucl. Med. Biol.* **21:** 151–156.

Frey, K. A., Koeppe, R. A., Kilbourn, M. R., Vander Borght, T. M., Albin, R. L., Gilman, S., and Kuhl, D. E. (1995). Reduction of presynaptic monoaminergic vesicles in the striata of Parkinsonian patients and in normal human aging. *J. Cerebr. Blood Flow Metab.,* **15:** S38.

Kilbourn, M. R., DaSilva, J. N., Frey, K. A., Koeppe, R. A., and Kuhl, D. E. (1993). *In vivo* imaging of vesicular monoamine transporters in human brain using [¹¹C]tetrabenazine and positron emission tomography. *J. Neurochem.* **60:** 2315–2318.

Kilbourn, M. R., Lee, L. C., Jewett, D. M., Vander Borght, T. M., Koeppe, R. A., and Frey, K. A (1995a). *In vitro* and *in vivo* binding of α-dihydrotetrabenazine to the vesicular monoamine transporter is stereospecific. *J. Cerebr. Blood Flow Metab.,* **15:** S650.

Kilbourn, M. R., Lee, L., Vander Borght, T., Jewett, D., and Frey, K. (1995b). Binding of α-dihydrotetrabenazine to the vesicular monoamine transporter is stereospecific. *Eur. J. Pharmacol.* **278:** 249–252.

Koeppe, R. A., Frey, K. A., Vander Borght, T. M., Kilbourn, M. R., Jewett, D. M., Lee, L. C., and Kuhl, D. E. (1995). Kinetic evaluation of [C-11]-dihydrotetrabenazine (DTBZ) by dynamic PET: A marker for the vesicular monoamine transporter. *J. Cereb. Blood Flow Metab.*, **15:** S651.

Lee, L. C., Sherman, P., and Kilbourn, M. R. (1994). *In vivo* structure-activity study of alkylated tetrabenazine derivatives. *J. Nucl. Med.* **35:** 84P.

Masuo, Y., Pelaprat, D., Scherman, D., and Rostene, W. (1990). [³H]Dihydrotetrabenazine: A new marker for the visualization of dopaminergic denervation in the rat striatum. *Neurosci. Lett.* **114:** 45–50.

Scherman, D., Boschi, G., Rips, R., and Henry, J.-P. (1986). The regionalization of [³H]dihydrotetrabenazine binding sites in the mouse brain and its relationship to the distribution of monoamines and their metabolites. *Brain Res.* **370:** 176–181.

Scherman, D., Raisman, R., Ploska, A., and Agid, Y. (1988). [³H]Dihydrotetrabenazine, a new *in vitro* monoaminergic probe for human brain. *J. Neurochem.* **50:** 1131–1136.

Scherman, D. (1986). Dihydrotetrabenazine binding and monoamine uptake in mouse brain regions. *J. Neurochem.* **47:** 331–339.

Schuldiner, S. (1994). A molecular glimpse of vesicular monoamine transporters. *J. Neurochem.* **62:** 2067.

Vander Borght, T. M., Kilbourn, M. R., Koeppe, R. A., DaSilva, J. N., Carey, J. E., Kuhl, D. E. and Frey, K. A. (1995a). *In vivo* imaging of the brain vesicular monoamine transporter, *J. Nucl. Med.*, **36:** 2252–2260.

Vander Borght, T. M., Sima, A. A. F., Kilbourn, M. R., Desmond, T. J., and Frey, K. A. (1995b). [³H]Methoxytetrabenazine: A high specific activity ligand for estimating monoaminergic neuronal integrity. *Neuroscience*, **68:** 955–962.

The Noncatechol Tracer 6-Fluoro-*m*-Tyrosine:

Extrastriatal Distribution of Dopaminergic Function

W. D. BROWN,[1] **O. T. DeJESUS,**[2] **S. E. SHELTON,**[3] **H. UNO,**[3] **D. HOUSER,**[3] **R. J. NICKLES,**[2]
S. J. SWERDLOFF,[2] **A. ROBERTS,**[2] **E. BAKER,**[2] **and J. E. HOLDEN**[2]

[1]*Department of Radiology and* [2]*Department of Medical Physics*
University of Wisconsin Medical School
Madison, Wisconsin 53792
[3]*Primate Center, University of Wisconsin*
Madison, Wisconsin 53792

Neurons that use Dopamine as their neurotransmitter synthesize it by the decarboxylation of the precursor L-*DOPA. Exogenous DOPA readily crosses the blood–brain barrier and is the classic treatment for the loss of dopamine in Parkinson's disease; its analog* ^{18}*F-6-fluoro-*L*-DOPA (FDOPA) follows the same neurochemical and neurophysiologic pathways, making it a successful PET tracer for this system. However, the usefulness of FDOPA is limited by the rapid peripheral formation of its methylated metabolite, which also freely crosses into the brain. The methylating enzyme requires a catechol as substrate. In this chapter, results are presented from PET scans in rhesus monkeys using a DOPA analog (*^{18}*F-6-fluoro-meta-tyrosine, FMT), which is not catecholic and not methylated and therefore has much higher specific-to-nonspecific activity in PET studies of the brain. This allows the delineation of areas of small concentrations of dopaminergic neurons and terminals. Because of the decarboxylating enzyme that acts on DOPA, FDOPA, and FMT present in all catecholaminergic and serotonergic neurons, small concentrations of nondopaminergic neurons are also demonstrated. This tracer may be particularly useful in evaluation of diseases such as schizophrenia, which involve extrastriatal dopamine systems.*

I. INTRODUCTION

^{18}F-6-fluoro-L-DOPA (FDOPA) is a well-established tracer for assessing the integrity of nigrostriatal neurons in Parkinson's disease and other movement disorders. However, because it is a catechol, it is rapidly metabolized throughout the body by catechol-*O*-methyl transferase (COMT) to the product 3-*O*-methyl-6-fluoro-DOPA, which can pass freely between plasma and all brain tissues. This metabolite adds error and complexity to the measurement of specific FDOPA uptake in the striatum and obscures lower concentrations of Dopaminergic cells and their terminals elsewhere in the brain.

Even though not all of the neurochemical determinants of FDOPA uptake have been firmly established, it is clear that decarboxylation is a necessary step. Therefore, noncatecholic analogs of DOPA that are not substrates to COMT (DeJesus, 1989) but are substrates to aromatic amino acid decarboxylase (AAAD) (Firnau, 1991) may provide tracer maps that more accurately represent the smaller densities of dopaminergic neurons found outside the striatum. This chapter discusses our initial experience with such a tracer, ^{18}F-6-fluoro-*meta*-tyrosine (FMT; see Fig. 1).

II. MATERIALS AND METHODS

Eight adult male rhesus monkeys (*Macaca mulatta*) were included in this study. Each underwent an MRI scan and a two-dimensional (2D) PET scan with the tracer FMT (148–185 MBq); these animals had pre-

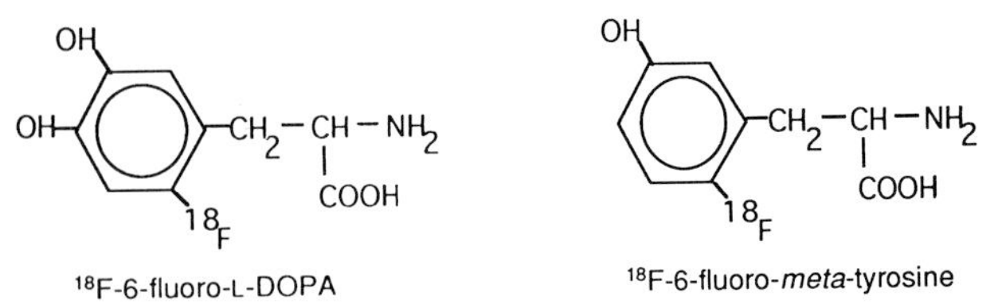

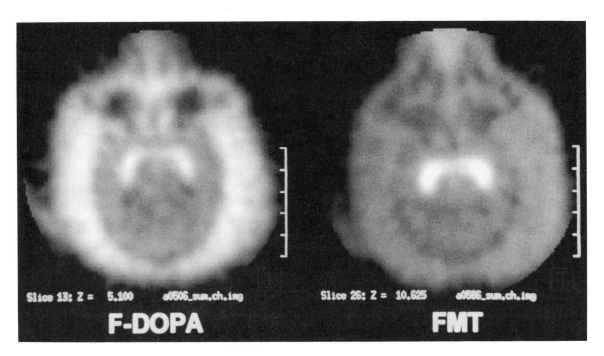

FIGURE 1 This figure shows the structures of 6-FDOPA and 6-FMT. 6-FDOPA is seen to have the ring structure with adjacent hydroxyl groups that is common to all catechols and required for *O*-methylation by COMT. The absence of a hydroxyl group at the 4 position in 6-FMT, therefore causes it not to be a COMT substrate.

viously undergone 6-fluoro-L-DOPA (FDOPA) PET scans as well, allowing direct comparison of the two PET tracers. A three-dimensional (3D) PET scan using FMT was also performed later on three of the animals. All scans were performed under general anesthesia administered by an experienced veterinarian, and the animals were pretreated with carbidopa 1 hour prior to injection of either PET tracer.

MRI imaging consisted of a 3D gradient-recalled echo with spoiler gradient ("SPGR") sequence reconstructed into coronal slices 1.3 mm in thickness. These scans were performed on a GE Advantage (1.5 Tesla) clinical MRI system. The 2D PET scans were performed on a CTI 831 scanner with an axial field of view of approximately 5 cm (four rings of detectors, seven reconstructed planes). Because the interslice distance

of 6.75 cm is large with respect to the structures being imaged, an "interleaved" scan was obtained after a 90 min dynamic study: from 90 to 120 min after injection, static imaging was performed in two bed positions offset by one-half of the slice separation, yielding 14 overlapping slices. The 3D PET scans were performed on a GE Advance scanner, with a 15 cm axial field of view and 4.25 cm interslice distance; these were also obtained 90–120 min after tracer injection.

Neuroanatomic analyses were performed by a neuroradiologist using a rhesus brain anatomic atlas (Kusuma, 1970) and the corresponding MRI image sets; MRI coregistration to 2D PET was used to help confirm tracer localization. The 3D PET scans obtained recently were not formally coregistered with MRI.

III. RESULTS AND DISCUSSION

Comparison of FMT with FDOPA scans demonstrated a marked decrease in nonspecific background activity, corresponding to the absence of FDOPA's major metabolite 3-*O*-methyl-DOPA (Fig. 2). In the monkey, FDOPA scans obtained 90–120 min after injection show activity in the extracranial muscles comparable to striatal activity. Nonspecific activity in the brain is lower, but still sufficient to prevent visualization of extrastriatal specific uptake.

FIGURE 2 Markedly decreased nonspecific activity in FMT images compared with FDOPA images in the same animal under the same scan conditions.

In contrast, FMT scans show a high specific-to-non-specific ratio. As expected, the highest concentration of this tracer was in the neostriatum. In the 2D scans the caudate nucleus and putamen could not be resolved; in some of the 3D image sets, the anterior limb of the internal capsule could be faintly visualized. At the axial level of the inferior striata, these structures are bridged by an area of moderate activity (approximately half of the peak striatal activity), extending through the hypothalamic region into the midbrain. Some specific activity was also present in the anteromedial temporal lobes, corresponding to the regions of the amygdala and pyriform (olfactory) lobes; the activity level was approximately one-fourth that of the striatal maximum. These are regions known to be innervated by the nigrostriatal and mesolimbic Dopaminergic systems (Nieuwenhuys, 1985).

Midbrain activity, however, was not limited to the Dopaminergic cell areas (the largest being the pars compacta of the substantia nigra) but was diffuse. In fact, activity was present throughout the brain stem, including the pontine tegmentum and (to our level of resolution) the entire medulla. Brain stem activity levels decreased steadily from about half the striatal peak in the midbrain to approximately one-third that of the striatal peak in the medulla. The cerebellum had the lowest activity in the brain, in the range 10–15% of striatal activity. Activity in the cerebral hemispheres was slightly higher, about 20% of peak striatal activity; no reproducible focality of uptake was discernible in the hemispheres.

Dopamine is the dominant monoaminergic neurotransmitter in the striatum, and Dopaminergic neurons may be responsible for much of the limbic, diencephalic, and mesencephalic uptake as well. However, the presence of specific FMT uptake diffusely through the brain stem, including large areas without Dopaminergic cell bodies or terminals, demonstrates accumulation in other monoamine neurons (Lloyd, 1972; Sourkes, 1979). This is to be expected since aromatic amino acid decarboxylase is present in serotonergic neurons as well as all catecholaminergic neurons. As recently discussed by Opacka-Juffry and Brooks (Opacka-Juffry and Brooks, 1995), exogenous DOPA and several of its analogs may accumulate in some or all of these cells. AAAD is not rate limiting in any of these neurons (Siegel *et al.*, 1994); unless affected by different cell membrane uptake site specificities, FMT would be expected to label catecholaminergic and serotonergic neurons equally well.

Lack of the 3-*O*-methyl metabolite after FMT administration will markedly simplify Dopaminergic PET scans performed for evaluation of the nigrostriatal system in patients with movement disorders. More striking, however, is the possibility that smaller concentrations of extrastriatal Dopaminergic terminals may be now measurable *in vivo* by PET, which may be important in studying diseases such as schizophrenia. Even the "confounding" specific accumulation of FMT in non-dopaminergic neurons may find eventual scientific or clinical use. Studies should be carried out soon to assess both the chemoarchitectural features and potential clinical significance of this tracer in the human brain.

Acknowledgment

This work was funded in part by NIA grant AG10217.

References

DeJesus, O. T., Mukherjee, J., and Appelman, E. H. (1989). Synthesis of o- and m-tyrosine analogs as potential tracers for CNS Dopamine. *J. Labelled Compd. Radiopharm.* **26:** 133–134.

Firnau, G., Chirakal, R., Nahmias, C., and Garnett, E. S. (1991). (^{18}F)-Fluoro-meta-tyrosine is a better PET tracer than (F18)-fluoro-L-DOPA for the delineation of Dopaminergic structures in the human brain. *J. Labelled Compd. Radiopharm.* **30:** 266–268.

Kusuma, T., and Mabuchi, M. (1970). "Stereotaxic Atlas of the Brain of Macaca fuscata." University Park Press, Baltimore.

Lloyd, K. G., and Hornykiewicz, O. (1972). Occurrence and distribution of aromatic L-amino acid (L-DOPA) decarboxylase in the human brain. *J. Neurochem.* **19:** 1549–1559.

Nieuwenhuys, R. (1985). "Chemoarchitecture of the Brain." pp. 11–19. Springer-Verlag, Berlin.

Opacka-Juffry, J., and Brooks, D. J. (1995). L-Dihydroxyphenylalanine and its decarboxylase: New ideas on their neuroregulatory roles. *Movement Disorders.* **10:** 241–249.

Siegel, G. J., Agranoff, B. W., Albers, R. W., and Mollnoff, P. B., eds. (1994). "Basic Neurochemistry," 5th ed. Raven Press, New York.

Sourkes, T. L. (1979). DOPA Decarboxylase (aromatic amino acid decarboxylase). *In* "The Neurobiology of Dopamine" (A. S. Horn, J. Korf, and B. H. C. Westerink, Eds.), pp. 123–132. Academic Press, London.

3

Quantification of Dopamine Receptors and Transporter in Rat Striatum Using a Small Animal PET Scanner

R. MYERS, S. P. HUME, S. ASHWORTH, A. A. LAMMERTSMA, P. M. BLOOMFIELD, S. RAJESWARAN, and T. JONES

PET Methodology Group
MRC Clinical Sciences Centre
Royal Postgraduate Medical School
Hammersmith Hospital
London, W12 0NN, United Kingdom

A dedicated small-diameter positron emission tomography (PET) scanner has been used to quantify binding of three positron-emitting tracers in rat striatum in vivo: [^{11}C]SCH 23390 (D$_1$ receptor antagonist), [^{11}C]raclopride (D$_2$ receptor antagonist), and the dopamine transporter ligand [^{11}C]RTI-121. As the sizes of the striatal regions of interest used for analysis are of the same order as the dimensions of a detector element (3–4 mm), slight differences in position of the rat within the scanner significantly affected the final images. Rats therefore were held in a perspex stereotaxic frame during scanning, thus abolishing movement and allowing precise positioning such that the striata were at the center of the field of view.

Data are reported from a total of 31 previously untreated rats scanned over a period of 17 months. In addition, for each radioligand, groups of three rats were scanned after pretreatment with a blocking dose of the stable compound. Specific binding was quantified from the kinetic data using a reference tissue compartment model, with the cerebellum as an indirect input function. The results demonstrate that regional time-radioactivity data acquired using small animal PET can provide reproducible and consistent quantitative information on pre- and postsynaptic dopaminergic function in rat striatum and that the system is sufficiently sensitive to allow the study of animal models of disease.

I. INTRODUCTION

A dedicated small-animal PET scanner was designed and built in collaboration with CPS (CTI PET Systems, Knoxville, TN) and its physical characteristics subsequently described (Bloomfield *et al.*, 1995). For the system to be of value in experimental studies, it must be sufficiently stable to permit serial scans and sensitive enough to detect reasonably small changes in radioligand binding.

The present study reports on the use of the system to quantify specific binding of three positron-emitting tracers in rat striatum *in vivo*: [^{11}C]SCH 23390 (D$_1$ receptor antagonist), [^{11}C]raclopride (D$_2$ receptor antagonist) (Playford and Brooks, 1992), and the recently described dopamine transporter ligand [^{11}C]RTI-121 (Brown *et al.*, 1994).

II. MATERIALS AND METHODS

The scanner comprises 16 bismuth germanate detector blocks, each cut into an array of 7 × 8 detectors, circumscribing a ring of diameter 115 mm and giving an axial field of view (FOV) of 50 mm. The transaxial resolution of the scanner was measured as 2.3 mm at full-width–half-maximum (FWHM) at the centre of the

FOV, and 3.5 mm at a 5 mm radial displacement. The axial slice width was 4.3 mm FWHM at the center of the FOV (Bloomfield *et al.*, 1995). All data were acquired within the energy thresholds 250–850 keV.

The scanner has no interplane septa, so all acquisitions are fully 3D. For these initial validation studies, 2D data sets were extracted by taking the 8 direct and 7 adjacent cross planes, giving a total of 15 planes of contiguous data. These data were reconstructed into an image volume by conventional filtered back projection using a ramp filter with a cutoff at 0.5 cycles per pixel. Using a zoom of 1.5 and reconstructing into an image volume of $128 \times 128 \times 15$ pixels, the pixel sizes were 0.47 mm in the X and Y directions, with a slice width of 3.125 mm. For initial studies, where a measured attenuation correction was performed, a transmission scan of 30 min duration was acquired using a rod source of ^{68}Ge, rotating at a radius of 50 mm. In later studies, no transmission scan was collected and attenuation correction was performed by applying a constant factor to striatum and cerebellum data (see later).

The ligands ($\sim$10 MBq) were injected via a catheterized tail vein into adult male Sprague–Dawley rats (270–310 g), maintained under isoflurane anaesthesia. Scan durations were 60 min ([^{11}C]raclopride) or 90 min ([^{11}C]SCH 23390 and [^{11}C]RTI-121), collected in 21 and 24 time frames, respectively, with frame lengths increasing progressively from 5 to 600 sec. Image manipulation was carried out using ANALYZE software (Robb and Hanson, 1991). For the purpose of analyses, image volumes were linearly interpolated in the Z dimension such that voxels had cubic dimensions (0.47 mm). Regions of interest (ROI) were positioned over the left and right striata and the cerebellum in horizontal projections and time-radioactivity curves generated. Figure 1 illustrates the sizes and positions of the ROI used; the striatal ROI were 4×8 pixels and the cerebellar ROI were 8×6 pixels. In a uniform, cylindrical phantom (30 mm diameter), mean pixel values from ROI of the same sizes as those used in the rat brain had coefficients of variation of <3%, at count rates comparable to those encountered during a typical scan.

It may be seen that the striatal ROI are on the same order as the dimensions of a detector element. This has profound implications for the positioning of the rat within the scanner. For example, the distribution of activity within the volume would differ depending on whether the striata were aligned with the center of an individual detector element or with the boundary between two elements, so that the activity was "shared" between two planes. In addition, even minimal head motion due to breathing was found to cause significant and systematic changes in the final dynamic images. Rats therefore were held in a perspex stereo-

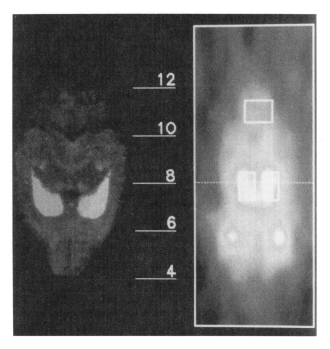

FIGURE 1   On the left, is shown an *in vitro* autoradiograph of a horizontal section of rat brain (bregma, −6 mm; interaural, 4 mm) exposed to [^{11}C]RTI-121 (10 nM, in 50 nM Tris-HCl buffer, pH 7.9, with 300 mM NaCl and 5 mM KCl) for 20 min at room temperature, washed (2×2 min) with ice-cold buffer, rinsed in ice-cold distilled water, and exposed to Hyperfilm-3H (Amersham, U.K.) for 1 hr. The image was digitized using a high-resolution CCD video camera and illustrates the orientation of the rat brain relative to the reconstructed planes of the tomograph. On the right, is a horizontal slice taken from an interpolated volume acquired using the small animal scanner 30–35 min following injection of [^{11}C]RTI-121. Both images are shown so that the brain is orientated "nose down" and with increasingly high radioactivity represented by pixel values of increasing intensity. Rectangular ROI are shown located over the regions of high activity corresponding to the striata and also over the region corresponding to the cerebellum. The high activity located in the intraorbital lachrymal glands can also be seen. The dotted line indicates the centre of the FOV (midplane 8) and the numbered lines mark the centers of the planes indicated.

taxic frame (Fig. 2) during scanning. The design of this was based on the commercial Kopf small-animal stereotaxic frame. The animal's upper incisors locate over a plastic tooth bar and plastic ear bars are located within the interaural canal such that the heights of the bregma and lambda skull points are equal (Paxinos and Watson, 1986). Rats orientated in this "flat-skull" position conform with the stereotaxic atlas of Paxinos and Watson (1986), provided that their body weights fall within the range 270–310 g. Use of this frame abolished movement during scanning and allowed precise positioning of the rat within the tomograph such that the striata were at the center of the FOV, that is, plane 8, as illustrated in Figure 1. Of the 15 reconstructed

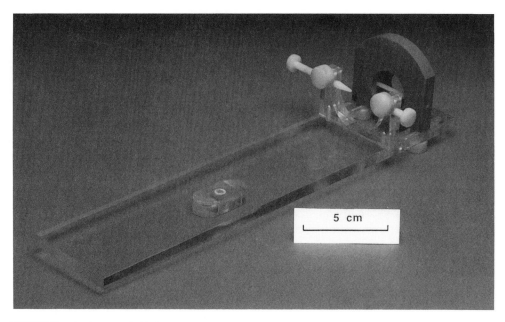

FIGURE 2 A photograph of the perspex stereotaxic frame used for holding rats in the tomograph during scanning. The animal's upper incisors locate over the plastic tooth bar and the plastic ear bars are located within the interaural canal. Anaesthetic is delivered via the unit holding the tooth bar.

planes of data from the tomograph, 8 lie within the 25 mm length of the rat brain. Location of the rat within stereotaxic space also allows objective placement of ROI, as the relative positions of tissues of interest, in this case the striata and cerebellum, are predictable and the sizes are known.

Specific binding was quantified from the kinetic data using a reference tissue compartment model, fitting for the binding potential (BP) with cerebellum as an indirect input function (Hume *et al.*, 1992). BP is defined as the ratio of rate constants to and from the specifically bound tissue compartment.

III. RESULTS AND DISCUSSION

Striatal binding potentials for all three radioligands in a total of 31 previously untreated rats, scanned over a period of 17 months, are shown in Figure 3. Each estimate of BP had an associated standard error of the order of 5% for [^{11}C]raclopride, 8% for [^{11}C]SCH 23390, and 14% for [^{11}C]RTI-121. The data show that the system was stable, showing no significant variation with time. The mean ± standard deviation value for BP for each radioligand is shown in Table 1. The coefficient of variation for each ligand was ~11%, which compares well with the value ~10% for clinical [^{11}C]-raclopride PET scans reported by Volkow et al. (1993).

A subset of the raclopride group ($n = 11$) was first processed with measured attenuation correction. Attenuation factors were calculated to be 16% for both the striatum and cerebellum of these rats. Based on this study, all other cerebellum and striatum data were multiplied by 1.16 to correct for attenuation.

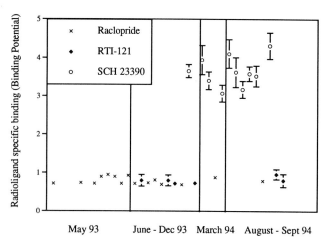

FIGURE 3 Striatal binding potentials in a total of 31 previously untreated rats scanned over a period of 17 months for [^{11}C]raclopride (×), [^{11}C]SCH 23390 (○), and [^{11}C]RTI-121 (◆). Vertical bars show the standard error associated with the BP. Where no error is shown it is within the dimensions of the symbol used.

TABLE 1 Binding Potentials (Mean ± Standard Deviation) from the Number of Rats Shown in Parentheses

	[¹¹C]raclopride	[¹¹C]SCH-23390	[¹¹C]RTI-121
Control	0.79 ± 0.09 (15)	3.64 ± 0.39 (10)	0.80 ± 0.09 (6)
Predosed	0.36 ± 0.03 (3)	0.35 ± 0.07 (3)	0.29 ± 0.06 (3)

In addition to the control animals, groups of three rats were scanned with each radioligand 5 min after pretreatment with a dose of stable compound sufficient to fully saturate the receptors. In each case, BP was reduced to ~0.3, that is, a factor of ~2 for [¹¹C]raclopride, ~3 for [¹¹C]RTI-121, and ~10 for [¹¹C]SCH 23390, indicating the sizes of the windows of specific binding within which changes can be detected.

That the dopaminergic system was used as the test bed for this study was due in part to the availability of appropriate ligands synthesized within the Unit for routine clinical use. In addition, earlier studies (Hume et al., 1992) had demonstrated the potential of PET to quantify [¹¹C]raclopride binding in rat striatum using a clinical tomograph. In the rat, the striata are relatively large compared with other brain structures and the specific binding of the dopaminergic ligands used is confined, to a great extent, to the striata. However, the effects of partial volume are significant when the sizes of the structures of interest are similar to the FWHM of the spatial resolution of the system (Hoffman et al., 1979). The cerebellum is surrounded by low-radioactivity tissues, avoiding contamination of the reference region by spillover of adjacent signal. Nonspecific accumulation of radioactivity does, however, occur within the intraorbital lachrymal glands (Hume et al., 1992 and visualized in Fig. 1, at the level of the striata), and the accumulation may contribute to the radioactivity measured in the striatal ROI. Such contamination may become proportionally greater when counts in the striatum are low. Using the line-spread function of the scanner, Lammertsma et al. (1993) estimated that the spillover fraction from the peak gland value was 0–3.5% in control rats scanned in a clinical PET camera (ECAT-953B, CPS, Knoxville, TN). Although similar calculations for the small animal PET are more difficult due to the variability of the line-spread function over the FOV (Bloomfield et al., 1995),

given the improved resolution of the small animal PET system, the spillover fraction in the present studies should be no worse than that measured for the 953B.

In conclusion, the results shown demonstrate that regional time–activity data acquired using a small animal PET system can provide reproducible and consistent quantitative information on pre- and postsynaptic dopaminergic function in rat striatum. Comparison of predosed and control data indicate that the system is sufficiently sensitive to allow the study of animal models of disease. The usefulness of the system for imaging radioligands or tracers with a more distributed binding pattern than those used in this study remains to be established.

References

Bloomfield, P. M., Rajeswaran, S., Spinks, T. J., Hume, S. P., Myers, R., Ashworth, S., Clifford, K. M., Jones, W. F., Byars, L. G., Young, J., Andreaco, M., Williams, C. W., Lammertsma, A. A., and Jones, T. (1995). The design and physical characteristics of a small animal positron emission tomograph. *Phys. Med. Biol.* **40:** 1105–1126.

Brown, D. J., Luthra, S. K., Brown, G. D., Carroll, F. I., Kuhar, M. J., Osman, S., Waters, S. L., and Brady, F. (1994). [¹¹C]RTI-121—A potential radioligand for PET studies of the dopamine transporter. *J. Labelled. Compd. Radiopharm.* **35:** 483–484.

Hoffman, E. D., Huang, S.-C., and Phelps, M. E. (1979). Quantitation in positron emission computed tomography: 1. Effect of object size. *J. Comput. Assist. Tomogr.* **3:** 299–308.

Hume, S. P., Myers, R., Bloomfield, P. M., Opacka-Juffry, J., Cremer, J. E., Ahier, R. G., Luthra, S. K., Brooks, D. J., and Lammertsma, A. A. (1992). Quantitation of carbon-11 labelled raclopride in rat striatum using positron emission tomography. *Synapse.* **12:** 47–54.

Lammertsma, A. A., Hume, S. P., Myers, R., Bloomfield, P. M., Rajeswaran, S., and Jones, T. (1993). RAT-PET: A bridge between ex vivo animal and in vivo patient studies. *In:* "Quantification of brain function: Tracer kinetics and image analysis in brain PET." Proceedings of Brain PET '93, Akita, Japan, 29–31 May, 1993. (K. Uemura, N. A. Lassen, T. Jones, and I. Kanno, Eds.), International Congress Series 1030, Tokyo, Japan.

Paxinos, G., and Watson, C. (1986). "The Rat Brain in Stereotaxic Coordinates." 2nd ed. Academic Press, London.

Playford, E. D., and Brooks, D. J. (1992). In vivo and in vitro studies of the dopaminergic system in movement disorders. *Cerebr. Brain Metab. Rev.* **4:** 144–171.

Robb, R. A., and Hanson, D. P. (1991). A software system for interactive and quantitative visualization of multidimensional biomedical images. *Australas. Phys. Eng. Sci. Med.* **14:** 9–30.

Volkow, N. D., Fowler, J. S., Wang, G.-J., Dewey, S. L., Schlyer, D., MacGregor, R., Logan, J., Alexoff, D., Shea, C., Hitzemann, R., Angrist, B., and Wolf, A. P. (1993). Reproducibility of repeated measures of carbon-11-raclopride binding in the human brain. *J. Nucl. Med.* **34:** 609–613.

Applicability of Experimental PET in Animal Models for the Interpretation of Incidental Findings in Human Stroke

W.-D. HEISS, K. WIENHARD, R. GRAF, J. LÖTTGEN, U. PIETRZYK, and R. WAGNER

Max Planck Institute for Neurological Research
University of Cologne Neurology Clinic
D-50931 Köln, Germany

A commercial high-resolution scanner designed for clinical PET studies was tested for its applicability to investigations of cerebral metabolism and blood flow in cats. CBF, $CMRO_2$, CBV, and CMR_{glc} were determined using ^{15}O-steady-state or bolus injection oxygen methods and ^{18}F-fluorodeoxyglucose (FDG). Metabolic and blood flow images of 14 contiguous, 3 mm PET slices were compared to histological sections in four control animals. In another 12 cats, hemodynamic and metabolic changes were followed by serial multitracer PET for 24 hr after permanent and 30 and 60 min occlusion of the left middle cerebral artery (MCA). The pattern and extent of the changes of the physiological variables were related to the final infarct verified in matched histological sections. At the scanner's spatial resolution (FWHM of 3.6 mm transaxial and of 4.0 mm axial), the gross anatomy of the cat's brain could be distinguished best in FDG images. The values of CBF, $CMRO_2$, and CMR_{glc} measured in cortex, white matter, and basal ganglia were in the range of common autoradiographic results. Immediately after MCA occlusion, there was widespread decrease in blood flow, but metabolism was preserved at values suggesting viable tissue. In permanent occlusion, the areas of increased oxygen extraction fraction (OEF) moved with time from the center to the periphery of the MCA territory, then OEF and CMR_{glc} subsequently declined, indicating transformation to the large infarcts later found in corresponding histologic sections. Reopening the MCA after 30 min induced short-lasting hyperperfusion and fast normalization of metabolism; no cortical infarcts were found. After 60 min occlusion, hyperperfusion lasted for extended periods, $CMRO_2$, OEF, and CMR_{glc} were permanently depressed, and large in-farcts were found. These results demonstrate that high-resolution PET is a valuable tool for clinically oriented experimental research.

I. INTRODUCTION

In acute neurological diseases, pathophysiological data can be acquired only incidentally at varying time points in the course of the clinical disorder, whereas the further development into a permanent defect or the recovery of normal function remains undetermined. To better understand the results of multitracer PET studies, such as in early stroke, reproducible animal experiments are necessary in which regional changes in physiologic variables can be followed from the vascular insult to the permanent defective state and then be related to histologic alterations.

II. METHODS

Adult cats were anesthetized with ketamine hydrochloride (25 mg/kg im), tracheostomized, immobilized with pancuronium bromide (0.2 mg/kg iv), and artificially ventilated. Anesthesia was continued with 0.8–1.5% halothane in a 70% N_2O/30% O_2 gas mixture. Physiological variables were kept in the normal range for awake cats; deep body temperature was maintained at 37–37.5°C. Four animals were studied repeatedly without further surgical procedures and served as controls. In 12 cats, the left MCA was exposed transorbitally and an implanted device (Graf *et al.*, 1986) was

16

used to occlude the MCA with a microdrive through the resealed orbit. In six cats the MCA was occluded permanently, in four cats the MCA was reopened after 30 min, and in four cats after 60 min.

Each cat underwent multiple consecutive PET studies. In animals with MCA occlusion, control measurements before and up to six measurements after occlusion (and reperfusion) were performed over an experimental period of 24 hr. For that purpose, cats were positioned with a head holder in the scanner gantry. Comparability among animals was achieved by the numerous 3.1 mm coronal tomographic slices across the cat's head, comprising the whole brain and permitting three-dimensional reconstruction and alignment to histological sections obtained in the same orientation. Correction of photon attenuation was carried out in each cat, using a transmission scan performed with rotating ^{68}Ge rod sources. For the assessment of cerebral blood flow (CBF), cerebral metabolic rate for oxygen ($CMRO_2$), oxygen extraction fraction (OEF), and cerebral blood volume (CBV), the steady-state ^{15}O continuous inhalation method or the bolus injection method was used (Baron et al., 1989). Cerebral glucose metabolic rate (CMR_{glc}) was measured after injection of 74 MBq ^{18}F-2-fluoro-2-deoxy-D-glucose (FDG) (Reivich et al., 1979).

Serial PET scanning was performed with a CTI Siemens ECAT EXACT HR tomograph, a commercial, clinical PET system that provides high-spatial resolution (Wienhard et al., 1994), yielding at the center of the FOV, a resolution of 3.6 mm transaxially and 4.0 mm axially. During each $C^{15}O_2$, $^{15}O_2$, and $C^{15}O$ or $H_2^{15}O$ scan, two arterial blood samples were taken (at the beginning and at the end of acquisition) for determination of blood gases and for whole blood and plasma radioactivity measurements in a well counter cross-calibrated to the camera. Their mean value was used for parametric image generation. During the FDG studies, eight blood samples were taken starting at tracer injection. Plasma radioactivity was used for CMR_{glc} calculations according to the model equation (Reivich et al., 1979). Furthermore, plasma glucose concentrations were measured.

At the end of the experiment, the animals were perfusion fixed with formalin (4%) and the brains were removed. Serial sections (stained with HE or Luxol Fast Blue) were matched individually with the various functional images to permit comparative assessment of infarcts. Data analysis was based on the parametric images from those 14 transaxial PET slices comprising the brain. For functional quantitation, regions of interest (ROIs) were placed in selected brain regions in relation to the corresponding histological sections. One set of ROIs was defined for each animal and used for all studies of that animal.

III. RESULTS

CBF and $CMRO_2$ images permitted the identification of the main anatomic and CBV images of the main vascular structures within the cat's head. Optimum spatial resolution was afforded by the CMR_{glc} images, which permitted clear distinction, say, of the caudate nucleus and olfactory bulb. The functional images were in good agreement with the matched histological sections, permitting easy identification of specific structures in a stereotactic atlas (Reinoso-Suárez, 1961). Despite the limited spatial resolution of the PET images compared to the size of a cat brain, physiological values could be obtained separately for compartments of mainly gray (cortex or basal ganglia) or white matter. These values can serve as a basis for among or within animal comparisons in a variety of experiments. The highest values for CBF, $CMRO_2$, and CMR_{glc} were measured in ROIs containing large proportions of basal ganglia or cortex, whereas the lowest values were found in ROIs of mainly white matter. The ratio between cortex or basal ganglia and white matter values ranged between 1.4 and 2.0.

The capability of the PET system to distinguish regional pathophysiological changes was tested using the MCA occlusion model. In all experimental animals, the arterial occlusion immediately reduced CBF to the respective supply territory below 30% of its control level, with a distinct but graded transition to surrounding brain tissue. Initially, $CMRO_2$ was less diminished, and consequently OEF was increased, thus indicating that oxygen supply was still sufficient to keep the tissue vital despite dense ischemia ("misery perfusion") (Fig. 1). With permanent MCA occlusion in the core of ischemia, both $CMRO_2$ and OEF eventually decreased, suggesting necrotic tissue transformation. Over the next 4–6 hr, this process spread from the center of the MCA territory to the region adjoining the core of ischemia. In this border zone, blood flow was initially impaired to a lesser degree and $CMRO_2$ was preserved. Within 18–24 hr, MCA infarction became complete, with blood flow and energy metabolism being equally reduced. At that time, the size of the ultimate infarct was reflected best by CMR_{glc} images. However, because of the functional deactivation of anatomically preserved tissue in the close vicinity of the infarct, the areas of metabolic impairment were always slightly larger than the necrotic zone on histological sections. In animals with large infarcts, within 24 hr, the ensuing

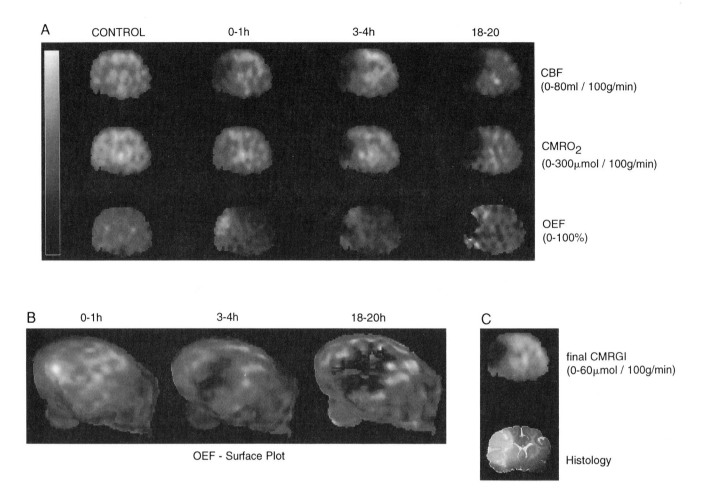

FIGURE 1   (A) Sequential quantitative PET images of an individual cat representing $CMRO_2$, CBF, OEF, before (control) and at three time points after left middle cerebral artery occlusion (0–1 hr, 3–4 hr, 18–20 hr). Progressive deterioration of oxygen consumption in the MCA territory corresponds with the spreading of the area with increased OEF and finally leads to hemodynamic and metabolic derangement of the contralateral hemisphere as well. (B) Reconstructed OEF surface views of the left hemisphere at the three time points, showing dynamic penumbra leading to progressive metabolic derangement. (C) PET image of CMR_{glc} representing the area of final glucose suppression at 18–20 hr after MCA occlusion and corresponding histological cross section showing the area of final infarction.

increase in intracranial pressure also impaired blood flow of the contralateral hemisphere, and the raised OEF indicated the development of whole-brain damage.

The quality of high-resolution PET images and the benefit of repeated multitracer studies is demonstrated by surface reconstructions of OEF. In all cats with permanent MCA occlusion, the ischemic penumbra, that is, the area of increased OEF, spread with time from the center to the borders of the ischemic MCA territory. In most instances, that misery perfusion condition was followed by a marked OEF drop, reflecting progressive impairment of blood flow and metabolism and suggesting transition to necrosis (Fig. 1). In one animal, the penumbra was reversible and the involved

cortex survived. Eventually, this cat suffered only a small persistent ischemic lesion of basal ganglia and internal capsule.

In the group with reversible MCA occlusion, CBF in the left cortex decreased to values between 20 and 40% in all animals, whereas $CMRO_2$ was reduced to 50–60% and, consequently, OEF increased to 130–140% of the preocclusion values, indicating viability of tissue. Reopening of the MCA after 30 min was followed by a short hyperperfusion with fast normalization of $CMRO_2$ and OEF. After 60 min of MCA occlusion, hyperperfusion lasted for extended periods—up to more than 6 hr—$CMRO_2$ as well as OEF were permanently depressed and $rCMR_{glc}$ was significantly reduced. Whereas large infarctions were present in cats after 60 min of MCA occlusion, no cortical infarcts were found after 30 min of occlusion.

IV. DISCUSSION

Previous PET studies in animals were used mainly to analyze the biodistribution and kinetics of new tracers developed for PET, to follow the distribution of tracers in the brain, and to image the brain uptake of labeled drugs and its inhibition. Mainly because of limitations with spatial resolution, physiological variables of animals under normal conditions were rarely studied with PET, and only a rough correlation of selected regions of interest with anatomical structures was achieved (Pinard *et al.*, 1993). In a few instances, the altered uptake of tracers was demonstrated in experimental lesions, for example, in focal edema following cold injury (Prenen *et al.*, 1989) or after thromboembolic stroke (De Ley *et al.*, 1988). Systematic investigations of altered physiology in acute experimental conditions like focal ischemia were limited by poor spatial resolution and therefore yielded rather global results. In several studies, the feasibility of repeated PET measurements in acute experimental focal ischemia was established in baboons (Pappata *et al.*, 1993; Sette *et al.*, 1993; Young *et al.*, 1995), but this approach was limited by the unfavorable spatial resolution of the equipment used and restriction to the first few hours after MCA occlusion, which in most instances prevented the evaluation of the development of permanent infarction and its histological verification. Our approach was designed to overcome these limitations and demonstrate that current high-resolution PET can be employed for serial studies of pathophysiologic changes in experimental focal ischemia of smaller animals like the cat. Due to the high resolution of the scanner (≤ 4 mm in all directions, Wienhard *et al.*, 1994), which still is coarse in relation to the fine anatomical details of the cat brain, regional changes of hemodynamic and metabolic measures could be assessed over time and the final brain lesions could be localized as a consequence of regional temporal pattern and in good agreement with the infarct as determined in histological serial sections. In transient MCA, occlusion of 60 min was established as the critical time window to cause large infarcts in the cat, despite (or because of) a significant and long-lasting hyperperfusion occurring in most of these animals after reopening of the vessel. These results, which help to interpret incidental find-

ings in acute human stroke, demonstrate that high-resolution PET is an efficient tool to investigate the pathophysiology of transient or persisting focal brain damage of various etiologies in experimental models and might also be a cost-effective means to evaluate therapeutic strategies.

References

Baron, J. C., Frackowiak, R. S. J., Herholz, K., Jones, T., Lammertsma, A. A., Mazoyer, B., Wienhard, K. (1989). Use of PET methods for measurement of cerebral energy metabolism and hemodynamics in cerebrovascular disease. *J. Cerebr. Blood Flow Metab.* **9:** 723–742.

De Ley, G., Weyne, J., Demeester, G., Stryckmans, K., Goethals, P., Van de Velde, E., and Leusen, I. (1988). Experimental thromboembolic stroke studied by positron emission tomography: Immediate versus delayed reperfusion in fibrinolysis. *J. Cerebr. Blood Flow Metab.* **8:** 539–545.

Graf, R., Kataoka, K., Rosner, G., and Heiss, W.-D. (1986). Cortical deafferentation in cat focal ischemia: Disturbance and recovery of sensory functions in cortical areas with different degrees of CBF reduction. *J. Cerebr. Blood Flow Metab.* **6:** 566–573.

Pappata, S., Fiorelli, M., Rommel, T., Hartmann, A., Dettmers, C., Yamaguchi, T., Chabriat, H., *et al.* (1993). PET study of changes in local brain hemodynamics and oxygen metabolism after unilateral middle cerebral artery occlusion in baboons. *J. Cerebr. Blood Flow Metab.* **13:** 416–424.

Pinard, E., Mazoyer, B., Verrey, B., Pappata, S., and Crouzel, C. (1993). Rapid measurement of regional cerebral blood flow in the baboon using ^{15}O-labelled water and dynamic positron emission tomography. *Med. Biol. Eng. Comput.* **31:** 495–502.

Prenen, G. H. M., Go, K. G., Paans, A. M. J., Zuiderveen, F., Vaalburg, W., Kamman, R. L., Molenaar, W. M., Zijlstra, S., *et al.* (1989). Positron emission tomographical studies of 1-^{11}C-acetoacetate, 2-^{18}F-fluoro-deoxy-D-glucose, and L-1-^{11}C-tyrosine uptake by cat brain with an experimental lesion. *Acta Neurochir. Wien* **99:** 166–172.

Reinoso-Suárez, F. (1961). Topographischer Hirnatlas der Katze. Darmstadt: E. Merck AG.

Reivich, M., Kuhl, D., Wolf, A., Greenberg, J., Phelps, M., Ido, T., Casella, V., Fowler, J., Hoffman, E., Alavi, A., Som, P., and Sokoloff, L. (1979). The ^{18}F-fluorodeoxyglucose method for the measurement of local cerebral glucose utilization in man. *Circ. Res.* **44:** 127–137.

Sette, G., Baron, J.-C., Young, A. R., Miyazawa, H., Tillet, I., Barré, L., Travère, J. M., Derlon, J. M., and MacKenzie, E. T. (1993). In vivo mapping of brain benzodiazepine receptor changes by positron emission tomography after focal ischemia in the anesthetized baboon. *Stroke* **24:** 2046–2058.

Wienhard, K., Dahlbom, M., Eriksson, L., Michel, Ch., Bruckbauer, T., Pietrzyk, U., and Heiss, W.-D. (1994). The ECAT EXACT HR: Performance of a new high resolution positron scanner. *J. Comput. Assist. Tomogr.* **18:** 110–118.

Young, A. R., Touzani, O., Baron, J.-C., Mezenge, F., Derlon, J.-M., MacKenzie, E. T. (1995). To reperfuse or not to reperfuse?: Quantitative volumes after middle cerebral artery occlusion in the baboon. *J. Cerebr. Blood Flow Metab.* **15,** Suppl. 1: S72.

The MOC Counter:

A Pharmacological Tool for the *in Vivo* Measurement of Ligand Occupancy Indices in the Human Brain

A. MALIZIA,[1,2] G. FORSE,[1] R. N. GUNN,[1] A. HAIDA,[1] L. SCHNORR,[1] S. RAJESWARAN,[1]
K. POOLE,[1] D. NUTT,[2] and T. JONES[1]

[1]*Neuroscience and Methodology Sections*
Clinical Sciences Centre, Royal Postgraduate Medical School
Hammersmith Hospital, London W12 0NN, United Kingdom
[2]*Psychopharmacology Unit, University of Bristol*
Bristol BS8 1TD, United Kingdom

We describe the development of a technique that has the potential to measure macroregional indices of drug delivery and occupancy using very low levels of radiation (<3.7 MBq). The initial experiments with the multiple organs coincidences counter (MOCC) are described in the context of answering some of the initial questions about the possible applications and the shortcomings of this instrument. Pilot data with [^{11}C] flumazenil (a benzodiazepine site marker), [^{11}C]diprenorphine (an opiate receptor marker), [^{11}C]RTI 55 (a dopamine and serotonin reuptake site marker) and [^{11}C]WAY 100635 are discussed as examples.

I. INTRODUCTION

The advent of computerized tomography of radioligands has resulted in the ability to investigate drug occupancy in tissues of interest and thus to provide a more direct pharmacokinetic measure of drug concentration in the target organs than the estimation of free drug in plasma.

When applied to pharmacology, the main objective is in obtaining a relative measure of occupancy change at the receptor site. This measure needs to be repeated in time to correlate the receptor kinetics with pharmacological, pathological, and physiological indices such as response to treatment, side effects, tolerance, displaceability by other agents, patterns of tissue-specific metabolism and changes in physiological parameters. This line of enquiry can be also extended to healthy volunteers, for drug discovery and development and for clinical pharmacological inquiry (Ritter and Jones, 1995).

However, some factors limit the *in vivo* use of radioligand: The doses of radiation used in SPECT/PET result in a maximum limit of two or three scans per year in patients and human volunteers. This is a severe limitation for repeated clinical measurement. In addition, healthy women cannot take part in these investigations as healthy controls. Women, however, have a ratio of at least 2:1 prevalence of common psychiatric conditions, therefore it would be cogent to assess pharmacokinetics in this half of the population. Further, in many PET centers the access to a camera is limited by competition with other research programs.

While investigating benzodiazepine-site kinetics with PET in a pulse chase experiment using [^{11}C]flumazenil and intravenous midazolam as a displacement agent, we observed that the head curve obtained by summing the counts from all the detectors contained enough information to provide us with a summary index of the proportional signal change across the various cortical areas that have significant benzodiazepine binding. At the peak of the decay-corrected curve, about 250,000 counts per second were recorded from the head having injected 220–270 MBq of [^{11}C]flumazenil. Hence, it was reasoned that by summing the signal from all the detectors, this global information could be collected by injecting much lower doses of radioactivity. In addition, because no tomographic information needed to be acquired, we thought it possible to undertake these experiments using simpler nonto-

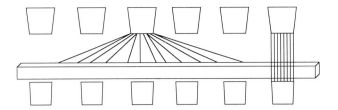

Field of view for singles v coincidences

FIGURE 1 Schematic representation of the whole body counter with detectors placed above and below the bed on which the subject lies. The lines in the diagram show the field of view for single photons or coincidences.

mographic information. To this end, we successfully adapted a whole-body gamma counter. This chapter briefly describes its function and characteristics and summarizes the experiments carried out with a range of tracers that illustrates its advantages and shortcomings.

II. THE MULTIPLE ORGANS COINCIDENCES COUNTER

The whole-body gamma counter consists of 12 large sodium iodide detectors spaced above and below a sliding bed on which the subject lies (Fig. 1). In pilot experiments it was determined that this system was not sensitive enough to detect a displacement of [11C]-flumazenil on the order of 20%, which had been previously recorded using the PET camera. This was due to the large field of view of the detectors (of the order of 50 cm), which resulted in photons being recorded from a large area of the body, thus diluting the specific signal from the head. This effect accounts for the fact that, in previous experiments in the whole-body counter, sizeable displacement had been observed only with very high doses of cold ligand. To avoid this problem two pairs of detectors were connected to count coincidences. As a result, this electronic collimation has significantly improved the sensitivity of the system to changes in specific signal due to pharmacological manipulation. We have called this system the *multiple organs coincidences counter* (MOCC).

Data collected to date suggests that displacements of about 10% can be easily detected but displacements calculated to be less than 5% of the signal are not distinguishable from control, tracer alone experiments. The pairs of detectors that count coincidences have a FWHM of 8 cm and a FWTM of 12 cm as measured with germanium point sources in the same geometry

as in the clinical studies. A MOCC injection of about 1% (2.4–3.7 MBq) of the dose of radioligand used for PET results in about 0.25% of the coincidences being detected from the head; therefore, the system has a comparable efficiency because the two detectors are recording from a lesser solid angle than the circular array in the PET camera. Detector dead time, due to high counts, is negligible up to about 12,000 coincidences per second, which is well above the range detected in our experiments. The geometry used to acquire the data has been standardized in terms of detector distances from the bed and their centers are placed in standard positions, derived from external anatomical markings. In addition, to correct for the different body sizes and possible differences in detector sensitivity, "attenuation" information is acquired by recording counts from a disk-shaped germanium source prior to each experiment, for each detector pair, with and without the subject in position. Initial blood activity measurements have demonstrated that little activity can be detected unless the samples are collected over a long period of time. This would result in unacceptable smoothing of the input function; in addition, metabolites cannot be measured at these concentrations with the available technology, therefore the measure would be a composite of parent and metabolites, which would be of limited use as an input function.

III. IS IT POSSIBLE TO OBTAIN AN INDEX OF OCCUPANCY USING THE MOCC?

Pulse chase experiments with [11C]flumazenil and cold flumazenil have indicated that it is possible to obtain an index of occupancy with this method. Seven healthy male volunteers took part in 12 experiments with [11C]flumazenil in the MOCC. On all occasions they were administered 2.4–3.7 MBq of radiotracer at the beginning of the experiment. Four experiments were of the tracer alone, and the others were pulse chase ones with doses of 2.5, 5, 7, 10, 12.5, 15, 20 and 40 μg/kg cold flumazenil administered between 20 and 30 min after the radiotracer. In all the displacement experiments, a change in slope was observed on the total head curve. An index of occupancy for the whole volume was obtained using spectral analysis (Cunningham and Jones, 1993) and a synthetic input function. This index was plotted versus the dose administered, as if it were an occupancy measure mimicking standard pharmacological plotting techniques (dose–occupancy, log dose–occupancy, double inverse, and Scatchard; Fig. 2). The index behaved as if it were a measure of occupancy, and inspection of the resulting

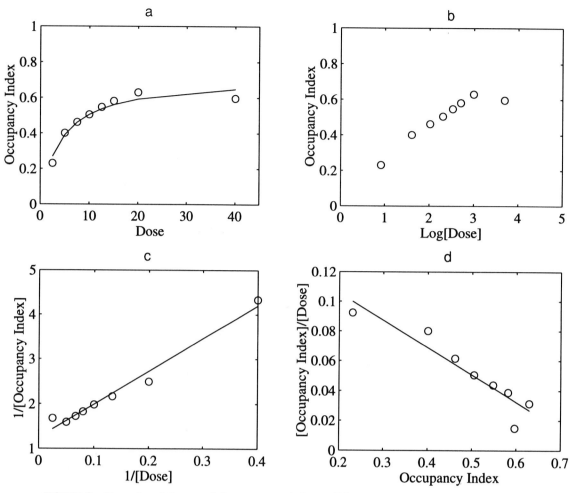

FIGURE 2   Examples of the use of the occupancy index as if it were an occupancy measure. (a) Dose μg/kg *v* index, (b) log dose μg/kg *v* log index, (c) double reciprocal, and (d) Scatchard-based (index *v* index/ dose μg/kg) plots of [¹¹C]flumazenil displacement by various doses of cold flumazenil.

plots indicates that 5–7 μg/kg of cold flumazenil displace about 50% of the signal.

IV. DOES THE COLLECTION OF INFORMATION FROM MULTIPLE ORGANS GIVE ADDITIONAL INFORMATION?

At present, we are recording information from two volumes. These can be anywhere in the body. All the data collected thus far refers to head and left chest. [¹¹C]diprenorphine (a nonselective μ, κ, and δ opiate marker (Jones *et al.*, 1994)); [¹¹C]WAY 100635 (a 5-HT1a receptor marker; (Pike *et al.*, 1995); and [¹¹C]-flumazenil studies suggest binding in the head but not in the left chest. The converse was found with [¹¹C]-MHED (*meta*-hydroxyephedrine) (Rosenspire *et al.*,

1990), a noradrenaline reuptake site marker. This is consistent with information from preclinical studies and provides some information on the biodistribution of the ligand. In addition, displacement experiments with [¹¹C]flumazenil and [¹¹C]diprenorphine have confirmed that none of the left chest signal could be displaced even at high doses of competing cold ligand. This is interpreted as lack of significant specific binding in the tissues observed (mainly heart and some lung). We have also recorded the information from the administration of [¹⁵O]-CO, which suggested a ratio of blood volume of 3 : 1 between the left chest and the head. In addition, because the time–activity curves from organs with no uptake resemble the total radioactivity blood time–activity curves we are in the process of attempting to devise a method to utilize this information as an input function (i.e., a reference tissue approach).

An experiment with [^{11}C]RTI-55 (Carroll *et al.*, 1995) has clearly demonstrated the potential uses of collecting information from more than one volume of interest. RTI-55 crosses the blood–brain barrier and binds to both serotonergic and dopaminergic reuptake sites. When clomipramine 10 mg iv (a tricyclic antidepressant with significant serotonergic reuptake inhibition) was administered during an [^{11}C]RTI-55 MOCC experiment, the counts in the head volume counterintuitively increased (Fig. 3(a)). However, inspection of the left chest curve (Fig. 3(b)) revealed that RTI-55 had been significantly displaced peripherally, probably from platelet and lung serotonin reuptake sites. The increased circulating RTI-55 had crossed the blood–brain barrier and bound probably both to nonspecific and dopaminergic reuptake sites in the brain. This conjecture was confirmed by injection of [^{11}C]RTI-55 after preloading with clomipramine. In this experiment, the head curve reached a higher number of counts more rapidly than when the tracer had been administered alone but the left chest curve declined more readily. Thus the collection of information from more than one anatomical volume can provide additional information that could be used to characterize a radiotracer behavior *in vivo*.

V. WHAT CONCLUSIONS CAN BE DRAWN FROM EXPERIMENTS WHERE THERE IS A FAILURE OF CHANGING A SIGNAL BY PHARMOCOLOGICAL MANIPULATION?

WAY 100635 is a very high affinity 5-HT$_{1A}$ antagonist. PET studies in human volunteers have demonstrated that it delineates brain areas where there is a high density of such receptors. These are widespread in the cortex but are especially concentrated in medial temporal structures and raphe nuclei (Pike *et al.*, 1995). Concurrently with PET experiments, we investigated this ligand in the MOCC. Initial studies demonstrated that, as expected, a signal was detectable from the head consistent with the finding that this ligand crosses the blood–brain barrier and binds in the brain. However, subsequent experiments where subjects were preloaded with either buspirone 30 mg (a 5-HT$_{1A}$ partial agonist) or pindolol 30 mg (a noradrenergic beta-blocker with significant 5-HT$_{1A}$ antagonism in humans) by mouth 3 hr prior to the administration of the radioligand did not show any change in signal. In this case a coherent interpretation of the data is not possible, as this technique does not provide enough information. The lack of observed effect could be due to either

the very high affinity of WAY-100635, dilution of the specific signal by a labeled metabolite that crosses the blood–brain barrier and thus obscures relatively small changes in occupancy, different radioligand metabolism induced by the competing agent, blood flow changes affecting delivery or to concurrent receptor affinity changes masking the decrease in number of sites available for binding.

VI. DISCUSSION

We have described the use of low doses of injected ligand for the detection of global changes in receptor occupancy by the administration of exogenous competing ligands. Even though this information could be collected in a PET camera by using very coarse or no reconstruction, we have modified an existing whole-body gamma counter to do this because of the time pressure on the existing PET resources. Although the use of the whole-body gamma counter denies any possible tomographic information, it has other advantages. It is possible to record information from more than one part of the body and also the radiochemical residuals of PET syntheses (typically tens of mCi) can be employed for up to two consecutive experiments without any additional synthesis. Apart from an index of drug occupancy in tissue, this technique could also be extended to provide repeated measures of enzymatic (e.g. MAO) and precursor processes (e.g., L-tryptophan) with disease progress.

The main disadvantages of this technique are the lack of tomographic information and the low levels of circulating ligand, which make detection of counts in blood difficult and the detection of metabolites not feasible with current techniques.

The assumptions underlying the displacement or preloading studies are that this ligand is widely distributed in the organ under study, that its metabolism is not changed by the competing agent, and that no changes in receptor affinity are induced during the experiment so that in any experiment the change in signal is solely due to changes in the available number of receptors.

Despite these limitations this technique has a number of advantages, which are a function of the very low doses of radioactivity administered and the opportunity to acquire data from more than one part of the body. The very low dose administered results in the possibility of conducting repeated examinations, which can probe the effects of medication changes and disease progress or map the relationship between receptor kinetic and dynamic measures in a dose ranging fashion.

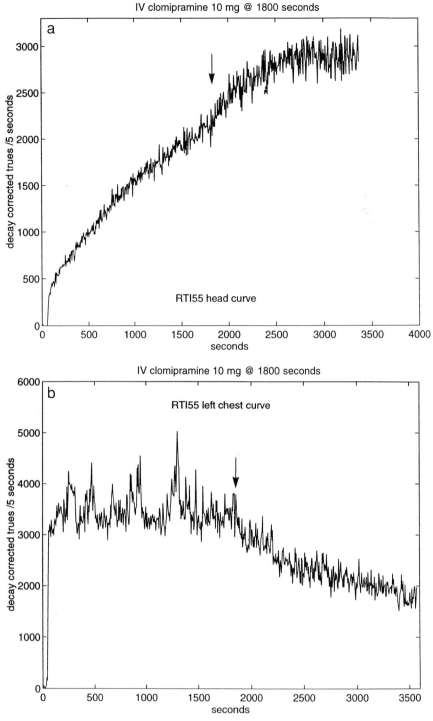

FIGURE 3   (a) Increase in [^{11}C]RTI-55 head signal after the administration of intravenous clomipramine. (b) Decrease in left chest [^{11}C]RTI-55 signal after the administration of intravenous clomipramine.

In addition, these low doses mean that it is acceptable for women volunteers to take part in these pharmacological studies, thus not excluding information from a very substantial and highly relevant part of the potential patient population. Further it will be possible to start examining the pharmacological properties of ligands that can be produced only in low yields of radioactivity to test whether they are taken up in the organ of interest and whether they can be displaced, thus confirming specific binding. For the latter, the caveat is that a negative experiment does not necessarily confirm that this is not feasible when tomographic information is available. The ability to acquire information from more than one volume is useful not only for total body kinetics and metabolism but also because it provides a potential way to acquire an input function for these studies.

Future studies should be directed at validating the use of this tool and exploring the possibility of also studying ligands that have a more limited cerebral or other organ distribution, for instance with D2 dopamine receptor markers such as raclopride. In addition, it will be worth exploring the administration of such low doses in the PET camera, which may enable investigators to carry out many repeated experiments in the same subject and perhaps also collect coarse tomographic information in the brain.

Acknowledgment

AM is a Wellcome training fellow.

References

Carroll, F. I., Kotian, P., Dehghani, A., Gray, J. L., Kuzemko, M. A., Parnham, K. A., Abraham, P., Lewin, A. H., Boja, J. W., and Kuhar, M. J. (1995). Cocaine and 3β- (4'-substituted phenyl) tropane 2β carboxylic acid ester and amide analogues. New high affinity and selective compounds for the dopamine transporter. *J. Med. Chem.* **38**, 379–388.

Cunningham, V. J., and Jones, T. (1993). Spectral analysis of dynamic PET studies. *J. Cerebr. Blood Flow* **13**:15–23.

Jones, A. K. P., Cunningham, V. J., Ha-Kawa, S. K., Fujiwara, T., Liyii, Q., Luthra, S. K., Ashburner, J., Osman, S., and Jones, T. (1994). Quantitation of [^{11}C]diprenorphine cerebral kinetics in man acquired by PET using presaturation, pulse-chase and tracer only protocols. *J. Neurosci. Methods* **51**: 123–134.

Pike, V. W., McCarron, J. A., Lammertsma, A. A., Hume, S. P., Poole, K., Grasby, P. M., Malizia, A. L., Cliffe, I. A., Fletcher, A., and Bench, C. J. (1995). First delineation of 5HT 1A receptors in living human brain with PET and [^{11}C]-WAY 100635. *Eur. J. Pharmacol.* **283**: R1–R3.

Ritter, J. M., and Jones, T. (1995). PET: A symposium highlighting its clinical and pharmacological potential. *TIPS* **16**: 117–119.

Rosenspire, K. C., Haka, M. S., Van Dort, M. E., Jewett, D. M., Gildersleeve, D. L., Schwaiger, M., and Wieland, D. M. (1990). Synthesis and preliminary evaluation of carbon-11-meta-hydroxyephedrine: A false transmitter agent for heart neuronal imaging. *J. Nucl. Med.* **8**: 1328–1334.

Autoradiography as a Tool for PET/SPECT Tracer Selection and Assessment

A. BIEGON
Pharmos Ltd.,
Kiryat Weizmann Science Park,
Rehovot, Israel

C. MATHIS
PET Facility,
Department of Radiology,
University of Pittsburgh,
Pittsburgh, Pennsylvania
15213

W. JAGUST
Lawrence Berkeley Laboratory
Center for Functional Imaging,
Berkeley, California 94720

Autoradiographic techniques have been used to study a number of neurotransmitter ligands to assess their use for in vivo imaging with PET or SPECT. This chapter reports results with several compounds with high affinity to the serotonin transporter in vitro. In vitro autoradiography with [³H]imipramine (IMI), performed at 4°C, resulted in a distribution of optical density reminiscent of the known distribution of serotonin transporters. However, ex vivo autoradiography resulted in a totally different pattern, with the highest tracer densities found in cortical and hippocampal regions. This binding was not displaceable in vivo, predicting that IMI would be useless as a PET tracer. Ex vivo autoradiography with paroxetine (PAR) revealed a distribution pattern reminiscent of, but not identical with, the in vitro distribution. Specifically, density values in cortical, hippocampal, and striatal regions were too high. Excess unlabeled PAR in vivo efficiently blocked tracer accumulation in serotonin rich regions such as the hypothalamus and raphe, but failed to completely block binding in the cortex, hippocampus, and striatum, predicting limited utility of PAR as an in vivo tracer. Finally, ex vivo autoradiography with INQUIP resulted in a distribution identical to that of serotonin transporters 6–12 hr after tracer injection in rats. In vivo binding was uniformly and specifically blocked by cotreatment with other known, selective serotonin uptake blockers. [¹²³I]INQUIP administered to rhesus monkeys was imaged by SPECT, with a distribution identical to that documented for serotonin transporters in primates. The tracer accumulation in primates was blocked by pretreatment with paroxetine; and it is now being developed for use in human studies. Thus, ex vivo autoradiography can predict tracer inad-equacies not apparent with cruder methods and is an important step in tracer development.

I. INTRODUCTION

The serotonin transporter is implicated in a number of neuropsychiatric disorders, including depression, Alzheimer's, and Parkinson's disease (e.g., Meltzer and Lowy, 1987; D'Amato *et al.*, 1987). The prototype tricyclic antidepressant imipramine, as well as several other antidepressants, have been found to label the serotonin transporter *in vitro* with affinity in the nanomolar or sub-n*M* range (e.g., Sette *et al.*, 1981; Habert *et al.*, 1985; d'Amato *et al.*, 1987). Many attempts have been made to synthesize and develop an *in vivo* tracer for the serotonin transporter based on these *in vitro* findings, but most of these tracers were unsuccessful *in vivo* (e.g., Maziere *et al.*, 1978; Berger *et al.*, 1979; Lasne *et al.*, 1989; Hume *et al.*, 1989; Kilbourn *et al.*, 1989; Hume *et al.*, 1991; Laruelle *et al.*, 1994). The studies summarized in this chapter demonstrate how autoradiography was used to understand the reason for these failures and finally to identify a promising ligand that specifically and selectively labels the serotonin transporter *in vivo*.

II. MATERIALS AND METHODS

Several compounds with high binding affinity and selectivity toward the serotonin transporter *in vitro* were evaluated. These included [³H]imipramine (IMI),

[³H]paroxetine (PAR) and [¹²⁵I]-5-iodo-6-nitro quipa-zine (INQUIP) (Mathis *et al.*, 1992, 1993). PAR and IMI were purchased from N.E.N. INQUIP was synthe-sized as described (Mathis *et al.*, 1992). Young adult male rats (Sprague–Dawley) or adult *Macaca mulatta* monkeys were used in the experiments.

Autoradiography

In vitro autoradiography of the various ligands was performed as previously described (Biegon and Rain-bow, 1983; Biegon, 1986, 1990). For *ex vivo* autoradiog-raphy, animals were injected iv with the radiolabeled drug (Biegon and Mathis, 1993; Biegon *et al.*, 1993). Excess unlabeled drugs (0.5–2 mg/kg PAR or 20 mg/kg IMI) were coinjected with the radioactive drug in some of the animals to assess nonspecific binding *in vivo*. The animals were sacrificed at the indicated times post injection. A blood sample was saved for direct counting of radioactivity in plasma. The brain was quickly removed from the skull. Samples of prefrontal cortex and cerebellum were also removed from rats brains for counting and chemical analysis. The brains were frozen in powdered dry ice. Twenty (rat) or 40 (monkey) μm sections were produced in a cryostat at −15°C and apposed to tritium sensitive film (³H-Hyperfilm from Amersham) for 4–16 weeks. Appro-priate commercial standards were coexposed with the brain sections. The films were developed by hand and the sections were then stained with cresyl violet for anatomical reference.

A. Image Analysis

A video-camera-based, computerized image analy-sis system (Apple Macintosh IICi computer using the IMAGE software from NIH) was used to quantify lev-els of radioactivity in various brain regions, identified with reference to the histologically stained sections and a rat or monkey brain atlas (Paxinos and Watson, 1986; Kusama and Mabuchi, 1970). Optical densities on film were translated into concentration units (fmol/mg pro-tein) using the standard curve, the specific activity of the drug, and an average ratio of 1 mg protein to 10 mg tissue wet weight.

B. Dissection

The animals (rats only) were injected and sacrificed as described, but their brains were dissected into sev-eral regions (prefrontal cortex, olfactory tubercule, hippocampus, hypothalamus, and cerebellum), which were weighed, solubilized (for tritium-labeled com-pounds), and counted.

C. Serotonergic Lesions

Serotonin terminals were lesioned in rats as pre-viously described, using intracerebroventricular injec-tions of 5,7-dihydroxytryptamine (5,7-DHT; e.g., Bie-gon and Rainbow, 1983) or intraperitoneal injections of parachloro amphetamine (PCA; e.g., Biegon *et al.*, 1993).

III. RESULTS AND DISCUSSION

In vitro autoradiography with 2 n*M* [³H]IMI, per-formed at 4°C (Biegon and Rainbow, 1983), resulted in a density reminiscent of the known distribution of serotonin transporters (Fig. 1). *In vitro* binding was efficiently blocked by coincubation with excess unla-beled IMI or by lesions of serotonin terminals. How-ever, injection of the ligand in rats followed by *ex vivo* autoradiography resulted in a different distribution (Biegon *et al.*, 1986), with the highest tracer densities found in cortical and hippocampal regions and the pi-neal, rather than in the raphe and hypothalamus (Fig. 1).

Ex vivo autoradiography with PAR (Biegon and Mathis, 1993) revealed a distribution pattern reminis-cent of, but not identical with, the *in vitro* distribution (De Souza and Kuyatt, 1987). Specifically, density val-ues in cortical, hippocampal, and striatal regins were too high relative to the known density of serotonin transporters in these regions (Table 1). Excess unla-beled PAR *in vivo* efficiently blocked tracer accumula-tion in serotonin rich regions such as the hypothalamus and raphe, but was considerably less effective in block-ing the *in vivo* binding in the cortex, hippocampus, and striatum. Similar results were seen in a dissection experiment. These results partially confirm and greatly expand those of previous *in vivo* experiments carried out on dissected samples only (Hashimoto and Goro-maru, 1990a,b; Scheffel and Ricaurte, 1990) and indi-cate a very limited use for paroxetine as an *in vivo* tracer in humans.

Ex vivo autoradiography with INQUIP resulted in a distribution identical to that of serotonin transporters 6–12 hr after tracer injection in rats. *In vivo* binding was uniformly and specifically blocked by cotreatment with excess unlabeled paroxetine or other serotonin uptake blockers; and selectively inhibited in terminal regions by pretreatment with PCA (Biegon *et al.*, 1993).

Based on the encouraging results in rats, the ligand was labelled with ¹²³I and tested in nonhuman primates. [¹²³I]INQUIP administered to rhesus monkeys was im-aged by SPECT, giving a good signal-to-noise ratio and the expected distribution pattern, which was blocked

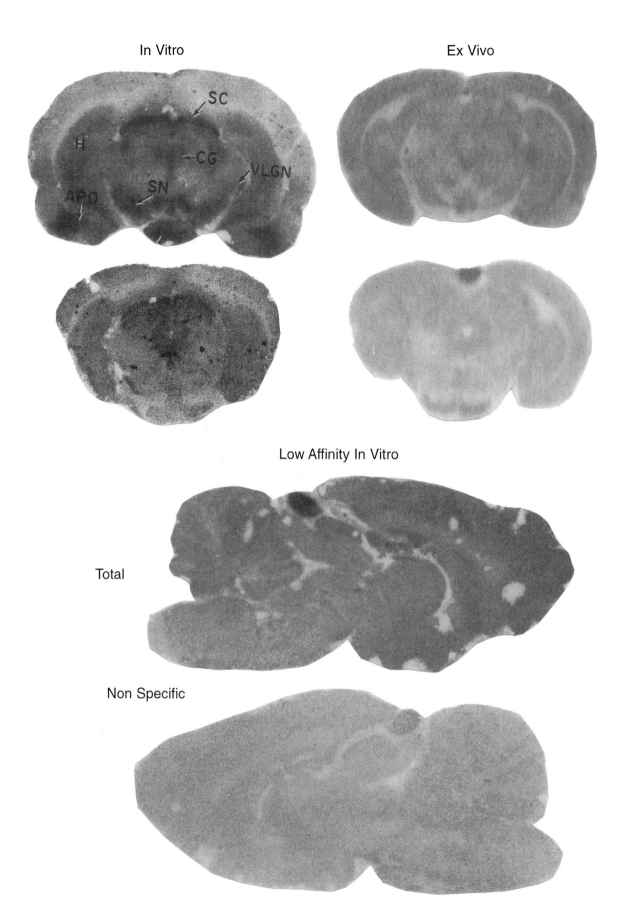

In Vitro

Ex Vivo

SC

H

CG

VLGN

SN

APO

Low Affinity In Vitro

Total

Non Specific

TABLE 1   Distribution of [³H]Paroxetine in the Rat Brain following iv Injection as Determined by *ex Vivo* Quantitative Autoradiography

Region	Total	Nonspecific	Specific	Total Cb	Ratio
Dorsal raphe nucleus	721 ± 72	196 ± 39	525	549	1.05
Interpeduncular nucleus	658 ± 110	185 ± 44	473	486	1.03
Pineal	609 ± 134	467 ± 70	142	438	**3.08**
Amygdala	510 ± 145	255 ± 51	325	338	1.0
Dorsomedial hypothalamic n.	482 ± 92	186 ± 51	296	310	1.05
Olfactory tubercule	434 ± 77	204 ± 34	230	262	1.14
Dorsal hippocampus, CA3	433 ± 87	269 ± 25	164	261	**1.38**
Ventral hippocampus, CA1	421 ± 71	264 ± 45	157	249	**1.58**
Superior colliculus, superficial layer	418 ± 29	167 ± 38	252	247	0.98
Ventromedial hypothalamic n.	388 ± 55	161 ± 43	227	216	0.95
Anterior cingulate cortex	386 ± 50	275 ± 45	111	214	**1.93**
Dorsal hippocampus, CA1	382 ± 29	297 ± 39	83	205	**2.48**
Globus pallidus	370 ± 39	180 ± 32	190	198	1.04
Frontal cortex	308 ± 63	209 ± 39	99	136	**1.37**
Caudate putamen	296 ± 52	198 ± 31	99	124	**1.25**
Occipital cortex	293 ± 39	225 ± 56	67	121	**1.81**
Cerebellum	172 ± 7	150 ± 15	22	0	—
Corpus callosum	130 ± 34	123 ± 34	7	—	—

Results are means ± standard deviation of three animals/group. *Total* = radioactivity (fmol/mg protein) in brain regions of animals injected with 3.7 MBq ³H paroxetine alone. *Nonspecific* = radioactivity in animals coinjected with labeled paroxetine and excess (0.5 mg/kg) unlabeled paroxetine; *Specific* = the difference between total and nonspecific binding; *Total Cb* = results of estimating specific binding by subtracting total cerebellar binding from total binding in all other brain regions (Scheffel and Hartig, 1989; Scheffel and Ricaurte, 1990); *Ratio* = ((Total Cb)/Specific) indicates the degree to which specific binding is overestimated in various regions, using the cerebellar concentrations as an index of nonspecific binding. For regions in which specific binding is overestimated by more than 20%, the ratio figure is in bold.

by pretreatment with paroxetine (Jagust *et al.*, 1993). *Ex vivo* autoradiography of INQUIP in some of the same monkeys (Biegon and Jagust, 1994; Fig. 2), injected with ¹²⁵I and ¹²³I labeled INQUIP, simultaneously, resulted in a distribution identical to the known distribution of serotonin transporters in primates (e.g., Cortes *et al.*, 1988). The tracer accumulation in primates was uniformly blocked by pretreatment with paroxetine in the *in vivo* SPECT images (Jagust *et al.*, 1993). These results support further development of INQUIP as a SPECT tracer in humans.

In summary, several compounds that bind to the serotonin transporter *in vitro* with high affinity and apparent specificity, failed to retain these characteristics on close inspection by autoradiography *in vivo*. The reason appears to be the presence in the brain of a large population of low (micromolar range) affinity sites for these ligands (Biegon and Samuel, 1979; Conway and Brunswick, 1985; Biegon, 1986). The low affinity sites are heterogeneously distributed in the brain, with high concentrations in the frontal cortex, hippocampus, and pineal. Therefore, when high concentrations of presynaptic aminergic ligands are seen in the frontal cortex, this is most always a sign of extensive

FIGURE 1   *In vitro* and *ex vivo* autoradiography of [³H]imipramine in the rat brain. Top, left: *In vitro* autoradiography (5 n*M* IMI, 4°C, coronal sections) at the levels of substantia nigra (SN) and dorsal raphe, which also contain the highest densities of binding sites. Nonspecific binding (not shown), determined in the presence of 100 μ*M* IMI, was low and uniform. Top, right: *Ex vivo* autoradiography 30 min after injection of IMI. Same anatomical levels as on the left. High concentrations of binding sites were found in cortex, hippocampus, and pineal. This binding was not displaceable *in vivo*. Bottom: *In vitro* autoradiography of low affinity binding of IMI (determned for 0.5 μ*M* ligand at 37°C, sagittal sections). The highest concentrations of binding sites were found in the frontal cortex, hippocampus, and pineal. This binding is displaceable *in vitro*. Nonspecific binding (coincubation with 100 μ*M* unlabeled drug) is low and uniform.

A

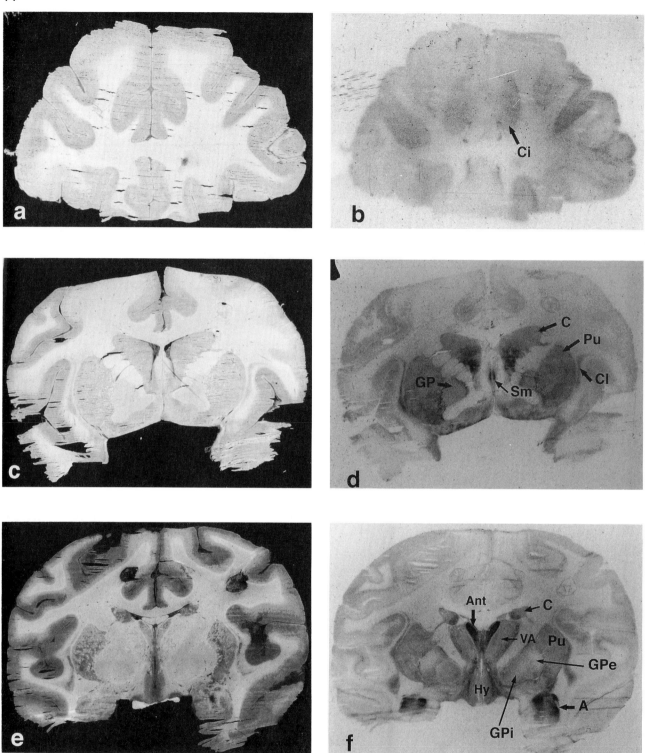

FIGURE 2 *Ex vivo* autoradiography of [¹²⁵I]INQUIP in the monkey brain. The illustrations show representative histology (a, c, e) and autoradiographic distribution of INQUIP binding sites (b, d, f) in a monkey injected with the radiotracer and killed 17 hr later. (2A) Anterior sections. (2B) Posterior sections. Abbreviations: A = amygdala, Ant = anterior thalamic nuclei, C = caudate, Ci = anterior cingulate cortex, Cl = claustrum, DR = dorsal raphe, GP = globus pallidus, GPe = external division of the globus pallidus, GPi = internal part of the globus pallidus, Hy = hypothalamus, IO = inferior olive, IP = interpeduncular nucleus, MR = median raphe, PU = putamen, Pul = pulvinar nucleus of the thalamus, SC = superior colliculus, St = striate cortex (visual cortex, area 17), V = cerebellar vermis.

B

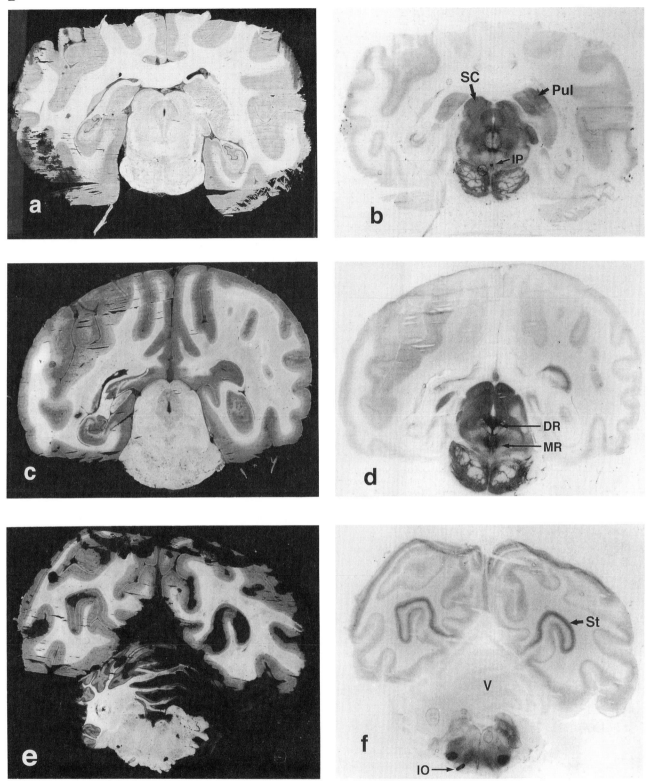

low affinity binding. In general, putative PET or SPECT tracers for specific receptors or transporters are most commonly selected on the basis of *in vitro* binding data, followed by *in vivo* brain distribution studies relying on dissection of brain regions in rodents. This methodology is crude and may produce misleading results. Different receptors, transporters, and enzymes may appear to share a similar distribution in the brain if the distribution is studied in a small number of relatively large brain regions. The development, in the early 1980s, of quantitative autoradiography facilitated the detailed quantitative mapping of the neuroanatomical distribution of such markers. For a PET/SPECT tracer to be truly specific and selective for a given brain constituent, the regional distribution of radioactivity in the brain *in vivo* must be identical to the known distribution of the same marker *in vitro*, and surgical or pharmacological manipulation known to specifically block or deplete binding using *in vitro* assays must be shown to be equally effective using *in vivo* assays. Over the last two decades, a number of putative receptor or transporter ligands were labeled with positron or gamma emitters and administered in humans or nonhuman primates only to be later proven inadequate for *in vivo* imaging due to lack of specificity or selectivity. The examples described here support our contention that the use of rodent *ex vivo* autoradiography relatively early in the evaluation and development process of radiopharmaceuticals provides unique and valuable information not provided by other, less sensitive techniques. The specific example we chose to describe was the search for an *in vivo* radioligand for imaging the serotonergic transporter, but our conclusions are applicable to other binding sites and systems as well.

Acknowledgment

Supported in part by NIH grant AG07793 to W. J. Jagust

References

Berger, G., Maziere, M., Knipper, R., Parent, C., and Comar, D. (1979). Automated synthesis of 11C-labeled radiopharmaceuticals: Imipramine, nicotine and methionine. *Int. J. Appl. Radiat. Isot.* **30**: 393.

Biegon, A., and Samuel, D. (1979). Binding of a labelled antidepressant to rat brain tissue. *Biochem. Pharmacol.* **28**: 3361–3366.

Biegon, A., and Rainbow, T. C. (1983). Distribution of imipramine binding sites in the rat brain studied by quantitative autoradiography. *Neurosci. Lett.* **37**: 209–214.

Biegon, A. (1986). Quantitative autoradiography in drug research: Tricyclic antidepressants. *In:* "Receptor Binding in Drug Research." pp. 477–486. Dekker, New York.

Biegon, A. (1990). Characterization and localization of binding sites for tricyclic antidepressants in rat and human brain. *In:* "Antidepressants: Thirty Years On." (B. Leonard and P. Spencer, Eds.), pp. 46–53. CNS Publishers, London.

Biegon, A., and Mathis, C. (1993). Evaluation of [³H]paroxetine as an in vivo ligand for serotonin uptake sites: A quantitative autoradiographic study in the rat brain. *Synapse* **13**: 1–9.

Biegon, A., Mathis, C. A., Hanrahan, S. M., and Jagust, W. J. (1993). [125I]5-iodo-6-nitroquipazine: A potent and selective ligand for the 5-hydroxytryptamine uptake complex II. In vivo studies in rats. *Brain Res.* **619**: 236–246.

Biegon, A., and Jagust, W. (1994). Autoradiography of primate brain serotonin terminals with [¹²⁵I]5-iodo-6-nitroquipazine. *Soc. Neurosci. Abstr.* **20**: 627.

Biegon, A., Eberling, J. L., Taylor, S. E., VanBrocklin, H. F. Jordan, S., Hanrahan, S. M., Roberts, J. A., Brennan, K. M., Mathis, C. A., and Jagust, W. J. (1995). In vivo studies of the serotonin transporter with 5-iodo-6-nitroquipazine. *Soc. Neurosci. Abstr.* **21**: 866.

Conway, P. G., and Bruswick, D. K. (1985). High- and low-affinity binding components from [³H]imipramine in rat cerebral cortex. *J. Neurochem.* **45**: 206–209.

Cortes, R., Soriano, E., Pazos, A., Probst, A., and Palacios, J. M. (1988). Autoradiography of antidepressant binding sites in the human brain: Localization using [³H]imipramine and [³H]paroxetine. *Neuroscience* **27**: 473–496.

d'Amato, R. J., Zweig, R. M., Whitehouse, P. J., *et al.* (1987). Aminergic systems in Alzheimer's disease and Parkinson's disease. *Ann. Neurol.* **22**: 229–236.

d'Amato, R. J., Largent, B. L., Snowman, A. M., and Snyder, S. H. (1987). Selective labeling of serotonin uptake sites in rat brain by [³H]citalopram contrasted to labeling of multiple binding sites by [³H]imipramine. *J. Pharmacol. Exp. Ther.* **242**: 364.

De Souza, E. B., and Kuyatt, B. (1987). Autoradiographic localization of 3H-paroxetine-labelled serotonin uptake sites in rat brain. *Synapse* **1**: 488–496.

Habert, E., Graham, D., Tahraoui, L., Claustre, Y., and Langer, S. Z. (1985). Characterization of [³H]-paroxetine binding to rat cortical membranes. *Eur. J. Pharmacol.* **118**: 107–114.

Hashimoto, K., and Goromaru, T. (1990a). Evaluation of ³H-paroxetine as a radioligand for in vivo study of 5-hydroxytryptamine uptake sites in mouse brain. *Radioisotopes* **39**: 335–341.

Hashimoto, K., and Goromaru, T. (1990b). Reduction of in vivo binding of [³H]paroxetine in mouse brain by 3,4-methylenedioxymethamphetamine. *Neuropharmacology* **29**: 633–639.

Hume, S., Myers, R., Manjil, L., and Dolan, R. (1989). Sertraline and paroxetine fail tests in vivo as 5HT reuptake site ligands for PET. *J Cerebr. Blood Flow Metab.* **9**(suppl 1): 117.

Hume, S. P., Pascal, C., Pike, V. W., *et al.* (1991). Citalopram: Labelling with carbon-11 and evaluation in rat as a potential radioligand for in vivo PET studies of 5HT reuptake sites. *Nucl. Med. Biol.* **18**: 339–351.

Jagust, W. J., Eberling, J. L., Roberts, J. A., Brennan, K. M., Mathis, C. A., Hanrahan, S. M., Van Brocklin, H., Roos, M., and Biegon, A. (1993). In vivo imaging of the 5-HT reuptake site in primate brain using SPECT and [¹²³I]-5-iodo-6-nitroquipazine. *Eur. J. Pharmacol.* **242**: 189–193.

Kilbourn, M. R., Haka, M. S., Mulholland, G. K., Jewett, D. M., and Kuhl, D. E. (1989). Synthesis of radiolabelled inhibitors of pre-synaptic monoamine uptake systems: [¹⁸F]GBR 13119 (DA), [¹¹C]nosoxetine (NE) and [¹¹C]fluoxetine (5HT). *J. Labelled Compd. Radiopharm.* **26**: 412.

Kusama, T., and Mabuchi, M. (1970). "Stereotaxic Atlas of the Brain of Macaca Fuscata." University of Tokyo Press, Tokyo.

Lasne, M. C., Pike, V. W., and Turton, D. R. (1989). The radiosynthesis of [N-methyl-^{11}C]sertraline. *Appl. Radiat. Isot.* **40:** 147.

Laruelle, M., Wallace, E., Seibyl, J. P., *et al.* (1994). Graphical, kinetic and equilibrium analyses of in vivo [^{123}I]beta-CIT binding to dopamine transporters in healthy human subjects. *J. Cerebr. Blood Flow Metab.* **14:** 982–994.

Mathis, C., Biegon, A., Taylor, S., Ennas, J., and Hanrahan, S. (1992). [^{125}I]5-I-6-nitro quipazine: A potent and selective ligand for the serotonin uptake complex. *Eur. J. Pharmacol.* **10:** 103–104.

Mathis, C. A., Taylor, S. E., Biegon, A., and Enas, J. D. (1993). [125I]5-iodo-6-nitroquipazine: A potent and selective ligand for the 5-hydroxytryptamine uptake complex I. In vitro studies. *Brain Res.* **619:** 229–235.

Maziere, M., Berger, G., and Comar, D. (1978). ^{11}C-clomiparamine: Synthesis and analysis. *J. Radioanal. Chem.* **45:** 453.

Meltzer, H. Y., and Lowy, M. T. (1987). The serotonin hypothesis of depression. *In* "Psychopharmacology: The Third Generation of Progress" (H. Y. Meltzer, Ed.), pp. 513–526. Raven Press, New York.

Paxinos, G., and Watson, C. (1986). "The Rat Brain in Stereotaxic Coordinate." 2nd ed. Academic Press, Sydney.

Scheffel, U., and Ricaurte, G. A. (1990). Paroxetine as an indicator of 3,4-MDMA neurotoxicity: A presynaptic serotonergic positron emission tomography ligand? *Brain Res.* **527:** 89–95.

Scheffel, V., and Hartig, P. R. (1989). In vivo labelling of serotonin uptake sites with [^{3}H] paroxetine. *J. Neurochem.* **52:** 1605–1612.

Sette, M., Raisman, R., Briley, M., and Langer, S. Z. (1981). Localization of tricyclic antidepressant binding sites on serotonin nerve terminals. *J. Neurochem.* **37:** 40–42.

7

Radioactive Metabolites of the 5-HT$_{1A}$ Receptor Radioligand, [*O-methyl-*[11]*C*]WAY-100635, in Humans

S. OSMAN,[1] J. A. McCARRON,[1] S. P. HUME,[1] S. ASHWORTH,[1] V. W. PIKE,[1] S. K. LUTHRA,[1]
A. A. LAMMERTSMA,[1] C. BENCH,[1,2] P. GRASBY,[1] I. A. CLIFFE,[3] and A. FLETCHER[3]

[1]*PET Methodology Group, MRC Clinical Sciences Centre*
Royal Postgraduate Medical School
Hammersmith Hospital, London W12 0NN, United Kingdom
[2]*Charing Cross and Westminster Medical School*
London W6 8RF, United Kingdom
[3]*Wyeth Research (U.K.) Ltd.*
Taplow, Maidenhead, Berkshire, SL6 OPH, United Kingdom

[O-methyl-[11]*C]WAY-100635 {[O-methyl-*[11]*C]N-2-(1-(4-(2-methoxypheny)-l-piperazinyl)-ethyl)-N-(2-pyridyl)-cyclohexanecarboxamide} is a promising radioligand for the study of 5-HT$_{1A}$ receptors in human brain with positron emission tomography (PET). Mathematical modeling of the acquired PET data requires a knowledge of radioligand metabolism. After iv injection of [O-methyl-*[11]*C]WAY-100635 in five healthy male volunteers, radioactivity was found to clear rapidly from plasma. Radioactivity in serial plasma samples was analyzed by solid phase extraction and reverse phase HPLC of the retained components. In all samples, a polar fraction of plasma radioactivity was not retained by the solid phase extraction column. High performance liquid chromatography (HPLC) analyses of retained radioactivity revealed three major components, of which unchanged radioligand is the least polar. Of the radioactivity in plasma, on average 94.9% was unchanged radioligand at 2.5 min after iv injection and 4.5% at 60 min. One radioactive metabolite was found to coelute with descyclohexanecarbonyl-WAY-100635 (WAY-100634). [*[11]*C]WAY-100634 represented 35% of the radioactivity in plasma at 10 min and 26% at 60 min. At 60 min, polar radioactive metabolites represented 70.5% of the radioactivity in plasma. WAY-100634 is known to have high affinity for 5-HT$_{1A}$ and α_1-adrenoceptors and higher extraction into rat brain than WAY-100635. Thus, [O-methyl-*[11]*C]WAY-100634 may contribute to nonspecific and specific binding in human brain in PET studies*

with [O-methyl-[11]*C]WAY-100635. We conclude that WAY-100635 labelled with carbon-11 in the amido carbonyl group might be the preferred for PET studies of 5-HT$_{1A}$ receptors in humans because [*[11]*C]WAY-100634 cannot be formed from this radioligand.*

I. INTRODUCTION

[*O-methyl-*[11]*C*]WAY-100635 {[*O-methyl-*[11]*C*]N-2-(1 - (4 - (2 - methoxypheny) - l - piperazinyl) - ethyl) - N - (2 - pyridyl)cyclohexanecarboxamide} has been shown to be an effective radioligand for studying brain 5-HT$_{1A}$ receptors in mice (Laporte *et al.*, 1994), rats (Hume *et al.*, 1994; Mathis *et al.*, 1994; Pike *et al.*, 1995a), and monkeys (Mathis *et al.*, 1994). Recently, it has also been shown to be the first promising radioligand for studies of 5-HT$_{1A}$ receptors in human brain with positron emission tomography (Pike *et al.*, 1995b,c).

The development of a meaningful mathematical model of PET data acquired from the use of a receptor radioligand in humans requires radioligand metabolism to be examined; for example, to assess whether labelled metabolites in plasma are able to cross the blood–brain barrier and contribute to specific and nonspecific binding and for certain models to establish a plasma input function (Cunningham and Lammertsma, 1995). With a view to modeling regional cerebral radioactivity uptake in PET studies of volunteers injected intravenously with [*O-methyl*-¹¹C]WAY-100635, in this study we have measured the plasma clearance of radioactivity and the percentages of radioactivity in plasma represented by unchanged radioligand and its radioactive metabolites in serial plasma samples.

II. MATERIALS AND METHODS

A. Materials

The reverse phase analytical HPLC column ("μ" Bondapak C18) was purchased from Anachem Ltd. HPLC grade methanol was purchased from Fisons Ltd. Ammonium formate and di-ammonium hydrogen phosphate were of analytical grade and purchased from BDH Ltd.

B. Radiosynthesis of [*O-methyl*-¹¹C]WAY-100635

[*O-methyl*-¹¹C]WAY-100635 was prepared within 50 min from the cyclotron production of carbon-11, by treating the corresponding *O*-desmethyl precursor with no carrier-added [¹¹C]iodomethane and purified by reverse phase HPLC (Pike *et al.*, 1995a). Typically, this radioligand had a specific radioactivity of 199.8 GBq/μmol (corrected to the end of radionuclide production) and radiochemical and chemical purities of 99.5 and 94.4%, respectively, as demonstrated by analytical HPLC on each preparation.

C. PET Studies with [*O-methyl*-¹¹C] WAY-100635 in Humans

Studies in healthy male volunteers were performed under approval from the Administration of Radioactive Substances Advisory Committee (U.K.) and the local Hammersmith Hospital Ethics Committee. All volunteers gave informed written consent. Five healthy male volunteers (age range from 28 to 41 years) were studied. The subjects were injected intravenously with a tracer dose of [*O-methyl*-¹¹C]WAY-100635 (approximately 330 MBq containing <10 μg of unlabeled WAY-100635). PET scans were performed parallel to the orbito–meatal line for 90 min using a brain PET scanner (CTI SIEMENS 953B; Knoxville, TN). The subjects underwent arterial cannulation for continuous monitoring of total blood radioactivity and sampling of selected blood for radioactive metabolite analysis.

D. Analysis of Radioactive Metabolites in Human Plasma

Analysis of radioactivity in human plasma samples was carried out using a semi-automated metabolite

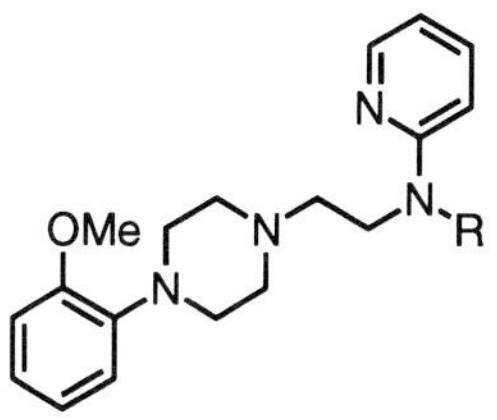

WAY-100635, R = cyclohexanecarbonyl
WAY-100634, R = H

FIGURE 1

analysis system described previously (Luthra *et al.*, 1993). Serial arterial blood samples were taken from volunteers at 2.5, 5, 10, 20, 40, and 60 min after intravenous injection of [*O-methyl*-¹¹C]WAY-100635 and centrifuged at 2000 g for 2 min to obtain cell-free plasma (CFP). An aliquot of CFP (1.0 ml) was spiked with nonradioactive WAY-100635 and its descyclohexanecarbonyl analog (WAY-100634; Fig. 1) and injected onto a solid-phase extraction (SPE) column (octadecylderivatised silica). The SPE column was then washed with 0.1 M diammonium hydrogen phosphate solution at 2 ml/min for 3 min to elute plasma proteins and very polar radioactive metabolites. Retained radioligand and its radioactive metabolites were eluted from the SPE column and onto a reverse phase HPLC column (μ-Bondapak C18, 30 × 0.78 cm inside diameter, 10 μ particle diameter) with methanol–0.1 M ammonium formate (70: 30 v/v) at a flow rate of 3 ml/min. The HPLC eluate was monitored for absorbance at 254 nm and radioactivity. Both detectors were linked to a PC-based integrator, allowing the data to be recorded, corrected for physical decay, and integrated. Aliquots from CFP, and the SPE and HPLC eluates were each collected and counted for radioactivity using a gamma counter (Compugamma 1272, LKB/Pharmacia) for calculation of the overall recovery of radioactivity from the analysis. Typically, recovery was 98%. The percentages of radioactivity in plasma represented by unchanged radioligand and its radiolabeled metabolites at known times after the administration of radioligand were calculated from the radioactivity measurements taken in HPLC and gamma counting.

III. RESULTS AND DISCUSSION

After intravenous administration of [*O-methyl*-¹¹C]WAY-100635 in all five human subjects the clearance of radioactivity from blood and plasma was rapid

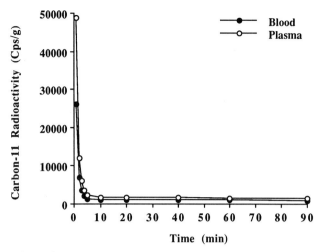

FIGURE 2 Clearance of radioactivity from blood and plasma after iv injection of [*O-methyl*-^{11}C]WAY-100635 into a healthy male volunteer. Similar data were obtained from four other healthy male volunteers.

(Fig. 2). The ratio of radioactivity in plasma to that in blood, expressed as radioactivity per gram, was about 0.6 at all time points, indicating that the cellular uptake of radioactivity was low. Similar results have been found in the rat with [*O-methyl*-^{3}H]WAY-100635 (Hume *et al.*, 1994).

Figure 3 shows a typical chromatogram from the HPLC analysis of human plasma taken 10 min after intravenous injection of [*O-methyl*-^{11}C]WAY-100635. Three major radioactive components were separated. The least polar component is unchanged radioligand (retention time, 9 min). The radioactive component with a retention time of 7 min coelutes with reference WAY-100634. The third component, eluting over 4–6

min, is more polar than WAY-100634 and has not been identified.

Figure 4 shows the percentage of radioactivity in human plasma represented by parent radioligand over the 60 min duration of a PET study, averaged from one study in each of the five volunteers. At 2.5 and 60 min after intravenous injection of radioligand, the values are 94.9% (SD ± 2.0%) and 4.6% (SD ± 1.0%), respectively. The values for the radioactive metabolite, [*O-methyl*-^{11}C]WAY-100634, are 31.0% (SD ± 16.9%) at 10 min and 25% (± SD 14.4%) at 60 min (Fig. 4). The polar radioactive metabolites found in the HPLC analysis increased from 1.2% at 2.5 min to 44% (SD ± 15.9%) at 60 min (Fig. 4). Additionally, the percentage of radioactivity in plasma represented by the very polar radioactive metabolites in the SPE eluate increased from 0.66% (SD ± 0.45%) at 2.5 min to 26.2% (SD ± 9.4%) by 60 min (Figure 4). This kinetic pattern suggests the possibility that some polar metabolites are formed sequentially from [*O-methyl*-^{11}C]WAY-100634. Qualitatively similar results were obtained in the same subjects studied after pretreatment with buspirone (30 mg oral) about 1 hr before injection of radioligand (data not shown).

The formation of [^{11}C]WAY-100634 was expected on the basis of results obtained with WAY-100635 and liver microsomes *in vitro* (C. Tio; personal communication). By contrast [^{11}C]WAY-100634 has not been detected in plasma after intravenous administration of [*O-methyl*-^{11}C]WAY-100635 into rats; only polar radioactive metabolites were observed in rat plasma (Hume *et al.*, 1994). WAY-100634 has high affinity for 5-HT$_{1A}$ and α_1-adrenoceptors *in vitro* (unpublished results). We have shown that after intravenous administration [*O-methyl* ^{11}C]WAY-100634 has a higher nonspecific uptake into the rat brain than [*O-methyl*-

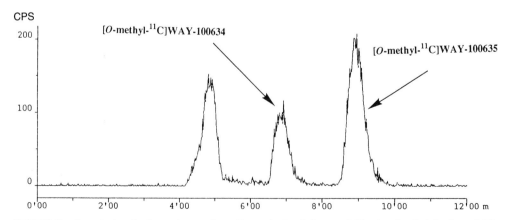

FIGURE 3 A typical radiochromatogram from the analysis of plasma at 10 min after iv injection of [*O-methyl*-^{11}C]WAY-100635 into a healthy male volunteer (see text for analytical details).

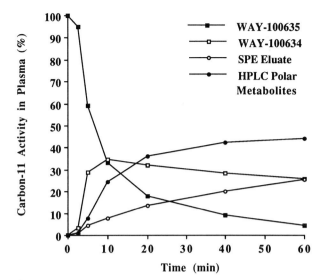

FIGURE 4 Distribution of radioactivity between parent radioligand and its metabolites in human plasma after iv injection of [O-methyl-¹¹C]WAY-100635 into a healthy male volunteer.

¹¹C]WAY-100635 (Hume *et al.*, 1994). This suggests that [*O-methyl* ¹¹C]WAY-100634 could contribute to nonspecific binding and perhaps also to specific binding in brain in PET studies with [*O-methyl*-¹¹C]WAY-100635 in humans and thereby complicate attempts to model data from the use of the radioligand.

We have developed a procedure for labeling WAY-100635 with carbon-11 in the carbonyl group (Pike *et al.*, 1995a). Carbonyl-labeled WAY-100635 cannot be metabolized to [¹¹C]WAY-100634 in humans and may therefore be preferred for PET studies of 5-HT$_{1A}$ receptors. Moreover, this radioligand is expected mainly to give cyclohexane derivatives as polar radioactive

metabolites, which should not enter brain or interact with 5-HT$_{1A}$ or other receptors. Work is now in progress to evaluate this radioligand.

References

Cunningham, V. J., and Lammerstma, A. A. (1995). Radioligand studies in brain: Kinetic analysis of PET data. *Med. Chem. Res.* **5**: 79–96.

Hume, S. P., Ashworth, S., Opacka-Juffry, J., Ahier, R. G., Lammertsma, A. A., Pike, V. W., Cliffe, I. A., Fletcher, A., and White, A. C. (1994). Evaluation of [*O-methyl*-¹¹C]WAY-100635 as an *in vivo* radioligand for 5-HT$_{1A}$ receptors in rat brain. *Eur. J. Pharmacol.* **271**: 515–523.

Laporte, A.-M., Lima, L., Gozlan, H., and Hamon, M. (1994). Selective *in vivo* labelling of brain 5-HT$_{1A}$ receptors by [³H]WAY-100635 in the mouse. *Eur. J. Pharmacol.* **271**: 505–514.

Luthra, S. K., Osman, S., Turton, D. R., Vaja, V., Dowsett, K., and Brady, F. (1993). An automated system based on solid phase extraction and HPLC for routine determination in plasma of unchanged [¹¹C]-L-deprenyl; [¹¹C]diprenorphine; [¹¹C]flumazenil; [¹¹C]raclopride and [¹¹C]Schering 23390. *J. Labelled. Compd. Radiopharm.* **32**: 518–520.

Mathis, C. A., Simpson, N. R., Mahmood, K., Kinahan, P. E., and Mintun, M. (1994). [¹¹C]WAY 100635: A radioligand for imaging 5-HT$_{1A}$ receptors with positron emission tomography. *Life Sci.* **55**: 403–407.

Pike, V. W., McCarron, J. A., Hume, S. P., Ashworth, S., Opacka-Juffry, J., Osman, S., Lammerstma, A. A., Poole, K. G., Fletcher, A., White, A. C., and Cliffe, I. A. (1995a). Pre-clinical development of a radioligand for studies of central 5-HT$_{1A}$ receptors *in vivo*—[¹¹C]WAY-100635. *Med. Chem. Res.* **5**: 208–227.

Pike V. W., Hume, S. P., McCarron, J. A., Ashworth, S., Opacka-Juffry, J., Lammertsma, A. A., Osman S., Bench, C. J., Poole, K. G., Grasby P., Malizia, A., Cliffe, I. A., Fletcher, A., and White, A. C. (1995b). [¹¹C]WAY-100635—A radioligand for the study of central 5-HT$_{1A}$ receptors *in vivo*. *J. Nucl. Med.* **36**: 58P.

Pike, V. W., McCarron, J. A., Lammertsma, A. A., Hume, S. P., Poole, K., Grasby P. M., Malizia, A., Cliffe, I. A., Fletcher, A., and Bench, C. J. (1995c). First delineation of 5-HT$_{1A}$ receptors in human brain with PET and [¹¹C]WAY-100635. *Eur. J. Pharmacol*, **283**: R1–R3.

[^{11}C]Nefopam as a Potential PET Tracer of Serotonin Reuptake Sites

Initial Findings in Living Pig Brain

DONALD F. SMITH,[1] ROBERT GLASER,[2] ANTHONY GEE,[3] and ALBERT GJEDDE[3]

[1]*Department of Biological Psychiatry, Psychiatric Hospital of Aarhus University, 8240 Risskov, Denmark*
[2]*Department of Chemistry, Ben-Gurion University of the Negev, Beersheva 84105, Israel*
[3]*PET Center, Aarhus University Hospitals, 8000 Aarhus C, Denmark*

Nefopam is a nonnarcotic analgesic drug with some antidepressant properties. Pigs were used to study the regional distribution and kinetics of radiolabeled nefopam in the brain using PET scanning. First, 550–860 MBq of [^{11}C]nefopam was administered intravenously; arterial blood samples were drawn at intervals thereafter. A Siemens Model HR 961 scanner equipped with a ECAT computer package was used for PET scanning and for reconstructing the pig brain image. [^{11}C]nefopam was found to cross the blood–brain barrier and enter the pig brain readily. Plasma curves showed that [^{11}C]nefopam may be metabolized rapidly in body tissues. Differences in the time course of [^{11}C]nefopam-derived radioactivity in pig brain regions suggest that the drug may be binding to serotonin uptake sites, as well as other receptors. However, displacement studies using a potent and selective 5-HT uptake inhibitor failed to provide conclusive proof that nefopam interacts selectively with the cerebral 5-HT transporter.

I. INTRODUCTION

Early detection, correct diagnosis, and proper treatment of neurological and mental disorders continues to be a challenge for medical science. It is, therefore, of interest to have new methods available for studying the status of cerebral neuropathways, preferably in the living human brain.

Numerous studies on affective disorders (i.e., unipolar and bipolar depression) have indicated that alterations in neuronal receptor systems related mainly to monoaminergic neurotransmitters (i.e., serotonin,

dopamine, and noradrenaline) are involved in the efficacy of antidepressant treatments. We are currently engaged in projects aimed at finding compounds that can be used as radiopharmaceuticals for studying, in particular, the serotonin reuptake site in living brain. In this chapter, we present our initial results using nefopam, a racemic nonnarcotic analgesic drug with some antidepressant properties (Glaser and Donnell, 1989; Glaser *et al.*, 1988; Glaser *et al.*, 1993), as a PET radioligand.

II. METHODS

A. Synthesis and Radiolabeling

Racemic *N*-desmethylnefopam HCl was prepared as described in detail elsewhere (Glaser *et al.*, 1993). Racemic *N*-desmethylnefopam HCl (1.2 mg) was alkylated with ^{11}C-methyl iodide in DMF (300 μl) at 130°C for 5 min using 0.5 mg NaOH as base. The crude product was purified by HPLC (Spherisorb 5ODS, 250 × 8 mm, ethanol : 0.05M ammonium formate (95 : 5), 4 ml/min). Racemic [^{11}C]nefopam was prepared and formulated ready for injection within 30 min after end of bombardment with a 20% decay-corrected radiochemical yield, specific activity of >50 GBq μmol^{-1} (1.3 Ci μmol^{-1}), and a radiochemical purity of >98 %.

B. Experimental Procedures

The project was approved by the Danish National Committee for ethics in animal research. Female Danish country bred pigs (Yorkshire Land Race) weighing

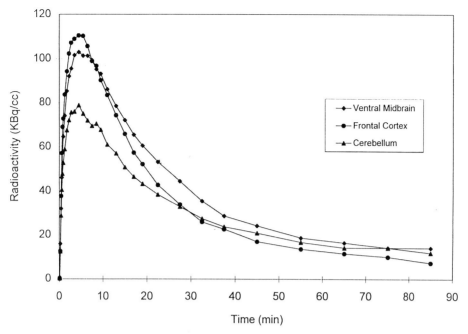

FIGURE 1   Time–activity curves for [^{11}C]nefopam-derived radioactivity in various regions in the living pig brain.

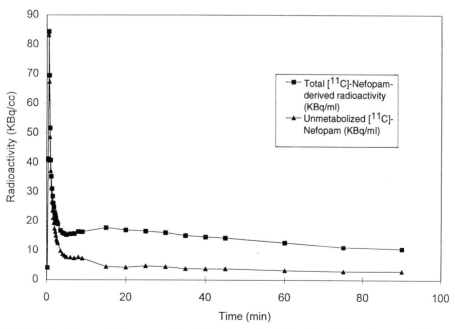

FIGURE 2   Time–activity curves for [^{11}C]nefopam-derived radioactivity and unmetabolized [^{11}C]nefopam radioactivity in the blood of pig.

39–44 kg were used. They were housed singly in stalls in a thermostatically controlled (20°C) animal colony with natural lighting conditions. The pigs had free access to water but were deprived of food for 24 hr prior to experiments.

The pigs were sedated with an im injection (3 ml/10 kg) of a mixture of midazolam (5 mg/10 kg) and ketamine HCl (100 mg/10 kg). After approximately 15 min, a catheter (1.2 mm Venflon 2) was installed in an ear vein through which an injection of ketamine HCl (1 ml/10 kg; 50 mg/10 kg) was administered. The pig was then intubated and isoflourane anesthesia was given by a Komesaroff anesthesia machine. Catheters (Avanti, size 4F–7F) were surgically installed in the right femoral artery and vein. Then, the pig was positioned in the scanner (Siemens Model HR 961) and the arterial catheter was flushed with 3–4 ml of heparin solution (20 IU/1 l isotonic saline). An iv infusion of isotonic saline (ca. 100 ml/hr) and of 5% glucose (ca. 20 ml/hr) was administered throughout each experiment.

Each pig was used for one to three dynamic scans, each lasting 90 min. Each scan consisted of 31 frames (6 × 10 sec, 4 × 30 sec, 7 × 1 min, 5 × 2 min, 4 × 5 min, 5 × 10 min). Scans were started upon an injection of racemic [11C]nefopam (radioactive dose 550–860 MBq) given via the femoral vein, followed immediately by a injection of heparin solution to flush the catheter. Physiological functions (i.e., blood pressure, heart rate, and expired air CO_2) were monitored continuously by a Siemens Sirecust 1281. At the end of experiments,

pigs were killed by an iv injection of 20 ml of saturated potassium chloride.

C. Data Analysis

Metabolite analysis was carried out after extraction of plasma from arterial blood samples in ethyl acetate alkalinized with sodium hydroxide. The extraction phase was transferred to a vial for determination of nefopam-derived radioactivity and [11C]-labeled metabolites by gamma counting. Brain image analysis was carried out using ECAT software version 7.0. Brain regions of interest (ROIs; cerebellum, ventral midbrain, and frontal cortex) were selected on the basis of a neuroanatomical atlas of the pig brain (Yoshikawa, 1968). For each region, radioactivity was calculated for the sequence of frames, corrected for the radioactivity decay of [11C] (20.3 min) and plotted versus time. The cerebellum was used as a control region for estimating nonspecific binding (Suehiro *et al.*, 1993). Computerized analysis of brain regional radioactivity was carried out using a two-compartmental model for estimating kinetic parameters for the distribution of [11C]nefopam and its [11C]metabolites in brain regions (Gjedde, 1990).

III. RESULTS AND DISCUSSION

Figure 1 shows time–activity curves for the regional distribution of [11C]nefopam-derived radioactivity in

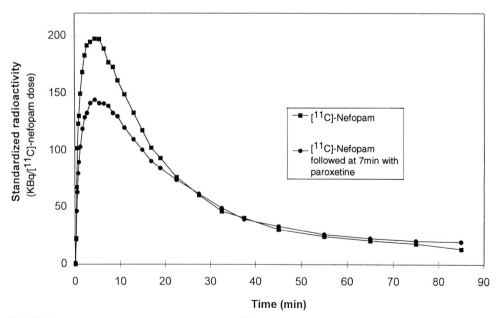

FIGURE 3 Standardized time–activity curves for [11C]nefopam-derived radioactivity in the frontal cortex of living pig brain without (squares) and with (circles) administration of paroxetine (5 mg/kg) after 7 min of the scan.

TABLE 1 Kinetic Parameters for the Regional Distribution of [^{11}C]Nefopam-Derived Radioactivity in the Living Pig Brain Using a Two-Compartment Model

		Kinetic parameters		
Treatment	Brain region	K_1 (ml/g/min)	k_2 (min^{-1})	Binding potential*
Control	Cerebellum	1.88 ± 0.44	0.19 ± 0.05	
	Ventral midbrain	1.88 ± 0.33	0.26 ± 0.05	−0.27
	Frontal cortex	0.84 ± 0.50	0.08 ± 0.06	0.06
Paroxetine	Cerebellum	1.10 ± 0.17	0.21 ± 0.04	
	Ventral midbrain	1.06 ± 0.29	0.14 ± 0.05	0.48
	Frontal cortex	1.10 ± 0.21	0.17 ± 0.04	0.24

Note. An iv injection of the potent and selective 5-HT uptake inhibitor paroxetine (5 mg/kg) was given 7 min after beginning the second scan.

* Binding potential = $[(K_1/k_2)_{ROI}/(K_1/k_2)_{CERE}] - 1$. A value greater than 1 indicates that more of the [^{11}C]nefopam-derived radioactivity was present in the region of interest (ROI; i.e., ventral midbrain or frontal cortex) than in the cerebellum (region of nonspecific binding).

the pig brain. The findings indicate that [^{11}C]nefopam crosses the blood–brain barrier and enters the pig brain readily. Apparent differences in the time course of [^{11}C]nefopam-derived radioactivity in the ventral midbrain and frontal cortex of the pig compared to the cerebellum suggest that the drug might be binding to serotonin uptake sites.

Plasma studies showed that [^{11}C]nefopam may be metabolized rapidly in body tissues (Fig. 2), which raises uncertainties concerning whether [^{11}C]nefopam or its metabolites or both were responsible for the radioactivity recorded in the brain regions. Further work using HPLC for studying the metabolism of nefopam in pigs is necessary to settle this issue.

In one experiment, the potent and selective 5-HT uptake inhibitor paroxetine (5 mg/kg) was administered iv 7 min after injection of [^{11}C]nefopam to determine whether paroxetine would displace nefopam from cerebral 5-HT uptake sites (Fig. 3). The results failed to provide conclusive proof that nefopam binds selectively at the cerebral 5-HT transporter, in that no marked difference in kinetic parameters was obtained in a two-compartmental model for the analysis of the data (Table 1). Moreover, the binding potential of [^{11}C]-nefopam in the pig frontal cortex versus the cerebellum was too low to suggest that the radioligand was specifically bound to the 5-HT transporter.

These findings indicate that *N*-desmethylnefopam can be successfully ^{11}C-labeled and that [^{11}C]nefopam can be used as a PET radioligand. The existence of only a very small amount (approximately 4 mg) of *N*-desmethylnefopam has precluded us from carrying out studies to characterize the radioligand further. Based on the present data, however, it is unlikely that [^{11}C]nefopam will prove to fulfill the criteria required for its use as a radiopharmaceutical for PET brain imaging (Sedvall *et al.*, 1986).

Acknowledgments

We thank the technical staff (Bente, Helle, John, and Søren) at the PET Center of Aarhus University Hospitals for their skillful assistance, as well as S. Geresh and J. Blumenfeld of the Dept. of Chemistry at Ben-Gurion University for preparing *N*-desmethylnefopam HCl.

References

Gjedde, A. (1990). Modeling of neuroreceptor binding of radioligands in vivo. *In:* "Quantitative Imaging of Neuroreceptors" (J. Frost and H. N. Wagner, Jr., Eds.), pp. 51–79. Raven Press, New York.

Glaser, R., and Donnell, D. (1989). Stereoisomer differentiation for the analgesic drug nefopam hydrochloride using modeling studies of serotonin uptake area. *J. Pharm. Sci.* **78:** 87–90.

Glaser, R., Frenking, G., Loew, G. H., Donnell, D., and Agranat, I. (1988). Stereochemistry and conformation in solution of nefopam hydrochloride, a benzoxazocine analgesic drug. *New J. Chem.* **12:** 953–959.

Glaser, R., Geresh, S., Blumenfeld, J., Donnell, D., Sugisaka, N., Drouin, M., and Michel, A. (1993). Solution- and solid-state structures of *N*-desmethylnefopam hydrochloride, a metabolite of the analgesic drug. *J. Pharm. Sci.* **82:** 276–281.

Sedvall, G., Farde, L., Persson, A., and Wiesel, F.-A. (1986). Imaging of neurotransmitter receptors in the living human brain. *Arch. Gen. Psychiatry* **43:** 995–1005.

Suehiro, M., Scheffel, U., Ravert, H. T., Dannals, R. F. Jr., and Wagner, H. N. Jr. (1993). [^{11}C](+)McN5652 as a radiotracer for imaging serotonin uptake sites with PET. *Life Sci.* **53:** 883–892.

Yoshikawa, T. (1968). "Atlas of the Brains of Domestic Animals." pp. 1–33. Academic Press, New York.

The Effect of Amine pKa on the Transport and Binding of Amphetamine Analogs in the Pig Brain

An *in Vivo* Comparison of β, β-Difluoro[*N-methyl-*^{11}*C*] Methamphetamine and [*N-methyl-*^{11}*C*]Methamphetamine Using PET

A. D. GEE,[1] **N. GILLINGS,**[1] **D. SMITH,**[1,2] **O. INOUE,**[3] **K. KOBAYASHI,**[3] and **A. GJEDDE**[1]

[1]*PET Centre, Aarhus University Hospital, 8000 Aarhus C, Denmark*
[2]*Department of Biological Psychiatry, Psychiatric Hospital of Aarhus University, 8240 Risskov, Denmark*
[3]*National Institute of Radiological Sciences, Chiba-shi, 260 Japan*

An in vivo comparison of two ^{11}*C-labeled amphetamine analogs,* β,β*-difluoro[N-methyl-*^{11}*C]methamphetamine (DiFMAMP) and [N-methyl-*^{11}*C]methamphetamine (MAMP), possessing different acid dissociation constants (pKa values ca. 8 and 10, respectively), was made to determine the importance of the amine pKa on the transport and binding of biogenic amines in vivo. The kinetics of the tracers were analyzed by a three-compartment model, where* K_1, k_2, k_3 *were described as the clearance, washout, and metabolism in tissue, respectively. Kinetic analyses were performed for seven regions of interest, including the basal ganglia, thalamus, brain stem, frontal cortex, temporal cortex, occipital cortex, and cerebellum. DiFMAMP showed a marked increase in blood–brain barrier permeability (*$K_1 = 0.82–1.7$ *ml* g^{-1} min^{-1}; $k_2 = 0.39–0.71$ min^{-1}*) compared to MAMP (*$K_1 = 0.43–0.67$ *ml* g^{-1} min^{-1}; $k_2 = 0.11–0.14$ min^{-1}*). Relative magnitudes of* K_1 *and* k_2 *for MAMP were respectively two- and four- to fivefold lower than corresponding values for DiFMAMP. Whereas MAMP possessed a degree of brain retention, DiFMAMP was rapidly washed out of the tissue (volumes of distribution for MAMP and DiFMAMP were 3.6–5.3 and 2.1–3.2, respectively). Estimates of the rate of metabolism in tissue were similar for both compounds (*$k_{3MAMP} = 0.005–0.007$ min^{-1}; $k_{3DiFMAMP} = 0.004–0.008$ min^{-1}*). The lower than expected* k_2 *values for MAMP indicate that the tracer an affinity for a polar (amine) binding site, homogeneously distributed in the brain, which is less able to bind amines with low pKa values.*

I. INTRODUCTION

Methamphetamine, a methylated analog of amphetamine, has been reported to possess a variety of pharmacological actions. Among these are the stimulation of catecholamine release at presynaptic noradrenaline and dopamine neurons, blockade of catecholamine reuptake, and a certain degree of agonist activity at dopamine and 5-HT receptors. Methamphetamine has been used in the treatment of narcolepsy, hyperkinesis, and obesity, but may be best known as a substance of abuse causing increased alertness and a sense of well-being. Chronic abuse can result in a psychoticlike state resembling schizophrenia that may not be reversed after the drug is withdrawn. This "amphetamine psychosis" has been used as an animal model of schizophrenia. Methamphetamine is known to rapidly enter the brain and accumulate in tissue. A long-term retention of this amine in the brain, and a high ratio of brain to plasma concentrations indicate that amphetamine is bound in brain tissue.

The brain retention and binding of amphetamine derivatives may be dependent on at least two pharmacophoric interactions: a polar (amine) recognition site and

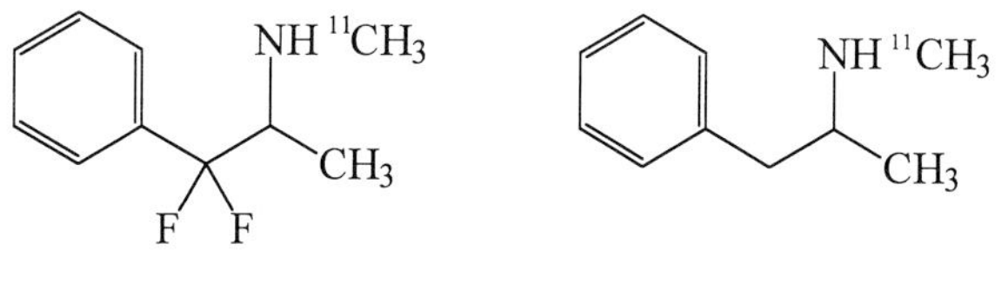

FIGURE 1   Structures and pKa values of MAMP and DiFMAMP.

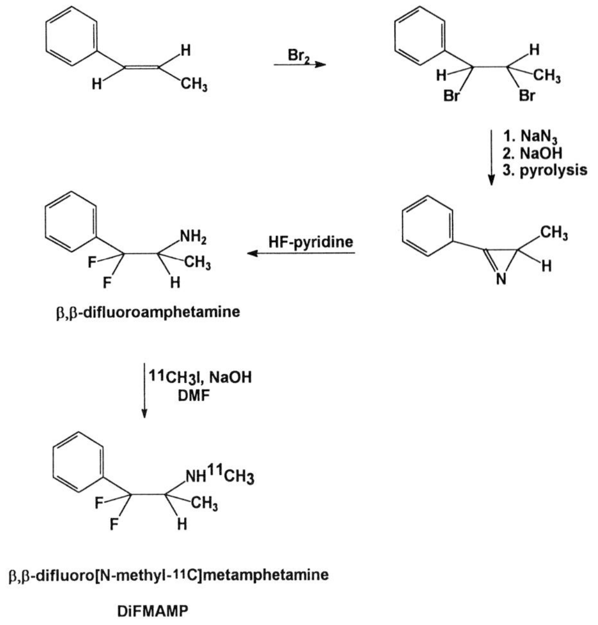

DiFMAMP
pKa ≈ 8

MAMP
pKa ≈ 10

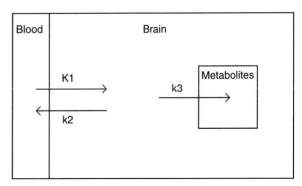

FIGURE 2   The synthesis of [^{11}C]DiFMAMP and its labeling precursor.

a lipophilic recognition site. To study these hypothesized interactions, we designed and synthesized [^{11}C] β,β-difluoromethamphetamine (DiFMAMP). Compared to methamphetamine (MAMP), at physiological pH, a greater proportion of DiFMAMP exists as the nonprotonated amine; that is, the β,β-difluoro substituted analog of MAMP has a lower acid dissociation constant or pKa (Fig. 1). The aim of this work was to compare the *in vivo* binding and kinetics of [^{11}C]MAMP (pKa 10) and [^{11}C]DiFMAMP (pKa 8) to provide information about the substrate selectivity of the proposed polar (amine) recognition site with respect to amine pKa.

II. MATERIALS AND METHODS

A. Tracer Synthesis

[^{11}C]DiFMAMP was synthesized by the alkylation of β,β-difluoroamphetamine with [^{11}C]methyl iodide in dimethylformamide (plus 10 μl 5M NaOH) at 120°C3 min, followed by preparative HPLC purification (Fig. 2). The labeling precursor was synthesized from 3-methyl-2-phenyl-1-azirine by treatment with polypyridinium hydrofluoride. [^{11}C]MAMP was synthesized by a modification of previously reported methods (Inoue, 1990; Shiue, 1994). [^{11}C]DiFMAMP or [^{11}C]MAMP were prepared and formulated ready for injection within 30 min after the end of bombardment (EOB) in 8% radiochemical yield (decay corrected to EOB) with a specific activity >50 GBq μmol^{-1} and a radiochemical purity >98%.

B. Scanning

Female pigs (40 kg, $N = 3$) were installed with catheters in the femoral artery and vein, anesthetized with isoflurane, and injected with 700–800 MBq [^{11}C]MAMP or [^{11}C]DiFMAMP intravenously. The order of injection of the two tracers was randomized in all three studies. Scans of 90 min duration (36 planes)

were performed, using an ECAT exact HR tomograph. Arterial plasma radioactivity concentrations were determined at 37 time points during the study in addition to 7 samples for the determination of plasma metabolites. Analysis of plasma metabolites was performed by the extraction of unmetabolized tracer from alkalinized arterial plasma (10 μl 50% NaOH) using ethyl acetate.

C. Data Analysis

Regions corresponding to the basal ganglia, thalamus, brain stem, temporal cortex, occipital cortex, frontal cortex, and thalamus were drawn using a histological pig brain atlas. The data was fitted to a three-

Blood	Brain
K1 →	Metabolites
← k2	k3 →

FIGURE 3   The three-compartment model used in this study.

A. D. Gee *et al.*

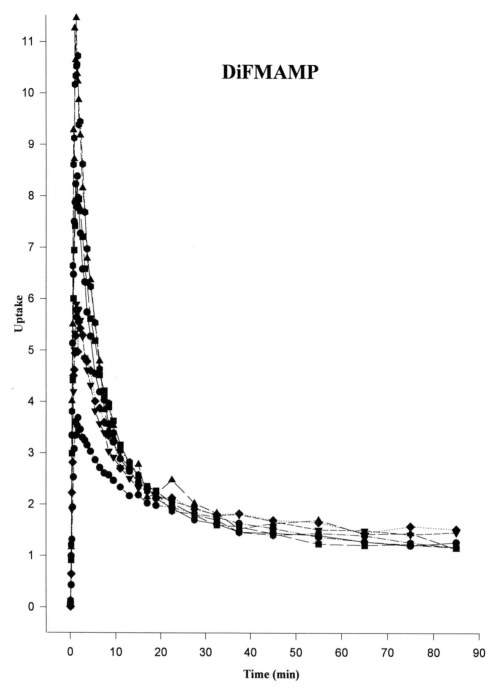

FIGURE 4 Normalized time activity curves for DiFMAMP and MAMP. ''Uptake'' is calculated as regional radioactivity concentration/Injected dose per body weight [(Bq/cc)/(Bq/g)].

compartment model (Fig. 3), where K_1, k_2, and k_3 are described as the clearance, washout, and rate of tracer metabolism in tissue, respectively. The parameters K_1, k_2, and k_3 were estimated by multilinear regression of the compartmental equations to the observed regional time–activity curves and metabolite-corrected arterial input function. K_1, k_2, and k_3 values for all regions were averaged from three separate studies.

III. RESULTS AND DISCUSSION

Normalized time activity curves for MAMP and DiF-MAMP (Fig. 4) show that both tracers rapidly enter the brain. Whereas DiFMAMP was rapidly washed out of brain tissue, MAMP was eliminated only slowly.

MAMP showed a slightly higher accumulation in subcortical regions compared to cortical regions and

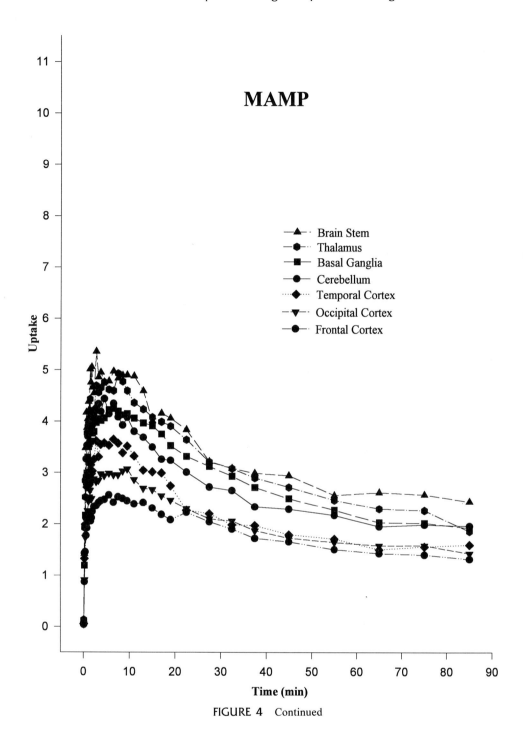

FIGURE 4 Continued

cerebellum. Estimates of K_1, k_2, and k_3 corresponding to the three-compartment model are shown in Table 1.

DiFMAMP exhibited a high rate of brain entry, with K_1 values ranging from 0.82–1.74 ml g^{-1} min^{-1} in the frontal cortex and brain stem, respectively. Comparative K_1 values for MAMP were generally twofold lower, ranging 0.43–0.67 ml g^{-1} min^{-1} in the frontal cortex and the basal ganglia, respectively.

The k_2 values for MAMP (range, 0.11–0.14 min^{-1}) were approximately four- to fivefold less than those of DiFMAMP (range, 0.39–0.71 min^{-1}).

The rate of tracer metabolism in tissue (k_3) was similar for both compounds (range, 0.004–0.08 min^{-1}).

With a pKa value of 10, MAMP exists to a great extent as the protonated amine at physiological pH, hence its entry across the blood–brain barrier is ex-

TABLE 1 Estimates of K_1, k_2, k_3, and Volume of Distribution for MAMP and DiFMAMP (Average Values from Three Studies)

Tracer	Region	K_1	k_2	k_3	VD
MAMP	Cerebellum	0.64	0.14	0.007	4.6
	Basal ganglia	0.55	0.11	0.007	5.0
	Brain stem	0.67	0.14	0.008	4.8
	Frontal cortex	0.43	0.12	0.006	3.6
DiFMAMP	Cerebellum	1.5	0.61	0.005	2.4
	Basal ganglia	1.5	0.50	0.004	3.0
	Brain stem	1.7	0.71	0.006	2.4
	Frontal cortex	0.82	0.39	0.008	2.1

pected to be somewhat slower than that of DiFMAMP with a pKa of 8. This was reflected by the higher K_1 values observed for DiFMAMP (ca. twofold greater than K_1 values for MAMP).

The four- to fivefold difference in the k_2 values of MAMP and DiFMAMP is, however, only partially attributable to the greater endothelial permeability of DiFMAMP. If the k_2 values of MAMP were governed by blood–brain barrier permeability alone, the k_2 values would be expected to be only twofold less than that of DiFMAMP. The lower than expected k_2 values for MAMP suggests that the tracer has a binding component in tissue that is not present in DiFMAMP.

These results cannot be explained by an increase in nonspecific binding due to a lipophilic interaction with brain tissue. In such a case, DiFMAMP would be expected to have lower k_2 values than MAMP. This binding interaction does, however, appear to be sensitive to the degree of amine protonation, with a greater retention of amines with high pKa values. These results indicate that the binding of amines in the brain may be due mainly to the hypothesized polar (amine) recognition site, which seems to be relatively homogenously distributed in the brain.

References

Inoue, O., Axelsson, S., Lundqvist, H., Oreland, L., and Langstrøm, B. (1990). Effect of reserpine on the brain uptake of carbon-11 methamphetamine and its N-propagyl derivative, deprenyl. *Eur. J. Nucl. Med.* **17**: 121–126.

Shiue, C.-Y., Shiue, G. G., Cornish, K. G., O'Rourke, M. F., and Sunderland, J. J. (1994). Regional distribution of (-)-[^{11}C]methamphetamine and (-)-3,4-methylenedioxy[^{11}C]methamphetamine in a monkey brain: Comparison with cocaine. *J. Labelled Compd. Radiopharm.* **35**: 528–530.

Tracer Selection Summary

MICHAEL R. KILBOURN
Division of Nuclear Medicine
Department of Internal Medicine
University of Michigan Medical School
Ann Arbor, Michigan 48109

The development of new radiopharmaceuticals for human brain PET imaging involves many steps. In the session "Tracer Selection," several authors made presentations that exemplified both the challenges and the successes in this important area of overall programs to PET image human neurochemistry.

For a variety of reasons—not the least being cost, ethics, and availability—most if not all new radiotracers are first subjected to intense *in vitro* and *in vivo* evaluation in animals prior to their introduction into clinical trials. Using appropriate methods, several of which were the subject of this session, animals models can provide invaluable insight into the potential applications of a new radiotracer.

Autoradiography, performed either *in vitro* or *ex vivo*, is a powerful tool for visualizing radiotracer distribution into specific binding sites. As shown by Biegon, Mathis, and Jagust (Chapter 6), the combination of *in vitro* and *ex vivo* autoradiography can identify both encouraging radiotracers (which should then be further pursued as imaging agents) and obviously poor possibilities. Drawing on their experiences with radiolabeled inhibitors of the neuronal serotonin transporter, they described examples of a "good" radiotracer, 6-nitro-iodoquipazine, and two poor *in vivo* radiotracers, paroxetine and imipramine.

Although autoradiography is an excellent method for determining radiotracer distributions, sometimes with great spatial resolution, it essentially provides only a snapshot of radiotracer distribution at one point in time. Construction of a kinetic curve would then require repetition of the experiment at various different times, which can be costly in both time and animals. Malizia *et al.* (Chapter 5) described a relatively simple alternative method for obtaining kinetic distribution data. They utilized a modified whole body counter, termed a *MOC* (multiple organs coincidences) *counter*,

which is a sensitive method for detecting radiotracer distribution in large areas. Use of such a simple device has advantages, in that low injected amounts of radioactivity are needed and repeated studies might be performed. Using [^{11}C]flumazenil as an example, a global change in radiotracer binding could be shown in the presence of a competing drug. However, the technique has significant disadvantages, chiefly a lack of spatial resolution and an inability to accurately determine a metabolite correction for blood radioactivity.

Finally, several groups presented data showing that PET scanners can be used successfully to detect changes in radiotracer distributions in an animal brain. A presentation by Myers *et al.* (Chapter 3) demonstrated that a small animal scanner can be built and used to image radiotracer kinetics in a small rat brain. Although successful at imaging radioligand binding in the striatum, the application of such an imaging method to smaller rat brain structures—such as the cortical areas, hippocampus, or such—remains questionable and will require even more efforts in the physics and engineering of PET scanners. In the subsequent presentation by Heiss *et al.* (Chapter 4), a clinical PET scanner was used to study an experimental cat model of a stroke, using a multiradiotracer imaging protocol. This exemplified that, for some applications, a special animal PET scanner may not be necessary and important work on animals can be completed using the new generation of human PET scanning equipment.

The aforementioned methods—autoradiography, coincidence counting, or PET imaging—provide information on the distribution of radioactivity following peripheral administration of a radiotracer. Interpretation of the meaning of this distribution requires, at the least, an understanding of the chemical nature of the radioactivity being detected. Two papers addressed the

47

importance of metabolism to the interpretation of PET studies. Osman *et al.* (Chapter 7) demonstrated the importance of the position of the radioactive label in a new radiotracer. [*O-methyl*-^{11}C]WAY-100635, labeled in a methyl group, was found to be metabolized *in vivo* in humans to a lipophilic metabolite, which likely contributed to the nonspecific brain uptake of radioactivity. The same radioligand, labeled in a carbonyl position, did not suffer such radioactive metabolites and therefore would be the superior agent for human PET studies of the receptor. Most important, this metabolism was species specific: lipophilic metabolites of the methyl labeled radioligand had not been seen in rats. This exemplifies the importance of considering species differences in metabolism and perhaps provides impetus for metabolism studies in primates before final radioligand selection.

In an example of how a prior knowledge of metabolism can be used to develop new, improved radiotracers, Brown *et al.* (Chapter 2) described the *in vivo* behavior of 6-fluoro-*m*-tyrosine. Detection of extrastriatal dopaminergic neurons is difficult with 6-fluoro-DOPA, due to the metabolism of the tracer by catechol-O-methyl transferase and the nonspecific distribution of the labeled metabolite. In constrast, 6-fluoro-*m*-tyrosine, being a noncatechol tracer of dopaminergic function, provided a means to detect nonstriatal dopaminergic innervation.

Thus, with proper knowledge of radiotracer metabolism and using any one of several methods of *in vivo* radiotracer distribution measurement, we can obtain *in vivo* data from which estimates are made of radiotracer binding sites densities. What do such data tell us, and can they be used to predict good radiotracers? Two papers addressed the issues of *in vitro* vs. *in vivo* distributions. Biegon *et al.* (Chapter 6) showed that *in vitro* and *in vivo* results with their new serotonin reuptake inhibitor, 6-nitro-iodoquipazine, were highly correlating and thus encouraging for further development as a human imaging agent. On the other hand, Kilbourn (Chapter 1) discussed several examples of such *in vitro–in vivo* correlations that, although linear and with good correlation coefficients, were insufficient in identifying a good vs. poor radiotracer. In particular, such correlations need to be normalized to maximal rates of binding both *in vitro* and *in vivo*; such correlation graphs then clearly indicate not only the linearity of the correlation, but more important, the relative dynamic ranges of the two methods.

As a theme for the subsequent informal discussion session, a handful of participants considered a proposal that PET imaging of biochemistry should now move into more complex procedures employing multiple radiotracers, pertubation of study conditions, or even a mixture of the two. Therefore, Bengt Langstrom supports combinations of radiotracers to examine several aspects of a physiological system; combinations of agents may provide insight not afforded by any single measure. Others propose that we may need to "perturb" the system, using either a pharmacological or a physiological stimulus, and determine if there are differences in the response of the system among individuals or between patient groups. It was pointed out that this would be, in a way, analogous to ongoing cerebral blood flow activation studies, and so the techniques and concepts developed in the latter (for example, statistics) could be applied.

The questions of multiple radiotracers and altering radiotracer distributions in the middle of a study are thought provoking and certainly would be a departure from the more strict, one-agent, full quantitative studies currently in vogue. Unfortunately, the ability to do such studies requires significant input from the imaging physics, instrumentation, modeling, quantitation, and statistics experts; and very few of those attended this breakaway session. Perhaps, in future meetings, these concepts can be brought up again, with adequate input from all sides of the questions.

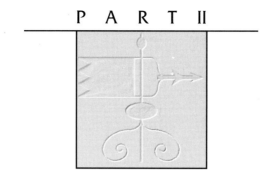

DATA ACQUISITION

11

Application of Simultaneous Emission and Transmission Scanning to Quantitative Cerebral PET

STEVEN R. MEIKLE, STEFAN EBERL, BRIAN F. HUTTON, PATRICK K. HOOPER, and MICHAEL J. FULHAM

The PET Department, Division of Medical Imaging Services
Royal Prince Alfred Hospital, Sydney, Australia

Accurate quantification of brain function with PET requires a separate transmission scan to correct for photon attenuation, which extends the duration of the study. Alternatively, emission and transmission measurements can be performed simultaneously, at the potential cost of bias due to increased scatter and dead time. We investigated the impact of simultaneous emission and transmission (SET) scanning on parameter estimation in tracer kinetic studies of the brain. Scatter and dead time correction errors in SET were measured as functions of the emission count rate. Net bias was used to predict distortion in FDG tissue curves and the effect on model parameter estimates. The effective scatter fraction for SET was <2% higher than usual at 30 kcounts · sec^{-1} (11.8 vs. 10.6%) but increased with decreasing emission count rate. In contrast, dead time correction error was −5% at 30 kcounts · sec^{-1} and became worse with increasing count rate. The net effect was to overestimate activity at low count rates and underestimate activity at high count rates. As a result, estimates of glucose metabolic rate using SET were lower than those from conventional acquisition and the bias was greater in gray matter than in white matter. However, in both cases the bias was small (<5% by simulation and <10% in a patient study) relative to measurement noise. We conclude that quantitative cerebral PET studies can be performed with acceptable bias and reduced study duration using SET.

I. INTRODUCTION

Accurate quantification of brain function with positron emission tomography (PET) requires a transmis- sion scan to correct for photon attenuation in the body. However, this extends the study duration and may result in attenuation artifacts due to misregistration of emission and transmission data (Huang *et al.*, 1979). In principle, these problems can be overcome by per- forming simultaneous emission and transmission (SET) measurements (Bailey *et al.*, 1987; Thompson *et al.*, 1989; Tung *et al.*, 1992; Tan *et al.*, 1993) but at the potential cost of bias and increased noise. We have implemented SET using unshielded rotating rod sources and applied the technique to whole body PET (Meikle *et al.*, 1995). Rod activity is kept relatively low (typically 50 MBq in total) to reduce dead time and randoms (Meikle *et al.*, 1993). Despite the use of low activity rods, the lack of shielding may make our SET method susceptible to scatter arising from the rod sources and dead time on adjacent detectors. The mag- nitude of bias due to these factors may determine the applicability of our SET method to quantitative brain imaging.

In this study, we investigated the impact of SET on accuracy of quantification in tracer kinetic studies of the brain. SET measurements were characterized in terms of scatter and accuracy of dead time correction and the measured bias was used to predict distortion in FDG tissue curves and the effect on model parame- ter estimates.

II. MATERIALS AND METHODS

SET was implemented on an ECAT 951R whole body tomograph (Siemens/CTI, Knoxville, TN), according to the method described for whole body studies (Meikle *et al.*, 1995). Except where stated, one or two rods, containing 50 MBq of ^{68}Ge/Ga in total, were used, the width of the sinogram window was seven projection bins (22 mm) per rod and the energy window was 250–850 keV.

A. Effective Scatter Fraction for SET

A baseline scatter fraction measurement was made using an elliptical water-filled cylinder (16 × 20 × 16 cm) approximating the human head. A 2 mm diameter line source containing 32 MBq ^{68}Ge/Ga was placed in the center of the phantom and emission data were acquired for 30 min. The scatter fraction (k) was calculated from projections parallel and orthogonal to the minor axis of the phantom, and the two values were averaged, with k defined in the usual way:

$$k = \frac{S_{em}}{C_{em} + S_{em}} \quad (1)$$

where S_{em} is the number of scattered coincidences arising from the emission source, obtained by integrating under the scatter tails within the boundaries of the phantom, and C_{em} is the number of unscattered coincidences.

To determine the additional scatter in SET measurements, blank and transmission scans of the head-sized phantom were acquired for 30 min. Data were recorded in both emission and transmission windows. A region of interest (ROI) was drawn around the boundaries of the phantom on the transmission sinogram and superimposed on the blank sinogram. The effective scatter fraction for SET then was calculated as

$$k_{SET} = \frac{S_{em} + S_{tr}}{C_{em} + S_{em} + S_{tr}}$$
$$\text{where } S_{tr} = T_{em} - (B_{em}/B_{tr})T_{tr} \quad (2)$$

Here, B and T refer to the blank and transmission coincidence rates within the ROI, respectively, and the subscripts refer to the respective windows. The ratio (B_{em}/B_{tr}) gives the fraction of transmission events that spill over into the emission window in the absence of scatter. Thus, S_{tr} is the increased scatter coincidence rate arising from the transmission sources. Note that k_{SET} varies as a function of emission count rate, whereas k is normally considered a constant. This variation in k_{SET} was calculated for count rates ranging from 1 to 50 kcounts · sec^{-1}.

B. Accuracy of Dead Time Correction

To assess the effect of SET on dead time correction, a 20 cm diameter cylinder containing a uniform concen-

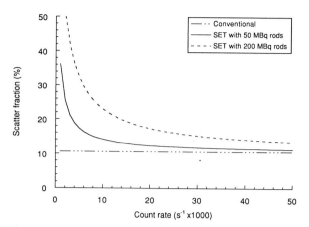

FIGURE 1 Effective scatter fraction for SET (k_{SET}) using 50 MBq and 200 MBq rod sources (solid and dashed curves, respectively) plotted against observed emission count rate. The scatter fraction measured for conventional (non-SET) imaging is also shown for comparison (dot–dashed curve).

tration of ^{18}F (160 kBq · ml^{-1} initially) was imaged over six half-lives (659 min) with alternating dynamic emission and SET frames. The scan commenced with a 5 min emission frame followed by a 5 min SET frame. The scanning sequence was repeated every 30 min throughout the study. After extracting emission data from SET frames, all emission frames (SET and non-SET) were corrected for dead time using a singles based method supplied by the vendor (Casey, 1992). The error in SET dead time correction was assessed by comparing corrected trues for SET and non SET frames.

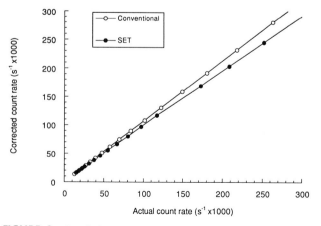

FIGURE 2 Dead time corrected emission count rate vs. actual count rate for conventional (non-SET) and SET imaging (open and closed circles, respectively).

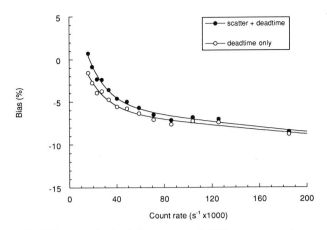

FIGURE 3 Bias in dead time corrected SET measurements as a function of observed emission count rate without (open circles) and with (closed circles) the effect of scattering from the rods included.

C. Effect of SET Bias on Parameter Estimates

The effect of SET bias on parameter estimates was investigated for the case of the three-compartment FDG model (Sokoloff *et al.*, 1977; Phelps *et al.*, 1979). An arterial input function, representing a rapid bolus administration, was simulated using a multiexponential model (Feng and Wang, 1993). Gray and white matter tissue time–activity curves were simulated using this input function and rate constants reported by Phelps *et al.* (Phelps *et al.*, 1979). The tissue curves so obtained were multiplied point by point by the net count rate-dependent bias calculated previously for SET studies. The simulated tissue curves were corrected for decay and integrated according to the following sampling schedule: 5×1 min, 5×2 min, and 15×5 min. Rate constants were then estimated by fitting the three-compartment FDG model to the simulated tissue curves. To calculate local cerebral metabolic rate of glucose utilization (lCMRGlu), plasma glucose concentration was arbitrarily set equal to $100 \text{ mg} \cdot \text{ml}^{-1}$ and the lumped constant was 0.42. Uncertainty in lCMRGlu values was estimated by repeating the curve fitting procedure 100 times, using simulated noise typical for a 15 mm diameter ROI, and calculating the standard deviation of the parameter estimates (Graham, 1993).

D. Patient Study

A dynamic [18F]FDG study was performed on a male patient with a superior frontal lobe tumor, using a modified protocol to verify our findings. A 10 min transmission scan was performed before administering 370 MBq of [18F]FDG intravenously to the patient. A 16 frame dynamic scan was then acquired over the next 81 min with alternating conventional and SET frames. Arterialized blood samples were taken throughout the study. Attenuation correction was applied to conventional emission frames using the preinjection data and to SET emission frames using the summed SET transmission data (total acquisition time = 33 min). All frames were reconstructed using filtered back projection with a 1D Hanning window cut off at the Nyquist frequency ($f_{\text{Nyq}} = 1.6 \text{ cycles} \cdot \text{cm}^{-1}$). Tissue curves were generated from ROIs enclosing the tumor and an area of normal cortical gray matter on the contralateral side. Kinetic parameters were estimated by fitting the tissue curves and the measured input function to the three-compartment FDG model.

III. RESULTS AND DISCUSSION

A. Effective Scatter Fraction for SET

The scatter fraction for conventional emission scanning was measured to be 12.1% and 9.1% for the 0° and 90° projections, respectively, giving an average of 10.6%. The value of k_{SET} as a function of emission count rate is shown in Figure 1, along with the conventional scatter fraction for comparison. Although k_{SET} is not much higher than the conventional scatter fraction at 30 kcounts · sec^{-1} (11.8% compared to 10.6%), it increases dramatically at low count rates. To demonstrate the effect of rod activity on k_{SET}, the values shown for 50 MBq rods were extrapolated to 200 MBq

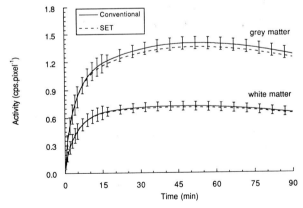

FIGURE 4 Simulated gray and white matter FDG tissue curves for conventional imaging (solid curves) and for SET (dashed curves), taking into account the bias due to scatter and dead time correction. The error bars indicate measurement noise (± 1 sd) given typical counting statistics and sampling schedule.

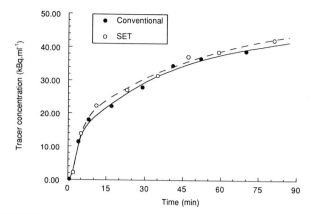

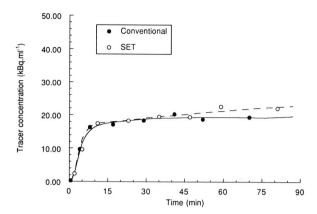

FIGURE 5 FDG tissue curves obtained from a region of normal cortical gray matter in a patient study, where acquisition frames were alternated between conventional (closed circles) and SET frames (open circles). The solid and dashed curves indicate the model fit to the conventional and SET data points respectively, using the three-compartment FDG model.

FIGURE 6 FDG tissue curves obtained from a tumor region in the same patient study as shown in Figure 5. The solid and dashed curves indicate the model fit to the conventional and SET data points, respectively, using the three-compartment FDG model.

rods (also shown in Fig. 1), which are typically used for conventional transmission scanning.

B. Accuracy of Dead Time Correction

Figure 2 shows the corrected count rate for SET and conventional acquisition plotted against actual count rate. The two curves are approximately linear and show good agreement over a large range of count rates but diverge with increasing count rate. The difference between these two curves gives the bias in dead time corrected SET measurements, which is plotted against count rate in Figure 3. This figure indicates that net bias in SET measurements (closed circles) is positive at low count rates (<20 kcounts $\cdot$ sec^{-1}) and negative at higher count rates, but the magnitude of bias is $\leq 5\%$ over the range 8–50 kcounts $\cdot$ sec^{-1}. Thus, the lack of physical shielding of transmission sources in our implementation of SET does not unduly affect

tomograph performance. This is primarily because of the use of relatively low rod source activity.

C. Effect of SET Bias on Parameter Estimates

Simulated tissue time–activity curves for gray and white matter are shown in Figure 4, indicating the predicted distortion due to bias in SET measurements. The error bars indicate measurement noise (± 1 standard deviation) for a 15 mm diameter ROI and typical image counting statistics and sampling schedule. The graph demonstrates that bias in SET is smaller than measurement noise in a typical tissue curve. Parameter estimates obtained by fitting the three-compartment FDG model to the simulated tissue curves are given in Table 1. The rate constant k_2, which was most affected by SET, was overestimated by 13% for gray matter and 16% for white matter. All other parameters agreed to

TABLE 1   Parameter Estimates for Simulated Conventional (Non-SET) and SET FDG Tissue Curves

	Gray matter			White matter		
	Non-SET	**SET**	**Bias**	**Non-SET**	**SET**	**Bias**
K_1 (ml $\cdot$ min^{-1} $\cdot$ ml^{-1})	0.103	0.107	+4%	0.054	0.058	+7%
k_2 (min^{-1})	0.133	0.149	+13%	0.111	0.128	+16%
k_3 (min^{-1})	0.063	0.063	+1%	0.045	0.047	+4%
k_4 (min^{-1})	0.0068	0.0063	−7%	0.0059	0.0056	−5%
lCMRGlu (ml $\cdot$ min^{-1} $\cdot$ 100g^{-1})	7.90	7.64	−3%	3.79	3.74	−1%

TABLE 2 Parameter Estimates Obtained from Conventional (Non-SET) and SET Patient Data

	Gray matter		Tumor	
	Non-SET	SET	Non-SET	SET
K_1 (ml · min^{-1} · 100g^{-1})	0.13 ± 0.01	0.117 ± 0.008	0.105 ± 0.006	0.12 ± 0.01
k_2 (min^{-1})	0.27 ± 0.07	0.16 ± 0.04	0.19 ± 0.03	0.22 ± 0.03
k_3 (min^{-1})	0.10 ± 0.03	0.06 ± 0.02	0.03 ± 0.02	0.029 ± 0.006
k_4 (min^{-1})	0.010 ± 0.004	0.007 ± 0.005	0.01 ± 0.01	0.005 ± 0.003
lCMRGlu (ml · min^{-1} · 100g^{-1})	8.4 ± 0.8	7.6 ± 0.9	3.7 ± 1.0	3.5 ± 0.4

within 10%. The bias in lCMRGlu estimates was −3% and −1% for gray matter and white matter, respectively. Therefore, bias in parameter estimates following SET acquisition is negligible compared with measurement uncertainty due to noise, which was estimated to be 15% (±1 SD) for gray matter and 19% (±1 SD) for white matter.

D. Patient Study

The tissue curves for normal cortical gray matter and tumor are shown in Figures 5 and 6, respectively. The estimated kinetic parameters are given in Table 2. There was good agreement between SET and conventional tissue curves and the estimates of lCMRGlu agreed to within 10% in both gray matter and the tumor. However, the trend in both sets of curves was for SET to slightly overestimate tracer concentration in the middle to late part of the study, which is in contrast to the simulation study. This suggests that either the scatter was higher or the bias in dead time correction was smaller than was estimated in the phantom measurements. Furthermore, the tumor curves appear to diverge at late times, but this is probably an artifact caused by sensitivity of the curve fitting procedure to noise in the data and relatively sparse sampling.

IV. SUMMARY

This chapter reports on the impact of SET on quantification in tracer kinetic brain studies with PET. We found that bias due to scatter and dead time correction work in opposite directions and that the bias is small (≤5%) over a large range of count rates typically encountered in kinetic studies. As a result, estimates of lCMRGlu obtained from SET data agreed with those from conventional data to within 5% in simulations and 10% in a patient study. Therefore, quantitative cerebral PET studies can be performed with acceptable bias

and reduced study duration using SET. Although we studied [^{18}F]FDG in this work, we believe the results can be applied to other tracers to determine the applicability of SET imaging.

Acknowledgments

The authors thank Dr. Michael Graham for the use of his parameter optimization software (P-Opt) and advice regarding estimation of parameter errors. We also acknowledge the input of Roger Fulton, Kevin Ho-Shon, Dagan Feng, and Dale Bailey to discussions on this work.

References

Bailey, D. L., Hutton, B. F., and Walker, P. J. (1987). Improved SPECT using simultaneous emission and transmission tomography. *J. Nucl. Med.* **28**: 844–851.

Casey, M. E. (1992). An analysis of counting losses in positron emission tomography. PhD thesis. University of Tennessee.

Feng, D., and Wang, X. (1993). A computer simulation study on the effects of input function measurement noise in tracer kinetic modeling with positron emission tomography (PET). *Comput. Biol. Med.* **23**: 57–68.

Graham, M. M. (1993). Errors associated with parameter estimation. *J. Nucl. Med.* **34**: 257P.

Huang, S. C., Hoffman, E. J., Phelps, M. E., and Kuhl, D. E. (1979). Quantitation in positron emission tomography: 2. Effect of inaccurate attenuation correction. *J. Comput. Assist. Tomogr.* **3**: 804–814.

Meikle, S. R., Bailey, D. L., Hooper, P. K. *et al.* (1995). Simultaneous emission and transmission measurements for attenuation correction in whole body PET. *J. Nucl. Med.* **36**: 1680–1688.

Meikle, S. R., Bailey, D. L., Hutton, B. F., and Jones, W. F. (1993). Optimisation of simultaneous emission and transmission measurements in PET. Conference Record of the 1993 IEEE Medical Imaging Conference, San Francisco. pp. 1642–1646.

Phelps, M. E., Huang, S.-C., Hoffman, E. J., Selin, C., Sokoloff, L., and Kuhl, D. E. (1979). Tomographic measurement of local cerebral glucose metabolic rate in humans with (F-18)2-fluoro-2-deoxy-D-glucose: Validation of method. *Ann. Neurol.* **6**: 371–388.

Sokoloff, L., Reivich, M., Kennedy, C., *et al.* (1977). The (^{14}C)-deoxyglucose method for the measurement of local cerebral glucose utilization: Theory, procedure and normal values in the conscious and anesthetized albino rat. *J. Neurochem.* **28:** 897–916.

Tan, P., Bailey, D. L., Meikle, S. R., Eberl, S., Fulton, R. R., and Hutton, B. F. (1993). A scanning line source for simultaneous emission and transmission measurements in SPECT. *J. Nucl. Med.* **34:** 1752–1760.

Thompson, C. J., Ranger, N. T., and Evans, A. C. (1989). Simultaneous transmission and emission scans in positron emission tomography. *IEEE Trans. Nucl. Sci.* **36:** 1011–1016.

Tung, C.-H., Gullberg, G. T., Zeng, G. L., Christian, P. E., Datz, F. L., and Morgan, H. T. (1992). Non-uniform attenuation correction using simultaneous transmission and emission converging tomography. *IEEE Trans. Nucl. Sci.* **39:** 1134–1143.

12

A New PET Camera for Noninvasive Quantitation of Physiological Functional Parametric Images
Headtome-V-Dual

HIDEHIRO IIDA, SHUICHI MIURA, IWAO KANNO, TOSHIHIDE OGAWA, and KAZUO UEMURA

Research Institute for Brain and Blood Vessels
Akita City, 010, Japan

Headtome-V-Dual is designed as our latest generation PET camera system; it covers the whole brain and whole myocardium simultaneously. The axial field of view (FOV) is 15 cm and 10 cm corresponding to the brain and heart scanners, respectively. The heart scanner can move axially to adjust distance between the brain and the heart in each study (minimum distance, two detector rings ≈10 cm). Each gantry consists of 112 units of two-dimensional position-sensitive detector blocks. Detector diameter is 84.7 cm. A unique data acquisition system is implemented, which consists of a large-scale data acquisition memory (1 GB) and a microprocessor that controls the data transfer and the numerical operation, enabling real-time weighted-integration data acquisition either in two- or three-dimensional acquisition modes. Thus, functional parametric images can be calculated rapidly without acquiring the dynamic data. Each microprogram is under control of a UNIX host computer, enabling software development to be flexible and easy. The coincidence path acceptance is designed to be variable in the axial direction, so that the sensitivity and axial spatial resolution can be optimized in each study protocol. In two-dimensional acquisition, observed in-plane spatial resolution was ≈4.0 mm full-width at half-maximum (FWHM) at the center FOV as measured by a Ge-68 line source in the air. The axial spatial resolution was ≈4.3 mm FWHM at the center of FOV. The sensitivity measured by a 20 cm⌀ cylindrical phantom was 5.95 and 4.05 kcps/kBq/ml for the brain and heart scanners, respectively. A dead time loss for a 14 cm⌀ cylindrical phantom was approximately 32% at concentration of 118 kBq, and 18% at 67 kBq. The peak noise-equivalent counts (NEC) were 120 and 80 kcps at 100 kBq/ml, respectively. It was found that this dual-PET system can be used to scan the brain and heart simultaneously. Use of the left ventricular time–activity curve as input function obviates the needs for arterial cannulation, which would be of great advantage in clinical use.

I. INTRODUCTION

PET is capable of providing quantitative biomedical and physiological functions *in vivo*. This is predicated on a mathematical-model based analysis for accurately measured arterial input function as well as regional radioactivity concentration in tissue. The arterial input function is usually determined by frequent or continuous sampling of the arterial blood from peripheral artery and is known to be an important source of errors (Iida *et al.*, 1986). In addition, the procedure of arterial cannulation is rather laborious and invasive, which is often a limiting factor in clinical studies.

Several attempts have been made to remove arterial cannulation in the determination of the arterial input function for quantitative PET studies. Use of a standardized input function and calibrating it with a minimal number of blood samples (either arterial or venous blood) is one of the simplified procedures for clinical use, and its validity has been demonstrated for slowly behaving tracers (Takikawa *et al.*, 1993; Iida *et al.*,

1994a and 1994b). However, because of the rapid kinetics, this is of a limited applicability for O-15 labeled compound studies (O-15 water and O-15 oxygen), as calculated physiological parameters are highly dependent on the shape of the input curve for these tracers (Iida *et al.*, 1986, 1988b, 1989, 1992b).

Tomographic scanning of the vasculature has been tested for several parts of the body to obtain a noninvasive arterial curve; for example, scanning the arm (radial or ulnar artery; Eriksson and Kanno, 1991), scanning the neck (carotid artery; Kanno *et al.*, 1991), and scanning the chest (cardiac chamber; Iida *et al.*, 1992a). Accurate determination of the input function requires the following four factors: (1) large recovery of the blood volume, (2) small spillover from surrounding tissue, (3) an established model to correct for the error sources mentioned previously, and (4) high statistics. Scanning the radial artery with a PET scanner, which may be performed using a small tomograph, may provide significant signal with little spillover from the soft tissue. However, the recovery coefficient appears to be too small (<0.1) to be corrected within acceptable accuracy (Iida *et al.*, 1992a). In addition, the long transit time in the arterial line makes the correction for dispersion difficult, unless arterial blood is continuously withdrawn. Scanning the neck (Kanno *et al.*, 1991), which may be performed by extending the axial FOV of the PET scanner, also demonstrated significant signal in the carotid artery. However, there was nonnegligible amount of spillover from the soft tissue, which was probably difficult to correct. In addition, the recovery coefficient was too small to be accurately corrected (≈0.1). Scanning the cardiac chamber (e.g., left ventricle) with a PET scanner was thought to be the only way of noninvasively determining the input function within acceptable accuracy. This provided large recovery (>0.8) with sufficient count statistics. Even though there may still be significant spillover from the myocardium, this can be corrected by a newly developed kinetic model (Iida, 1992a).

Based on these considerations, we have designed our new generation PET camera, Headtome-V-Dual, to simultaneously cover the whole brain and whole myocardium. This scanner provides not only the simultaneous quantitation of physiological functions both in brain and heart, but also the noninvasive input function, thus enabling the noninvasive quantitation of biomedical and physiological parametric maps without arterial cannulation. It was also intended to install a unique data acquisition system that was successfully developed in our previous scanner (Iida *et al.*, 1995a) for a rapid calculation of parametric rate constant images without dynamic data acquisition. The aim of this chapter is to evaluate the physical performance of the

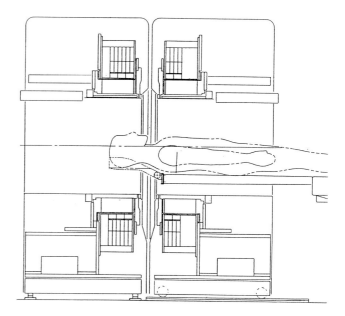

Akita   Noken

FIGURE 1   Cross-sectional view of the Headtome-V-Dual scanner.

Headtome-V-Dual PET scanner as a clinical investigative tool.

II. MATERIALS AND METHODS

A. Scanner Design

The scanner was designed to cover the brain and heart simultaneously. The cross-sectional view of the Headtome-V-Dual scanner is shown in Figure 1. The axial field of view of this scanner is 15 cm and 10 cm, corresponding to the brain and heart scanners, respectively. The heart gantry can move axially to adjust the distance between brain and heart in each study. The minimum distance between the detector rings of the two gantries is ≈10 cm, so that most subjects can place their arms between the gantries. The brain scanner can move perpendicular to the bed axis (perpendicular to the figure), allowing a separate use of each scanner as two independent machines. Each gantry consists of 112 units of two-dimensional position-sensitive detector blocks. Detector diameter is 850 mm. The septa can be retracted for three-dimensional (3D) data acquisition. The physical geometry is summarized in Table 1.

B. Data Acquisition System

The front-end data acquisition system consists of large scale acquisition memories (1 GB) and a micro-

TABLE 1 Physical Aspect of Headtome-V-Dual

	Brain	Heart
BGO detector size	3.8 mm × 6.25 mm × 30 mm	
Detectors per block	48 (6 × 8)	
Blocks per ring	336	224
Slice spacing	3.125 mm	
Number of slices	47	31
Axial FOV	150 mm	100 mm
Septa length	55 mm	
Gantry diameter	850 mm	

TABLE 2 Physical Performance of Headtome-V-Dual

	Brain	Heart
Inplane resolution	≈4.0 mm FWHM at center	
Axial resolution	≈4.3 mm FWHM at center	
Scatter (2D)	13%	
Peak NEC (2D)	120 kcps at 100 kBq/ml	80 kcps at 100 kBq/ml
Peak NEC (3D)	109 kcps at 24 kBq/ml	73 kcps at 24 kBq/ml
Sensitivity (2D)	5.95 kcps/kBq/ml	4.05 kcps/kBq/ml
(3D)	45.9 kcps/kBq/ml	21.6 kcps/kBq/ml

processor that controls the data collection in histogram mode, data transfer, and the arithmetic operation. Each microprogram for these operations is directly controlled by a UNIX host computer, enabling flexible and easy software development. This system is also capable of acquiring multiple weighted-integration sinograms in real time for 2D or 3D modes. The acquired multiple sinograms, weighted by time-dependent functions, are transferred to a UNIX workstation and then reconstructed to generate weighted–integrated tomographic images. According to the algorithm published previously (Iida *et al.*, 1995a; Alpert *et al.*, 1984), parametric rate-constant images can be calculated rapidly. It should be noted that this calculation process does not require dynamic frame data acquisition. The coincidence path acceptance is designed to be variable in the axial direction, so that the sensitivity and axial spatial resolution can be optimized for each study protocol (Fig. 2).

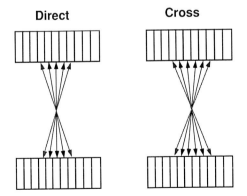

Direct **Cross**

FIGURE 2 Variable axial coincidence path acceptance (ACPA) in 2D acquisition with nonretracted septa. Sensitivity and noise-equivalent count (NEC) increase as the ACPA increases up to seven and eight rings, corresponding to direct and cross planes, respectively. ACPA of five and six are selected for typical O-15 compound studies for the brain.

III. RESULTS AND DISCUSSION

The physical performance of the Headtome-V-Dual is summarized in Table 2. In 2D acquisition, observed in-plane spatial resolution was ≈4.0 mm full-width at half-maximum at the center of the FOV, as measured by a Ge-68 line source in air. The axial spatial resolution was ≈4.3 mm FWHM at the center of the FOV. The sensitivity and the peak noise-equivalent count (NEC, $(\alpha T)^2/(T + 2fR)$), from Strother *et al.* (1990), increased with increasing axial coincidence path acceptance (ACPA) up to seven and eight rings, corresponding to direct and cross planes, respectively. The sensitivity measured with a 20 cmϕ cylindrical phantom was 5.95 (45.9) and 4.05 (21.6) kcps/kBq/ml for the brain and heart scanners in the 2D (3D) acquisition modes, respectively (ACPA, five and six for direct and cross planes, respectively). A dead time loss for a 14 cmϕ cylindrical phantom was approximately 32% (18%) at 118 (67) kBq/ml. The peak NEC values were 120 (109) and 80 (73) kcps at 93 (24) kBq/ml, corresponding to the brain and the heart scanners in 2D (3D) data acquisition mode, respectively (Fig. 3).

This study demonstrates that the physical performance of Headtome-V-Dual is suitable for scanning the brain and heart simultaneously. Relatively flat characteristics of NEC around the peak in 2D acquisition is an important feature for the dual-PET use, as the counting rate in each gantry might be quite different and might have a large dynamic range.

Simultaneous scanning of brain and heart has several advantages for clinical use. Use of the left ventricular time–activity curve as the input function obviates the need for arterial cannulation. This avoids the risk of vasospasm or hemorrhage. In addition, the mental stress to the subject due to the arterial cannulation can be removed, which would be particularly important for a neurological study. Furthermore, the amount of withdrawn blood is not a limiting factor for long data

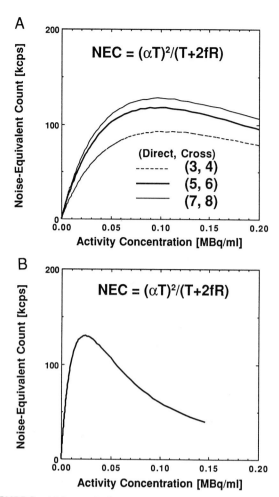

$$NEC = (\alpha T)^2/(T+2fR)$$

(Direct, Cross)
(3, 4)
(5, 6)
(7, 8)

FIGURE 3 Noise-equivalent count (NEC) as a function of radioactivity concentration with septa (A) and with retracted septa (B). For the nonretracted septa mode (2D), data are plotted for three different axial coincidence path acceptance; that is, three and four rings (dashed line), five and six rings (bold solid line), and seven and eight rings (thin solid line), corresponding the direct and cross planes, respectively.

and therefore direct measurement of the metabolized water is not required.

Recent studies demonstrated that the use of O-15 labeled compounds is also capable of providing several fundamental physiological functions in the myocardium, and these parameters were suggested to be clinically useful; for example, regional myocardial blood flow (Iida *et al.*, 1988; Bergmann, 1988), water perfusable tissue fraction (Iida *et al.*, 1991), and oxygen extraction fraction and oxygen metabolism (Iida *et al.*, 1995). Therefore, simultaneous measurement of these functional parameters both in brain and heart might be of clinical interest. However, the outcome of combining all of this information is still unknown, and further investigation is needed.

The dual-PET system might be advantageous particularly for O-15 compound studies. Arterial cannulation has been a limiting process for the O-15 water and O-15 oxygen protocols. Relatively long transit time in the arterial line in the arm makes the correction for delay and dispersion difficult, and these were known to be significant sources of errors in the estimated physiological parameters (Iida *et al.*, 1986, 1988). Because of a shorter transit time from the left ventricle to the brain than that from the left ventricle to the radial artery, the correction for delay and dispersion would be more accurate by scanning the heart. It should also be noted that, with a short half-life of O-15, removal of arterial cannulation would increase significantly the throughput of the study.

The advantage of our data acquisition system is not only the capability of real-time weighted-integration, but also the flexibility in developing software for new clinical protocols. The data acquisition memory can be accessed from a UNIX workstation even during the data acquisition, enabling the on-line monitoring of the acquisition memory, and easy collection of multiple sinograms with different scan modes, such as multiple weighted-integration sinograms, static and conventional dynamic frame data, or static scans and gated scans. These programs may minimize the time for off-line data analysis and may be helpful in increasing the throughput of the study.

The minimum scan duration is 1.0 sec for each frame in the dynamic scan mode. This provides sufficiently precise temporal resolution in monitoring the arterial input function with use of the heart PET scanner. Sinograms may be acquired only for areas that cover the mid-ventricular slices, and these sinograms may be added together, and reconstructed, so that the input function may be determined from the minimum amount of tomographic data. Simultaneously, tomographic data may be acquired for whole axial FOV with the real-time weighted-integration mode or a static scan

acquisition, and thus kinetic analysis can be performed for relatively long scanning periods with full measurement of the input curve. It should also be noted that the whole body PET scan can be performed more efficiently with the two gantries.

Small recovery of the left ventricular chamber ($\approx$0.8) and spillover from the myocardial signal into the left ventricular chamber can be corrected according to a method validated previously (Iida *et al.*, 1992a). The O-15 oxygen inhalation study requires determination of metabolized O-15 water component in the arterial blood in addition to the O-15 oxygen concentration time–activity curve. This can be estimated from the whole blood curve according to the mathematical model that was validated previously (Iida *et al.*, 1993), mode otherwise. Functional tomographic images can then be calculated for the whole heart with sufficiently precise slice separation.

Quantitative aspects of the 3D acquisition mode are, however, unknown. The NEC falls quickly at >0.3 MBq/ml, and therefore simultaneous scanning brain and heart in 3D requires further investigation. Although artifacts due to Compton scatter may be compensated by an empirical cross-calibration procedure, it would be highly desirable to develop a correction technique for the scatter.

References

Alpert, N. M., Eriksson, L., Chang, J. Y., Bergstrom, M., Litton, J. E., Correia, J. A., Bohm, C., Ackerman, R. H., and Taveras, J. M. (1984). Strategy for the measurement of regional cerebral blood flow using short-lived tracers and emission tomography. *J. Cereb. Blood Flow Metab.* **4**: 28–34.

Bergmann, S. R., Fox, K. A., Rand, A. L., McElvany, K.D., Welch, M. J., Markham, J., and Sobel, B. E., (1989). Noninvasive quantitation of myocardial blood flow in human subjects with oxygen-15-labeled water and positron emission tomography. *J. Am. Coll. Cardiol.* **14**: 639–652.

Erikkson, L., and Kanno, I. (1991). Blood sampling devices and measurements. *Med. Prog. Tech.* **17**: 249–257.

Iida, H., Kanno, I., Miura, S., Murakami, M., Takahashi, K., and Uemura, K. (1986). Error analysis of a quantitative cerebral blood flow measurement using $H_2^{15}O$ autoradiography and positron emission tomography, with respect to the dispersion of the input function. *J. Cereb. Blood Flow Metab.* **6**: 536–545.

Iida, H., Kanno, I., Takahashi, A., Miura, S., Murakami, M., Takahashi, K., Ono, Y., Shishido, F., Inugami, A., Tomura, N., Higano, S., Fujita, H., Sasaki, H., Nakamichi, H., Mizusawa, S., Kondo, Y., and Uemura, K. (1988a). Measurement of absolute myocardial blood flow with $H_2^{15}O$ and dynamic positron emission tomography: Strategy for quantification in relation to the partial-volume effect. *Circulation.* **78**: 104–115.

Iida, H., Higano, S., Tomura, N., Shishido, F., Kanno, I., Miura, S., Murakami, M., Takahashi, K., Sasaki, H., and Uemura, K. (1988b). Evaluation of regional difference of tracer appearance time in cerebral tissues using [^{15}O] water and dynamic positron emission tomography. *J. Cereb. Blood Flow Metab.* **8**: 285–288.

Iida, H., Kanno, I., Miura, S., Murakami, M., Takahashi, K., and Uemura, K. (1989). A determination of the regional brain/blood partition coefficient of water using dynamic positron emission tomography. *J. Cereb. Blood Flow Metab.* **9**: 874–885.

Iida, H., Rhodes, C. G., de Silva, R., Yamamoto, Y., Jones, T., and Araujo, L. I. (1991). Myocardial tissue fraction—Correction for partial volume effects and measure of tissue viability. *J. Nucl. Med.* **32**: 2169–2175.

Iida, H., Rhodes, C. G., de Silva, R., Araujo, L. I., Bloomfield, P. M., Lammertsma, A. A., and Jones, T. (1992a). Use of the left ventricular time-activity curve as a noninvasive input function in dynamic oxygen-15-water positron emission tomography. *J. Nucl. Med.* **33**: 1669–1677.

Iida, H., Kanno, I., and Miura, S. (1992b). Rapid measurement of cerebral blood flow with positron emission tomography. (CIBA Foundation Symposium 163, Exploring brain functional anatomy with positron emission tomography); pp. 23–42. Wiley, Chichester.

Iida, H., Jones, T., and Miura, S. (1993). Modeling approach to eliminate the need to separate arterial plasma in oxygen-15 inhalation positron emission tomography. *J. Nucl. Med.* **34**: 1333–1340.

Iida, H., Itoh, H., Bloomfield, P. M., Munaka, M., Higano, S., Murakami, M., Inugami, A., Eberl, S., Aizawa, Y., Kanno, I., and Uemura, K. (1994a). A method to quantitate cerebral blood flow using a rotating gamma camera and iodine-123 iodoamphetamine with one blood sampling. *Eur. J. Nucl. Med.* **21**: 1072–1084.

Iida, H., Itoh, H., Nakazawa, M., Hatazawa, J., Nishimura, H., Onishi, Y., and Uemura, K. (1994b). Quantitative mapping of regional cerebral blood flow using Iodine-123-IMP and SPECT. *J. Nucl. Med.* **35**: 2019–2030.

Iida, H., Bloomfield, P. M., Miura, S., Kanno, I., Murakami, M., and Uemura, K. (1995a). Effect of real-time weighted integration system for rapid calculation of functional images in clinical positron emission tomography. *IEEE Trans. Med. Image* **14**: 116–121.

Iida, H., Rhodes, C. G., Araujo, L. I., Yamamoto, Y., de Silva, R., Ph.D., Maseri, A., and Jones, A. (1995b). Non-invasive quantification of regional myocardial metabolic rate of oxygen using $^{15}O_2$ inhalation and positron emission tomography: Theory, error analysis and application in man. *Circulation,* in press.

Kanno, I., Iida, H., Miura, S., and Murakami, M. (1991). Noninvasive measurement of input function by dynamic neck scan for quantitative brain PET using [O-15] water. *J. Nucl. Med.* **32** (suppl), p 1003.

Strother, S. C., Casey, M. E., and Hoffman, E. J. (1990). Measuring PET scanner sensitivity: Relating countrates to image signal-to-noise ratios using noise equivalent counts. *IEEE Trans. Nucl. Sci.* **37**: 783–788.

Takikawa, S., Dhawan, V., Spetsieris, P., Robeson, W., Chaly, T., Dahl, R., Margouleff, D., and Eidelberg, D. (1993). Noninvasive quantitative fluorodeoxyglucose PET studies with an estimated input function derived from a population-based arterial blood curve. *Radiology* **188**: 131–136.

Development of an On-Line Blood Detector System for PET Studies in Small Animals

SHARON ASHWORTH, ALEX RANICAR, PETER M. BLOOMFIELD, TERRY JONES, and ADRIAAN A. LAMMERTSMA

PET Methodology Group, Cyclotron Unit, MRC Clinical Sciences Centre
Royal Postgraduate Medical School
Hammersmith Hospital, London W12 ONN, United Kingdom

This study reports on the development of a dedicated on-line blood detection system and its preliminary application, in conjunction with a dedicated small animal PET scanner, to the measurement of glucose metabolism (CMR_{glu}) in the rat brain. The β^+ detector was composed of a shielded block of NE102A scintillating plastic (5 × 5 × 38 mm), with a 1.6 mm diameter longitudinal hole, through which an arterial catheter was passed. The detector was optically coupled to a single 38 mm photomultiplier tube and standard NIM electronics were used to shape, gate, and process the signal output. An ALT-386SX laptop PC was used to record the logic pulses. Ten male Sprague–Dawley rats were used, five of whom were fed ad lib (fed) and five whose food was withdrawn overnight (fasted). Each rat was given [^{18}F]-fluoro-deoxyglucose (~19 MBq) iv and a 60 min dynamic scan was performed. Arterial blood was allowed to flow freely through the on-line β^+ detector at intermittent predetermined time intervals, throughout the study period. In addition, blood samples were collected manually and measured in a well counter, cross-calibrated with the scanner. There was good correlation between the blood curve, as measured by the on-line detector, and the discrete blood samples. The on-line detector provided marked improvement in the definition of the peak. Plasma curves were generated and brain time–radioactivity curves were fitted to a two-tissue compartmental model using standard nonlinear regression techniques. Assuming a lumped constant of 0.58, CMR_{glu} was 0.6 ± 0.1 and 0.7 ± 0.1 (mean ± standard deviation) for fed and fasted animals, respectively.

I. INTRODUCTION

Quantification of specific binding of a positron emitting ligand in rat brain using positron emission tomography is possible if a reference tissue exists within the field of view, which can be used as an indirect input function (Hume *et al.*, 1992). In the absence of such a tissue, quantification is possible only if the plasma input function is available.

The present study describes a sensitive on-line detection system for monitoring trace concentrations of radioactivity within rat arterial blood. It also reports on the preliminary application of this system, in conjunction with a prototype small animal PET scanner (Bloomfield *et al.*, 1995), to the measurement of glucose metabolism (CMR_{glu}) in the rat brain.

II. MATERIALS AND METHODS

A. On-Line Detection System

The β^+ detector was composed of a rectangular block of polished NE102A scintillating plastic (5 × 5 × 38 mm) (NE Technology Ltd., United Kingdom) with a 1.6 mm diameter longitudinal hole, through which an arterial catheter (0.5 mm ID, 1.0 mm OD) was passed, giving a detectable volume of blood in the field of view of 0.00746 ml. Black polytetrafluoroethylene (PTFE) tubing was selected for the arterial catheter to protect the detector from exposure to external light and to eliminate possible ligand cohesion to the inside of the tubing. The detector was optically coupled to a matched photomultiplier tube, type 6097A (Thorn EMI, United Kingdom). The signal output was shaped, gated, and processed by standard NIM electronics and photons with energies greater than 35 keV were collected. An ALT-386SX laptop computer (Amstrad, UK) was used to record the logic pulses over 1 sec intervals.

Shielding of the detector was provided by 4 cm thick, light tight, lead rings. The detector assembly was positioned on a vertically adjustable base adjacent to the scanner bed. This permitted the detector to be positioned as close as possible to the rat, minimizing the length of tubing (35 cm) and consequently the delay and dispersion on the blood curves.

B. PET Scanning

Ten male Sprague–Dawley rats (Harlan and Olac Ltd., Bicester, United Kingdom) were used (body weights, 248–316 g). Five of the animals were allowed free access to food and water until the time of the experiment (fed) and the remaining five animals had their food withdrawn overnight (fasted).

Each rat had a polythene catheter (0.58 mm ID, 0.96 mm OD) inserted into a tail vein while under isoflurane anesthesia (mixed with oxygen and nitrous oxide). At the same time, a PTFE catheter was inserted into the tail artery for blood withdrawal. Rats were stereotaxically positioned in the camera (Myers *et al.*, 1996, Chapter 3) and a 30 min transmission scan performed, using a rotating external ^{68}Ge line source. The transmission scan was used to correct subsequent emission scans for attenuation. [^{18}F]fluorodeoxyglucose (~19 MBq) was injected iv and a dynamic scan performed over 60 min with frame lengths progressively increasing from 5 to 300 sec. Arterial blood was allowed to flow freely through the on-line detector for the first minute following tracer injection and then at intermittent predetermined time intervals throughout the study period. In addition, at set times, blood samples were collected manually. Plasma and whole blood ^{18}F radioactivities of these samples were determined in a NaI(TI) well counter, cross-calibrated with the scanner. Plasma concentrations of stable glucose were measured using a glucose analyzer, model 2300 stat plus (Yellow Springs [Ohio] Instrument Co., USA).

The blood time–radioactivity curves obtained using the on-line detector were scaled to the samples and plasma curves were generated, essentially as described previously (Lammertsma *et al.*, 1991). Scans were reconstructed using a ramp filter at Nyquist cutoff frequency, resulting in a transaxial resolution of 2.34 mm FWHM at the center of the field of view. Each image was reconstructed into a 128×128 matrix with a voxel size of $0.47 \times 0.47 \times 3.13$ mm. Analyze software (Robb and Hanson, 1991) was used to select and sample a region of interest (ROI) at the center of the brain (3×3 mm). The corresponding tissue time–radioactivity curves were fitted to both reversible and irreversible two-tissue compartment models using standard nonlinear regression techniques, including parameters for delay and blood volume. CMR_{glu} was calculated using the fitted rate constants, assuming a lumped constant of 0.58 (Lear and Ackerman, 1989).

III. RESULTS AND DISCUSSION

A. Blood Curve

A typical blood curve, as measured by the on-line detection system, is shown in Figure 1. There is good correlation between the blood curve and the separately measured discrete blood samples, indicating that the blood curve is an accurate measure of the radioactivity present within the blood over time. No attempt was made to characterize the peak of the blood curve by discrete samples. It is clear, however, that a major advantage of the on-line detection system is the accurate definition of this peak as a result of the detector's high temporal resolution.

B. Plasma Input Function

For kinetic analysis of the data, the whole blood curve is required to fit for the intravascular component (blood volume). However, the delivery to the tissue depends on the arterial plasma concentration. In contrast to [^{18}F]fluorodeoxyglucose studies in humans, in rats the plasma to whole blood ratio changes as a function of time. An example is given in Figure 2, where the open circles represent the plasma to whole blood ratio as determined from the discrete samples. Also shown (solid line) is the best (multiexponential function) fit to the data. The plasma time-radioactivity curve, obtained by multiplying the on-line blood curve with this function is shown in Figure 3. It is clear that both the shape and the height of plasma and whole blood curves are quite different. Therefore, both should be obtained for subsequent use in the kinetic analysis of tissue data.

C. Plasma Glucose Concentration

The rats with free access to food had a plasma glucose concentration of 14.9 ± 3.1 mmol/liter (mean $\pm$ SD) at the time of the experiment. Fasted rats, how-

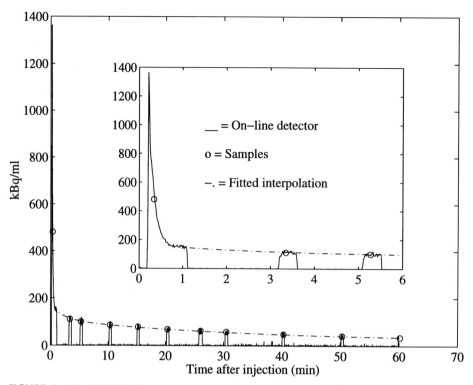

FIGURE 1 A typical blood curve, as measured by the on-line blood detector (solid line), with the dot–dashed line representing the exponential interpolation between bleeding periods. The discrete blood samples are indicated by the open circles.

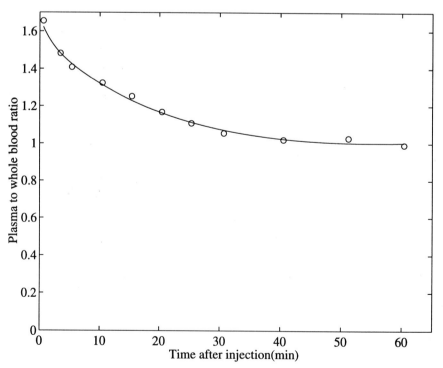

FIGURE 2 The ratio of plasma to whole blood radioactivity for each discrete sample (open circles), together with the multiexponential fit to these data (solid line).

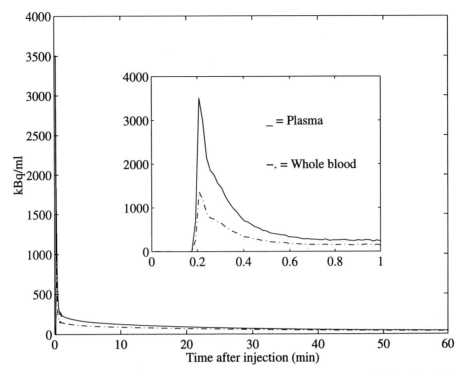

FIGURE 3   A plasma time–radioactivity curve (solid line), obtained by multiplying the whole blood curve (dot–dashed line) by the multiexponential function from Figure 2.

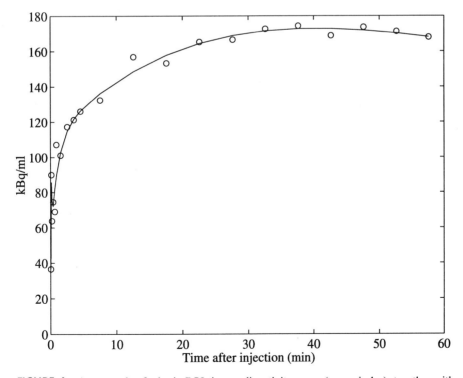

FIGURE 4   An example of a brain ROI time–radioactivity curve (open circles), together with the best fit of these data to the reversible two-tissue compartment model (solid line).

ever, had a much lower plasma glucose concentration of 7.7 ± 1.3 mmol/liter. These values correspond to those previously reported for anaesthetised rats (Ingvar *et al.*, 1980). In all of the animals, plasma glucose concentration remained stable throughout the period of the scan.

D. Mathematical Modeling

In all studies, the reversible two-tissue compartment model provided significantly better fits than the irreversible two-tissue compartment model (i.e., $k_4 = 0$), as determined by the Akaike (1974) and Schwarz (1978) criteria. An example of a brain ROI time–radioactivity curve, together with the best fit of these data to the reversible two-tissue compartment model is shown in Figure 4. As previously reported (Ingvar *et al.*, 1980), CMR_{glu} did not differ between fed and fasted animals, being 0.6 ± 0.1 and 0.7 ± 0.1 (mean ± standard deviation), respectively, consistent with previously reported values (Cremer *et al.*, 1988; Hargreaves *et al.*, 1986).

IV. CONCLUSION

Due to the high temporal resolution of the on-line blood detection system described, it is possible to accurately measure the plasma input function required for the quantification of global CMR_{glu} in the rat brain using PET.

Acknowledgments

The authors wish to thank J. Opacka-Juffry, K. Clifford, and the members of the blood lab for all their input into this work.

References

Akaike, H. (1974). A new look at the statistical model identification. *IEEE Trans. Automat. Contr.* **19:** 716–723.

Bloomfield, P. M., Rajeswaran, S., Spinks, T. J., Hume, S. P., Myers, R., Ashworth, S., Clifford, K. M., Jones, W. F., Byars, L. G., Young, J., Andreaco, M., Williams, C. W., Lammertsma, A. A., and Jones, T. (1995). The design and physical characteristics of a small animal positron emission tomograph. *Phys. Med. Biol.* **40:** 1105–1126.

Cremer, J. E., Seville, M. P., and Cunningham, V. J. (1988). Tracer 2-deoxyglucose kinetics in brain regions of rats given kainic acid. *J. Cereb. Blood Flow Metab.* **8:** 244–253.

Hargreaves, R. J., Planas, A. M., Cremer, J. E., and Cunningham, V. J. (1986). Studies on the relationship between cerebral glucose transport and phosphorylation using 2-deoxyglucose. *J. Cereb. Blood Flow Metab.* **6:** 708–716.

Hume, S. P., Myers, R., Bloomfield, P. M., Opacka-Juffry, J., Cremer, J. E., Ahier, R. G., Luthra, S. K., Brooks, D. J., and Lammertsma, A. A. (1992). Quantitation of carbon-11-labelled raclopride in rat striatum using positron emission tomography. *Synapse.* **12:** 47–54.

Ingvar, M., Abdul-Rahman, A., and Siesjö, B. K. (1980). Local cerebral glucose consumption in the artificially ventilated rat: Influence of nitrous oxide analgesia and of phenobarbital anaesthesia. *Acta Physiol. Scand.* **109:** 177–185.

Lammertsma, A. A., Bench, C. J., Price, G. W., Cremer, J. E., Luthra, S. K., Turton, D., Wood, N. D., and Frackowiak, R. S. J. (1991). Measurement of cerebral monoamine oxidase B activity using L-[^{11}C]deprenyl and dynamic positron emission tomography. *J. Cereb. Blood Flow Metab.* **11:** 545–556.

Lear, J. L., and Ackerman, R. F. (1989). Regional comparison of the lumped constants of deoxyglucose and fluorodeoxyglucose. *Metab. Brain Dis.* **4:** 95–104.

Myers, R., Hume, S. P., Ashworth, S., Lammertsma, A. A., Bloomfield, P. M., Rajeswaran, S., and Jones, T. (1996). Quantification of dopamine receptors and transporter in rat striatum using a small animal PET scanner. *In*: "Quantification of Brain Function in PET" (R. Myers, V. Cunningham, D. Bailey, and T. Jones, Eds.). Academic Press, San Diego. (This volume.)

Robb, R. A., and Hanson, D. P. (1991). A software system for interactive and quantitative visualisation of multidimensional biomedical images. *Austral. Phys. Eng. Sci. Med.* **14:** 9–30.

Schwarz, G. (1978). Estimating the dimension of a model. *Ann. Statist.* **6:** 461–564.

14

Noninvasive Determination of Arterial Input of ^{15}O Tracers, Using a Dual Cutaneous β-Detector Set above the Radial Artery

M. ITOH,[1] H. WATABE,[2] M. MIYAKE,[2] S. HAGISAWA,[1] T. FUJIWARA,[1] R. IWATA,[3] T. IDO,[3] and T. NAKAMURA[2]

[1]*Division of Nuclear Medicine*
[2]*Division of Radioprotection*
[3]*Division of Radiopharmaceutical Chemistry*
Cyclotron Radioisotope Center, Tohoku University
Sendai, 980-77, Japan

As the clinical use of PET technology grows, so does the demand for noninvasive measurement of cerebral blood flow (CBF). We have developed a compact radiation monitor composed of dual β-detectors suitable for detection of radiation from superficial tissue. One detector was placed over the wrist above the radial artery to monitor arterial radioactivity while another was placed on an adjacent skin area to measure the background. The monitor worked fairly well except on obese subjects, for whom an arterial count curve was not recoverable. We developed a model to restore the arterial input function comparing the two-detector response with time that incorporated the superficial tissue flow, mainly of skin and the subcutaneous tissue. Twenty-four studies on five normal volunteers were conducted with [^{15}O]-water slow bolus injections, which were controlled by an automatic injection system. A significant correlation was obtained between the calculated CBF using restored input function by our system and the CBF using an actual arterial input curve by arterial cannulation. Further refinement of the procedures that include the calibration of restored arterial input to well counter and accurate correction of dispersion in the restored arterial input may increase the accuracy of this noninvasive method.

I. INTRODUCTION

^{15}O-labeled radiotracers are commonly used in positron tomography. Regional cerebral blood flow is accurately measured with injections of [^{15}O]-water. However, quantitative determination of CBF requires arterial cannulation to get an input function. This can be a burden to both patients and physicians. We developed a γ-ray miniature probe for tumor localization using a 9 mm $\varnothing$ BGO crystal and photomultiplier (Watabe et al., 1993). For recording noninvasive arterial radioactivity counting, we proposed a dual counting system attachable over the wrist capable of subtracting background radiation (Fares et al., 1993). Configurations of the counting system, model solutions and clinical results are presented.

II. SYSTEM CONFIGURATION AND THEORY

Two thin plastic scintillators (8 mm × 20 mm × 1 mm each) were mounted on a dual-photomultiplier tube (PMT, Hamamatsu R1548, Japan). The detection window was covered with thin aluminum foil to allow maximum β-ray penetration. The energy window was adjusted above the 511 keV γ-ray peak with an open upper threshold to reject annihilation γ-rays. The PMT output was amplified and stored in a memory (NAIG, Japan) that was connected to a DOS computer (PC9801VX, NEC, Japan). These detectors monitor radioactivity in the skin. The system configurations and outlook of a detector are shown in Figures 1 and 2.

This method requires a comparison of three different time–activity curves; that is, a standard or group averaged arterial input collected by invasive monitoring,

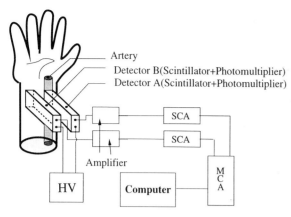

FIGURE 1   System configurations: The system is composed of a pair of plastic scintillators mounted on a photomultiplier tube. The energy window was adjusted above 511 keV by single channel analyzers to reject annihilation γ rays. MCA memory serves as a data storage. The detector was positioned over a wrist with one detector just over the radial artery and the other over the tissue next to it.

$Ca'(t)$, and cutaneous β count profiles, one obtained over radial artery and the other from the adjoining skin (Fig. 3). Cutaneous β activity is composed of the arterial component and the tissue component. If the former is negligible in the skin radioactivity curve, $f_2(t)$, it may be explained on the assumption that tissue constitutes a single compartment as follows:

$$f_2(t) = C_f \cdot f \cdot Ca(t) \otimes \exp[-(f + \lambda)t] \qquad (1)$$

where $Ca(t)$ is a real arterial input; f and λ are tissue blood flow and physical decay of ^{15}O, respectively; C_f

is the calibration factor that relates to the efficiency of the detector and effective volume of the detection; and $\otimes$ denotes the operation of convolution. Since cutaneous monitoring over the radial artery records radioactivity of artery and the interstitium, its response, $f_1(t)$, may be expressed as follows:

$$f_1(t) = C_f\{\alpha \cdot \Phi \cdot Ca(t) + (1 - \Phi) \cdot f \cdot Ca(t) \qquad (2)$$
$$\otimes \exp[-(f + \lambda)t]\}$$

where α and Φ correspond to the count recovery of blood count relative to the skin and the fraction of blood volume in the effective volume of the detection, respectively. We assume the two detectors are already calibrated to a standard β source and have the same sensitivity. The unknowns of C_f and f may be determined by a least-squares approach in equation (1) using $Ca'(t)$, instead of the true input function.

Inserting equation (1) into equation (2), we get

$$f_1(t) = C_f \cdot \alpha \cdot \Phi \cdot Ca'(t) + (1 - \Phi) \cdot f_2(t) \qquad (3)$$

Equation (3) is simplified by substituting $C_f \cdot \alpha \cdot \Phi$ with A and $1 - \Phi$ with B:

$$f_1(t) = A \cdot Ca'(t) + B \cdot f_2(t) \qquad (4)$$

The least-squares estimation for equation (4) may give values for A and B, and finally the individual arterial input function scaled by $Ca'(t)$ may be restored as follows:

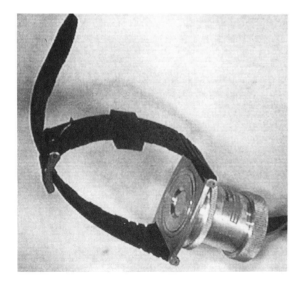

FIGURE 2   Outlook of a newly designed detector: The detector is so compact that it is fixed over the wrist using a watchband.

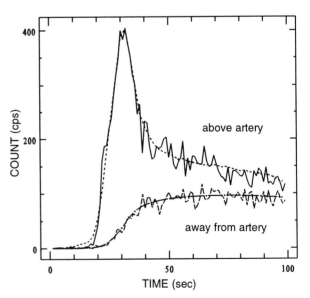

FIGURE 3   Response profiles of β-detectors attached to the wrist: The upper and lower curves were obtained from the detectors above the radial artery and over adjoining skin, respectively. The dotted lines depict the fitting results using equations (1) and (4) for a standard input function.

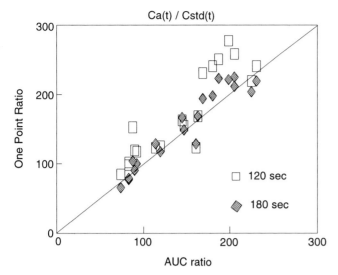

FIGURE 4 Plots of height ratio between arterial input functions by arterial invasive monitoring ($Ca(t)$) and a standard input function (Cstd(t)) for β detector calibration. The area under the curve ratio (abscissa) was more accurately predicted by a one-point blood sampling at 180 sec ($\diamond$) than 120 sec ($\square$) after injection. These one-point calibration factors were used as the factor C in equation (5) to restore arterial input functions calibrated to the well counter. The diagonal line indicates the line of identity.

$$Ca(t) \approx C\{f_1(t) - B \cdot f_2(t)\}/A \qquad (5)$$

where C is a scaling factor that relates the standard input function to the well counter count rates. This was determined by taking one blood sample (arterial count was used in this study) at the end of each experiment. We found that the sampling point at 180 sec after injection was superior to readings at 120 sec (Fig. 4).

III. SUBJECTS AND METHODS

Twenty-four studies were carried out with five young male volunteers aged 21–32 years, of which three runs were discarded because of failure in data recording. Arterial blood radioactivity was directly monitored by arterial cannulation into the cubital artery of the opposite arm. An arterial β detector with a 50 mm thick lead shield counted radioactivity in the cannula through which blood was withdrawn at speed of 4.0 ml/min by using a mechanical pump (Nakagawa Seikodo, Japan). A standard input function was generated by averaging these arterial data after normalization by the area under the curve and time–shift adjustment by using the cross-correlation peak. Positron emission tomography was carried out with about 1100 MBq of [^{15}O]-water injected in 20 sec by an autoinjector (Anzai Medical, Japan) followed by 10 ml of saline flush at

the same speed. Cerebral blood flow was calculated according to Lammertsma et al. (1989) with delay and dispersion correction according to Iida et al. (1986).

IV. RESULTS AND DISCUSSION

A phantom experiment using a water-filled acrylic box and 2.7 kBq ^{22}Na point source revealed that the β component could be detected over the surface up to 7 mm, which is close to the maximum range of ^{15}O of 9 mm. One example of collected β count curves of a clinical case is shown in Figure 3. The detector over the radial artery recorded a sharper rise in the count in the early phase of the experiment. Subtraction between these two curves, according to equation (5), restored arterial input function successfully (Fig. 5), which was very close to the actual arterial curve recorded through an arterial draining line. The higher peak and faster down slope in the restored input function compared to the actual arterial curve (without dispersion correction) suggested less dispersion. However, in our calculation of CBF, the difference in dispersion rate was ignored and fixed at 0.1 sec^{-1}, the value for the dispersion correction of arterial curves currently used in our laboratory.

Equation (1) gives estimates of skin blood flow using a cutaneous β detector. It was 0.42 ± 0.24 ml/g/min, slightly increasing in the course of the study (Fig. 6). This flow value for the skin seems reasonable when we consider its physiological role as heat and moisture regulator and being at the high level of cellular prolifer-

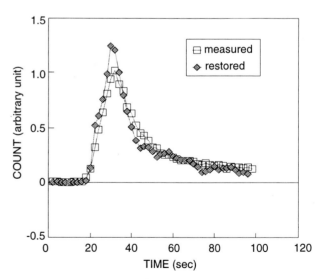

FIGURE 5 Restored arterial input function ($\diamond$) by applying equation (5) for the β-detector data shown in Figure 3. The actual input function ($\square$) is also shown. Note that the effect of dispersion within the draining line was minimized in the restored data.

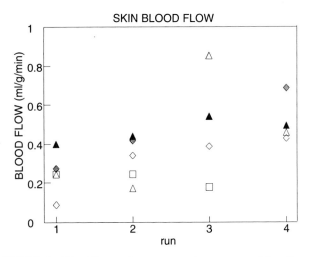

FIGURE 6   Blood flow to the cutaneous tissue measured four times at 10 min intervals by using a β-detector placed over the wrist. The markers track individual subjects.

ation. It is known that blood flow to the skin changes in relationship to the mental state. Mental tension causes constriction of arterioles and reduces blood flow to the skin. Therefore, the slight increase of blood flow to the skin that we observed during the course of the study might reflect mental relaxation. We calculated cerebral blood flow by using three different input functions: the restored input solved by equation (5), a standard input, and the real arterial input recorded by an arterial β detector. The average blood flow to the brain calculated by each method was compared in Figure 7. CBF calculated by the restored or standard input functions were significantly correlated with the values by the invasive method, with correlation coefficients of 0.66 and 0.74

for the former and the latter, respectively. When the difference in the CBF calculated by using the invasive input functions and the restored or the standard input functions were related to the corresponding averages according to Bland and Altman (1986), the noninvasive methods tended to underestimate the CBF by -10.4 ± 7.4 and -9.6 ± 6.9 (ml/100 g/min) for the restored and standard input functions, respectively. The calibration between the restored flow and well counter rate is crucial. We applied a one-point blood sampling 180 sec after injection for the calibration. Counts of restored input function at a later phase were not reliable because the subtraction between two detector response curves were carried out at a low count level. Therefore, we calibrated the one-point blood count to the standard input function. The restored input function can be correlated to the standard function through equation (5). Although the one-point calibration was validated in Figure 4, errors in the calibration directly reduces the accuracy of our method. We used arterial sampling for the calibration, and therefore, our method can still be classified as invasive. We suspect venous sampling may possibly substitute for arterial sampling when taken at very late phase of the study because the radioactivity in the body reaches an equilibrium.

In conclusion, a dual β-counting system may be applicable for a clinical CBF study as a device for noninvasive measurement of arterial input function. However, the increased distance between the radial artery and the skin surface due to, say, obesity, limits its detection. In such cases the use of a standard input function may be a choice as long as the injection of [^{15}O]-water is mechanically controlled at the same

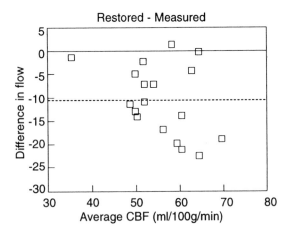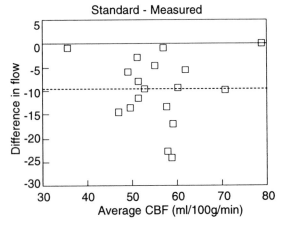

FIGURE 7   Relation between whole brain average blood flow (ml/100 g/min) calculated using the restored (left) and the standard (right) input functions. The differences in CBF between the noninvasive method and the invasive method are plotted against the corresponding averages. The dotted lines indicate the average of differences.

speed and the cardiovascular state of the subjects remains within normal range.

Acknowledgments

The authors wish to express their gratitude to Professor Y. Fares for valuable suggestions and to Professor H. Fukuda of the Department of Functional Imaging, Research Institute for Aging and Cancer; Professor H. Sasaki of the Department of Gerontology, School of Medicine, Tohoku University for supporting the study.

References

Fares, Y., Itoh, M., Watabe, H., and Ghista, D. N. (1993). 18-FDG in diabetes mellitus. *Nucl. Instrum. Phys. Res.* **B79:** 936–941.

Bland, J. M., and Altman, D. G. (1986). Statistical methods for assessing agreement between two methods of clinical measurement. *Lancet* **Feb. 8,** 307–310.

Iida, H., Kanno, I., Miura, S., *et al.* (1986). Error analysis of a quantitative cerebral blood flow measuring using $H_2^{15}O$ autoradiography and positron emission tomography, with respect to the dispersion of input function. *J. Cereb. Blood Flow Metab.* **6:** 536–545.

Lammertsma, A. A., Frackowiak, R. S. J., Hoffman, J. M., *et al.* (1989). The $C^{15}O_2$ build-up technique to measure regional cerebral blood flow and volume of distribution of water. *J. Cereb. Blood Flow Metab.* **9:** 461–470.

Watabe, H., Nakamura, T., Takahashi, H., *et al.* (1993). Development of a miniature gamma-ray endoscopic probe for tumor localization in nuclear medicine. *IEEE Trans. Nucl. Sci.* **40(2):** 88–94.

Dispersion Correction for Automatic Sampling of O-15-Labeled H₂O and Red Blood Cells

M. VAFAEE, K. MURASE, A. GJEDDE, and E. MEYER

Positron Imaging Laboratories
McConnell Brain Imaging Centre and Montreal Neurological Institute
McGill University, Montreal, Quebec, Canada H3A 2B4

*The external dispersion characteristics of an automatic blood sampling system (ABSS) were evaluated by comparing the manually sampled arterial blood curve, Ca(t), measured proximally to the ABSS, with that from the ABSS, g(t), using data from cerebral blood flow (CBF) and oxygen metabolic (CMR$_{O_2}$) studies. The tracers were H$_2^{15}$O and ^{15}O–O$_2$, respectively. Five normal volunteers were studied in each series. The two blood curves were assumed to be related to each other by an unknown dispersion function, d(t), via the convolution g(t) = Ca(t) * d(t). The dispersion function, d(t), was obtained by deconvolution of this equation using Fourier transforms. It was then fitted by a double exponential function of the form d(t) = [a/τ$_1$] exp(−t/τ$_1$) + [(1 − a)/τ$_2$] exp(−t/τ$_2$). For the CBF data (H$_2^{15}$O), a single exponential function with a dispersion time constant of τ = 5.0 ± 0.5 sec provided a satisfactory fit. For the CMR$_{O_2}$ data (^{15}O–O$_2$), a double exponential function with dispersion time constants τ$_1$ = 1.32 ± 0.06 sec and τ$_2$ = 0.82 ± 0.05 sec gave the best fit. The blood withdrawal rate was 7.5 ml/min, the external catheter length 20 cm, and its inner diameter 2.05 mm. We suggest that the difference in the external dispersion characteristics of the two tracers is related to the fact that, for H$_2^{15}$O, the label is approximately uniformly distributed between the plasma and the RBC phases of the blood whereas for ^{15}O–O$_2$, it is restricted to the RBC fraction. We, therefore, conclude that the dispersion characteristics of ABSSs must be separately evaluated for each tracer.*

I. INTRODUCTION

Quantification of physiological functions with positron emission tomography (PET) requires knowledge of the arterial radioactivity concentration. Automated blood sampling systems (ABSSs) increase the accuracy of this measurement, particularly for short-lived tracers such as oxygen-15 ($t_{1/2} \sim 2$ min), by reducing the sampling interval to a fraction of a second. They, however, require correction for tracer delay between the arterial puncture site (e.g., the radial artery) and the external radiation detector (external delay) and for the tracer bolus distortion occuring in the sampling catheter leading to the detector (external dispersion) (Vafaee *et al.*, 1993).

We have evaluated the external dispersion characteristics of an ABSS by comparing the manually sampled blood curve at the level of the radial artery, proximal to the ABSS, Ca(t), with that measured by the ABSS, g(t), for blood data obtained during CBF and CMR$_{O_2}$ studies using as tracers, respectively, H$_2^{15}$O, where the label is approximately uniformly distributed in the plasma and red blood cell (RBC) fractions, and ^{15}O–O$_2$, in which case RBCs are exclusively labeled. We characterized the distortion of the blood radioactivity curve brought about by the ABSS by means of a dispersion function that was different for each of the two tracers while, at a fixed blood withdrawal rate, a single external tracer delay was measured.

II. MATERIALS AND METHODS

The degree of distortion in the curve shape of the manually sampled arterial input function, $C_a(t)$, due to the withdrawal catheter of the ABSS is described by the convolution

$$g(t) = Ca(t) \otimes d(t) \qquad (1)$$

where $g(t)$ is the output from the ABSS and $d(t)$ is the impulse response, or dispersion function, of the ABSS (Iida et al., 1986).

Five sets of manual and automatic blood curve pairs from CBF ($H_2^{15}O$) and CMR_{O_2} ($^{15}O-O_2$) PET studies were used. The ABSS was operated at a blood withdrawal rate of 7.5 ml/min and a sampling interval of 0.5 sec. The transit time of blood between the manual sampling site and the detector of the ABSS (external delay) was measured to be 4.5 sec. All blood curves were corrected for radioactive decay. The amplitudes of the manual and automatic curve pairs were calibrated with respect to each other, and the automatic curves were shifted to the left on the time scale by the measured external delay.

The dispersion function, $d(t)$, was then obtained by deconvolution of equation (1), using Fourier transforms:

$$d(t) = F^{-1} \left[\frac{F[g(t)]}{F[Ca(t)]} \right] \qquad (2)$$

where F stands for the Fourier transform operation and F^{-1} for its inverse.

The mono-exponential model proposed by Iida et al. (1986),

$$d(t) = (1/\tau) \exp(-t/\tau) \qquad (3)$$

with a single dispersion time constant, τ, as well as its double-exponential extension (Yeung et al., 1992):

$$d(t) = [a/\tau_1] \exp(-t/\tau_1) + [(1 - a)/\tau_2] \exp(-t/\tau_2) \qquad (4)$$

with two dispersion time constants, τ_1 and τ_2, were tested to fit $d(t)$ by means of nonlinear least-squares regression.

With the dispersion time constants known from the fit and using Laplace transforms, the dispersion corrected input function could be calculated:

$$\overline{Ca}(t) = \{(\tau_1 + \tau_2)/[a(\tau_2 - \tau_1) + \tau_1]\} g(t) + \{\tau_1\tau_2/[a(\tau_2 - \tau_1) + \tau_1]\} (dg/dt) \qquad (5)$$

and compared to the manually sampled curve, $Ca(t)$. The corresponding expression for the mono-exponential model is

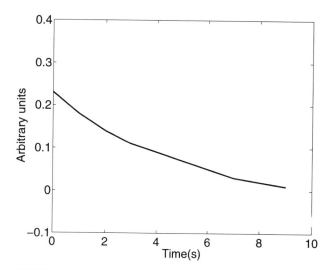

FIGURE 1   Dispersion function, $d(t)$, resulting from the deconvolution of the manual input function, $Ca(t)$, with the automatically sampled curve, $g(t)$, obtained from a CBF study using $^{15}O-H_2O$ as a tracer.

$$\overline{Ca}(t) = g(t) + \tau(dg/dt) \qquad (6)$$

The dispersion time constant, τ, of the external sampling catheter had previously been determined, using the mono-exponential model, by fitting the step response function measured by the ABSS to the expression

$$y = 1 - \exp(-t/\tau) \qquad (7)$$

A radioactive mixture of sugar and water with the same viscosity as blood had been used for that purpose.

III. RESULTS AND DISCUSSION

The results of the deconvolution of equation (1) are demonstrated with two examples shown in Figures 1 and 2 for the cases of a CBF study and a CMR_{O_2} study. Here, $d(t)$ is plotted as a function of time. For CBF studies with $^{15}O-H_2O$ as a tracer (Fig. 1), the distortion in $Ca(t)$ brought about by the ABSS may be adequately described by a mono-exponential dispersion function with a single dispersion time constant, τ. This is illustrated by the excellent match of $\overline{Ca}(t)$ and $Ca(t)$ for the corresponding CBF blood data set shown in Figure 3. The average τ from the five CBF data pairs shown in Table 1 is 4.90 ± 0.65 sec. Interestingly enough, this value is very similar to the one obtained from the step function response measurements using a sugar–water solution; namely, 5.0 ± 0.65 sec. The CBF values calculated either with $\overline{Ca}(t)$ or $Ca(t)$ did not differ by

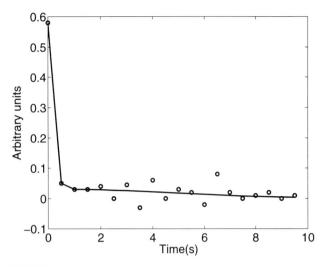

FIGURE 2   Dispersion function, $d(t)$ (circles), resulting from the deconvolution of the manual input function, $Ca(t)$, with the automatically sampled curve, $g(t)$, from a CMR_{O_2} study using $^{15}O-O_2$ as a tracer, fitted to a double-exponential model (line).

TABLE 1   External Dispersion Time Constants of ABSS for CBF ($^{15}O-H_2O$) and CMR_{O_2} ($^{15}O-O_2$) Studies

	$^{15}O-H_2O$	$^{15}O-O_2$ (RBCs)		
Study	τ [sec]	a^*	τ_1 [sec]	τ_2 [sec]
1	5.5	0.30	1.30	0.80
2	4.5	0.40	1.35	0.75
3	5.0	0.25	1.40	0.85
4	5.5	0.35	1.25	0.80
5	4.0	0.30	1.40	0.90
Mean ± SD	4.90 ± 0.65	0.33 ± 0.05	1.32 ± 0.06	0.82 ± 0.05

* Amplitude of first term in dispersion function (equation (4)).

more than 5%. Figure 2 shows the dispersion function obtained in the case of a CMR_{O_2} study with the tracer $^{15}O-O_2$. The appearance of this display suggests that a double exponential dispersion model is required here. The five pairs of dispersion time constants, τ_1, τ_2, obtained by fitting the double-exponential model of equation (4) to the CMR_{O_2} data are shown in Table 1 together

with their means as well as the weighting factor, a. Figure 4 illustrates the substantial mismatch between $\overline{Ca}(t)$ and $Ca(t)$ when the mono-exponential dispersion correction is applied to the CMR_{O_2} data. With this correction, the CMR_{O_2} values calculated either with $\overline{Ca}(t)$ or $Ca(t)$ differed by more than 20% whereas, with the double-exponential correction, they were within 5% of each other. The improved match between $\overline{Ca}(t)$ and $Ca(t)$, particularly in the peak region, when using the double-exponential model, is illustrated in Figure 5.

We attribute the observation that the dispersion characteristics of the ABSS are different for $^{15}O-H_2O$ and $^{15}O-O_2$ to the fact that the ^{15}O label is quite uni-

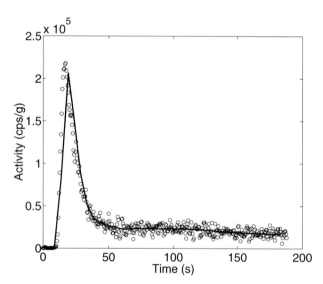

FIGURE 3   Comparison of a decay, delay, and dispersion corrected automatic blood curve (circles) with the corresponding manual one (line) from a CBF study using $^{15}O-H_2O$ as a tracer. A single dispersion time constant of $\tau = 5.0$ sec was sufficient to correct the automatic curve.

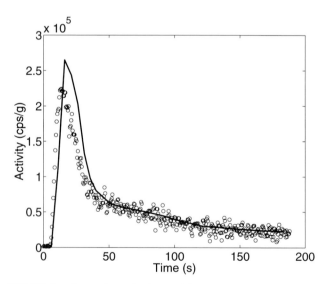

FIGURE 4   Comparison of a decay, delay, and dispersion corrected automatic blood curve (circles) with the corresponding manual one (line) from a CMR_{O_2} study using $^{15}O-O_2$ as a tracer. Note that a single dispersion time constant of $\tau = 5.0$ sec was not sufficient to provide a satisfactory match between the peak regions of the two curves.

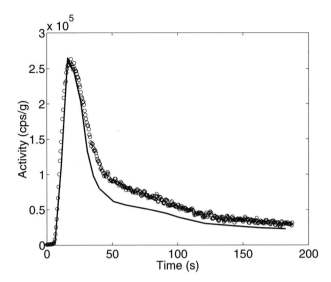

FIGURE 5 Comparison of a decay, delay, and dispersion corrected automatic blood curve (circles) with the corresponding manual one (line) from the same CMR_{O_2} study as in Figure 4, but using two dispersion time constants, $\tau_1 = 1.3$ sec and $\tau_2 = 0.8$ sec, which allowed us to properly match the peak regions of the two curves.

formly distributed in the plasma and RBC phases in the case of $^{15}O-H_2O$ but $^{15}O-O_2$ is labeling RBCs exclusively, due to the high affinity of molecular oxygen for hemoglobin. It is known that plasma and RBCs have different flow characteristics, with RBCs having a tendency to accumulate in the center of the vessels. Furthermore, a certain fraction of the RBCs might be slowed down by sticking to the walls of the sampling catheter, although the hematocrits measured at the manual arterial sampling site and at the distal end of the ABSS did not differ significantly.

Whichever phenomenon is responsible for our observation, the important conclusion to be drawn from this study is that, to avoid significant quantification errors in the analysis of PET studies, the external delay and dispersion characteristics of automated blood sampling systems have to be evaluated individually for each tracer rather than derived from tests with uniformly labeled radioactive solutions. If this is not possible for practical reasons, effects related to the proportioning of the label between the plasma and red blood cell fractions have to be carefully examined.

Acknowledgments

This work was supported by MRC (Canada) grant SP-30 and the Isaac Walton Killam Fellowship Fund of the Montreal Neurological Institute.

References

Vafaee, M., Meyer, E., and Gjedde, A. (1993). O-15 water and O-15 labeled red blood cells require separate external dispersion corrections. *J. Nucl. Med.* **34:** 51P.

Iida, H., Kanno, I., Miura, S., Murakami, M., Takahashi, K., and Uemura, K. (1986). Error analysis of a quantitative cerebral blood flow measurement using O-15 H₂O autoradiography and positron emission tomography, with respect to the dispersion of the input function. *J. Cerebr. Blood Flow Metab.* **6:** 536–545.

Yeung, W. T., Lee, T.-L., Del Maestro, R. F., Kozak, R., Bennett, J. D., and Brown, T. (1992). An adsorptiometry method for the determination of arterial blood concentration of injected iodinated contrast agent. *Phys. Med. Biol.* **37:** 1741–1758.

16

Scatter Correction for Brain Receptor Quantitation in 3D PET

D. W. TOWNSEND, J. C. PRICE, B. J. LOPRESTI, M. A. MINTUN, P. E. KINAHAN, F. JADALI, D. SASHIN, N. R. SIMPSON, and C. A. MATHIS

PET Facility, Department of Radiology
University of Pittsburgh Medical Center
Pittsburgh, Pennsylvania 15213

The recent development of 3D PET has shown that, after correcting for a threefold increase in scatter, the sensitivity of a multiring scanner can be increased by a factor of 5 when operated with septa retracted. However, the acquisition, reconstruction, and analysis of 3D data sets necessitates new approaches to detector efficiency normalization, attenuation and scatter correction, image reconstruction, and absolute quantitation. The 3D mode of operation is of particular interest in receptor ligand studies, where increased sensitivity can be used to (1) significantly reduce the injected dose, (2) increase image signal-to-noise ratio to improve reproducibility of results, or (3) follow brain kinetics of short-lived tracers over longer time periods. To date, despite these advantages, 3D PET has been little used for receptor imaging because of valid concerns about quantitative aspects of the technique. However, the growth in the number of radiolabeled ligands available to PET provides the required incentive to address such concerns. We have used the benzodiazepine receptor ligand [^{11}C]flumazenil to explore the quantitative potential of 3D PET. Data are presented for five normal subjects, each of whom was injected twice with high specific activity [^{11}C]flumazenil and imaged in 2D (septa extended) and 3D (septa retracted) on separate occasions. Based on a two-compartment fit, results show that, compared with 2D, scatter-corrected 3D estimates of ligand distribution volume are unbiased and have significantly reduced intersubject variability, particularly in brain regions with low receptor density.

I. INTRODUCTION

The retraction of septa from a multiring PET scanner allows the tomograph to be operated in 3D (volume) mode [Townsend *et al.*, 1991; Cherry *et al.*, 1991]. As a result of both the overall increase in the number of active lines of response (LORs) and the elimination of the shadowing effect of the septa, 3D acquisitions have six to eight times greater sensitivity than 2D. However, the absence of septa also results in an increase in scatter by a factor of 3 so that after scatter subtraction the net increase in sensitivity is a factor of 5. As a consequence of the cylindrical geometry of the scanner, the increase in sensitivity is spatially variant, reaching a maximum at the center of the axial field of view with an almost linear decrease toward the edges. The signal-to-noise ratio follows a similar trend.

All PET studies can, in principle, benefit from this significant increase in sensitivity. However, the accompanying increase in scatter and randoms, and the spatially variant sensitivity, raises well-founded concerns about the quantitative accuracy of 3D PET scans and emphasizes the need for careful validation. Such considerations are especially important for ligand studies, where accurate quantitation is essential; and in practice the majority of 3D PET scans performed to date have been nonquantitative, such as [^{15}O]water activation studies.

Even though it is important to ensure accurate detector efficiency normalization and correction for attenuation, the high level of scatter in 3D places particular emphasis on an effective and accurate scatter correction procedure. Recently, a number of different 3D scatter correction techniques have been proposed, and in this article we focus on two methods: the dual-energy window (DEW) approach as implemented by Grootoonk *et al.* (1992), and the convolution–subtraction method (CON) proposed by Bailey and Meikle (1994). The two techniques have been validated previously with phantom data and some comparative studies performed (Townsend *et al.*, 1994). In this chapter, we present a study with the Utah scatter phantom and investigate the performance of the two correction algorithms when applied to scatter from activity outside the field of view.

Finally, we explore the quantitative potential of 3D PET, and in particular the efficacy of the two scatter correction procedures, when applied to neuroreceptor ligand studies. We use [^{11}C]flumazenil, a ligand for imaging central benzodiazepine receptors [Mazière *et al.*, 1983; Koeppe *et al.*, 1991; Price *et al.*, 1993]. Data were acquired in both 2D (septa extended) and 3D (septa retracted) for five normal subjects, and a two-compartment fit to tissue time–activity curves was performed for 2D and 3D, with and without scatter correction. In each case, the mean and variance of the volume of distribution across the five subjects were determined for different brain regions. The variability of the 2D estimates is compared to that of the 3D estimates, with and without scatter correction.

II. MATERIALS AND METHODS

All phantom and human data were acquired on a Siemens/CTI ECAT 951R/31 whole body PET scanner, which has an axial field of view of 10.8 cm. Spatial resolution is 5–6 mm in all three spatial directions. The scatter fraction measured with a line source in the center of a 20 cm water cylinder is 12% (2D) and 41% (3D), with a lower energy threshold of 250 keV.

A. Phantom Data

The Utah phantom (Fig. 1) consists of a cylinder 20 cm in diameter and 15 cm in length, containing four compartments: (1) an annulus 15 cm long, 2 cm thick, with an outside diameter of 20 cm; (2) an inner cylinder 15 cm long and 18 cm in diameter; (3) a small cylinder 10.5 cm long and 4.5 cm diameter; and (4) a shorter cylinder 5.5 cm long and 4.5 cm diameter. A fifth cylindrical compartment, 10 cm long and 20 cm in diameter, is attached to one end of the phantom to provide out-of-field activity when required. The phantom has been

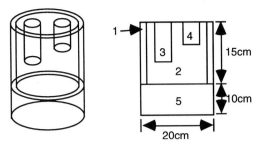

FIGURE 1 Schematic of the Utah phantom showing the five fillable chambers as described in the text.

designed to have a high degree of inhomogeneity both axially and transaxially so as to challenge the different scatter-correction methods.

We present two studies with the Utah phantom: in the first, the entire water-filled phantom contains uniform activity with the exception of the short cylinder (4), which contains only water, and chamber 5, which is empty. The fraction of scattered (mispositioned) events in the image can then be estimated from the mean value in a region of interest (ROI) placed on the short (cold) cylinder expressed as a fraction of the activity in the inner cylinder (2). In the second study, the annulus (1) contains approximately four times the activity in the inner cylinder (2) to simulate increased cortical uptake. In addition, the long cylinder (3) contains twice the background activity to simulate uptake in subcortical structures. As in the first study, cylinder 4 contains only water, and the scatter fraction is estimated as the ratio of the counts in this cold cylinder to the counts in the background cylinder (2). In both studies, data were acquired in 2D and 3D and reconstructed without scatter correction. The 3D data were also reconstructed with the DEW and CON corrections.

Finally, an important effect that can influence accurate quantitation is that of scatter from activity *outside* the field of view. In principle, the DEW method can correct for this effect because the second energy window potentially incorporates such information, whereas the convolution–subtraction approach assumes that all activity is in the field of view. To demonstrate the effect of scatter from activity outside the field of view, a small point source of low activity (to minimize randoms) was placed centrally within a 20 cm diameter cylinder containing water (no activity). The cylinder was positioned within the scanner such that it filled the entire 10 cm axial field of view. The point source was positioned on axis, 2.5 cm *outside* the scanner field of view. Data were acquired in 3D and reconstructed without scatter correction and with both the DEW and CON correction techniques. For all three conditions (no correction, DEW, and CON), a region of interest equal to the size of the phantom was placed on each reconstructed slice and the ROI average estimated and plotted as a function of slice number.

B. Human Data

Five normal subjects were injected on two separate occasions with high specific activity ^{11}C-labeled flumazenil (~260 MBq, 5.6 GBq/μmol) and imaged in 2D (septa extended) on one occasion and in 3D (septa retracted) on the other occasion. For each study, 20 dual-energy window time frames were acquired, comprising 6 frames of 20 sec, 2 of 30 sec, 2 of 90 sec, 3 of 180 sec, 1 of 300 sec, 5 of 600 sec, and finally 1 of 1200 sec. In 3D, a total of 424 MB of data were collected over the 90 min study duration. The 3D studies were reconstructed without scatter correction, and with both the DEW and CON correction techniques. To be consistent with earlier studies, the 2D data were not corrected for scatter. Both 2D and 3D data were reconstructed with the same pixel size (2.17 × 2.17 mm) and the same smoothing window and frequency cut-off. For each subject, the first 15 time frames of the 2D study were summed to form a reference image for the alignment of both the 2D and 3D image sets. The first 15 time frames of the 3D study with DEW scatter correction were summed and the 3D DEW summed image aligned to the 2D summed image. The alignment parameters were then used to align both the 3D CON images and the 3D images without scatter correction. Thus, the same ROIs could be applied to the realigned 2D and 3D data sets. To obtain absolute tissue activity concentrations, cross-calibration of the scanner with the well counter was performed, using a 20 cm diameter uniform cylinder. In each case in 3D, both the flumazenil data and the corresponding calibration cylinder were corrected for scatter using the same correction technique. The use of the same scatter correction parameters (e.g., scatter fraction) for both the brain and the cylinder may result in a slight undercorrection of the cylinder.

The plasma time–activity curves were sampled every 6 sec for the first 2 min for a total of 35 time points (in 90 min) and corrected for the presence of radiolabeled metabolites. Tissue time–activity curves were generated for regions of interest placed on the occipital cortex (OC), frontal cortex (FRT), cerebellum (CER), thalamus (THAL), and pons (PONS). Distribution volumes (K_1/k_2) were determined using a two-compartment model that accounted for blood volume (Koeppe *et al.*, 1991; Lassen *et al.*, 1995). For subse-

Table 1   Measurements with the Utah Phantom—ROI Mean Values Relative to the Activity in the Inner Cylinder (2)

Chamber	Annulus (1)	Inner cylinder (2)	Long cylinder (3)	Short cylinder (4)
Study a				
Well counter	0.99	1.0	1.03	0 (water)
2D	0.85	1	0.99	0.09
3D	0.84	1	1.01	0.21
3D (DEW)	0.92	1	0.99	0.02
3D (CON)	0.88	1	1.01	0.07
Study b				
Well counter	3.16	1.0	1.88	0 (water)
2D	2.49	1	1.65	0.14
3D	2.18	1	1.54	0.34
3D (DEW)	2.95	1	1.77	0.02
3D (CON)	2.77	1	1.72	0.10

Note. Results are shown for two activity distributions: (a) similar activity in all chambers except for the short cylinder, which contains only water; and (b) increased activity in the annulus (1) and the long cylinder (3). DEW indicates the dual-energy window approach, and CON, the convolution–subtraction method.

quent analysis, the regional distribution volumes were normalized to the pons (ROI/PONS). The mean and standard deviation of the normalized distribution volumes over the five volunteers were determined for each of the four brain regions and for each of the four conditions (2D, 3D without scatter correction, 3D DEW, and 3D CON).

III.   RESULTS AND DISCUSSION

As shown in Table 1, in the first phantom study, which corresponds to a uniform 20 cm diameter cylinder with a cylindrical cold region inside, the mispositioned scatter events represented a 9% background in 2D and 21% in 3D, as estimated from the ratio of the ROI mean in the cold cylinder (4) to the mean of the large inner cylinder (2). After scatter correction, this background was reduced to 2% (DEW) and 7% (CON), which is less than the scatter background in 2D. The second phantom study represented a more challenging situation for the scatter correction techniques. The mispositioned events fraction increased to 14% in 2D and 34% in 3D. However, both scatter correction techniques perform well in reducing the background to 10% or less. The DEW is also particularly effective at recov-

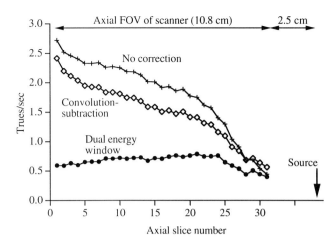

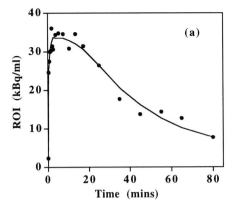

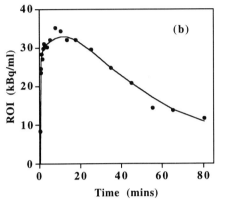

FIGURE 2 The mean count rate for an ROI placed on each of the 31 reconstructed image slices for the ECAT 951R. There is no activity in the FOV and the counts arise from scatter from a source outside the FOV, as indicated. The dual-energy window technique appears to correct for this effect.

FIGURE 3 Time–activity plots for an occipital region of interest for (a) 2D (septa extended), no scatter correction; and (b) 3D (septa retracted), scatter corrected using the DEW method. The curve fits are based on a two-compartment, two-parameter (plus blood volume) model. The residual sum of squares for the data from 14–90 mins (after normalizing the data to the peak observed value) is .023 (2D) and .007 (3D DEW).

ering the correct ratio for the annulus to background, with a value of 2.95 compared to the well counter value of 3.16; the ratio without scatter correction is 2.18.

The DEW approach also performs well in correcting for scatter from activity outside the field of view, as shown in Figure 2. The mean for an 8 cm diameter circular ROI placed centrally on each of the 31 transaxial slices was plotted as a function of axial slice number. Since there was no activity within the field of view (FOV), the mean of each ROI should ideally be 0. When no scatter correction is performed, the ROI mean increases with increasing distance from the source. A similar trend was observed after convolution–subtraction scatter correction. However, the DEW correction (lower curve) significantly reduced the effect of scatter *throughout* the axial FOV, even though the scatter originates entirely from activity outside the FOV.

The results from the phantom studies clearly demonstrate the superior performance of the DEW approach in correcting for scatter from activity both inside and outside the field of view, although a correction technique that requires a measurement from a second energy window may potentially introduce additional noise into the reconstructed image. In addition, collecting a second energy window doubles the acquisition memory and disk space requirements for the study.

An illustration of the quality of the human data obtained with [11C]flumazenil in 2D and 3D is shown in Figure 3, for one of the five volunteers. The mean of two regions of interest placed on the occipital cortex is plotted as a function of time from the start of the

scan. The curves are the result of a two-compartment, two-parameter (plus blood volume) fit to the data points. Graphs are shown for (a) 2D (septa extended), and (b) 3D (septa retracted) scatter corrected by the DEW method. The improved statistical quality of the 3D data, particularly at intermediate time points (14–90 min), is reflected in a residual sum of squares of .023 in 2D compared with .007 for 3D DEW; the residuals were determined after normalizing the data to the peak observed value. Of potentially more significance are the data for the pons, which is used as a measure of nonspecific binding in flumazenil studies. The time–activity curves for such small structures with low tracer uptake are typically noisy. As shown in Figure 4 for the same subject as in Figure 3, the 3D DEW data (Fig. 4(b)) for the pons are considerably less noisy at intermediate times than the corresponding 2D study (Fig. 4(a)). The residual sum of squares (14–90 min) for the pons is .037 (2D) and .009 (3D DEW).

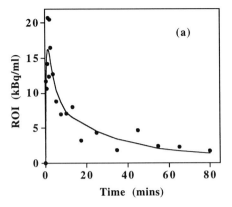

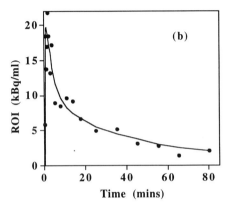

FIGURE 4 Time–activity plots for the pons for (a) 2D (septa extended), no scatter correction; and (b) 3D (septa retracted), scatter corrected using the DEW method. The curve fits are based on the two-compartment, two-parameter (plus blood volume) model. The residual sum of squares for the data from 14–90 mins (after normalizing the data to the peak observed value) is .037 (2D) and .009 (3D DEW).

The overall results obtained from the five subjects are summarized in Figure 5. The distribution volume (K_1/k_2) for each brain region is normalized to the corresponding value for the pons. The ratios for the 2D studies show a similar variability of 17–22% for all brain regions examined because in 2D the signal-to-noise ratio is fairly constant throughout the imaging field of view. In our study, the relatively large variability compared with previous studies which had a comparable number of subjects (Koeppe *et al.*, 1991) is due to the low injected activity (260 MBq). The ratios from the 3D studies reconstructed without scatter correction show a significant bias (23% lower) relative to 2D with a reduced variability of 10%—a factor of 2 less than 2D. With the exception of the thalamus, the normalized distribution volume for the 3D DEW is only 3–5% lower than the corresponding 2D estimate; the thalamus is 25% lower. The 3D DEW has a slightly reduced variability of 9% compared to 3D without scatter correction, whereas the convolution–subtraction has in-

creased variability (13.5%). The variability of the 3D DEW values was a factor of 2.4 lower than the 2D values, with only a small overall bias of 3–5%.

On average, the K_1 values from the 3D DEW data were generally higher than the average 2D values by about 9%, whereas the k_2 values were within $\pm 6\%$, across regions. For the thalamus, however, the difference in distribution volume was attributed to a 13% larger k_2 from the 3D DEW data compared with 2D; the K_1 value was only 2% smaller. The average parameters for the 3D CON data were consistently smaller than the 2D values for both K_1 and k_2 by about 15% across regions, with the greatest difference again observed for the thalamus, which had a 24% reduction in K_1 and a 10% reduction in k_2.

These results suggest that DEW is, in general, an effective method to correct for the high levels of scatter in 3D PET ligand studies. Correction for scatter from activity outside the field of view appears to be incorporated in the DEW approach. The convolution–subtraction method is also able to correct effectively for scatter from activity within the field of view but not for scatter from activity outside. However, for most brain studies, the contribution from activity outside the field of view is likely to be small, particularly for the new scanners with an axial length of 15 cm, enough to cover the whole brain. When applied to the [^{11}C]-flumazenil studies, both correction procedures effectively remove the bias introduced by scatter. In addition, the variability of the 3D estimates is a factor of 2.4 less than the corresponding estimates from the 2D studies, although for small centrally located structures with low receptor density, such as the thalamus, the reduction in variability can be up to a factor of 3.

The main difficulties with the human studies are the small number of subjects, the absence of a "gold standard" against which to compare the 3D estimates, and the normal physiological variability introduced by performing the 2D and 3D studies on different days. However, the aim of this work has been to demonstrate that 3D can provide unbiased estimates of fitted parameters with reduced variability compared to 2D. The estimates from the 2D data (uncorrected for scatter) were chosen as the "gold standard" because they represent the currently accepted values. In addition, although it is probable that part of the intrasubject variability is due to normal physiological changes, Holthoff *et al.* (1991) reported a maximum 3.5% change in normalized distribution volume for test–retest studies performed in 2D on the same day. The reduced variability of the 3D estimates is consistent with the expected improvement in the statistical quality of the 3D data.

Much work still remains before all the quantitation issues relating to 3D PET are satisfactorily resolved.

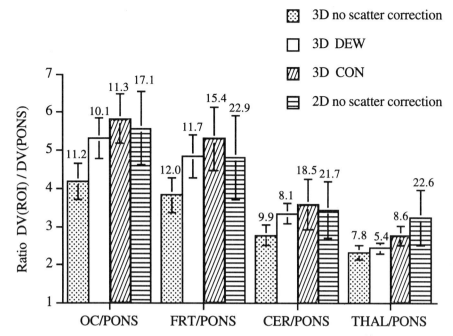

FIGURE 5 Distribution volumes normalized to the pons for the uptake of [¹¹C]-flumazenil. The mean (±1 SD) is shown for five normal subjects. The figure above each bar is the coefficient of variation over the five subjects. Data are shown for 2D, 3D without scatter correction, and 3D with both CON and DEW scatter corrections.

Nevertheless, this study has shown that effective scatter correction techniques exist that can reduce the bias due to mispositioned events to below 5% in both phantom studies and ligand studies in normal volunteers, without compromising the statistical advantages of 3D PET.

Acknowledgments

The authors thank Sylke Grootoonk (MRC Cyclotron Unit, Hammersmith Hospital) for supplying the implementation of the DEW scatter correction, and Dale Bailey (MRC Cyclotron Unit, Hammersmith Hospital) for the CON scatter correction program.

References

Bailey, D. L., and Meikle, S. R. (1994). A convolution-subtraction scatter correction method for 3D PET. *Phys. Med. Biol.* **39:** 412–424.

Cherry, S. R., Dahlbom, M., and Hoffman, E. J. (1991). Three-dimensional positron emission tomography using a conventional multislice tomograph without septa. *J. Comput. Assist. Tomogr.* **15:** 655–668.

Grootoonk, S., Spinks, T. J., Jones, T., Michel, C., and Bol, A. (1992). Correction for scatter using a dual energy window technique with a tomograph operating without septa. IEEE 1991 Medical Imaging Conference Record, 1569–1573.

Holthoff, V. A., Koeppe, R. A., Frey, K. A., Paradise, A. H., and Kuhl, D. E. (1991). Differentiation of radioligand delivery and

binding in the brain: Validation of a two-compartment model for [¹¹C]-flumazenil. *J. Cereb. Blood Flow Metab.* **11:** 745–752.

Koeppe, R. A., Holthoff, V. A., Frey, K. A., Kilbourn, M. R., and Kuhl, D. E. (1991). Compartmental analysis of [¹¹C]-flumazenil kinetics for the estimation of ligand transport rate and receptor distribution using positron emission tomography. *J. Cereb. Blood Flow Metab.* **11:** 735–744.

Lassen, N. A., Bartenstein, P. A., Lammertsma, A. A., Prevett, M. C., Turton, D. R., Luthra, S. K., Osman, S., Bloomfield, P. M., Jones, T., Patsalos, P. N., O'Connell, M. T., Duncan, J. S., Andersen J., and Vanggaard (1995). Benzodiazepine receptor quantification in vivo in humans using [¹¹C]-flumazenil and PET: Application of the steady-state principle. *J. Cereb. Blood Flow Metab.* **15:** 152–165.

Mazière, M., Prenant, C., Sastre, J., Crouzel, M., Comar, D., Hantraye, P., Kaisima, M., Guibert, B., and Naquet, R. (1983). ¹¹C-RO 15 1788 et ¹¹C-flunitrazepam, deux coordinats pour l'etude par tomographie par positons des sites de liaisons des benzodiazepines. *CR Acad. Sci. (Paris)* **296:** 871–876.

Price, J. C., Mayberg, H. S., Dannals, R. F., Wilson, A. A., Ravert, H. T., Sadzot, B., Rattner, Z., Kimball, A., Feldman, M. A., and Frost, J. J. (1993). Measurement of benzodiazepine receptor number and affinity in humans using tracer kinetic modeling, positron emission tomography, and [¹¹C]-flumazenil. *J. Cereb. Blood Flow Metab.* **13:** 656–667.

Townsend, D. W., Geissbuhler, A., Defrise, M., Hoffman, E. J., Spinks, T. J., Bailey, D. L., Gilardi, M.-C., and Jones, T. (1991). Fully three-dimensional reconstruction for a PET camera with retractable septa. *IEEE Trans. Med. Imaging* **MI-10:** 505–512.

Townsend, D. W., Choi, Y., Sashin, D., Mintun, M. A., Grootoonk, S., and Bailey, D. L. (1994). An investigation of practical scatter correction techniques for 3D PET. *J. Nucl. Med. Suppl.* **35(5):** 50P.

17

Implementation of 3D Acquisition, Reconstruction, and Analysis of Dynamic [^{18}F]Fluorodopa Studies

JAMES S. RAKSHI,[1] DALE L. BAILEY,[1] PAUL K. MORRISH,[1] and DAVID J. BROOKS[1,2]

[1]MRC Cyclotron Unit, Hammersmith Hospital
London W12 ONN, United Kingdom
[2]Institute of Neurology, Queen Square
London, United Kingdom

The aim of this study was to implement quantitative 3D PET [^{18}F]fluorodopa studies, and compare the results with our previous protocol using 2D PET. The approach has been validated using phantom studies. The data are corrected for scatter with a convolution-subtraction method prior to reconstruction, and the blood data and reconstructed images are calibrated in $kBq \cdot ml^{-1}$. Eight normal subjects were scanned in 3D and eight different normals scanned in 2D. All scans were analyzed using standard regions of interest and the multiple time graphical analysis method, with occipital reference tissue as the input function to determine the striatal influx rate constant (K_i^o). The mean K_i^o values of the putamen and the caudate in the 3D group were 0.017 ± 0.002 min^{-1} and 0.016 ± 0.002 min^{-1}, respectively, as compared to the 2D group of 0.012 ± 0.003 min^{-1} and 0.013 ± 0.003 min^{-1}, respectively. The average coefficient of variation in the K_i^o estimates for the putamen and caudate were 12.7% and 11.7% for 3D and 24.8% and 25.0% for 2D, respectively. Three normal subjects were scanned twice in 3D to assess reproducibility. The mean K_i^o difference, that is, the mean difference in the K_i^o values, between the first and second scans in the same normal subject was 4.8% (range 2.5–7.5%) for putamen and 8.8% (range 8–10.5%) for the caudate. We attribute the differences in K_i^o values between the two groups to the greater sensitivity and higher resolution (and hence lower partial volume effect) of the 3D scanner. Implementation and quantification of 3D [^{18}F]fluorodopa PET demonstrates improved precision and reproducibility in the assessment of the functional integrity of the presynaptic dopaminergic system.

I. INTRODUCTION

In positron emission tomography (PET), 3D scanning has a great sensitivity advantage over 2D acquisitions. Initial measurements of the potential data improvement with the use of 3D acquisition and reconstruction techniques appeared in the literature approximately five years ago (Bailey *et al.*, 1991a; Cherry *et al.*, 1991). These techniques were rapidly applied to nonquantitative studies of cerebral blood flow using H$_2$^{15}O with the aim of improving the signal-to-noise ratio in the data to detect focal activations (Bailey *et al.*, 1993; Cherry *et al.*, 1993; Silbersweig *et al.*, 1993; Watson *et al.*, 1993). However, reports of quantitative 3D scanning have been slow to appear as corrections for scatter, attenuation, and detector normalization and calibration required further development. In addition, logistical issues such as data set size and reconstruction times have hindered the introduction of 3D methods more widely. We have implemented quantitative 3D [^{18}F]fluorodopa studies on an ECAT 953B neuroscanner (CTI/Siemens, Knoxville, Tennessee) and compared the results with 2D [^{18}F]fluorodopa studies acquired with our previous generation whole body PET scanner, an ECAT 931–08/12 (CTI, Knoxville, Tennessee). The aim of

---

this chapter is to present the methods that have been implemented, the results obtained, and to compare the 3D data with that obtained with our previous 2D protocol.

II. METHODS

A. Data Acquisition and Reconstruction

The 3D data sets were acquired on an ECAT 953B, the performance characteristics of which have been documented previously (Bailey, 1992; Spinks *et al.*, 1992). The energy window used in all studies was 380–850 keV. Reconstruction was done by using a 3D filtered back-projection/reprojection algorithm (Kinahan and Rogers, 1989; Townsend *et al.*, 1989). The filter used for the initial 2D estimates was a ramp filter with a cut-off at the Nyquist frequency, and the generalized Colsher filter (Colsher, 1980) was used in the 3D back projection with a rectangular window cutoff at the Nyquist frequency. With these parameters, the reconstructed resolution is approximately isotropic within the head with an average resolution of 6 mm full-width at half-maximum (FWHM) or better. Prior to reconstruction the data were corrected for scattered photons by an iterative convolution–subtraction method (Bailey and Meikle, 1994) with a scatter fraction of 0.32 and a mono-exponential scatter function of $0.084\ cm^{-1}$. The data were calibrated in units of activity per unit volume by multiplication with a "reconstructed count rate in air" conversion factor, determined using a method previously described for measuring the absolute sensitivity of a tomograph (Bailey *et al.*, 1991b), but where the factor is derived from reconstructed images with identical zoom, windowing, and so forth as the patient studies. The calibration factor has units of $counts \cdot sec^{-1} \cdot kBq^{-1}$ and so, when the reconstructed images ($counts \cdot sec^{-1} \cdot pixel^{-1}$) are divided by this factor they have units of $kBq \cdot pixel^{-1}$.

The 2D data that have been used for the comparisons were acquired on the ECAT 931 tomograph. The 2D data sets were reconstructed with a standard filtered back projection algorithm with a ramp filter and Hann window cutoff at 0.5 of the Nyquist frequency. This results in reconstructed resolution of ~8–9 mm FWHM transaxially and ~7–8 mm FWHM axially (Spinks *et al.*, 1988). The absolute sensitivities in air of the two tomographs are $32.3\ kcps \cdot MBq^{-1}$ for the 953B in 3D and $3.9\ kcps \cdot MBq^{-1}$ for the 931 in 2D (Bailey *et al.*, 1991b). The scatter fraction for the 953B is 0.32 (380–850 keV energy window), and for the 931 it is 0.15 (250–850 keV). The 2D data were not scatter corrected.

All studies included on-line arterial sampling that outputs a count rate every second (Ranicar *et al.*, 1991). In addition, seven arterial samples were withdrawn for (1) calibration of the on-line arterial system by cross-calibration against a NaI(Tl) well counter, (ii) determination of plasma:whole blood [^{18}F]fluorodopa ratio, and (3) determination of radio-labeled parent and metabolites in plasma.

B. Validation

To test the accuracy of the entire process of 3D data acquisition, reconstruction, and analysis, a validation experiment to simulate a patient study was performed on the ECAT 953B. A 20 cm diameter perspex cylinder containing ^{18}F in water (concentration at start = 3.7 $kBq \cdot ml^{-1}$) was placed in the scanner, with the count rate at the start of the acquisition matched to approximately that at the peak of a patient [^{18}F]fluorodopa 3D scan (~100 kcps). Arterial tubing was connected to luer locks fitted to the top of the cylinder, and the cylinder's solution was passed through the on-line counter and back to the cylinder in a closed loop, simulating a blood input curve. Discrete samples were withdrawn at the same frequency as in a patient study and used to calibrate the on-line detector. Dynamic frames were acquired at the same sampling rates used in a patient scan. The metabolite fraction was assumed to be 0 and the plasma fraction 1. Perhaps uniquely in kinetic analyses, with the multiple time graphical analysis approach (Rutland, 1979; Gjedde, 1981; Patlak *et al.*, 1983), it is possible to analyze this simple validation experiment, where the input function's concentration is in equilibrium with the tissue response curve. The results of this experiment should yield a regression line with a slope (K_i) of 0.0 and intercept (V_o) of 1.0.

C. Normal Subjects

Sixteen normal subjects in total were scanned. Eight normal subjects were scanned in 3D mode on the ECAT 953B and eight different normal subjects were scanned in 2D mode on the ECAT 931 scanner. Three subjects were scanned twice in 3D, 4–6 weeks apart, and were given half the normally administered dose of [^{18}F]fluorodopa per scan. Another normal subject had both a 3D and 2D scan one year apart, again having half the normal dose on each occasion (i.e., approximately 80 MBq per scan).

All normal subjects had a routine neurological examination and no evidence of rest tremor, rigidity, or bradykinesia was found. None of the volunteers was taking any medication. Ethical approval for these stud-

TABLE 1   The Results from the
Validation Experiment

Input function	K_i	$V_o \pm$ COV
Reference region	0.00016	$1.006 \pm 10.5\%$
On-line sampling	0.000022	$0.966 \pm 10.3\%$

Note. The data were acquired and reconstructed in 3D. The values shown are derived from functional K_i maps via pixel-by-pixel fitting of the calibrated images, from a large single region encompassing virtually all of the phantom. In this experiment the true K_i value $= 0.0 \, \text{min}^{-1}$ and the true $V_o = 1.0 \, \text{ml.ml}^{-1}$.

ies was granted by the ethical committee of the Royal Postgraduate Medical School and written informed consent was obtained from all volunteers before each scan, after a full explanation of the procedure.

D. Scanning Protocol

All subjects (except the normal subject who had both a 3D scan and a 2D scan) received 100 mg of carbidopa and 400 mg of the catechol-O-methyltransferase (COMT) inhibitor entacapone (OR-611; Orion Pharmaceuticals, Espoo, Finland) 1 hr before the study and 50 mg of carbidopa shortly before tracer injection. A 22-gauge arterial cannula was inserted into the radial artery (after subcutaneous infiltration with bupivacaine 1%), and a venous line was inserted for tracer injection. The subjects were positioned such that the orbito–meatal line was parallel to the transaxial plane of the tomograph and head position was monitored throughout the scan. A 10 min 2D transmission scan was performed prior to tracer injection (acquired using retractable ^{68}Ga/^{68}Ge sources). The 3D subjects received approximately 80 MBq (except for two who received

~150 MBq each) and the 2D subjects received between 120 and 175 MBq of [^{18}F]fluorodopa by intravenous infusion over 30 sec.

Continuous arterial sampling was performed (Ranicar *et al.*, 1991) and discrete arterial samples were taken at 5, 10, 20, 30, 45, 60, and 90 min for calibration purposes and metabolite estimation by the alumina separation method, to calculate the plasma activity due to unmetabolized [^{18}F]fluorodopa (Boyes *et al.*, 1986).

The 3D emission scans were acquired in 25 frames (4×1 min, 3×2 min, 3×3 min, 15×5 min) and 2D scans were acquired in either 25 (same frame rates as 3D) or 31 frames, with an increased number of shorter, earlier frames in the 31 frame protocol. Total scan duration for all scans was 94 min. In the 3D method the images are reconstructed into 31 planes of slice separation 3.4 mm, and in 2D the same axial field of view is reconstructed into 15 planes of slice separation 6.4 mm.

E. Data Analysis

Analysis of data was performed on Sun Sparc workstations (Sun Microsystems, Mountain View, California) using in-house software written in IDL (Research Systems, Inc, Boulder, Colorado). Region of interest (ROI) analysis was performed using standardized regions of a 10 mm diameter circular ROI for each caudate and a 10×24 mm elliptical ROI for each putamen sample aligned to the long axis of the putamen. These regions were placed manually by visual inspection with reference to a stereotaxic atlas (Talaraich and Tournoux, 1988) on three combined planes encompassing the striatum in 3D and two combined planes in 2D, which gives approximately equivalent total axial coverage (~18 mm). Two circular regions of 32 mm diameter were defined for the tissue input function (T_o) in the

TABLE 2   The Results Comparing the Mean ($\pm$SD) of the Influx Rate Constants,
Coefficients of Variation, and Mean Right–Left Difference in Uptake Rate
Constants in Eight Normal Subjects Scanned in 3D with a Different Eight Normal
Subjects Scanned in 2D

Region of interest	Parameter	3D	2D
Putamen	Number of subjects	8	8
	K_i^o (min^{-1})	0.017 ± 0.002	0.012 ± 0.003
	COV	12.6%	25.2%
	Mean R–L K_i^o difference	3.6%	8.4%
Caudate	K_i^o (min^{-1})	0.016 ± 0.002	0.013 ± 0.003
	COV	11.9%	25.0%
	Mean R–L K_i^o difference	5.0%	17.2%

TABLE 3 The Mean Percentage Differences in K_i^o for Repeated Studies in 3D of Three Normal Subjects

| | Putamen K_i^o (min^{-1}) | | | Caudate K_i^o (min^{-1}) | | |
Subject	Scan 1	Scan 2	Mean difference	Scan 1	Scan 2	Mean difference
1	0.0175	0.0189	7.5%	0.0166	0.0175	8.0%
2	0.0191	0.0195	2.5%	0.0177	0.0181	8.0%
3	0.0169	0.0167	4.5%	0.0165	0.0186	10.5%

Note. The mean percent difference values are calculated separately for the right and left putamen and caudate, then averaged. The K_i^o values are the average of the left and right putamen and caudate, respectively, for each scan.

occipital lobes in the same planes as those used for the striatal regions and averaged. Mean counts per pixel were measured for each region of interest in the last 14 frames, corresponding to the period 25–94 min after injection, for the striatal regions, and for the entire study for the tissue input function. The [^{18}F]fluorodopa influx rate constant (K_i^o) was then calculated for caudate and putamen using the multiple time graphical analysis method. For the purposes of this study the metabolite-corrected plasma input function has not been used. All scans were analyzed by a single experienced observer.

III. RESULTS AND DISCUSSION

A. Validation Experiment

For the analysis, the data were treated in the same way as the human data and summed over three planes before the analysis. Input functions were tested from both a reference region in the phantom and from the on-line sampling of the activity concentration. The results are shown in Table 1. The values were derived from large regions drawn on K_i maps and V_o images obtained via pixel-by-pixel analysis of the combined planes. These results suggest that attenuation and scatter correction, normalization, and calibration of the various measuring devices was accurate, as well as confirming the accuracy of the software.

B. Normal Subjects

Table 2 demonstrates that the mean K_i^o values for the putamen and the caudate were found to be higher in 3D (on the ECAT 953B) than in 2D (on the ECAT 931) by 29% and 20%, respectively. In addition, the variation in K_i^o values about the mean, expressed as the average coefficient of variation (COV), were halved

for the putamen and the caudate in 3D compared to 2D, suggesting a tighter range with 3D. As a further measure of *intrasubject* precision, we compared the right and left putamen and right and left caudate K_i^o values in each normal subject, because we would expect these to be very similar in normal subjects. This showed that the mean putamen and caudate K_i^o differences between the right and left sides was less in 3D (3.6%, putamen; 5.0%, caudate) than in 2D (8.4%, putamen; 17.2%, caudate).

Figure 1 shows two different normal subjects, one scanned in 2D and the other in 3D. The figure shows plane-by-plane K_i^o maps, where the better definition in 3D is well demonstrated, even with only half the administered dose of [^{18}F]fluorodopa.

C. Reproducibility

To date, three normal subjects have been scanned twice to measure reproducibility. The differences in the average putamen and caudate K_i^o values between the two scans are shown in Table 3. The overall mean variation is 4.8% for the putamen and 8.8% for the caudate.

D. Discussion

The major advantage of 3D PET over 2D PET is the greater sensitivity, which results in better data quality. Not only does this contribute an obvious improvement in signal-to-noise ratio, but it allows higher frequency cutoff windows to be used in the reconstruction process to achieve higher resolution in the final images without significantly compromising the data. This, along with the increased intrinsic resolution as a consequence of smaller detectors in the ECAT 953B scanner, leads to a reduction in the partial volume effect and is, we believe, the major contributory factor for the higher K_i^o

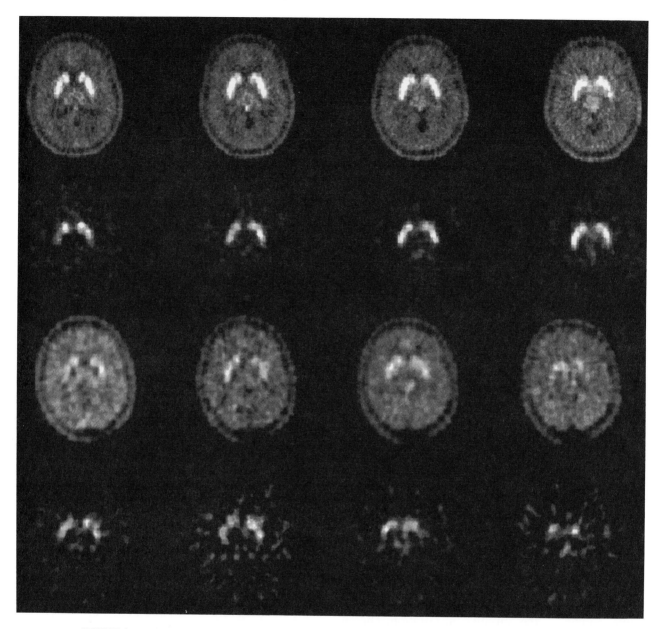

FIGURE 1   The top row shows a 3D summed image of the data from 25–90 min, which are the data used in the analysis, for reference. The next row shows the corresponding K_i^o maps from the pixel-by-pixel graphical analysis. The bottom two rows show the same for the 2D data. The 3D data differ from the 2D data in two respects: Only half the dose of [^{18}F]fluorodopa was administered as for the 2D scan, and as the plane thickness is less than in 2D, less volume was sampled per plane. The comparison on a plane-by-plane basis of 3D and 2D dopa scans reflects the improvement in image quality of the 3D data.

values in 3D. These advantages can be seen clearly in the improved image quality and better definition of striatal boundaries as well as the much lower standard errors in the *y*-estimate in the graphical analysis. The 3D method has also demonstrated excellent reproducibility on repeated measures in the same individual with a mean difference in K_i^o values between scans of 4.8% for the putamen and 8.8% for the caudate in three

normal subjects. These encouraging results using 3D in normal subjects have been achieved using typically half of the dose of [^{18}F]fluorodopa used with the subjects in 2D, and therefore the use of the usual dose of [^{18}F]fluorodopa in 3D would be expected to realize even greater improvements.

The development and quantification of 3D acquisition in [^{18}F]fluorodopa studies should permit us to more accurately follow small changes in the striatum over time, for example, monitoring progression in Parkinson's disease, more clearly discriminating between normality and early Parkinson's disease, monitoring neuroprotective therapies, and allowing closer examination of other regions of the brain of interest in dopamine synthesis and transmission. The enhanced precision and reproducibility of 3D PET has been shown to offer distinct advantages in assessing the functional integrity of the presynaptic dopaminergic system. 3D acquisition and reconstruction should result in similar improvements with other ligands, especially those labeled with the shorter lived ^{11}C, to produce data that has greater sensitivity and accuracy in assessing *in vivo* functional integrity of metabolic pathways.

Acknowledgments

The authors are grateful to their data manager, Leonard Schnorr, for preparation of the data for this study. JSR is supported by Smith Kline Beecham.

References

Bailey, D. L. (1992). 3D acquisition and reconstruction in positron emission tomography. *Ann. Nucl. Med.* **6**(3): 123–130.

Bailey, D. L., Jones, T., Spinks, T. J., Gilardi, M.-C., and Townsend, D. W. (1991a). Noise equivalent count measurements in a neuro-PET scanner with retractable septa. *IEEE Trans. Med. Imag.* **10**(3): 256–260.

Bailey, D. L., Jones, T., and Spinks, T. J. (1991b). A method for measuring the absolute sensitivity of positron emission tomographic scanners. *Eur. J. Nucl. Med.* **18**: 374–379.

Bailey, D. L., Jones, T., Watson, J. D. G., Schnorr, L., and Frackowiak, R. S. J. (1993). Activation studies in 3D PET: Evaluation of true signal gain. "Quantification of Brain Function: Tracer Kinetics and Image Analysis in Brain PET." (K. Uemera, N. Lassen, T. Jones, and I. Kanno, Eds.), pp. 341–350. Excerpta Medica, Amsterdam.

Bailey, D. L., and Meikle, S. R. (1994). A convolution-subtraction scatter correction method for 3D PET. *Phys. Med. Biol.* **39**(3): 411–424.

Boyes, B. E., Cumming, P., Martin, W. R. W., and McGeer, E. G. (1986). Determination of plasma [^{18}F]-6-fluorodopa during positron emission tomography: Elimination and metabolism in carbidopa-treated subjects. *Life Sci.* **39**: 2243–2252.

Cherry, S. R., Dahlbom, M., and Hoffman, E. J. (1991). 3D PET using a Conventional Multislice Tomograph without Septa. *J. Comput. Assist. Tomogr.* **15**: 655–668.

Cherry, S. R., Wood, R. P., Hoffman, E. J., and Mazziotta, J. C. (1993). Improved detection of focal cerebral blood flow changes using three-dimensional positron emission tomography. *J. Cereb. Blood Flow Metab.* **13**(4): 630–638.

Colsher, J. G. (1980). Fully three-dimensional positron emission tomography. *Phys. Med. Biol.* **25**: 103–115.

Gjedde, A. (1981). High- and low-affinity transport of D-glucose from blood to brain. *J. Neurochem.* **36**: 1463–1471.

Kinahan, P. E., and Rogers, J. G. (1989). Analytic 3-D image reconstruction using all detected events. *IEEE Trans. Nucl. Sci.* **NS-36**: 964–968.

Patlak, C. S., Blasberg, R. G., and Fenstermacher, J. D. (1983). Graphical evaluation of blood-to-brain transfer constants from multiple-time uptake data. *J. Cereb. Blood Flow Metab.* **3**(1): 1–7.

Ranicar, A. S. O., Williams, C. W., Schnorr, L., et al. (1991). The on-line monitoring of continuously withdrawn arterial blood during PET studies using a single BGO/photomultiplier assembly and non-stick tubing. *Med. Prog. Technol.* **17**: 259–264.

Rutland, M. D. (1979). A single injection technique for subtraction of blood background in ^{131}I-hippuran renograms. *Br. J. Radiol.* **52**: 134–137.

Silbersweig, D. A., Stern, E., Frith, C. D., et al. (1993). Detection of thirty-second cognitive activations in single subjects with positron emission tomography: A new low-dose H$_2$^{15}O regional cerebral blood flow three-dimensional imaging technique. *J. Cereb. Blood Flow Metab.* **13**(4): 617–629.

Spinks, T. J., Jones, T., Bailey, D. L., et al. (1992). Physical performance of a positron tomograph for brain imaging with retractable septa. *Phys. Med. Biol.* **37**(8): 1637–1655.

Spinks, T. J., Jones, T., Gilardi, M. C., and Heather, J. D. (1988). Physical performance of the latest generation of commercial positron scanners. *IEEE Trans. Nucl. Sci.* **35**(1): 721–725.

Talaraich, J., and Tournoux, P. (1988). "Co-Planar Stereotactic Atlas of the Human Brain: 3-Dimensional Proportional System: An Approach to Cerebral Imaging." Thieme, Stuttgart.

Townsend, D. W., Spinks, T., Jones, T., et al. (1989). Three dimensional reconstruction of PET data from a multi-ring camera. *IEEE Trans. Nucl. Sci.* **36**(1): 1056–1065.

Watson, J. G. D., Myers, R., and Frackowiak, R. S. J., et al. (1993). Area V5 of the human brain: Evidence from a combined study using positron emission tomography and magnetic resonance imaging. *Cereb. Cortex* **3**(2): 79–94.

18

Quantitation of the [^{18}F]Fluorodopa Uptake in the Human Striata in 3D PET with the ETM Scatter Correction

R. TRÉBOSSEN, B. BENDRIEM, A. FONTAINE, V. FROUIN, and P. REMY

CEA, Service Hospitalier Frederic Joliot
Orsay 91406, France

The 3D acquisition mode is attractive for [^{18}F]fluoro-dopa studies because the sensitivity improvement is maximum for radioactive sources located in central planes, which is usually the case for the human striata. However, the image quantitation in that mode must be assessed, due to a nearly threefold increase in scattered coincidences. We report our first results of [^{18}F]-fluorodopa studies performed in two normal volunteers in both 2D and 3D modes. The 3D mode without scatter correction leads to an underestimation of the [^{18}F]-fluorodopa uptake in the striata when compared with the 2D mode. The ETM scatter correction helps to recover more quantitative values of the tracer uptake in the striata. This study also brings some insights on the strategy for the ROI analysis in 3D: the parameter estimation for such small structures seems to be more sensitive to the ROI type in 3D than in 2D.

I. INTRODUCTION

[^{18}F]fluorodopa studies are characterized by low statistic images due to the low amount of radioactive tracer usually injected to the patients: In our PET center such studies are currently performed using an intravenous injection of 74–222 MBq (2–6 mCi) [^{18}F]fluorodopa (Remy, 1995). The pixel noise is propagated to the estimation of the [^{18}F]fluorodopa uptake in the striata. The most common method for estimating these parameters is the Patlak graphical analysis (Patlak, 1985), which uses the ratio of tracer concentration in the striata to the concentration in a region of nonspecific binding (Remy, 1995). In this case, the parameter estimation also depends on the contrast between the

two regions. The striata are central structures in the brain that are most often axially centered in the tomograph for the data acquisition. The 3D acquisition mode is thus attractive for [^{18}F]fluorodopa studies because the sensitivity improvement is maximum for central planes (Cherry, 1991). However, the image quantitation in that acquisition mode must be assessed due to a nearly threefold increase in scattered coincidences (Cherry, 1991; Spinks, 1992). Here, we report our first results of [^{18}F]fluorodopa studies performed in two normal volunteers in both the tomographic (2D) and the volumetric (3D) acquisition modes. The quantitation of 3D acquisitions has been compared with that of 2D acquisitions. In the 3D mode, we have measured the [^{18}F]fluorodopa uptake in the striata without scatter correction and with the estimation of true method (ETM) for scatter correction (Bendriem, 1994).

II. MATERIALS AND METHODS

The study was conducted on an ECAT 953B under different statistical conditions. One subject, which we refer to as *volunteer 1*, was injected with 189 MBq (5.1 mCi) of [^{18}F]fluorodopa for the 2D examination and with 44 MBq (1.2 mCi) for the 3D scan, performed 7 weeks after the 2D one. The second normal volunteer (*volunteer 2*) was injected with 237 MBq (6.4 mCi) of [^{18}F]fluorodopa for the 2D acquisition and with 133 MBq (3.6 mCi) for the 3D scan acquired 1 week after the 2D examination. In each acquisition mode, a nine time frame dynamic scan was acquired over 90 min. In 2D, no scatter correction was applied and images were reconstructed using a ramp filter with a 0.5 cycles/

pixel cutoff frequency and a Hanning apodizing window. These parameters are routinely used.

The ETM used to correct 3D scans for scatter is based on a dual-energy window acquisition (Bendriem, 1994). Briefly, a sinogram of true unscattered coincidences is acquired in a high-energy window (e.g., 550 keV and 650 keV energy settings) in addition to the standard sinogram acquired with regular energy settings (250 keV and 650 keV). An estimate of the true unscattered counts acquired in the standard large energy window is computed from the high energy window sinogram. This estimate is subtracted from the total sinogram to produce a sinogram of scattered counts in the large window, which is then smoothed and subtracted from the sinogram acquired in the standard window.

In 3D, images were reconstructed using the filtered back projection with a reprojection algorithm (PRO-MIS from the Geneva package; Townsend, 1991). A Colsher filter and a Hamming apodizing window were used. Data were corrected for dead time, normalization, and attenuation. The normalization factors were calculated from a blank scan of the rotating rod sources acquired on the direct planes with the septa extended (Defrise, 1991). The 3D attenuation correction factors were computed from a transmission image obtained in the 2D mode with the septa extended (Townsend, 1991).

A. Data Analysis

For each subject, a MRI scan from a 0.5 T imager was used for 3D registration with the PET images obtained in 2D and in 3D modes (Mangin, 1993). Regions of interest (ROIs) were defined on the MRI and then reported on the corresponding PET images so that ROIs at the same anatomical location were used for comparison of the 2D and the 3D modes. ROIs of 10 mm diameter were defined on the striata (one on the caudate and three on the putamen) on four adjacent planes where they appear. The ROI concentrations were then averaged over these planes, thus providing an average of 4 ROIs for the caudate (left and right) and 12 ROIs for the putamen (left and right). The time–activity curves were extracted and the [^{18}F]fluorodopa uptake in the striata was determined using the Patlak analysis with the occipital activity concentration as a nonspecific input function. The occipital activity concentration was measured in 25 mm diameter ROIs defined on the same slices as the striata ROIs. This analysis is currently used for the follow-up of grafted parkinsonian patients with [^{18}F]fluorodopa (Remy, 1995). The effects of the ROI size and shape were analyzed by comparing anatomical ROIs with the small

2D acquisition mode with septa: 5.1 mCi injected, 1.5 hour images.

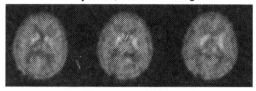

3D acquisition mode with septa:1.2 mCi injected, 1.5 hour images.

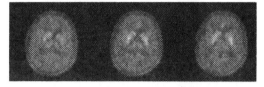

without scatter correction.

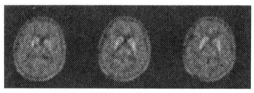

with the ETM scatter correction.

FIGURE 1   [^{18}F]fluorodopa study performed in 2D and in 3D PET for the same human volunteer.

circular ROIs. The anatomical ROIs were defined on the MRI following the edges of the caudate and the putamen on the four contiguous slices on which circular ROIs had been drawn. The same occipital ROIs were used for both anatomical and circular ROI analysis.

III. RESULTS AND DISCUSSIONS

Visual screening of the images indicates that the delineation between the caudate and the putamen is easier in the 3D acquisition mode than it is in the 2D mode (Fig. 1). It also shows a better contrast between the striata and the surrounding regions of the brain, especially the ventricles, when the ETM scatter correction is performed. It should be noted that the in-plane practical resolution measured at the center of the tomograph is more degraded in 2D than in 3D due to the apodizing windows used in the reconstruction (9 mm FWHM in 2D and 6 mm FWHM in 3D).

The values of [^{18}F]fluorodopa uptake (K_i) in the striata calculated using circular ROIs in 3D with and without the ETM correction and in 2D are presented in

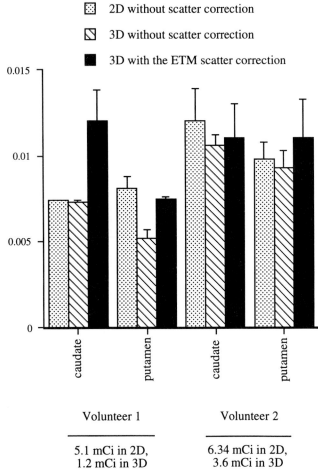

☒ 2D without scatter correction

◺ 3D without scatter correction

■ 3D with the ETM scatter correction

Volunteer 1

Volunteer 2

5.1 mCi in 2D,
1.2 mCi in 3D

6.34 mCi in 2D,
3.6 mCi in 3D

FIGURE 2   [^{18}F]fluorodopa uptake (K_i, min^{-1}) measured in 2D PET and in 3D PET for two human volunteers using circular ROIs defined on the MRI.

Figure 2. In 3D, the high number of scattered coincidences significantly reduces the contrast between the striata and the occipital leading to smaller K_i values than in 2D. For volunteer 1, the K_i value in the caudate is similar in both the 2D and the 3D modes but in the putamen, K_i is 36% lower in the 3D mode than in 2D mode. For volunteer 2, the mean difference between the 2D and the 3D modes is 12% for the caudate and 5% for the putamen.

The ETM scatter correction improves the contrast between the striata and the occipital regions, thus providing higher values of the [^{18}F]fluorodopa uptake than without scatter correction in the 3D mode (Fig. 2). For volunteer 1, the ETM correction allows us to recover most of the quantitation loss in the putamen in 3D but the uptake measured in the caudate is 1.6 times the uptake calculated from a 2D scan. For volunteer 2, in 3D with the ETM correction, K_i in the caudate is equal to 95% of the 2D value while in the putamen it is 12% higher. The higher K_i value measured in the caudate (volunteer 1) and in the putamen (volunteer 2) in 3D with the ETM correction could result from the better resolution of the 3D mode images. Such better resolution is achievable thanks to the higher sensitivity of the 3D acquisition mode. For volunteer 1, in the 3D mode, K_i in the putamen is 25% lower than in the caudate, and that difference is accentuated with the ETM. Such disparity between the caudate and the putamen, not observed in the 2D acquisition, is under investigation. It should also be noted that the present parameter comparison is based on the assumption that the physiological process of [^{18}F]fluorodopa uptake in the striata does not vary with time. The period between the 2D and the 3D scans was longer for volunteer 1 than for the other and this assumption may not be true for volunteer 1.

The quantitation loss observed in the 3D mode is more important when K_i are extracted from anatomical ROIs than when they are extracted from circular ROIs (Fig. 3, top). For both subjects, this effect is significant for the caudate (14% and 29% decrease) and the putamen (44% and 19% decrease). As the same occipital region is used for the calculation of K_i, it reflects that the radioactive concentration measured in such small structures is more sensitive to the contrast with the surrounding tissues for anatomical ROIs than for circular ROIs. Moreover, the caudate is to be affected more by partial volume effect than the putamen because that structure is located near the ventricles where there is no [^{18}F]fluorodopa fixation. A slight mispositioning of large ROIs is therefore more critical than for the putamen. The mispositioning of the ROIs on PET images could result from the 3D registration, whose precision is on the order of the MRI resolution (1 mm).

When the ETM correction is applied, nearly no differences are found with the 2D values in the putamen for both volunteers (Fig. 3, bottom). The use of anatomical ROIs reduces the differences in K_i between the 2D mode and the 3D acquisitions corrected for scatter with the ETM. Smaller K_i variations with the ROI definition were expected for the putamen than for the caudate because three circular ROIs were used for the putamen and only one for the caudate. Part of the differences between small and large ROIs could be attributed to the residual scatter component recorded in the high-energy window, not handled in the correction scheme. It could also be induced by a shift of the head position in the tomograph between both scans although a mask molded to the subject was used to restrain the head. It is well known that the radioactive concentration measurement is affected by the position of small structures inside the tomographic slice and that this effect is less

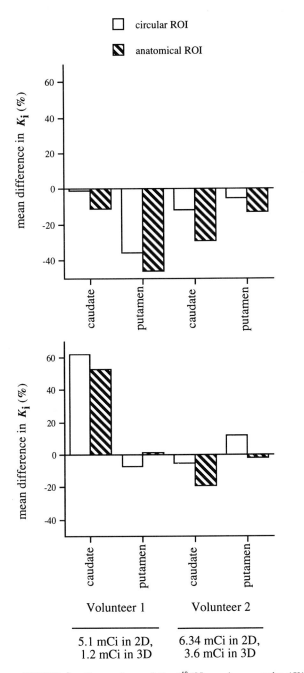

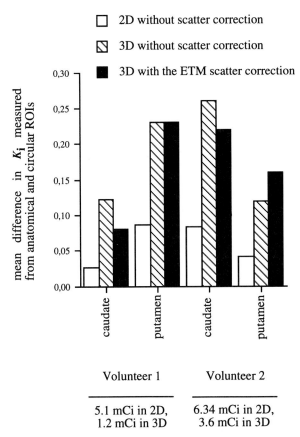

FIGURE 4   Comparison of the (^{18}F)fluorodopa uptake (K_i) extracted from anatomical ROIs and from circular ROIs in the 3D PET and in 2D PET for two human volunteers. The differences are divided by the K_i obtained with circular ROIs.

FIGURE 3   Comparison of the [^{18}F]fluorodopa uptake (K_i) measured in 3D PET and 2D PET for two human volunteers. Top: 3D mode without scatter correction; bottom: 3D mode with the ETM scatter correction.

pronounced for a large ROI (Bendriem, 1991). In 3D PET with the ETM scatter correction, we have also recently found that the recovery coefficients of spheres inserted in a cold cylinder are more sensitive to an axial shift of the spheres than in 2D.

The comparison of K_i measured using circular ROIs with K_i extracted from anatomical ROIs in 2D PET shows a higher variation with the ROI selection in the caudate than in the putamen for volunteer 1 but the reverse is observed for volunteer 2 (Fig. 4). The variations of K_i with the ROI definition are less important in 2D PET without scatter correction than they are in 3D without scatter correction. The ETM correction reduces the differences with the ROI selection in 3D but they remain higher than those noticed in 2D. The trends observed in 3D with the ETM correction are consistent with those observed in 2D for both volunteers, indicating that for such small structures the measurement of the tracer concentration is more dependent on the ROI size and shape in 3D than in 2D, which is consistent with the higher contrast observed in 3D mode.

The improvement of the K_i values measured in 2D and in 3D PET for small circular ROIs is obtained at the expense of a greater dispersion in the linear fit. The correlation coefficient of the linear fits is nearly similar in 2D and in 3D without scatter correction for these studies, indicating an improvement of the noise with regard to the injected activity. However, based on the analysis of the correlation coefficient, it appears that the ETM scatter correction increases the dispersion of the points. This might be due to the noise added by the correction scheme. Such a situation may be improved by an optimization of the filtering process in the ETM technique.

The 3D acquisition mode without scatter correction leads to an underestimation of the [^{18}F]fluorodopa uptake in the striata compared with the 2D mode. Therefore, these kinds of dynamic studies require correction for scatter to be quantitative. The ETM scatter correction helps to recover more quantitative values of the tracer uptake in the striata. Our data illustrate that, for an injected activity decreasing from 237 MBq to 133 MBq (a factor 2), the use of the 3D mode is as quantitative as the 2D mode without a significant degradation of the linear fit. Another implication of this work concerns the imaging of the striata for parkinsonian patients: The use of 3D acquisitions could compensate the decrease in contrast between the striata and the nonspecific binding region for a similar amount of radioactive tracer. This study also brings some insights on the strategy for the ROI analysis in the 3D mode.

References

Bendriem, B., Dewey, S. L., Schlyer, D. J., Wolf, A. P., and Volkow, N. D. (1991). Quantitation of the human basal ganglia with positron emission tomography: A phantom study of the effect of contrast and axial positioning. *IEEE Trans. Med. Imag.* **10:** 216–222.

Bendriem, B., and Trébossen, R. (1994). A PET scatter correction using simultaneous acquisitions with low and high lower energy thresholds. Proceedings of IEEE Medical Imaging Conference, San Franscisco, pp. 1779–1783.

Cherry, S. R., Dahlbom, M., and Hoffman, E. J. (1991). 3D PET using a conventional multislice tomograph without septa. *J. Comput. Assist. Tomogr.* **15** (4): 655–668.

Defrise, M., Townsend, D.W., Bailey, D., Geissbuhler, A., Michel, C., and Jones, T. (1991). A normalization technique for 3D PET data. *Phys. Med. Biol.* **36:** 939–952.

Mangin, J.-F., Frouin, V., Bloch, I., Bendriem, B., and Lopez-Krahe, J. (1993). Fast nonsupervised 3D registration of PET and MR images of the brain. *J. Cereb. Blood Flow Metab.* **14:** 749–762.

Patlak, C. S., and Blasberg, R. (1985). Graphical evaluation of blood-to-brain transfer constants from multiple-time uptake data. Generalizations. *J. Cereb. Blood Flow Metab.* **5:** 584–590.

Remy, P., Samson, Y., Hantraye, P., Fontaine, A., Defer, G., Mangin, J.-F., Fénelon, G., Gény, C., Ricolfi, F., Frouin, V., N'Guyen, J.-P., Jeny, R., Degos, J.-D., Peschanski, M., and Cesaro, P. (1995). Clinical correlates of [^{18}F]fluorodopa uptake in five grafted parkinsonian patients. *Ann. Neurol.* **38:** 580–588.

Spinks, T. J., Jones, T., Bailey, D. L., Townsend, D. W., Grootoonk, S., Bloomfield, P. M., Gilardi, M.-C., Casey, M. E., Sipe, B., and Reed, J. (1992). Physical performance of a positron tomograph for brain imaging with retractable septa. *Phys. Med. Biol.* **37** (8): 1637–1655.

Townsend, D., Geissbuhler, A., Defrise, M., Hoffman, E. J., Spinks, T. J., Bailey, D., Gilardi, M.-C., and Jones, T. (1991). Fully three-dimensional reconstruction for PET camera with retractable septa. *IEEE Trans. Med. Imag.* **10:** 505–512.

CHAPTER

19

3D PET Activation Studies with an $H_2^{15}O$ Bolus Injection

Count Rate Performance and Dose Optimization

S. HOLM,[1] I. LAW,[2] and O. B. PAULSON[2]

[1]Department of Nuclear Medicine
[2]Department of Neurology
Rigshospitalet, The National University Hospital, Copenhagen, Denmark

The quality of PET activation studies is limited by count rate performance of equipment and effective dose allowed to subjects. Higher radiation dose estimates for $H_2^{15}O$ have accentuated the need for optimization. We use a whole body PET scanner (Advance, General Electric) in 3D mode. For bolus water studies we collect one 90 sec frame starting 20 sec after injection. During acquisitions, true and random counts are stored in 1 sec intervals, and noise equivalent count (NEC) curves are calculated inserting estimated values for the random count fraction (0.32) and scatter (0.25). Using six normal volunteers, we studied the dependency of NEC on activity, injecting the bolus (25–1600 MBq) with the subjects in a resting condition, eyes closed and room lights dimmed. The 50–800 MBq exams were duplicated with the subjects' eyes open and the room lights on. Another four volunteers were exposed to 8 Hz flicker stimulation. Supplementary decay experiments, performed on the Capintec brain with and without added extra-FOV activity modeling the human body, clearly demonstrated effects of extra-FOV single counts on dead time and random counts, reducing both the optimal activity and the maximum NEC value by 60%. In humans, the calculated NEC vs. normalized activity after injection shows a broad maximum around the value at 800 MBq. Plotting instead NEC per MBq against MBq yields an efficiency measure. The maximal value of this measure for activity approaching 0 is about 48 kcounts/MBq. The measured data serve as guidelines in the choice of bolus size: More than 400 MBq in one bolus has only a limited positive effect on NEC; dose fractioning below 100 MBq to maximize total study NEC also provides little benefit.

I. INTRODUCTION

The quality of PET studies is ultimately determined by the number of counts that can be acquired under the limitations set by the count rate performance of the equipment and the effective dose allowed to the subjects. Recent higher radiation dose estimates for $H_2^{15}O$ (Smith et al., 1994; Brihaye et al., 1995) combined with increasingly complex activation study paradigms have only further accentuated the need for high sensitivity and optimization of the dose utilization. A major step forward in PET scanner design and use has been the introduction of full 3D acquisition and reconstruction by retraction of septa and utilization of a large angle of acceptance across detector rings (Townsend et al., 1991; Cherry et al., 1991; Spinks et al., 1992; Cherry et al., 1993), a development now becoming practical thanks to the performance and price improvements for computer hardware in general. Because the pioneering efforts were made on brain-dedicated scanners with smaller aperture and more shielding in the front, little attention has been paid to the effects of, say, body activity on the brain scans. When using commercially available 3D body scanners, the presence of often quite high activities outside, but close to, the field of view (FOV) causes a significant increase in single counts and consequently increase in dead time and random counts. In this study these effects were adressed directly in human activation studies over a wide range of doses (count rates), and a phantom model was developed that showed much better agreement with the human data than the simple brain phantom.

II. MATERIALS AND METHODS

We used an ADVANCE whole body PET scanner (General Electric Medical Systems, Milwaukee, Wisconsin), which has previously been described (DeGrado *et al.*, 1994). It has 18 detector rings with 672 elements each (in 6 × 6 blocks) and produces 35 image slices covering 15 cm axially with a 55 cm diameter transaxial field of view within the 59 cm aperture. The "3D" (septa retracted) acquisition and reconstruction is fully integrated in hardware and software and in routine use for activation studies. In our configuration of the scanner, it allows continuous sampling of 10 sec frames, up to 300 frames on a disk (9 GB), and reconstruction in absolute units with all corrections in less than 9 min per frame. During acquisition, count rates (prompts and delays) from total axial field of view (AFOV) are stored every second. From these measured values we calculate true counts (Trues = Prompts − Delays) including scatter, random counts (= Delays), and total counts = Prompts + Delays = 2 × Randoms + Trues (including scatter). The total is by design limited to 5 Mcps (well above normal use). From the estimated Trues and Randoms we further calculate the noise equivalent counts (NEC; Strother *et al.*, 1990) by the formula

$$NEC = [Trues \times (1 - SF)]^2 / (Trues + 2 \times f \times Randoms)$$

where $f = 0.32$ is the fraction of the projection covered by a brain or a brain phantom, and $SF = 0.25$ is the estimated (assumed) scatter fraction. The value of SF has a major influence on the absolute value of NEC but, because it is a factor only in the numerator, it has no implication for the shape of the NEC curve or its optimization as a function of dose. We have studied count rates during C-11 decay over 15 half-lives in the Capintec brain phantom. Recognizing the problem of predicting performance of dynamic human studies with activity outside the FOV from static phantoms inside the scanner, we also made count rate recordings during human bolus injections of O-15 labeled water as will be described. NEC during a scan was here calculated pointwise as a function of time and integrated over the scanning time. Guided by the observed human data, we made a phantom model combining the brain phantom in the scanner and an elliptical torso phantom outside the FOV with the appropriate slices of the Rando–Alderson tissue equivalent whole body phantom. The active torso contained five times the activity present in the FOV.

A. Human Studies

Two groups of young, healthy volunteers have been studied:

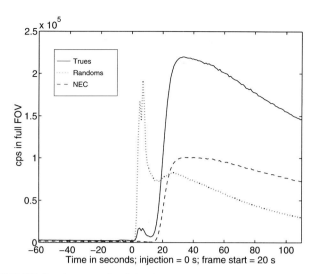

FIGURE 1   An example of the observed count rates from the scanner (summed over all detectors) following the injection of a 200 MBq bolus of $H_2^{15}O$ at $t = 0$. Scanning is performed from $t = 20$ to $t = 110$. The randoms in this graph are from the total FOV, before multiplication with the factor $f = 0.32$ in the formula for NEC.

1. Six subjects had a total of 12 injections (25–1600 MBq), ramping up the activity in steps of a factor 2. The 50–800 MBq were duplicated baseline–stimulated sequences, where the two states were with closed eyes and dimmed light versus open eyes and full light. Only count rates are shown from this experiment. Activity values were normalized to standard weight of 70 kg, but no other corrections (like heart rate, blood pressure) are considered in the data analysis.

2. Four subjects had 10 injections (50–800 MBq), ramping up and down. The stimulus was an 8 Hz flickering checkerboard during the first 60 sec after injection, and the baseline–stimulus sequence was randomized at each activity level and individual. The activation response was evaluated in gross "visual cortex ROIs," defined from the 400 MBq difference images and expressed as percentage increase relative to the rest of the brain.

III. RESULTS AND DISCUSSION

The count rates from a 200 MBq injection are shown in Figure 1. The injection was given at $t = 0$. Less than 2% background is left from the previous injection. At about $t = 5$ sec, there are peaks, mainly in random counts, that we ascribe to the bolus passing through the arm vein close to the FOV before entering the heart. At this activity level (200 MBq), the peak in Trues (actually scatter) is an order of magnitude less

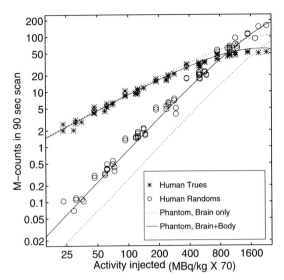

FIGURE 2 Comparison of human data (points, integrated from 90 sec scans) and phantom studies (curves, made from 10^4 points of decay study) plotted as a function of "injected" activity (see text for the details of scaling). A brain phantom alone matches the human Trues rate quite well but the corresponding Randoms rate is a factor of 4 too low. The addition of the body phantom does not change the Trues rate (including scatter) by more than 5% but makes the Randoms rate curve fit the human data considerably better, proving that extra-FOV activity is an important factor.

than the peak of the randoms. When comparing magnitudes of the early peaks to the brain counts, it should be recalled that the full bolus is traversing the arm vein, but only about 10–15% goes to the brain in the main peak that rises after approximately 20 sec.

When the human count rate data points for trues and randoms are plotted together with the phantom data (Fig. 2), it is evident that the brain phantom alone is a very poor model but the combined phantom agrees well. The randoms rate increased by a factor of 4 with the body activity present, but the additional scatter changed the trues rate by only less than 5%. The only visible change in trues is at the higher count rates, where dead time is important. The (phantom) curves shown are actually not fitted to the (human) data points. They are plotted as measured but with a shift along the activity axis to relate nominal activity injected and average activity present in the scanner from $t = 20$ to $t = 110$ sec, and a shift (simple factor of 90) along the counts axis corresponding to the 90 sec integration time in the human study. The activity shift factor was calculated as an assumed average fraction of tracer (cardiac output) going to the brain (0.13) corrected for decay from $t = 0$ (0.69) and average washout from $t = 20$ (0.70) to the midpoint ($t = 65$ sec) of the sampling period. For consistency with Figure 5, the conversion

of activity is made for the phantom data rather than the human. At very high activity levels, the agreement is imperfect. This is to be expected because the nonlinear changes during the measuring period in humans is not accounted for in the simple averaging. In Figure 3, NEC curves are displayed for the two situations. With the brain phantom alone, the max-point of the NEC curve, as found by a second-order polynomial fit, was (182 MBq, 500 kcps). In the combined model described, the max-point was (72 MBq, 190 kcps). Though presented here as only global values, the effect is not uniform over the axial direction but increases with distance from the front shield. Therefore, the values quoted should not be taken too literally as optimal.

The measured activation response for the four volunteers was fairly constant at about 25% in reconstructed activity at the five different activity doses. The values tended to spread more at the low end, and the average value dropped by 10% at the 800 MBq value. An example of the image quality as a function of dose is shown in Figure 4.

Finally, Figure 5 shows (a) the NEC as a function of injected (normalized) dose and (b) an efficiency measure, NEC per MBq injected. The maximum value of NEC integrated over a 90 sec scan following the bolus injection is located around 800 MBq. The value at this point is in all cases higher than the values at 400 MBq and 1600 MBq. The maximum is very flat, however,

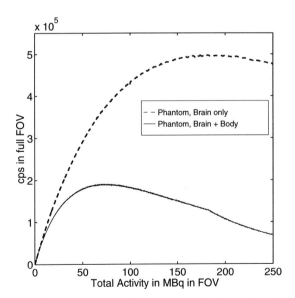

FIGURE 3 NEC curves calculated pointwise from the phantom data shown in Figure 2 (10^4 points). The abscissa in this graph, unlike those in Figures 2 and 5, is the activity actually present in the FOV. The maximum of the curve for brain phantom alone is 500 kcps at 182 MBq. With the body phantom included the result is only 190 kcps at 72 MBq.

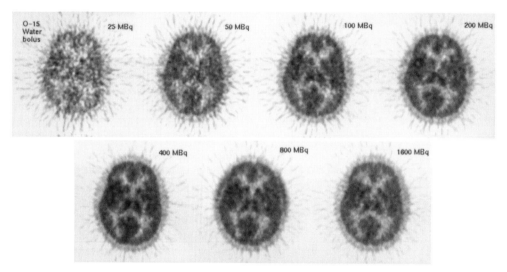

FIGURE 4   Example of image quality as a function of injected activity 25–1600 MBq for a single volunteer in a resting state.

and the activation study points to a possible (though small) reduction in signal from 400 to 800 MBq. With a shorter measuring period than 90 sec the optimum must be expected to shift against lower values because, for a given nominal dose injected the average activity in the scanner is higher. It must also be anticipated that inaccuracies in normalization and dead time corrections become more important as the count rate increases, although phantom images have been shown to maintain their quality and contrast (relative values) well beyond the saturation in total count rate. Extrapolation of effi-

ciency to zero activity gives 48 kNECs/MBq injected. At 500 MBq the value is down to 50% of that.

IV. CONCLUSION

The phantom studies with and without extra-FOV activity as well as the observed count rates during human injection have shown that the dead time and Randoms caused by extra-FOV single counts can be very

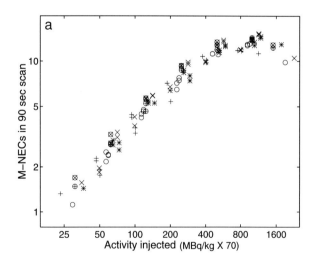

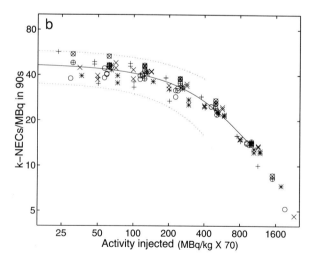

FIGURE 5   (a) Individually calculated values for NEC plotted as a function of injected activity. (b) The same data measurements as in (a) but with ordinates divided by activity to yield a measure of the efficiency by which the dose is utilized. A fit to these data points is included (with 95% confidence interval).

important in this body scanner configuration when the septa are out (3D mode). The 3D mode significantly lowers the maximum value of NEC, and the activity at which this maximum occurs. The effect certainly becomes less important when the activity has to be decreased for other reasons, such as for a large number of injections. Scatter from outside FOV is much less of a problem, although sources localized close to the scanner may still be important and difficult to correct for. A possible but not very practical solution to the problem of extra-FOV could be a removable shielding insert limiting the aperture to 25–30 cm.

For a single examination, the optimal bolus dose (the highest signal-to-noise ratio) in the ADVANCE scanner is obtained around 400 MBq, which gives an effective dose of 0.5 mSv. Fractioning of the dose can increase the total NECs acquired, but at 100 MBq, the gain of a further split (in two) is only 8% (15% by infinite fractioning). Fractioning below 100 MBq is, therefore, not recommended unless required by other considerations.

Acknowledgments

The authors thank the technical staff of the cyclotron, directed by Dr. Mikael Jensen, for the precise and timely delivery of the prescribed $H_2{}^{15}O$ doses, and the technology staffs of both the Nuclear Medicine and Neurology Departments for assisting with the human studies.

References

Brihaye, C., Depresseux, J. C., and Comar, D. (1995). Radiation dosimetry for bolus administration of oxygen-15-water. *J. Nucl. Med.* **36:** 651–656.

Cherry, S. R., Dahlbom, M., and Hoffman, E. J. (1991). 3D PET using a conventional multislice tomograph without septa. *J. Comput. Assist. Tomogr.* **15:** 655–668.

Cherry, S. R., Woods, R. P., Hoffman, E. J., and Mazziotta, J. C. (1993). Improved detection of focal cerebral blood flow changes using three-dimensional positron emission tomography. *J. Cereb. Blood Flow Metab.* **13:** 630–638.

DeGrado, T. R., Turkington, T. G., Williams, J. J., Stearns, C. W., Hoffman, J. M., and Coleman, R. E. (1994). Performance characteristics of a whole-body PET scanner. *J. Nucl. Med.* **35:** 1398–1406.

Smith, T., Tong, C., Lammertsma, A. A., *et al.* (1994). Dosimetry of intravenously administered oxygen-15 labelled water in man: A model based on experimental human data from 21 subjects. *Eur. J. Nucl. Med.* **21:** 1126–1134.

Spinks, T. J., Jones, T., Bailey, D. L., Townsend, D. W., Grootonk, S., Bloomfield, P. M., Gilardi, M.-C., Casey, M. E., Sipe, B., and Reed, J. (1992). Physical performance of a positron tomograph for brain imaging with retractable septa. *Phys. Med. Biol.* **37:** 1637–1655.

Strother, S. C., Casey, M. E., and Hoffman, E. J. (1990). Measuring PET scanner sensitivity: Relating count rates to image signal-to-noise ratios using Noise Equivalent Counts. *IEEE Trans. Nucl. Sci.* **37:** 783–788.

Townsend, D. W., Geissbuhler, A., Defrise, M., Hoffman, E. J., Spinks, T. J., Bailey, D., Gilardi, M.-C., and Jones, T. (1991). Fully three-dimensional reconstruction for a PET camera with retractable septa. *IEEE Trans. Med. Imag.* **MI-10:** 505–512.

20

Optimization of Noninvasive Activation Studies with O-15-Water and 3D PET

NORIHIRO SADATO,[1] RICHARD E. CARSON,[2] MARGARET E. DAUBE-WITHERSPOON,[2]
GREGORY CAMPBELL,[3] MARK HALLETT,[1] and PETER HERSCOVITCH[2]

[1]Human Motor Control Section, Medical Neurology Branch
[2]PET Department, Clinical Center
[3]Biometry and Field Studies Branch
National Institute of Neurological Disorders and Stroke
National Institutes of Health, Bethesda, Maryland 20892

To maximize the sensitivity of noninvasive activation studies with O-15-water and three-dimensional PET, we investigated the effects of varying the injected dose, speed of injection, and scan duration. A covert word generation task was used in four subjects with bolus injections of 92.5–1110 MBq of O-15-water. The noise equivalent count (NEC) for the whole brain peaked at an injected dose of 444—555 MBq. A 370 MBq injection gave an NEC of 92.4 ± 2.2% of the peak value. The significance of activation and the size of the activated area in Broca's area decreased as scan time increased from 60 to 120 sec. Therefore, we selected a 1 min scan using 370 MBq for bolus injections. We then performed simulation studies to evaluate the effect on signal-to-noise ratio (S/N) of longer scan duration with slow tracer infusions. Using a measured arterial input function obtained with a bolus injection, new input functions for longer duration injections were simulated. Combining noise information derived from Hoffman brain phantom studies with simulated tissue count data allowed calculation of the S/N for a given CBF change. Simulations showed an equivalent S/N for a 60 sec scan with a bolus injection and a single longer scan with a slow infusion, given the same injected dose. This permits investigators to customize scanning parameters for different activation paradigms while maintaining the S/N.

I. INTRODUCTION

In activation studies, the signal-to-noise (S/N) ratio of the quantitative CBF or tissue radioactivity measure-ment is important, because the significance of activation is measured by the increment of CBF or tissue counts divided by the standard deviation (SD) of the pixel (Kanno *et al.*, 1991). Few systematic evaluations have been made of the effects of the injection method and scan duration on the S/N of O-15-water activation studies, particularly with 3D PET, which has different noise characteristics than 2D PET. In this study, we employed human measurements and simulation studies to evaluate the effect of the injection dose, injection speed, and scan duration on the S/N of tissue activity changes due to a given CBF change.

II. MATERIALS AND METHODS

A. *In Vivo* Study

Subjects were four right-handed volunteers (three men, one woman) aged 22–65 years. Three subjects had 10 scans (5 resting and 5 task scans), performed at 10 min intervals. Varying amounts of O-15-water [92.5, 185 (× 2), 277.5 (× 2), 370 (× 2), 462.5, 555 (× 2) MBq] were injected as a bolus. To evaluate the S/N at a high dose range, one subject received 12 scans (6 resting and 6 task scans), with bolus O-15-water doses of 185, 370, 555, 740, 925, and 1110 MBq, each injected twice. The activation task consisted of a letter fluency task (Rueckert *et al.*, 1994) during which subjects were required to generate as many words as they could that began with a given letter without overtly pronouncing the words.

Dynamic scans (60 sec + 30 sec × 2) were acquired

with a GE Advance tomograph (Waukesha, Wisconsin) with the interplane septa retracted and a large axial acceptance angle. This scanner acquires 35 slices with interslice spacing of 4.25 mm. Its physical characteristics have been described by DeGrado *et al.* (1994). A 10-min transmission scan using two rotating Ge-68 sources was performed for attenuation correction. Then, 60, 90, and 120 sec images were generated from the dynamic frames. All images were aligned on a voxel-by-voxel basis using a 3D automated algorithm (AIR) (Woods *et al.*, 1992).

The following formula was used to calculate noise equivalent counts:

$$\text{NEC} = \frac{[T(1 - SF)^2}{(T + 2fR)}$$

where T equals the true counts (unscattered + scattered), R the random counts, SF the scatter fraction (0.35), and f the fraction of the field of view (FOV) subtended by the head (0.36) (Strother *et al.*, 1990). To determine the regionally specific effects of the letter fluency task, intersubject analysis was performed with statistical parametric mapping using software from the Wellcome Dept. of Cognitive Neurology, London (Friston *et al.*, 1989–1994) implemented in Matlab (Mathworks Inc. Sherborn, Massachusetts). Following realignment, all images were transformed into a standard stereotactic space (Talairach and Tournoux, 1988) with a 10 mm FWHM isotropic Gaussian kernel. The threshold was determined with three-dimensional Bonferroni-type correction to keep the false-positive rate at the defined level ($P < 0.05$) for the entire brain (Worsley *et al.*, 1992).

B. Simulation Studies

We performed simulations to evaluate the effect on S/N of longer scan durations with slow tracer infusions. The data on image noise as a function of local radioactivity were obtained by scanning a brain phantom. Then, simulations were used to predict the tissue radioactivity that would be observed with slow tracer infusions. Combining the measured phantom noise data with the predicted tissue data allowed calculation of the S/N corresponding to specified changes in rCBF.

1. Simulated Input Functions and Tissue Activity

An rCBF study performed with a bolus injection of O-15-water was used to obtain a representative arterial input function $b(t)$ and a quantitative rCBF image for use in the simulation study. The rCBF image was calculated from dynamic PET data and the arterial input function by fitting for CBF and partition coefficient (μ).

Input functions corresponding to slow infusions of T min duration, $b_T(t)$, were calculated with a decay correction:

$$b_T(t) = \frac{1}{T} \int_{t-T}^{t} b(u) \, du$$

where $b(t)$ is the decay-corrected input function obtained with a bolus injection. These functions were scaled to keep the injected dose of O-15-water constant, independent of T.

The PET tissue count value ($c_{S,T}$) for a scan duration of S min with a slow infusion of T min was then calculated:

$$c_{S,T} = \frac{1}{S} \int_{t_0}^{t_0+S} k_1[b_T(t) \exp(-\lambda t)] \otimes \exp(-k_2 t) \, dt$$
$$k_1 = F, \qquad k_2 = F/\mu + \lambda$$

where F is the regional CBF; μ, the partition coefficient (0.8); λ, the physical decay constant of O-15; t_0 the scan start time, and $\otimes$ represents the convolution operation. For each CBF value from $F = 0$ to 100 ml/(min · 100 ml) in steps of 5 ml/(min · 100 ml), the PET value $c_{S,T}$ was calculated. This lookup table $c_{S,T} = G_{S,T}(F)$ was approximated by a fourth-order polynomial equation for each value of S and T.

2. Estimation of Whole Brain Radioactivity

A histogram of rCBF for the whole brain was generated from the rCBF image data to obtain the volume of brain [$w(F_i)$, cc] in which the rCBF value was F_i. Tissue radioactivity corresponding to each rCBF value was calculated from the lookup table. Whole brain radioactivity $C_{S,T}$ (MBq) was then calculated with the following formula:

$$C_{S,T} = \Sigma \, G_{S,T}(F_i)w(F_i)$$

3. Pixel SD Evaluation

We then determined the pixel standard deviation that would be observed with different experimental conditions of flow, injection duration, and scan length. The 3D scans were performed with a Hoffman brain phantom (Hoffman *et al.*, 1990) initially filled with 370 MBq of C-11-bicarbonate solution. Consecutive scans were acquired as the activity decayed. The whole brain mean of each image was normalized to a global mean radioactivity of 37 kBq/ml. A subtraction image was generated from paired images with the closest whole brain radioactivity. The percentage coefficient of variation (%COV) of subtracted images was calculated with pooled variance across the whole brain with adjustment for acquisition time. The %COV of the difference images was taken as a measure of the average noise due to count statistics. The %COV was then plotted against averaged total radioactivity (MBq) in the phantom to obtain the relationship between whole brain radioactivity and %COV (COV(x)). The standard deviation of pixels with tissue activity c obtained by a T min scan with slow infusion of S min is then

$$SD_{S,T} = \frac{COV(C_{S,T})c}{\sqrt{T}}$$

4. Pixel S/N Corresponding to a Given Percentage Change in rCBF

The error propagation factor (EPF) from flow (F) to tissue count (c) is calculated with the lookup table $G_{S,T}(F)$:

$$EPF = (dc/c)/(dF/F)$$
$$= [dG_{S,T}(F)/dF] (F/c)$$

The fractional change of tissue activity ($\Delta c/c$) corresponding to a given fraction of change in rCBF of F ($\Delta F/F$) is

$$\frac{\Delta c}{c} = EPF \frac{\Delta F}{F}$$

when $\Delta F/F$ is small. The signal-to-noise ratio in a pixel (S/N$_{pix}$) for a change in tissue activity Δc is

$$S/N_{pix} = \Delta c/SD$$
$$= EPF \left(\frac{\Delta F}{F}\right) \left(\frac{1}{COV(C_{S,T})}\right)\sqrt{T}$$

The S/N$_{pix}$ corresponding to a 5% change in rCBF ($\Delta F/F = 0.05$) at $F = 80$ ml/(min $\cdot$ 100 ml) with various values of S and T were calculated.

III. RESULTS AND DISCUSSION

A. In Vivo Study

A linear relationship between the injected dose and whole brain radioactivity was noted. With a bolus injection and a 60 sec scan, the mean activity in the brain during the 60 sec scan (including decay) was 5.3 ± 0.6% (mean ± SD, N = 4) of the total injected dose. The NEC from human studies reached a plateau around 22.2 MBq of whole brain radioactivity, which is equivalent to a 444 MBq injection, whereas the NEC of the Hoffman brain phantom data reached its peak at 136.9 MBq in the field of view. When plotted against the injected dose, a 370 MBq injection gave an NEC of 92.4 ± 2.2% of the peak value at an injected dose of 444–555 MBq. The ratio of NEC measured in the human brain to that in the Hoffman brain phantom showed a linear decrease as whole brain radioactivity

TABLE 1 Regional Effects of Covert Word Generation in Broca's Area

Scan duration	Local maximum {x, y, z mm}	Region size	z-Score
60 sec	−38, −2, 32	76	5.93
	−46, 12, 20	7	4.67
	−46, 26, 20	14	4.55
90 sec	−36, −4, 28	34	5.20
	−46, 12, 20	21	5.01
120 sec	−48, 26, 16	7	5.24

increased ($y = 1.247 - 0.016\ x$, $r^2 = 0.917$). A main difference between the phantom and human studies is the effect of radioactivity outside of the brain in the human studies.

The ratio of NEC/whole brain radioactivity was negatively related to whole brain radioactivity ($y = 213.4 - 3.5\ x$; $r^2 = 0.94$). This finding indicates that overall multiple scans with split doses may yield better images than a single scan, given the same total injected dose. This is because dead time and random effects can be reduced with fractionated smaller doses (Cherry et al., 1993; Silbersweig et al., 1993).

Group analysis showed consistent activation in Broca's area in 60, 90, and 120 sec scans. Both the maximal z-score and extent of activation in Broca's area decreased as scan time increased (Table 1). Apparently, the benefit of the reduced noise of longer scans was canceled out by the increased nonlinear relationship between the CBF and tissue activity. Therefore, to detect changes in rCBF (or tissue activity) by a bolus method and 3D PET, we chose a 370 MBq injection with a 60 sec scan.

B. Simulation Study

With a bolus injection, peak S/N$_{pix}$ was seen with a scan duration of 1 min. For each injection duration of 1, 2, and 3 min, a scan duration (2, 3, and 3 min, respectively) produces a peak S/N$_{pix}$ equivalent to that of bolus injection. Therefore the investigator may choose the injection duration without paying a price in statistical noise. This relationship held over a wide range of injected doses (370–1,110 MBq). The slow infusion method has the advantage of averaging possible fluctuations of rCBF during the task period, as the contribution weights cover a larger time period (Iida et al., 1991). On the other hand, in the bolus injection procedure, the distribution of tissue activity is determined by the first 20 sec; hence the response may vary depending on the timing of the peak of the O-15-water input (Iida *et al.*, 1991; Hurtig *et al.*, 1994).

References

Cherry, S. R., Woods, R. P., Hoffman, E. J., and Mazziotta, J. C. (1993). Improved detection of focal cerebral blood flow changes using three-dimensional positron emission tomography. *J. Cereb. Blood Flow Metab.* **13**: 630–638.

DeGrado, T. R., Turkington, T. G., Williams, J. J., Stearn, C. W., Hoffman, J. M., and Coleman, R. E. (1994). Performance characteristics of a whole-body PET scanner. *J. Nucl. Med.* **35**: 1398–1406.

Friston, K. J., Passingham, R. E., Nutt, J. G., Heather, J. D., Sawle, G. V., and Frackowiak, R. S. J. (1989). Localisation in PET images: Direct fitting of the intercommissural (AC-PC) line. *J. Cereb. Blood Flow Metab.* **9**: 690–695.

Friston, K. J., Frith, C. D., Liddle, P. F., Dolan, R. J., Lammertsma, A. A., and Frackowiak, R. S. J. (1990). The relationship between global and local changes in PET scans. *J. Cereb. Blood Flow Metab.* **10**: 458–466.

Friston, K. J., Frith, C. D., Liddle, P. F., Frackowiak, R. S. J. (1991). Comparing functional (PET) images: The assessment of significant change. *J. Cereb. Blood Flow Metab.* **11**: 690–699.

Friston, K. J., Worsley, K. J., Frackowiak, R. S. J., Mazziotta, J. C., and Evans, A. C. (1994). Assessing the significance of focal activations using their spatial extent. *Hum. Brain Mapping* **1**: 210–220.

Hoffman, E. J., Cutler P. D., Digby W. M., and Mazziotta J. C. (1990). 3-D phantom to simulate cerebral blood flow and metabolic images for PET. *IEEE Trans. Nucl. Sci.* **37**: 616–620.

Hurtig, R., Hichwa, R., O'Leary, D., Noles Ponto, L., Narayana, S., Watkins, G., and Andreasen, N. (1994). Effects of timing and duration of cognitive activation in [15O] water PET studies. *J. Cereb. Blood Flow Metab.* **14**: 423–430.

Iida, H., Kanno, I., Miura, S. (1991). Rapid measurement of cerebral blood flow with positron emission tomography. *Ciba Foundation Symp.* **163**: 23–27.

Kanno, I., Iida H., Miura S., and Murakami, M. (1991). Optimal scan time of oxygen-15-labeled water injection method for measurement of cerebral blood flow. *J. Nucl. Med.* **32**: 1931–1934.

Rueckert, L., Appollonio, I., Grafman, J., Jezzard, P., Johnson, R. J., Le Bihan, D., and Turner, R. (1994). Magnetic resonance imaging functional activation of left frontal cortex during covert word production. *J. Neuroimaging* **4**: 67–70.

Silbersweig, D. A., Stern, E., Frith, C. D., Cahill, C., Schnorr, L., Grootoonk, S., Spinks, T., Clark, J., Frackowiak, R., and Jones, T. (1993). Detection of thirty-second cognitive activations in single subjects with positron emission tomography: A new low-dose $H_2{}^{15}O$ regional cerebral blood flow three-dimensional imaging technique. *J. Cereb. Blood Flow Metab.* **13**: 617–629.

Strother, S. C., Casey, M. E., and Hoffman, E. J. (1990). Measuring PET scanner sensitivity: Relating countrates to image signal-to-noise ratios using noise equivalent counts. *IEEE Trans. Nucl. Sci.* **37**: 783–788.

Talairach, J., and Tournoux, P. (1988). "Co-Planar Stereotactic Atlas of the Human Brain." Thieme, New York.

Woods, R. P., Cherry, S. R., and Mazziotta, J. C. (1992). Rapid automated algorithm for aligning and reslicing PET images. *J. Comput. Assist. Tomogr.* **16**: 620–633.

Worsley, K. J., Evans, A. C., Marrett, S., and Neelin, P. (1992). A three-dimensional statistical analysis for CBF activation studies in human brain. *J. Cereb. Blood Flow Metab.* **12**: 900–918.

Data Acquisition Summary

LARS ERIKSSON

Department of Clinical Neurophysiology, Karolinska Hospital/Institute, Stockholm, Sweden

The data acquisition part of positron emission tomography concerns optimization procedures to normalize data; to correct for scattered coincidences; to make accurate corrections for attenuation, dead time, and random coincidences; to solve data storage problems; and to make accurate determinations of the input function to correctly quantify dynamic PET data.

The data acquisition session contained seven oral contributions and four poster presentations. With one exception the presentations of the oral session were focused on quantitation problems of 3D PET. The exception was a presentation by S. Meikle *et al.* from the Sydney PET group (Chapter 11), concerning the methodological advantages by simultaneously measuring both transmission and emission data as a way to shorten scan duration. The results were based on phantom studies combined with simulated uptake for [^{18}F]FDG. The bias introduced by the technique was small ≤5%, but varies as a function of the count rate. The glucose metabolic rate will be underestimated relative to conventional acquisitions. A question was asked whether this technique also could be used for 3D PET, but the author answered that other attenuation techniques may be more profitable, such as the one suggested by deKemp and Nahmias using a point source and recording single counts in the attenuation measurement; that is, a more "CT"-like scheme.

Within the scientific PET community possible designs of future 3D PET systems have been discussed. With 3D PET, a large axial extension is especially important because the 3D sensitivity increases with the square of the axial extension. Within the European collaboration, an axial extension as large as 80 cm has been discussed (C. Michel, task group meeting, January 30–31, 1995, CERN), thus covering a major part of the human body. The system may be electronically sectioned into N different, independently operated parts. In this mode, the system may be seen as N simultaneously operated 3D PET cameras, N probably being a small number, $N \leq 4$. Within a selected section, a sensitivity optimization technique suggested by Dahlbom *et al.* (IEEE TNS, 1995, submitted) could be used, which automatically, on a frame-by-frame basis, selects an effective axial extension to optimize the performance in a noise equivalent count rate (NEC) sense.

The Akita group (Iida *et al.*; Chapter 12), has taken the first step in the realization of such a futuristic large axial extension system by the design and construction of the Headtome-V-Dual, having two simultaneously operated sections ($N = 2$): one with a 15 cm axial extension, and one with a 10 cm axial extension. The system is based on block detector technology and gives a spatial resolution of around 4 mm both transaxially and axially. The two sections, however, cannot be combined into one large ($N = 1$) 25 cm axial extension system. The two sections are currently used to simultaneously measure the activity distribution from both the brain and the heart. In dynamic studies, the information from the heart may provide the input function; for example, the left ventricular time–activity information. In the following discussion it was pointed out that this technique to measure the input function may be limited to blood flow studies, because in kinetic receptor studies, the metabolite corrections in plasma still requires arterial blood samples. However, other problems related to the input function, such as time delays and dispersion, are more easily solved using the left ventricular time–activity information.

The Copenhagen PET group (Holm, Law, and Paulson; Chapter 19) reported on a dose optimization study with the GE Advance system, operated in the 3D mode. The study was based on different dose administrations of $H_2{}^{15}O$ delivered with the bolus technique. The results showed that single dose administrations above 400–500 MBq provided no gain in a NEC sense, due to the increased number of random coincidences and the reduction in the true coincidence rate due to dead time limitations. It was also shown that dose fractionation below 100 MBq provides little benefit. Users of Ecat Exact HR systems have a similar experience. In the following discussion solutions to limit the random rate were discussed. One obvious way to do this is to fractionate the dose into smaller administrations. Other ways may be to use external shielding to minimize radiation from parts of the patient outside the FOV. Still another suggestion may be to include a limited number of septa ("2.5 D septa," C. Michel) to reduce random incidents and scatter.

The influence of scatter corrections in 3D activation studies was discussed by the Pittsburgh group (T. Nichols, not submitted for publication). It was found that the difference in z-score between images corrected and not corrected for scatter was negligible.

The chapter from the Pittsburgh group on brain receptor quantitation in 3D PET was discussed (D. Townsend *et al.*; Chapter 16). The scatter correction capability of different scatter correction schemes (convolution, dual-energy window (DEW), and modeling) had been investigated with the Utah phantom; all schemes giving results in fair agreement with the actual activity concentrations in the different compartments. It was, however, shown that the DEW technique may provide additional scatter information from activity outside the FOV, not directly available with the other techniques. The actual receptor study was based on [^{11}C]flumazenil in five normal subjects, studied with both 2D PET and 3D PET on different occasions. The good correlation between ROIs evaluated from 2D and 3D images indicated that the difficulties with the 3D technique now can be controlled and the benefits of the much higher sensitivity in 3D PET are now available in kinetic receptor studies.

The two following papers in the session addressed the same problem but with a different tracer, [^{18}F] fluorodopa.

The Hammersmith group (J. Rakshi *et al.*, Chapter 17) presented a 2D–3D comparison using [^{18}F]fluorodopa. In this chapter maps of the parameter K_i were used. After scatter correction in 3D, the ROI values taken from the K_i maps were in fair agreement with the "gold standard" values obtained in 2D, again showing the quantitation capability of 3D. The coefficient of variation in the K_i maps was 14% in 2D and 5% in 3D, showing the much higher sensitivity in 3D.

Chapter 18 was from the Orsay group (R. Trébossen *et al.*) using a DEW technique for the scatter correction

in 3D PET called *estimation of true method* (ETM), where one of the energy windows is set at the high-energy portion of the 511 keV photo peak to give data essentially free from scatter. For the comparison between 2D and 3D, the tracer uptake in the striata was determined from Patlak analysis using the occipital activity as input function, giving uptake values K_i. With the 3D scatter correction the regional K_i values in 2D and in 3D were in fair agreement, indicating the quantitation capability of 3D PET. As pointed out in the discussion, the "gold standard" 2D values were not scatter corrected. This will, however, change only slightly the 2D K_i values, the scatter fraction being small in 2D.

For determination of kinetic parameters in dynamic PET, an accurate determination of the input function is crucial. Different aspects of input function determinations were discussed in three of the four poster presentations, two of these dealt with actual devices: Chapter 13 discussed an automatic blood sampling system for small animals to be operated in conjunction with an animal PET scanner (S. Ashworth *et al.*, Hammersmith); and Chapter 14 discussed a device for noninvasive determinations of the input function for $H_2{}^{15}O$ blood flow measurements (M. Itoh *et al.*, Tohoku University, Sendai). Both devices used plastic scintillators to record the activity concentration in arterial blood, by detecting the positrons. In the animal system an arterial line was sensed. The other system used two plastic scintillators to externally record positrons over the radial artery and over nearby tissue.

Corrections for dispersion and delay are important for true quantitation of the input function. The Montreal group (M. Vafaee *et al.*; Chapter 15) examined the differences in dispersion corrections for the tracer concentration in blood from $H_2{}^{15}O$ blood flow studies and $^{15}O_2$ oxygen consumption studies. The dispersion correction function was, in the case of blood flow, well described by a single exponential function but, for the $^{15}O_2$ data, a double-exponential function was needed. They concluded that the dispersion characteristics should be evaluated for each tracer.

Chapter 20 dealt with an optimization problem for activation studies with $H_2{}^{15}O$, similar to the one already discussed by S. Holm *et al.* from the Copenhagen group. In addition to NEC calculations to determine the optimum dose, the authors (N. Sadato *et al.*, NIH) used the z-score to determine the optimum time duration for the study. They found that the NEC peaked around 440–550 MBq administrations and that the z-score evaluation favored a 60 sec duration of the study before a 90 or 120 sec scan. The actual choice for activation studies became 370 MBq (92% of the peak NEC) and the uptake of the $H_2{}^{15}O$ was followed for

TABLE 1 Ecat Exact HR; A Comparison Between 2D and 3D with ACSII and System 7.0 Software (T. Bruckbauer *et al.*)

Study	Comment		Results	Check	Remarks
Resolution	Transaxial	2D	3.6 mm	OK	
		3D	3.6 mm	OK	
	Axial	2D	4.0 mm	OK	Better than 3D at center
		3D	4.5 mm	OK	Better slice definition than 2D
Scatter	20 cm cyl	2D	12% *SF* 350 keV	OK	Scatter corrections 2D accurate
	20 cm cyl	3D	38% *SF* 350 keV	OK(?)	CTI scatter correction OK for static imaging; short frames may cause problems
Count rate	20 cm cyl	2D	Saturation@ 300 kBq/mL	OK	Good dead time correction $\leq$ 110 kBq/ml
	20 cm cyl	3D	Saturation@ 40 kBq/mL	OK	Good dead time correction $\leq$ 20 kBq/ml
Plane activity or axial uniformity	20 cm cyl	2D		OK	There are systematic deviations, however small ($\leq$ 2%)
	20 cm cyl	3D		OK	There are systematic deviations, however small ($\leq$ 2%)
Image uniformity	20 cm cyl	2D	$\leq$2%	OK	Measured with the phantom placed at the center of the camera
	20 cm cyl	3D	$\leq$2% (center) $\leq$2% (5 cm off-center)	OK	Measured with the phantom placed at the center of the camera and at 5 cm off-center
Frame-to-frame variations in a study of 10 frames by 10 sec	20 cm cyl	2D	<2%	OK	Same as the statistical variations
	20 cm cyl	3D	<3%		Larger than the statistical variations (<1%)

60 sec. Simulations showed, in addition, that this gave a S/N ratio equivalent to a 2 min scan with a 1 min slow injection of the 370 MBq $H_2{}^{15}O$.

Problems in Quantitation of 3D PET

The breakaway session had approximately 25–30 participants. It was found that almost all the participants had access to a PET camera with 3D capabilities. Of these 50% sometimes used the 3D capability but only 10% used the 3D capability in daily routine. As an example to illustrate problems to be considered before 3D PET can become a tool in clinical routine, Table 1 summarizes the 3D performance of the Ecat Exact HR scanner. The data in Table 1 imply that quantitative studies with the Ecat Exact HR can be performed in 3D, especially if long time frames are used. Kinetic studies with short frames (10 sec or less) may suffer from a slightly varying scatter fraction due to uncertainties of the normalization of the modeled scatter correction, thus increasing the errors in the selected regions of interest. The short frame scatter fraction uncertainties must first be solved before the Ecat Exact HR system covers all aspects on 3D clinical PET.

The transaxial resolution is approximately the same in 2D and 3D. However, the axial resolution, at least in the HR scanner, is approximately 10% worse in 3D than in 2D, probably due to the septa shielding in the 2D mode of operation.

For scatter inside the FOV, scatter correction techniques exist, which with sufficient accuracy remove the scatter component from the image data. Modeling techniques, for example, the CTI scatter correction, however, may have a normalization problem because model data is fitted to the actual data, which for short frames are noisy, making the fit unstable, as indicated in Table 1. Assuming the scatter distribution to be Gaussian and fitting a Gaussian distribution to the scatter part of the projection data suffers from the same problem; that is, unstable fits to noisy data. A problem that remains to be solved is the presence of out-of-FOV scatter. This question has been addressed by the Pittsburgh group (Chapter 16). Their data indicate that the DEW technique may provide a better estimate of large out-of-FOV scatter contributions than the other existing scatter correction techniques.

Overwhelmingly, 3D experiences come from cerebral blood flow activation studies. For the creation of maps of significance and the analyses of the data with the SPM technique, scatter correction is not necessary.

The data size problem was discussed. There are, however, experiences especially from Ecat Exact HR users, that data compression can be used to a large extent to reduce both the data size and the time needed for a 3D image reconstruction. As an example, experiences from the Max Planck Institute in Cologne show

that 152 MB of original data may be compressed down to 11.5 MB with only small degradation of the spatial resolution in the case of brain studies. The reconstruction time for such a data set is around 5 min. The new large 24 cm axial FOV 3D PET system constructed for Hammersmith by Siemens/CTI will use list mode to record data as a way to store only actual data and to give short time frames of <1–2 sec.

References

Dahlbom, M., Eriksson, L., and Wienhard, K. (1994). Design study of future 3-PET systems. *Conf. Rec. 1994 IEEE Nucl. Sci. Symp.* **4:** 1667–1671.

Bruckbauer, T., Wienhard, K., Hansen, S., Eriksson, L., Blomquist, G., Dahlbohm, M., and Casey, M. E. (1995). Evaluation of the ECAT EXACT HR with ACS II for clinical routine 3D measurements. *Conf. Rec. 1995 IEEE Nucl. Sci. Symp. in press.*

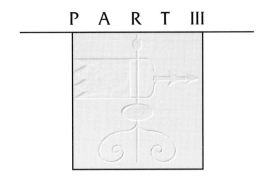

PART III

DATA PROCESSING

22

Sinogram Recovery of Dynamic PET Using Principal Component Analysis and Projections onto Convex Sets

JEFFREY T. YAP,[1] CHIEN-MIN KAO,[1] MALCOLM COOPER,[1] CHIN-TU CHEN,[1] and MILES WERNICK[2]

[1]*Franklin McLean Memorial Research Institute, Department of Radiology*
The University of Chicago, Chicago, Illinois 60637
[2]*Department of Electrical and Computer Engineering*
Illinois Institute of Technology, Chicago, Illinois

Positron emission tomography (PET) is typically limited by poor spatial resolution due to the finite size of the detector elements and Poisson noise due to nuclear count statistics. Noise becomes particularly limiting in dynamic studies with low count rates per individual frame. Unfortunately, most resolution enhancement schemes amplify high-frequency noise. Furthermore, tomographic reconstruction using simple filtered back projection (FBP) requires filtering out high-frequency information to prevent further amplification of noise. Thus, a trade-off between spatial resolution and noise is usually made in the reconstruction. We have previously used principal component analysis (PCA) to extract the relevant temporal kinetics while removing the noise from dynamic PET images. By applying this technique to raw projection data, the noise is removed prior to reconstruction, thus permitting preservation and enhancement of high-frequency spatial information. The method of projection onto convex sets (POCS) has been used to form a deblurred sinogram by utilizing additional detector wobble motion measurements and prior knowledge of the PET system's spatial response function. However, in low-count dynamic studies, this results in noise amplification. The combined methods of PCA and POCS have been applied to dynamic monkey neuroreceptor PET studies to reduce the noise and improve the spatial resolution. Consequently, this improves both the accuracy and precision of the estimation of the related kinetic parameters as compared to the known values obtained from postmortem radioassay. The specific binding and ratio of striatum/cerebellum were improved by factors of approximately 1.6 and 2, respectively.

I. INTRODUCTION

Dynamic positron emission tomography (PET) typically produces images with relatively poor spatial resolution and high noise levels. Unfortunately, many resolution enhancement schemes amplify noise, and conversely, many noise reduction techniques also degrade spatial resolution. Therefore, a trade-off between spatial resolution and noise is usually made in the tomographic reconstruction. Until recently, the finite size of detectors has had the largest contribution to the spatial resolution (Derenzo *et al.*, 1993). Thus, most efforts at improving resolution have been based on reducing the size of detector elements. However, this requires a large increase in the number of detector elements and thus a large increase in the cost of the scanner. Furthermore, sensitivity is often sacrificed with smaller detector elements. We have approached this problem by utilizing the method of projections onto convex sets (POCS) to deblur sinograms by incorporating wobble motion measurements of large detector elements and knowledge of the PET system's spatial response function (Wernick and Chen, 1992). This provides significant improvement in resolution without requiring hardware modification.

We have applied principal component analysis

(PCA), a statistical technique for the analysis and reduction of multidimensional data, to extract the significant temporal variations from dynamic PET images while removing the noise (Barber, 1980). The PCA results in a set of new variables, known as *principal components* (PCs), that are ordered on the basis of the amount of data variance they account for. Typically, most of the useful information can be extracted in the first few components. The remaining PCs can then be ignored to remove the unwanted variations from the analysis. In this regard, it may be construed as a means of improving the signal-to-noise ratio in tomographic data sets (Yap *et al.*, 1992). In the present study, we have combined PCA and POCS to both reduce noise and improve the spatial resolution of dynamic PET images.

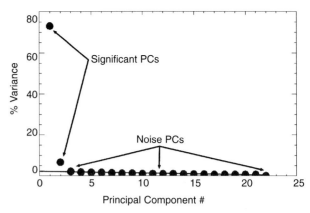

FIGURE 1   Plot of the percentage variance accounted for by each principal component.

II. MATERIALS AND METHODS

A. Data Acquisition

The methods of PCA, POCS, and combined PCA/POCS were applied to a dynamic monkey brain PET study using [^{18}F]fallypride, a dopamine D-2 radioligand recently developed by Mukherjee *et al.* (1993). Twenty-two consecutive 2.2 min image frames were acquired using a PETT VI tomograph in wobble mode (Ter-Pogossian *et al.*, 1982).

B. Principal Component Analysis

We previously used PCA to extract the statistically significant temporal variations from dynamic PET neuroreceptor images (Yap *et al.*, 1994). An approximation of the image sequence is formed by these PCs that has reduced noise while retaining the fundamental characteristics of the original data. This analysis has now been applied to the raw projection data, enabling resolution recovery prior to the tomographic reconstruction.

The raw dynamic PET data consists of a four-dimensional (3D spatial and 1D temporal) data set measuring the time evolution of the 3D volume of projection data. For each discrete 2D image plane, the data can be considered as the set of time–activity curves for all measurements in space. Thus, the 3D data set for each slice can be represented mathematically by a 2D matrix formed from the row vectors of each individual projection measurement's time–activity curve:

$$[\mathbf{X}]_{n \times p} = \begin{bmatrix} \mathbf{x}_1^T \\ \mathbf{x}_n^T \end{bmatrix} = \begin{bmatrix} x_{11} & x_{1p} \\ x_{n1} & x_{np} \end{bmatrix} \qquad (1)$$

where n is the number of measurements per image slice, p is the number of time frames, and $\mathbf{x}_i^T$ is the time–activity curve of the ith measurement. To reduce background effects and improve the sensitivity of the principal components, each time–activity curve is centered about its mean and normalized to unit variance (Jolliffe, 1986).

Assuming the data can be described by the linear combination of a limited number of functions, the mth order approximation of the sequence is given by

$$[\mathbf{X}]_{n \times p} \cong [\tilde{\mathbf{X}}^m]_{n \times p} \qquad \text{for } m \leq p \qquad (2)$$

where

$$[\tilde{\mathbf{X}}^m]_{n \times p} = [\mathbf{A}]_{n \times m}[\mathbf{B}]_{p \times m}^T \qquad (3)$$

The goal of PCA is to find a reduced set of m basis functions, $\mathbf{b}$, that can be multiplied by weighting coefficients, $\mathbf{a}$, to approximate the data $[\mathbf{X}]_{n \times p}$. These m PCs represent an optimal set of basis vectors that span an m-dimensional subspace of the original n-dimensional data. The tomographic reconstruction of the columns of $[\mathbf{A}]$ represent the principal component images and the rows of $[\mathbf{B}]$ represent their associated time functions. $[\mathbf{A}]$ and $[\mathbf{B}]$ are readily computed from the singular value decomposition (SVD) of the correlation matrix $[\mathbf{X}^T\mathbf{X}]$ (Press *et al.*, 1986).

C. Projection onto Convex Sets

Traditionally, raw projection data has been rebinned into sinograms using bilinear interpolation. In this approach, additional measurements obtained by detector wobble motion are used merely to improve the sampling of the object. However, if an estimate of the system response function is also known, then these measurements can be used to define a system of equa-

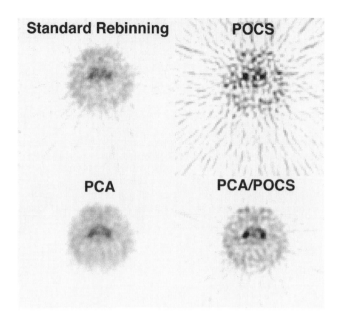

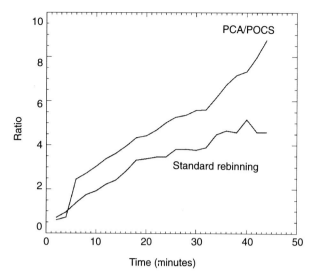

FIGURE 3   Plot of the ratio of average striatum/cerebellum activity vs. time.

FIGURE 2   Comparison of single image frame using standard rebinning, POCS, PCA, and combined PCA/POCS.

tions that can be solved to produce a deblurred sinogram.

It can be shown that in the absence of noise with an approximately depth-independent point spread function (PSF), each discrete projection measurement at a particular time frame is given by

$$x_{ij} = h_{ij}^T u_i \qquad (4)$$

where x_{ij} is the raw projection measurement at a given distance ρ_j and angle θ_i, $\mathbf{h}_{ij}$ is the effective discrete PSF, and $\mathbf{u}_{ij}$ is the ideal uniformly sampled projection. Thus, by knowing or estimating the spatial response function of the detector system, a set of linear equations can be defined by equation (4), which can then be solved using the method of projections onto convex sets (Youla and Webb, 1982; Sezan and Stark, 1982). Each measurement defines a convex set to which the ideal projection belongs. Therefore, $\mathbf{u}_{ij}$ must lie within the intersection of these convex sets. In POCS, $\mathbf{u}_{ij}$ is known to obey a set of n constraints, where the recursive estimate is obtained by sequentially projecting (in the linear algebra sense) the current estimate onto all of the sets describing the convex constraints:

$$\hat{u}^{(n+1)} = P_m P_{m-1} \cdot \ldots \cdot P_1 \hat{u}^{(n)} \qquad (5)$$

where P_k is the projection operator for the kth convex set. In the presence of noise, the measurement constraints defined by equation (4) become inconsistent and thus additional *a priori* constraints such as nonnegativity are employed.

III. RESULTS AND DISCUSSION

The PCA of the dynamic neuroreceptor data identifies two statistically significant PCs that are easily distinguished from the plateau of noise PCs obtained by plotting the relative eigenvalues in Figure 1. The reconstruction of the approximated image sequence using only these two PCs reduces the noise with no apparent effect on spatial resolution. POCS processing alone results in improved resolution at the cost of noise amplification. However, POCS applied after PCA shows notable resolution recovery without resulting in amplification of noise (Fig. 2). As a direct result, the estimation of specific binding and the ratio of striatum/cerebellum activity were improved by factors of approximately 1.6 and 2, respectively, when compared to the known values obtained from postmortem radioassay (Fig. 3).

The combined PCA/POCS method both reduces noise and improves spatial resolution in dynamic PET images, with consequent improvements in the accuracy and precision of quantitative measures. Since both the PCA and POCS are computationally efficient linear methods and are applied to the projection data, filtered back projection can be used to reconstruct the images with minimal increase in computation.

References

Barber, D. C. (1980). The use of principal components in the quantitative analysis of gamma camera dynamic studies. *Phys. Med. Biol.* **24**(2): 385–395.

Derenzo, S. E., Moses W. W., Huesman, R. H., Budinger, T. F. (1993). Critical instrumentation issues for resolution smaller than 2mm, high sensitivity brain PET. *In* "Quantification of Brain Function: Tracer Kinetics and Image Analysis in Brain PET" (K. Uemura *et al.*, Eds.), pp. 25–37. Excerpta Medica, Amsterdam.

Jolliffe, I. T. (1986). Principal Component Analysis, pp. 1–39. Springer-Verlag, New York.

Mukherjee, J., Yang, Z.-Y., Das, M. K., Kronmal, S., Brown, T., and Cooper, M. (1993). [^{18}F]fallypride as an improved pet radiotracer for dopamine D2 receptors. *J. Nucl. Med.* **34**(5): 243.

Press, W. H., Flannery, B. P., Teukolsky, S. A., and Vetterling, W. H. (1986). "Numerical Recipes, the Art of Scientific Computing," pp. 52–64. Cambridge Univ. Press, Cambridge.

Sezan, M. I., and Stark, H. (1982). Image restoration by the method of convex projections: Part 2—applications and numerical results. *IEEE Trans. Med. Imag.* **1**(2): 95–101.

Ter-Pogossian, M. M., Ficke, D. C., Hood, J.T., Yamamoto, M., and Mullani, N. A. (1982). PETT VI: A positron emission tomograph utilizing cesium fluoride scintillation detectors. *J. Comput. Assist. Tomogr.* **6**: 125–133.

Wernick, M. N., and Chen C.-T. (1992). Superresolved tomography by convex projections and detector motion. *J. Opt. Soc. Am.* **9**(9): 1547–1553.

Yap, J. T., Treffert J. D., Chen, C.-T., and Cooper, M. (1992). Image processing of dynamic images with principal component analysis. *Radiology* **185**: 177.

Yap, J. T. , Chen, C.-T., Cooper, M., and Treffert, J. D. (1994). Knowledge-based factor analysis of multidimensional nuclear medicine image sequences. *Proc. SPIE*, **2168**: 289–297.

Youla, D. C., and Webb, H. 1982. Image restoration by the method of convex projections: Part 1—theory. *IEEE Trans. Med. Imag.* **1**(2): 81–94.

Minimum Cross-Entropy Reconstruction of PET Images Using Prior Anatomical Information Obtained from MR

BABAK A. ARDEKANI,[1] **MICHAEL BRAUN,**[1] **BRIAN HUTTON,**[2] **and IWAO KANNO**[3]

[1]*Department of Applied Physics, University of Technology*
Sydney, New South Wales 2007, Australia
[2]*Department of Medical Physics, Westmead Hospital*
Westmead, New South Wales, 2145, Australia
[3]*Department of Radiology and Nuclear Medicine*
Research Institute for Brain and Blood Vessels
Akita City, Akita 010, Japan

The cross-entropy or directed divergence, $S(\mathbf{u},\mathbf{v})$, is a measure of "distance" between two vectors, $\mathbf{u}$ and $\mathbf{v}$, with positive components and is given by

$$S(\mathbf{u}, \mathbf{v}) = \sum_i [u_i \ln\left(\frac{u_i}{v_i}\right) - u_i + v_i]$$

We propose to reconstruct PET images using prior anatomical information obtained from magnetic resonance (MR) images of the same subject by minimizing a weighted sum:

$$J(\mathbf{x}; \beta) = S(\mathbf{y}, A\mathbf{x}) + \beta S(\mathbf{x}, \mathbf{p}) \qquad (0 \le \beta < \infty)$$

$S(\mathbf{y}, A\mathbf{x})$ is the cross-entropy between the emission data, $\mathbf{y}$, and the forward projection, $A\mathbf{x}$, of the PET image $\mathbf{x}$. $S(\mathbf{x}, \mathbf{p})$ is the cross-entropy between the PET image, $\mathbf{x}$, and a prior image, $\mathbf{p}$, which incorporates prior anatomical information. The parameter β determines how closely the estimated image $\mathbf{x}$ follows the emission data and the prior model. When $\beta = 0$, the problem reduces to minimizing $S(\mathbf{y}, A\mathbf{x})$, which is equivalent to the maximum likelihood (ML) image reconstruction. When $\beta \rightarrow \infty$, the emission data are ignored and the solution tends toward the prior image, $\mathbf{p}$. Details of implementation of this algorithm are presented as well as test reconstructions for simulated data. The performance of the algorithm is evaluated with respect to errors in the anatomical model obtained from MR. We conclude that this method provides significant improvement in the quality of reconstructed images as compared to the ML and techniques that use generic priors. The algorithm also displays robustness with respect to errors in prior anatomical information.

I. INTRODUCTION

The increasing availability of multimodality data, as well as the continuing advances in anatomical image segmentation (Liang *et al.*, 1993; Ardekani *et al.*, 1994) and anatomical–functional image registration (Pelizzari *et al.*, 1989; Woods *et al.*, 1993; Ardekani *et al.*, 1995), have prompted investigations into the problem of reconstruction of emission tomography images using prior anatomical information. Almost all of the reported approaches use the Bayesian estimation technique and introduce prior anatomical information into the reconstruction process by means of Gibbs priors (Leahy and Yan, 1991; Gindi *et al.*, 1993; Ouyang *et al.*, 1994). These methods estimate pixel values as well as the so-called line sites introduced by Geman and Geman (1984). Line sites are random variables, either binary (0 or 1) or continuously varying in the interval [0,1], which estimate the presence of an "edge" between two adjacent pixels. During the reconstruction process, a low line site value (edge unlikely) penalizes differences between the pixels, whereas a high value allows differences between them. Prior anatomical information incorporated by encouraging the formation of high-value line sites where anatomical boundaries are believed to exist. Although excellent reconstructions of simulated data were reported using Bayesian estimation with Gibbs priors incorporating line sites, some difficulties occur when dealing with line sites. Line sites may converge faster than the image intensities and reach stable but incorrect values in the first few iterations (Leahy and Yan, 1991). If the line sites are treated as binary variables, the objective function of the Bayesian estimation problem becomes nondifferentiable, causing difficulties in optimization. Elaborate relaxation methods have to be used to overcome this problem (Gindi *et al.*, 1993). When treated as continuous variables in the interval [0,1], convergence to 0 or 1 is not in general guaranteed (Ouyang *et al.*, 1994), and again some form of relaxation is necessary to ensure convergence (Leahy and Yan, 1991). In certain cases, line sites render the posterior objective function nonconvex with obvious numerical disadvantages.

In this chapter, we present a method whereby PET images are reconstructed by minimizing a weighted sum of two cross-entropy terms. The first term is the cross-entropy between the measured emission data and the expected emission data. The expected emission data are obtained by the forward projection of the estimated PET image. If we consider this term alone, the problem is equivalent to the ML estimation with Poisson likelihood function (Shepp and Vardi, 1982; Lange and Carson, 1984). The second cross-entropy term measures the distance between the estimated PET image and an *a priori* model for the PET image. Prior anatomical information obtained from MR images is coded in the *a priori* image model. An attractive feature of the algorithm presented in this chapter is its simplicity.

The use of cross-entropy priors in reconstruction of emission tomography images has been proposed previously (Liang *et al.*, 1989; Nunez and Llacer, 1990; Byrne, 1993). However, the use of MR as a source of prior anatomical information was not considered. The proposed approach incorporates MR data into the cross-entropy prior. Furthermore, we derive two complementary iterative algorithms that allow arbitrary weightings on the two sources of information available in PET image reconstruction: the measured emission data and the *a priori* image model.

II. THEORY

The cross-entropy $S(\mathbf{u}, \mathbf{v})$ between two vectors $\mathbf{u}$ and $\mathbf{v}$ with positive components is defined as follows:

$$S(\mathbf{u}, \mathbf{v}) = \sum_i [u_i \ln\left(\frac{u_i}{v_i}\right) - u_i + v_i] \qquad (1)$$

This can be considered as a form of "distance" between $\mathbf{u}$ and $\mathbf{v}$, although it does not have all the properties required to be a distance measure in the strict mathematical sense. We propose to reconstruct PET images by minimizing the following objective function:

$$J(\mathbf{x}; \beta) = S(\mathbf{y}, A\mathbf{x}) + \beta S(\mathbf{x}, \mathbf{p}) \qquad (0 \le \beta < \infty) \quad (2)$$

where $\mathbf{x} = \{x_j\}$ is the PET image to be reconstructed, $\mathbf{y} = \{y_i\}$ is the measured emission data, $\mathbf{p} = \{p_j\}$ is an *a priori* model for the PET image that incorporates prior anatomical information obtained from MR images of the same patient, and β is a constant. $A = \{a_{ij}\}$ is the forward projection probability matrix with elements a_{ij} representing the probability that a photon pair emitted at pixel j is recorded by detector pair i. The vector $A\mathbf{x}$ represents the forward projection of image $\mathbf{x}$ that is the expected value of the emission data vector. It can be shown that the objective function in equation (2) is strictly convex with respect to $\mathbf{x}$ and therefore the necessary and sufficient conditions for a global minimum are given by the Kuhn–Tucker conditions:

$$\frac{\partial J}{\partial x_j} = 0 \qquad \text{for } x_j > 0 \qquad (3)$$

$$\frac{\partial J}{\partial x_j} > 0 \qquad \text{for } x_j = 0 \qquad (4)$$

When the constant factor β is 0, the problem reduces to that of minimizing the cross-entropy term $S(\mathbf{y}, A\mathbf{x})$, which, as pointed out by Byrne (1993), is equivalent to the ML reconstruction. It is well known that when this minimization is performed using the expectation maximization (EM) method, the resulting reconstruction becomes increasingly noisy (Levitan and Herman, 1987; Snyder and Miller, 1985). This occurs because the algorithm tends to "overfit" the noisy emission data. For nonzero β, minimizing $J(\mathbf{x}; \beta)$ in equation (2) gives a solution that, although fitting the measured emission data $\mathbf{y}$, is not too distant from the *a priori* model of the image $\mathbf{p}$. In the extreme case when $\beta \to \infty$, the emission data is ignored and the solution defaults to $\mathbf{p}$.

To arrive at an iterative formula for optimization of $J(\mathbf{x}; \beta)$ in equation (2), let us first consider the case where $\beta = 0$. In this case, the EM algorithm for minimization of $S(\mathbf{y}, A\mathbf{x})$ is given as follows:

$$x_j^{(n+1)} = \frac{x_j^{(n)}}{\sum_i a_{ij}} \sum_i \frac{y_i a_{ij}}{\sum_k x_k^{(n)} a_{ik}} \qquad (5)$$

The EM iterative formula can also be written as follows:

$$x_j^{(n+1)} = x_j^{(n)} - \frac{x_j^{(n)}}{\sum_i a_{ij}} \frac{\partial J(\mathbf{x}; 0)}{\partial x_j}\bigg|_{\mathbf{x} = \mathbf{x}^{(n)}} \qquad (6)$$

This equation suggests an iterative formula for the case of $\beta \neq 0$, where $J(\mathbf{x}; \beta)$ replaces $J(\mathbf{x}; 0)$ in equation (6). Substituting the expression for $\partial J(\mathbf{x}; \beta)/\partial x_j$ and expanding yields

$$x_j^{(n+1)} = \frac{x_j^{(n)}}{\sum_i a_{ij}} \left[\sum_i \frac{y_i a_{ij}}{\sum_k x_k^{(n)} a_{ik}} - \beta \ln \left(\frac{x_j^{(n)}}{p_j} \right) \right] \quad (7)$$

The algorithm given by equation (5) has two useful properties. First, the positivity constraints $x_j > 0$ are automatically satisfied for positive initial conditions $x_j^{(0)} > 0$. Second, at each iteration, the total number of counts in the image equals the number of detected counts; that is, $\sum_j x_j = \sum_i y_i$. However, the algorithm given by equation (7) does not, in general, have either of these properties. The crucial positivity condition is satisfied only when

$$\sum_i \frac{y_i a_{ij}}{\sum_k x_k^{(n)} a_{ik}} > \beta \ln \left(\frac{x_j^{(n)}}{p_j} \right) \quad (8)$$

This condition will be violated when β is large. Therefore, the iterative formula (7) cannot be used with an arbitrarily large weighting on the prior image $\mathbf{p}$. For such cases, a second iterative equation is derived based on the Kuhn–Tucker condition given in equation (3). Setting the partial derivative of J with respect to x_j to 0, we obtain

$$\frac{\partial J}{\partial x_j} = \sum_i a_{ij} - \sum_i \frac{y_i a_{ij}}{\sum_k x_k a_{ik}} + \beta \ln \left(\frac{x_j}{p_j} \right) = 0 \quad (9)$$

By solving for x_j in $\ln(x_j/p_j)$, the following iterative formula emerges:

$$x_j^{n+1} = p_j \exp \left[\frac{-1}{\beta} \left(\sum_i a_{ij} - \sum_i \frac{y_i a_{ij}}{\sum_k x_k^{(n)} a_{ik}} \right) \right] \quad (10)$$

The solution (10) satisfies the positivity constraint for all β. It can be seen that, when $\beta \rightarrow \infty$, it yields $x_j = p_j$, as expected. However, due to the exponential form of the solution, this algorithm diverges for small values of β. Thus, the iterative formulas (7) and (10) are complementary, each suited to the situation for which the other fails.

III. METHODS

The algorithms presented in this chapter were evaluated using simulated data. The simple phantom shown in Figure 1(a) was chosen. The activity in the background was set to 0. The activity ratio of the three nonzero regions was set to $6:2:1$ (1 is the activity of the outer rim). Forward projections of the phantom were computed, and Poisson noise was added to each projection to simulate the emission data vector $\mathbf{y}$. The forward projection matrix A was based solely on the geometry of the detection system and did not account for factors such as attenuation and scatter. Approximately 1 million counts were generated. The simulated data were then reconstructed using the ML–EM algorithm (equation (5)) and the minimum cross-entropy algorithms of equations (7) and (10), which we shall denote as *MXE1* and *MXE2*, respectively. The prior anatomical information used in the MXE1 and MXE2 algorithms consists of region boundaries as shown in Figure 1(b). To evaluate the performance of the algorithm with respect to errors in the prior information, we also reconstructed the phantom image using the incorrect boundaries shown in Figure 1(c).

At each iteration the prior image model $\mathbf{p}$ was set to a smoothed version of the image from the previous iteration. The smoothing operation was an edge-preserving one where the smoothing was confined within the regions defined by anatomical boundaries (Figs. 1(b) or 1(c)).

IV. RESULTS AND DISCUSSION

The reconstruction results for the simulated emission data of the phantom in Figure 1(a) are shown in Figure 2. Figure 2(a) shows the ML–EM reconstruction, which is characteristically noisy. Figure 2(b) shows the reconstruction obtained by using the MXE1 algorithm and $\beta = 0.5$ without anatomical information. The noise is greatly reduced in this case. However, there is an apparent loss of resolution in the image compared to the ML–EM reconstruction. Figures 2(c) and 2(d) show the MXE1 and MXE2 reconstructions with $\beta = 0.5$, respectively, using the correct anatomical boundaries of Figure 1(b). It can be seen that, although noise is effectively suppressed in these images, image resolution is being preserved. It is interesting to note that the MXE1 and MXE2 reconstructions appear practically identical. However, the two algorithms have a complementary nature. MXE1 fails when β is large (>1.5 for the present simulation study) because condition (8) is violated. On the other hand, MXE2 can readily handle arbitrarily large β but fails for small β (<0.3 for the present simulation study). This suggests that the MXE1 and MXE2 algorithms can be used together in problems where one algorithm alone could

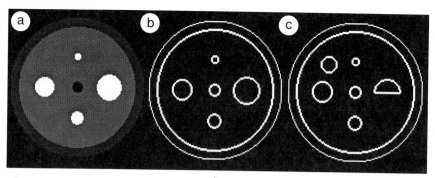

FIGURE 1   (a) Simulated phantom. (b) Correct region boundaries. (c) Incorrect region boundaries.

fail. For example, we could use the MXE1 algorithm but revert to MXE2 whenever condition (8) is not satisfied. It can be easily shown that MXE2 is stable when condition (8) is not satisfied. The two algorithms could also operate independently on different portions of the image. This would have an application when a large β is assigned to one part of the image, in order to stress prior information, although the reconstruction of the remaining part of the image relies more heavily on the emission data (i.e., β is small).

Figure 3 shows the root mean square (rms) error between the phantom of Figure 1(a) and the reconstructions of Figure 2 as a function of the number of iterations. It can be seen that, for $\beta = 0.5$, MXE2 converges faster than the MXE1 algorithm. However, their final rms errors are the same. It is interesting to note that the minimum rms errors of the MXE1 and MXE2 reconstructions occur at early iterations, and the rms value converges to a somewhat higher value than the minimum. However, examination of the image at the minimum rms value revealed a bias larger than that of the final image.

Figures 4(a) and 4(b) show the MXE1 and MXE2 reconstructions obtained when using the incorrect prior boundaries of Figure 1(c). Both algorithms dis-

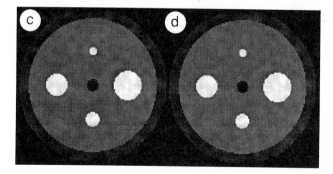

FIGURE 2   Reconstructions obtained after 80 iterations. (a) ML; (b) MXE1 ($\beta = 0.5$) without using any prior boundaries; (c) MXE1 ($\beta = 0.5$) using the correct region boundaries of Figure 1(b); (d) MXE2 ($\beta = 0.5$) using the correct region boundaries of Figure 1(b).

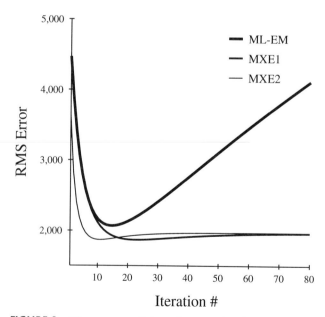

FIGURE 3   The rms error distance between the phantom of Figure 1a and the reconstructions of Figures 2(a), 2(c), and 2(d) vs. the number of iterations.

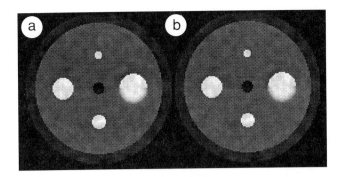

FIGURE 4 Reconstructions obtained after 80 iterations. (a) MXE1 reconstruction ($\beta = 0.5$) using the incorrect region boundaries of Figure 1(c); (b) MXE2 ($\beta = 0.5$) using the incorrect region boundaries of Figure 1(c).

play robustness with respect to errors in the prior anatomical information. That is, false MR boundaries do not create false edges in the reconstructed PET image, and an edge in the PET image is still reconstructed even when the corresponding MR boundary is missing.

In conclusion, we have presented a method of PET image reconstruction that introduces prior anatomical information obtained from MR images of the same subject. Two algorithms have been given that can be used together, allowing the placement of arbitrary weighting on the two sources of information available in PET image reconstruction; namely, the measured emission counts and the *a priori* image model. Simulation studies showed that the use of prior anatomical knowledge significantly improves the quality of reconstructed images. The algorithms were shown to be robust with respect to inaccuracies in prior anatomical boundaries.

References

Ardekani, B. A., Braun, M., Kanno, I., and Hutton, B. F. (1994). Automatic detection of intradural spaces in MR images. *J. Comput. Assist. Tomogr.* **18:** 963–969.

Ardekani, B. A., Braun, M., Hutton, B. F., Kanno, I., and Iida, H. (1995). A fully automatic multimodality image registration algorithm. *J. Comput. Assist. Tomogr.* **19:** 615–623.

Byrne, C. L. (1993). Iterative image reconstruction algorithms based on cross-entropy minimization. *IEEE Trans. Image Proc.* **2:** 96–103.

Geman, S., and Geman, D. (1984). Stochastic relaxation, Gibbs distributions, and the Bayesian restoration of images. *IEEE Trans. Pattern Anal. Machine Intell.* **6:** 721–741.

Gindi, G., Lee, M., Rangarajan, A., and Zubal, I. G. (1993). Bayesian reconstruction of functional images using anatomical information as priors. *IEEE Trans. Med. Imag.* **12:** 670–680.

Lange, K., and Carson, R. (1984). EM reconstruction algorithms for emission and transmission tomography. *J. Comp. Assist. Tomogr.* **8:** 306–316.

Leahy, R., and Yan, X. (1991). Incorporation of Anatomical MR Data for Improved Functional Imaging with PET. *In:* "Information Processing in Medical Imaging" (A. C. F. Colchester and D. J. Hawkes, Eds.), pp. 105–120. Springer-Verlag, New York.

Levitan, E., and Herman, G. T. (1987). A maximum *a posteriori* probability expectation maximization algorithm for image reconstruction in emission tomography. *IEEE Trans. Med. Imag.* **16:** 185–192.

Liang, Z. (1993). Tissue classification and segmentation of MR images. *IEEE Eng. Med. Biol.* **12:** 91–85.

Liang, Z., Jaszczak, R., and Greer, K. (1989). On Bayesian image reconstruction from projections: Uniform and nonuniform *a priori* source information. *IEEE Trans. Med. Imag.* **8:** 227–235.

Nunez, J., and Llacer, J. (1990). A fast Bayesian reconstruction algorithm for emission tomography with entropy prior converging to feasible images. *IEEE Trans. Med. Imag.* **9:** 159–171.

Ouyang, X., Wong, W. H., Johnson, V. E., Hu, X., and Chen, C. T. (1994). Incorporation of correlated structural images in PET image reconstruction. *IEEE Trans. Med. Imag.* **13:** 627–640.

Pelizzari, C. A., Chen, G. T. Y., Spelbring, D. R., Weichselbaum, R. R., and Chen, C. T. (1989). Accurate three-dimensional registration of CT, PET, and/or MR images of the brain. *J. Comput. Assist. Tomogr.* **13:** 20–26.

Shepp, L. A., and Vardi, Y. (1982). Maximum likelihood reconstruction for emission tomography. *IEEE Trans. Med. Imag.* **1:** 113–122.

Snyder, D. L., and Miller, M. I. (1985). The use of sieves to stabilize images produced with the EM algorithm for emission tomography. *IEEE Trans. Nucl. Sci.* **32:** 3864–3872.

Woods, R. P., Mazziotta, J. C., and Cherry, S. R. (1993). MRI-PET registration with automated algorithm. *J. Comput. Assist. Tomogr.* **17:** 536–546.

MR-Guided PET Reconstruction and Problems with Anatomical Misinformation

B. LIPINSKI,[1] H. HERZOG,[1] E. ROTA KOPS,[1] W. OBERSCHELP,[2] and H. W. MÜLLER-GÄRTNER[1]

[1]*Institute of Medicine, Research Center*
Jülich 52425, Germany
[2]*Institute of Applied Mathematics*
Aachen, Germany

In this chapter, we describe two algorithms for PET reconstruction that incorporate anatomical information into the reconstruction process. Both algorithms are based on the ML–EM algorithm, into which anatomical information can be included easily by taking into account the anatomical knowledge as a so-called a priori distribution.

The difference between the two algorithms is the way in which they model this distribution. The Markov–GEM algorithm uses a Gibbs distribution, whereas the Gauss–EM uses a Gaussian distribution. Both algorithms are based on the assumption that the radioactivity is distributed homogeneously within anatomical regions that are separable by segmentation of the MR data.

The resulting images show a considerable noise reduction and an improved delineation of borders. Furthermore, we tested the algorithms for effects of erroneous (e.g., incomplete or misregistered) anatomical information by means of simulated and physical phantoms.

Even though the Gauss–EM algorithm is superior in its use of accurate anatomical information, it is not stable in the case of defective a priori distribution, with changes in the reconstructed activity of up to 50%. The Markov–GEM yielded only small errors in the case of anatomical misinformation.

I. INTRODUCTION

Even though PET is a unique imaging tool for examining (patho)physiology and (patho)biochemistry *in*

vivo, it suffers from inherent problems, such as a poor signal-to-noise ratio, relatively low resolution, and partial volume effects. By incorporating high-resolution MRI information of the same object into the reconstruction process of the PET images, some of these problems can be overcome. Several groups have applied this approach to simulated and physical phantoms (Gindi, 1993; Leahy and Yan, 1991; Ouyang *et al.*, 1994; Ardekani *et al.*, 1993). For nonpatient data, these algorithms usually result in a noise reduction and improvement in the border delineation. If such algorithms are applied to patient data, one has to be aware of problems that can arise in the case of erroneous anatomical information.

In this chapter, we present the two methods that have been developed by our group and demonstrate the effect of erroneous anatomical data.

II. MATERIALS AND METHODS

The maximum likelihood–expectation maximization (ML–EM) algorithm (Shepp and Vardi, 1982) assumes the projection data to be Poisson distributed and calculates the image as a maximum likelihood estimation by the following iterative procedure:

$$\lambda_i^{(n+1)} = \lambda_i^{(n)} \sum_j \frac{p_{ij} y_j}{\sum\limits_k p_{kj} \lambda_k^{(n)}} \tag{1}$$

where n is the index of iteration, λ_i the unknown activity concentration in pixel i, and y_j is the number of coincidences registered in the detector pair j; p_{ij} denotes the probability that an event occurring in pixel i is recorded in the detector pair j.

Anatomical information can be incorporated in the ML–EM approach as so-called *a priori* information. The distribution of the *a priori* information together with the distribution of the measured data yields the so-called *a posteriori* distribution, which should be maximized by the reconstruction algorithm.

A. The Markov–GEM Algorithm

The Markov–GEM algorithm considers locally homogenous regions within the anatomical regions. Markov fields are appropriate to model interaction between neighboring pixels in the image space. Whereas Markov fields use a description of conditional distributions, we preferred the Gibbs formulation, which has proven to be equivalent to Markov fields (Griffeath, 1976). The following potential function is used for our Gibbs distribution:

$$V_C(\lambda) = \ln\left(\cosh|\lambda_i - \lambda_j|\right) \qquad (2)$$

where λ_i and λ_j are the intensity values of neighboring pixels.

Together with the Poisson distribution of the projection data the *a posteriori* distribution is obtained, which is then maximized, using an EM type algorithm, as suggested by Green (1990), that did not take into account different tissue components (Lipinski, 1995):

$$\lambda_i^{(n+1)} = \frac{\lambda_i^{(n)}}{1 + \beta \frac{\partial}{\partial \lambda_i} \sum_c V_C(\lambda^{(n)})} \sum_j \frac{y_j p_{ij}}{\sum_k p_{kj} \lambda_k^{(n)}} \qquad (3)$$

B. The Gauss–EM Algorithm

The Gauss–EM algorithm assumes global homogeneity inside the anatomical regions. All the pixels of an anatomical region are considered to have a Gaussian distribution around the same mean value:

$$p(\lambda) = c \cdot \exp\left[\frac{\gamma}{2}(\lambda - m)^T H(\lambda - m)\right] \qquad (4)$$

where m is the previously calculated mean activity, c is a constant, and γ is a parameter corresponding to the inverse standard deviation of the Gaussian distribution. The mean values are to be calculated in a preprocessing step for each anatomical segment; for example, by using the ML–EM algorithm for regions instead of pixels (Carson, 1986). Together with the Poisson distribution of the projection data, one obtains the *a posteriori* distribution. The EM algorithm for maximization of the *a posteriori* function results in the following formula (Levitan and Herman, 1987; Lipinski, 1995):

$$\lambda_i^{(n+1)} = \frac{\gamma H_{ii} m_i - 1 + \sqrt{(\gamma H_{ii} m_i - 1)^2 + 4\gamma H_{ii} \lambda_i^{(n)} \sum_j \frac{p_{ij} y_j}{\sum_k p_{kj} \lambda_k^{(n)}}}}{2\gamma H_{ii}} \qquad (4)$$

C. Anatomical Misinformation

When applying this approach to real patient data, errors in the anatomical *a priori* information have to be expected because of either an inaccurate segmentation of the MRI data or a misregistration between the MRI and PET data sets of the order of 2–3 mm. In this work the effects of such problems were intensively studied.

III. RESULTS AND DISCUSSION

A general finding for both algorithms was a noise reduction and an improvement in the delineation of the borders compared to the ML–EM algorithm. Using the Shepp–Logan phantom, noise reductions of up to 50% for the Gauss–EM and 30% for the Markov–GEM algorithm were obtained (Fig. 1).

A. Incomplete *a Priori* Information

To simulate complete and incomplete *a priori* MRI information, a cylindrical phantom consisting of six small cylinders, filled with different concentrations of radioactivity, was used both in its original form and with one of the small circles removed. The images were reconstructed for both cases, using both the Markov–GEM algorithm and the Gauss–EM algorithm (Fig. 2). For the Markov–GEM algorithm, the data reconstructed in the area of the missing region differed by only 1% when incomplete instead of complete *a priori* information was used. In the latter case, the border of the circle was slightly sharper. The Gauss–EM algorithm yielded a decrease in activity of about 10% in the area of the missing region when the anatomical information was incomplete, because the mean values of the Gauss distribution for the missing MRI region and its surroundings are assumed to be the same. Therefore, large errors in both the activity values and shape of the missing object resulted.

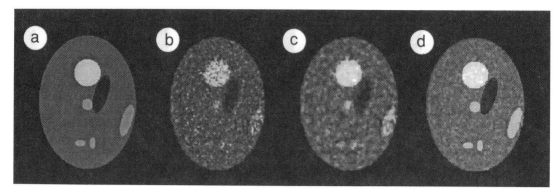

FIGURE 1   Shepp–Logan phantom: (a) anatomical information, reconstructed images obtained with (b) the ML–EM algorithm, (c) the Markov–GEM algorithm, and (d) the Gauss–EM algorithm.

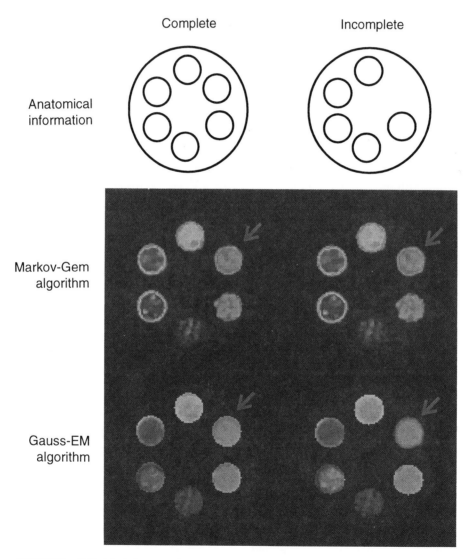

FIGURE 2   Cylindrical phantom with six small cylindrical inserts was reconstructed with complete and incomplete anatomical information, using the Markov–GEM and the Gauss–EM algorithm.

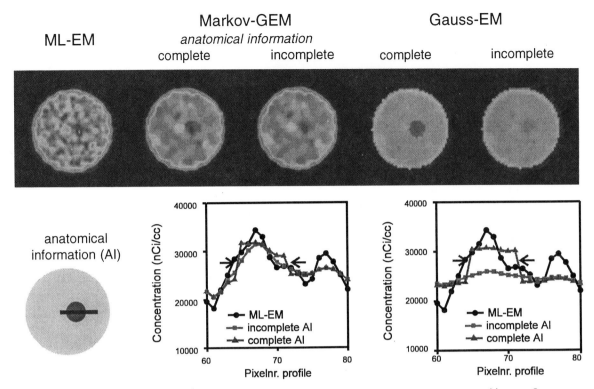

FIGURE 3 Simulated phantom with a small cylinder placed in a larger one. Upper row: reconstructed images. Lower row: anatomical information with profile indicated (left), profiles obtained with the Markov–GEM algorithm (middle), and the Gauss–EM algorithm (right).

A second experiment investigated the influence of incomplete anatomical information, when the concentrations of neighboring areas differed only slightly. The simulated phantom consisted of a small circle ($r = 10$ mm) placed excentrically in a larger one ($r = 40$ mm). The ratio of concentrations in the two circles was $6:5$. The configuration was reconstructed with the ML–EM algorithm, the Markov–GEM algorithm, and the Gauss–EM algorithm (Fig. 3). The MRI-guided algorithms were applied with and without knowledge about the inner circle. In the image obtained with the ML–EM algorithm, it is difficult to delineate the inner circle because of the high noise level. The Markov–GEM algorithm is superior to the conventional ML–EM algorithm, because the inner circle can be recognized for both complete and incomplete *a priori* information. The profiles defined across the inner circle reveal sharp edges for complete, and smooth edges for incomplete, *a priori* information. Using the Gauss–EM algorithm with incomplete information, the inner circle can hardly be recognized. As seen in the profiles, the values within the inner circle are only slightly higher than those outside.

Using incomplete *a priori* information, we obtained stable results with the Markov–GEM but not the Gauss–EM.

B. Incorrectly Registered *a Priori* Information

The influence of an incorrect registration was investigated using a 2D Hoffman phantom that was scanned with PET using ^{18}F and with MRI after having filled the phantom with cold water. The position of the MRI data set relative to the PET coordinate system was shifted in steps from 1 mm to 5 mm. For each position the Markov–GEM and the Gauss–EM algorithms were applied. ROIs marked in white and gray matter allowed the effect of the incorrect registration to be assessed. Using the Markov–GEM algorithm only small changes are seen in the intensity as a function of the shift (Fig. 4). Shifts of more than 2 mm produced no additional change, because the connection between the anatomical and functional space was lost. In the diagram for the Gauss–EM algorithm a steady change of the ROI means is found. The values for white and gray matter converge with unacceptable errors for a shift of 5 mm.

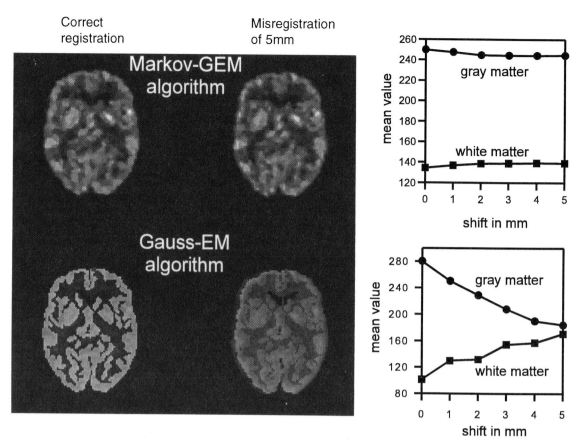

FIGURE 4   Images were acquired using a 2D Hoffmann brain phantom and reconstructed with the Markov–GEM (top) and Gauss-EM algorithm (bottom), with correctly registered anatomical information (left) and with misregistration of 5 mm (middle). Diagrams on the right display ROI means inside the gray matter and the white matter.

IV. CONCLUSION

The two approaches for MRI-guided iterative image reconstruction developed by our group show improved noise reduction and edge definition. For accurate *a priori* information, the Gauss–EM algorithm is superior to the Markov–GEM algorithm; however, in the presence of anatomical misinformation, the Gauss–EM algorithms produced unacceptable errors, whereas the Markov–GEM algorithm proved to be stable.

References

Ardekani, B. A., Braun, M., and Hutton, B. F. (1993). Improved quantification with the use of anatomical information in PET image reconstruction. *In*: "Quantification of Brain Function." Proceedings of Brain PET '93 Akita (K. Uemura, N. A. Lassen, T. Jones and A. Inugami, Eds.), pp. 351–359. Excerpta Medica, Amsterdam.

Carson, R. E. (1986). A maximum likelihood method for region-of-interest evaluation in emission tomography. *J. Comput. Assist. Tomogr.* **10**: 654–663.

Gindi, G., Lee, M., Rangarajan, A., and Zubal, I. G. (1993). Bayesian reconstruction of functional images using anatomical information as priors. *IEEE Trans. Med. Imag.* **12**(4): 670–680.

Green, P. J. (1990). Bayesian reconstructions from emission tomography data using a modified EM algorithm. *IEEE Trans. Med. Imag.* **9**(1): 84–93.

Griffeath, D. (1976). Introduction to random fields. *In*: "Denumberable Markov Chains" (A. Knapp, J. Kemeny, and L. Snell, Eds.), pp. 425–458. Springer, New York.

Leahy, R., and Yan, X. (1991). Incorporation of anatomical MR data for improved functional imaging with PET. *In* "Information Processing in Medical Imaging" (A. C. F. Colchester and D. J. Hawkes, Eds.), pp. 105–120. Springer, New York.

Levitan, E., and Herman, G. T. (1987). A maximum *a-posteriori* probability expectation maximization algorithm for image reconstruction in emission tomography. *IEEE Trans. Med. Imag.* **6**(3): 185–192.

Lipinski, B. (1995). Rekonstruktion von positronen-emissions-tomographischen Bildern unter Einbeziehung anatomischer Information. Ph.D. Thesis. RWTH Aachen, Germany.

Ouyang, X., Wong, W. H., Johnson, V. E., *et al.* (1994). Incorporation of correlated structural images in PET image reconstruction. *IEEE Trans. Med. Imag.* **13**(4): 627–640.

Shepp, L. A., and Vardi, Y. (1982). Maximum likelihood reconstruction for emission tomography. *IEEE Trans. Med. Imag.* **1**(2): 228–238.

25

Automatic 3D Regional MRI Segmentation and Statistical Probability Anatomy Maps

A. C. EVANS, D. L. COLLINS, and C. J. HOLMES

Montreal Neurological Institute, McGill University
McConnell Brain Imaging Centre
Montreal, Canada H3A 2B4

In the rapidly growing field of human brain mapping, the use of a standardized, or stereotaxic, coordinate space is a central factor in the interpretation and comparison of results from different centers. The use of some variant of the Talairach space is almost universal, but this procedure has a number of weaknesses arising because it (1) is derived from an unrepresentative single 60-year-old female brain, (2) ignores left–right hemispheric differences, and (3) has variable slice separations, up to 4 mm. We have previously reported the creation of a 305-member, finely sampled averaged MRI volume that can be used alongside the Talairach atlas. Although visually indicative of the anatomical variability across the young normal population usually scanned in brain mapping experiments, this data set did not express that variability quantitatively. Such information requires the accurate and reproducible labeling of all voxels in any given structure for each brain within the MRI ensemble. Manual labeling is prohibitively time consuming and error prone. We, therefore, describe an automated procedure for 3D labeling of individual brain structures based on the nonlinear deformation of individual MRI volumes to match a previously labeled target volume, followed by numerical inverse transformation of the labels to the native MRI space. Subsequent processing allows these labels to be mapped into stereotaxic space, now using a simple linear transformation, and combined to generate probability maps for the location of each predefined structure. The procedure is described, along with validation experiments and selected examples of such maps. The general principle described is applicable to any scale and any object that can be defined within the target volume. Importantly, because the labels themselves take no part in the image-matching process, any number of labeling schemes, representing different brain atlas formulations, can coexist and their corresponding probability maps generated from a single determination of the mapping transformation.

I. INTRODUCTION

The quantitative comparison of functional and structural brain image data across subjects requires a common, so-called stereotaxic, coordinate frame with respect to which the spatial variability of corresponding features from different individuals can be expressed. Since that positional variability will depend on the degrees of freedom (DOF) allowed for mapping the image data from its original, native space into stereotaxic space, it is essential that the stereotaxic transformation be well-defined and reproducible. For simplicity and ease of use of interpretation, it is also desirable that the transformation have as few DOF as possible while accounting for most of the positional variability. The problem of *quantifying* anatomical variability is thus considered to be distinct from the practical issue of *removing* anatomical variability. In the latter task, the goal is to render all brains identical after transformation, a goal that, in principle, could require as many DOF as there are independent samples in the data volume. Numerous nonlinear methods have been employed to increase the stereotaxic correspondence among different brains (e.g., Evans *et al.*, 1991; Roland *et al.*, 1994; Minoshima *et al.*, 1994). Unfortunately, because they vary in the number of effective DOF, any direct comparison of residual anatomical variability is difficult, if not impossible, and quotations for anatomical variability have little absolute meaning.

A related but separate problem is the accurate identification, or labeling, of ''correspondent'' points that are to be optimally aligned within the constraints of the stereotaxic transformation's allowed DOF. There is never an exact one-to-one mapping between two brains, even at the gross morphological level, owing to, for instance, multiple sulcal patterns, and at a finer spatial scale, the notion of correspondence becomes meaningless. The quantification of neuroanatomical variability is then an empirical process that is useful provided the positional uncertainty in labeling any point is small compared with the true positional variability among individuals. This uncertainty–variability trade-off varies widely, with deep gray structures and ventricular features being much easier to define than cortical features. Typically, structural labeling has been a manual process that, although likely to be more accurate than automated procedures for any one version of labeling within a single brain, will be less precise (reproducible) within that brain, less systematic across brains, and more time consuming. Also, the labeling scheme will differ among investigators, introducing further methodological inconsistencies that will mask the true neuroanatomical variability being sought.

We have considered these issues in defining a strategy for the creation of a probabilistic atlas of human neuroanatomy. The strategy uses automated techniques for 3D regional image segmentation and nonlinear volume deformation and comprises two conceptual stages, *labeling* and *stereotaxy*, as schematically illustrated in Figure 1. For the labeling stage, the native data is matched to a previously labeled target volume, already resident in stereotaxic space, using a 3D nonlinear deformation that will be described. The inverse transformation is used to map the voxel labels, defined on the target volume, back on to the native volume. Each newly labeled native volume can then be transformed into some simply defined coordinate frame so that the spatial variability in size, shape, or centroid location of any individual structure with respect to that coordinate frame–transformation pair can be quantified in the stereotaxy stage. The first stage allows unlimited DOF in matching a labeling template, or atlas, with the native image volume. The second allows only linear stereotaxic transformation of the labeled volume when quantifying anatomical variability. Note that it is not essential to the labeling process that the target volume and its associated labels be resident in stereotaxic space, merely convenient for purposes of implementation and later image comparison. The two perspectives, linear stereotaxy and nonlinear labeling, are

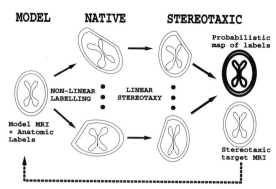

FIGURE 1 Schematic of principles underlying creation of probabilistic neuroanatomy maps. The labeling and stereotaxy steps can be considered to be independent operations. The result of the labeling step is the transfer of anatomic labels from a target space to the native space of the source data set. A subsequent stereotaxic mapping can be applied to investigate the spatial variability of those labels with respect to a well-defined coordinate frame. In practice, as indicated by the dotted line, the target volume and the stereotaxic target volume are in the same space, although this is not strictly necessary. Also in practice, a nine-parameter transformation is applied for stereotaxic mapping and probabilistic map creation.

combined within the concept of probabilistic neuroanatomical atlases. Here, large ensembles of brain image data are first labeled in their native space and then mapped into some stereotaxic space using a limited number of degrees of freedom, such as a 9- or 12-parameter affine transform. The likelihood of any structure label occuring at any stereotaxic voxel gives rise to a statistical probability anatomy map (SPAM) for each structure that, when expressed for all structures, gives rise to a probabilistic anatomical atlas.[1]

The perspective of segmentation as registration followed by delineation yields one powerful advantage, that of *atlas-independent* segmentation. The geometric contours defined on the target image volume are not used to determine the match between the source and target volumes. The nonlinear transformation is established by matching the two volumes directly. Therefore, any atlas defined in the target space can be used for segmentation. This allows the coexistence of multiple atlases, each of which is simultaneously mappable to the native MR image volume without the need to recalculate the nonlinear matching transformation. The underlying structure of the MRI is used as a frame,

---

[1]This rationale does not conflict with the notion of nonlinear stereotaxic mapping. The latter has the pragmatic goal of improved alignment of individual morphological features in the pursuit of increased signal from multisubject functional activation experiments rather than the quantitative characterization of individual anatomical differences being discussed here.

onto which the atlas contours are mapped. Thus, any structure can be defined in the atlas and need not follow edges present in the tomographic image volume. For example, functional neuroanatomy areas, whose limits can be inferred from the underlying anatomical substrate, can be incorporated into the atlas definitions without affecting the spatial transformation defined by the algorithm.

II. METHODS

A. Algorithm

The procedure for automatic segmentation, termed ANIMAL (automated nonlinear image matching and anatomical labeling; Collins *et al.*, 1995a, 1995b), builds up a 3D nonlinear deformation field by sequential linear matching of many small data cubes in one volume to the other volume. These cubes are arranged in a 3D grid to fill the volume and each cube can move only within a range defined by the grid spacing. The algorithm is applied iteratively in a multiscale hierarchy, so that image blurring and cube size are reduced after each grid pass. The initial fit is obtained rapidly because only lower spatial frequencies and gross distortions are considered, but later iterations at finer scales become increasingly computationally intensive as finer details are matched. ANIMAL can be terminated at any intermediate spatial scale if faster, approximate results are satisfactory. The algorithm is an extension of a previously reported linear method for stereotaxic normalization (Collins *et al.*, 1994). Here, we concentrate on the use of this nonlinear extension for automatic labeling of brain structures. Both linear and nonlinear registration procedures rely on the extraction of geometrically invariant features from the original volumetric images. We have chosen to use blurred versions of the image intensity and image gradient magnitude as features that are independent of the original position, scale, and orientation of one data set with respect to the other. These features are calculated by convolution of the original data with zeroth and first-order 3D isotropic Gaussian derivatives. Convolution with such an operator maintains linearity, shift invariance, and rotational invariance in the detection of features (tar Haar Romeny *et al.*, 1991; Koenderink and van Doorn, 1987). We use the full-width at half-max, FWHM = 2.35σ) of this Gaussian kernel as the parameter to measure the spatial scale.

The optimization procedure used to recover the best spatial transformation is accomplished in a hierarchical multiscale fashion. Registration is performed at different spatial scales, starting with very blurred data and increasing detail by using less blurred images, refining the registration at each stage. As well as increasing the speed of calculation, compared with performing all operations at the finest scale, this strategy avoids local minima in the objective function hypersurface. The linear component of the required spatial mapping is found by estimating the best affine transformation matrix that maximizes the similarity of invariant features extracted from both target and source volumes, described in detail in Collins *et al.* (1994). The feature similarity criterion used can be selected from a set including (1) cross-correlation, (2) minimum variance of feature ratio (Woods *et al.*, 1993), (3) z-score. All results reported here used cross-correlation as the similarity criterion. The remaining nonlinear morphological differences are again estimated with a hierarchical multiscale strategy. The approach is an extension of the linear registration method, except that now the target volume is a small cubic neighborhood of the whole brain. Also, only three translational parameters are varied to obtain optimal neighborhood similarity, using a simplex optimization procedure. The process is applied to all parts of the brain volume, with successive cubes being recursively selected by stepping through every node of the entire volume in a 3D grid pattern (Collins *et al.*, 1995a, 1995b). The size of the cube at each scale step is set at 1.5 FWHM with a node spacing set at 0.5 FWHM in each direction. After each scale step, the three translational parameters at each node define a 3D nonlinear deformation field, representing the nonlinear component of intersubject neuroanatomical variability.

B. Validation

The performance of the ANIMAL algorithm has previously been validated against experimental or digital brain phantom data and manual labeling of MRI data (Collins *et al.*, 1995a; Sorlie *et al.*, 1995). Some representative work, included for illustration, used a digital brain phantom created by identifying different structures and tissue types from an MR data set of a single volunteer. The volume is sampled on a $1 \times 1 \times 1$ mm³ matrix and covers the entire head. The resulting labeled volume could then be endowed with the appropriate contrast for each tissue type, and Rayleigh noise added, to resemble a true MRI acquisition. This 3D data set provides a gold standard with which to evaluate the linear registration algorithm. It should be noted that it does not matter that some voxels from the original MRI data may have been mislabeled. The labeled volume is now a phantom defined as *truth* that, even though no different in principle than a simple geometric phantom, closely mimics the convoluted nature of a real brain

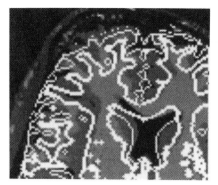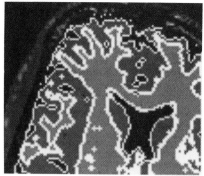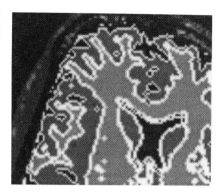

FIGURE 2 Segmentation of digital brain phantom. Three transverse images of the 3D digital brain phantom through the ventricles at the level of the basal ganglia are shown with the contours of the resulting segmentation superposed. The underlying image, the same in each case, was derived by application of a 3D thin-plate spline deformation to the initial brain phantom volume. The contours, defined initially on the unwarped volume, were then mapped to the warped volume in three ways. They correspond to the head of the caudate, the lateral ventricles, and the gray and white matter boundaries. On the left, the contours are mapped through the linear transformation only. In the center are the correctly warped contours, generated by mapping the original atlas contours through the known TPS transformation. On the right are the contours resulting from the ANIMAL segmentation. Almost no difference is visible between the two rightmost sets of contours.

and whose intensities and noise characteristics match those dealt with in MRI. An arbitary 3D distortion was applied to the T_1-weighted data using a thin-plate spline (TPS) transformation to produce a topologically equivalent, but spatially warped target data set. Noise of 10%, corresponding to the typical signal-to-noise ratio of our MRI scanner, was added to the source volume. In addition to the voxels classified as gray or white matter, the voxels contained in five anatomical structures (head of left and right caudate, lateral and third ventricles) were manually identified on the original unwarped phantom data. Application of the known TPS transformation to the labeled voxels identified corresponding voxels in the TPS-warped volume. ANIMAL was then applied to map the original volume to the TPS-warped volume with the goal of identifying the same voxels in the TPS-warped volume. The results were evaluated by calculating the percent difference, δ, and the percent overlap, Δ, between the known voxels within each TPS-warped structure and those identified by ANIMAL.

C. Statistical Probability Anatomy Maps

1. Comparison with Manual Labeling

As described previously, a primary motivation for the development of the ANIMAL algorithm is the need for automatic labeling of individual brain structures in each of a set of 3D MRI volumes and ultimately the automatic generation of probability maps for each structure. The utility of the algorithm for this was eval-

uated by statistical comparison of SPAMs for the frontal cortex labeled in 10 individual MRI volumes, generated by manual labeling or by ANIMAL. Individual volumes were collected as 160 1-mm thick contiguous slices with a 3D gradient-echo T_1-weighted sequence ($T_R/T_E = 18/10$ msec). Manual labeling was performed using a triplane display with real-time update of the transverse, sagittal, and coronal planes through a manually driven 3D cursor. At each voxel, the manual and automated SPAMs were compared by calculation of a z-statistic of the form

$$z = \left| \frac{P_a - P_b}{\sqrt{P(1-P)(1/N_a + 1/N_b)}} \right| \qquad (1)$$

where P_a, P_b and N_a, N_b are probabilities and subject numbers at each voxel and

$$P = \frac{N_a P_a + N_b P_b}{N_a + N_b} \qquad (2)$$

2. Generation of SPAMs for Multiple Regions

ANIMAL was applied as illustrated in Figure 1 to a total of 45 normal MRI volumes, obtained from young normal volunteers using the same pulse sequence. The 3D spatial transformation between each volume and the target volume was first obtained. A set of 3D neuroanatomical regions, both deep gray structures and lobar cortex zones, were labeled within the target volume by a trained neuroanatomist (CJH). The inverse spatial transformations were applied to label each volume in its native space. Finally, a nine-parameter linear stereo-

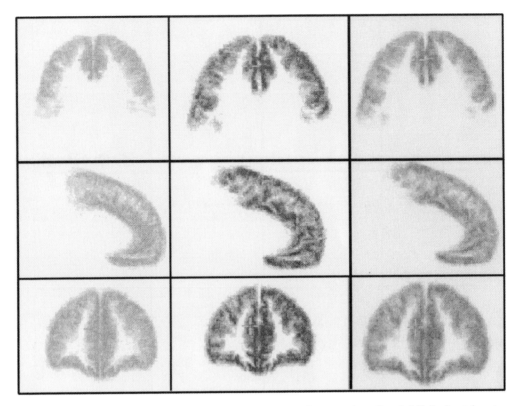

FIGURE 3   Visual comparison between manual and automatic generation of probabilistic frontal cortex from 10 brains. The left column shows three orthogonal cuts through the probabilistic map for frontal cortex derived from manual labeling of frontal cortex in 10 MRI volumes from young normal volunteers. The middle column shows corresponding cuts through the ANIMAL-generated equivalent. (Note that each panel has independent pan–zoom capability and so images in the left and middle columns may look incompatible. When images are combined, as in the rightmost column, pan–zoom parameters are identical.)

taxic transformation was applied to the individually labeled MRI volumes, now using a 305-MRI average MRI volume as the target for ANIMAL, running in linear mode (Evans *et al.*, 1992, 1993, 1994; Collins *et al.*, 1994).

III. RESULTS

As Figure 2 shows, the structures in the TPS-warped data are outlined well by the ANIMAL-warped contours, when compared to a simple nine-parameter linear transformation. Since a preclassified data set was used to create the brain phantom, the set of gray matter and white matter voxels were known and the overlap indices could be evaluated in the same way for the tissue classes as for the brain structures. Table 1 shows that on average, δ was reduced by more than half, from 4.2% to 1.7%, and Δ was improved 38%, from 70.4% to 97.0% when comparing nonlinear to linear matching.

Figure 3 compares the the manual and automated SPAMs for the frontal cortex from 10 subjects. Figure 4 shows the statistical z-field expressing significant differences between the two, thresholded at $z = 2.0$ and $z = 3.0$. The z-field is shown after convolution of the

TABLE 1   Segmentation Results for Brain Phantom

Structure	Linear		Nonlinear	
	δ	Δ	δ	Δ
Caudate	1.3%	65.7%	4.9%	96.4%
Ventricle	7.0%	77.6%	−0.0%	99.1%
Gray	3.4%	72.0%	1.0%	97.0%
White	5.0%	66.1%	−0.7%	95.6%
Average	4.2%	70.4%	1.7%	97.0%

Note. This table shows the percent volume difference, δ, and the percent volume overlap, Δ, for the individual structures defined on the digital brain phantom and segmented from a manually warped data set. These values are normalized to the true structure volume.

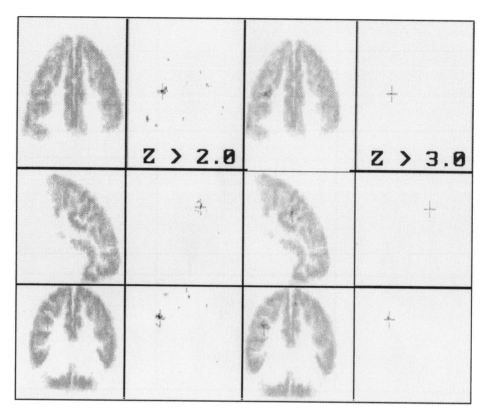

FIGURE 4 The z-statistic map for differences between manual and automatic generation of probabilistic frontal cortex from 10 brains. Statistical comparison of manual- and ANIMAL-generated probability maps for the frontal cortex where the z-statistic used is defined in equation (1). The z-map, smoothed with a 2 mm–FWHM 3D-Gaussian kernel, is thresholded at $z = 2.0$ and $z = 3.0$. Interleaved columns show the ANIMAL-generated probability map for comparison. The 3D cursor, defining the intersection of the three orthogonal planes displayed, is located on the single region exceeding the $z = 2.0$ threshold. No regions in the z-field exceeded $z = 3.0$.

original SPAMs with a 2 mm FWHM 3D Gaussian kernel, because the z-field should carry no signal spatial frequencies higher than the cutoff resolution used for the ANIMAL algorithm. The deformation field derived for each source volume applies equivalently to all internal structures. Hence, any new label can be defined in the target space and used to label the corresponding structure in each source MRI volume without a time-consuming recalculation of the deformation field. Figures 5, 6, and 7 show SPAMs for the frontal cortex, temporal cortex, and caudate nucleus, each derived from application of the procedure outlined in Figure 1 to 45 MRI volumes.

IV. DISCUSSION

The automatic segmentation method presented here reverses the standard segmentation strategy, from the matching of geometric contours directly to image data to regional labeling through nonlinear image deformation. The structures identified by this method are comparable to those segmented manually; and the experimental results on both simulated and real MRI data have shown that the method is accurate and robust (see Figs. 2, 3, and 4). The ANIMAL algorithm allows a mapping of any previously defined segmentation scheme onto individual MRI volumes so that this information can be obtained in a reproducible fashion. Once the deformation field has been defined, it is possible to use the strategy outlined in Figure 1 to generate any number of SPAMs for structures predefined in the target volume as illustrated by the selected examples in Figures 5, 6, and 7. It must be acknowledged that the automated approach may never be able to match human capabilities for outlining the finest details of individual brain structures, particularly in areas of high variance for location, sulcal pattern, or surface detail. It remains to be seen whether the objectivity and precision of an automated approach outweighs this de-

AVERAGE   PROBABILISTIC
MRI   FRONTAL CORTEX   OVERLAY

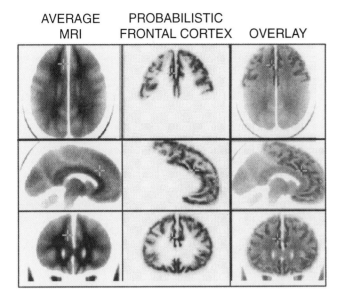

FIGURE 5 Probabilistic frontal cortex from 45 brains. Triplane display through the ANIMAL-generated probability map, derived from 45 individual MRI volumes, for frontal cortex (middle column), the 305-member average MRI (left column), and the overlay of the two (right column). Note pan–zoom comments for Figure 3.

AVERAGE   PROBABILISTIC
MRI   CAUDATE NUCLEUS   OVERLAY

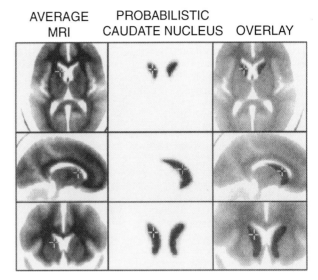

FIGURE 7 Probabilistic caudate nucleus from 45 brains. Triplane display through the ANIMAL-generated probability map, derived from 45 individual MRI volumes, for the caudate nucleus (middle column), the 305-member average MRI (left column), and the overlay of the two (right column). Note pan–zoom comments for Figure 3.

creased ability to delineate fine structures when investigating possible group differences between normal subjects or patients.

The goal of a probabilistic 3D description of normal neuroanatomy will take many years to achieve. It is most probable that the major components, that is, the

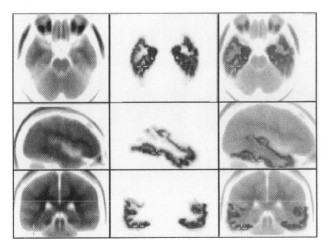

FIGURE 6 Probabilistic temporal cortex from 45 brains. Triplane display through the ANIMAL-generated probability map, derived from 45 individual MRI volumes, for temporal cortex (middle column), the 305-member average MRI (left column), and the overlay of the two (right column). Note pan–zoom comments for Figure 3.

target volumes and features, the matching and segmentation procedure, and the database being segmented, will all be repeatedly updated during that time. However, technical improvements in computers and brain imaging equipment combined with the knowledge gained at each iteration should produce an accelerating cycle. The work described here is part of a broader program to create a probabilistic atlas of human neuroanatomy by the International Consortium for Brain Mapping (ICBM, Mazziotta *et al.*, 1995). This effort will combine large numbers of normal MRI volumes with smaller numbers of high-resolution (100 micron) macrocryotome volumes in a stereotaxic space. These data will be labeled anatomically in different ways, and statistical maps of structural variance will be generated in ways similar to that described here. Functional information will be added as voxel attributes as well as pointers to nonvoxel databases. The ICBM perspective is that any single segmentation scheme, or atlas, will always be unacceptable to some sectors of the scientific community or become obsolete with time. Therefore it is vital that an automated regional labeling be independent of the specific form of parcellation employed so that many atlases can be applied simultaneously to any given brain. The segmentation strategy employed with the ANIMAL algorithm offers that independence.

Acknowledgments

We wish to thank Dr. Keith Worsley for advice on statistical matters as well as Peter Neelin, David MacDonald, and Greg Ward for help in data processing. The authors would like to express their appreciation for support from the Canadian Medical Research Council (SP-30), the McDonnell–Pew Cognitive Neuroscience Center Program, the U.S. Human Brain Project (HBP), NIMH, and NIDA. This work forms part of a continuing project of the HBP-funded International Consortium for Brain Mapping to develop a probabilistic atlas of human neuroanatomy.

References

Collins, D., Holmes, C., Peters, T., and Evans, A. (1995a). Automatic 3d model-based neuroanatomical segmentation. *Hum. Brain Mapping,* **3:** 190–208.

Collins, D. L., Evans, A. C., Holmes, C., and Peters, T. M. (1995b). Automatic 3D segmentation of neuro-anatomical structures from MRI. *In:* "Information Processing in Medical Imaging (IPMI)" (Bizais, Y., Barillot, C., and Paola, R. D., Eds.), pp. 139–152. Kluwer, Dordrecht, The Netherlands.

Collins, D. L., Neelin, P., Peters, T. M., and Evans, A. C. (1994). Automatic 3D inter-subject registration of MR volumetric data in standardized talairach space. *J. Comput. Assist. Tomogr.* **18**(2): 192–205.

Evans, A. C., Collins, D. L., Mills, S. R., Brown, E. D., Kelly, R. L., and Peters, T. M. (1993). 3d statistical neuroanatomical models from 305 mri volumes. *In:* Proc. IEEE-Nuclear Science Symposium and Medical Imaging Conference, pp. 1813–1817.

Evans, A. C., Collins, D. L., and Milner, B. (1992). An MRI-based stereotactic atlas from 250 young normal subjects. *Soc. Neurosci. Abstr.* **18:** 408.

Evans, A. C., Dai, W., Collins, D. L., Neelin, P., and Marrett, T. (1991). Warping of a computerized 3-D atlas to match brain image volumes for quantitative neuroanatomical and functional analysis. *In:* Proceedings of the International Society of Optical Engineering: Medical Imaging V, Vol. 1445, San Jose, California. SPIE.

Evans, A. C., Kamber, M., Collins, D. L., and MacDonald, D. (1994). An mri-based probabilistic atlas of neuroanatomy. *In:* "Magnetic Resonance Scanning and Epilepsy" (Shorvon, S., Ed.), pp. 263–274. Plenum, New York.

Koenderink, J., and van Doorn, A. (1987). Representation of local geometry in the visual system. *Biol. Cybern.* **55:** 367–375.

Mazziotta, J. C., Toga, A. W., Evans, A. C., Fox, P. T., and Lancaster, J. (1995). A probabilistic atlas of the human brain: Theory and rationale for its development. *Neuroimage* **2:** 89–101.

Minoshima, S., Koeppe, R., Frey, K., and Kuhl, D. (1994). Anatomic standardization: Linear scaling and nonlinear warping of functional brain images. *J. Nucl. Med.* **35**(9): 1528–1537.

Roland, P., Graufelds, C., Wahlin, J., Ingelman, L., Andersson, M., Ledberg, A., Pedersen, J., Ackerman, S., Dabringhaus, A., and Zilles, K. (1994). Human brain atlas: For high-resolution functional and anatomical mapping. *Hum. Brain Mapping,* 173–184.

Sorlie, C., Collins, D., Worsley, K., and Evans, A. (1995). Neuroanatomical variability: A quantitative study of young normal brains in stereotaxic space. *Hum. Brain Mapping,* in press.

tar Haar Romeny, B., Florack, L. M., Koenderink, J. J., and Viergever, M. A. (1991). Scale space: Its natural operators and differential invariants. *In:* "Information Processing in Medical Imaging." (A. C. F. Colchester and D. J. Hawkes, Eds.), p. 239. Wye, UK. IPMI.

Woods, R., Mazziotta, J., and Cherry, S. (1993). MRI-PET registration with automated algorithm. *J. Comput. Assist. Tomogr.* **17:** 536–546.

Difference Image vs Ratio Image Error Function Forms in PET–PET Realignment

ABRAHAM Z. SNYDER

Department of Neurology and Neurosurgery
Washington University School of Medicine
St. Louis, Missouri 63110

A mathematical analysis of common modality image registration is presented. Two alternative formulas are compared for computing registration error, the basis of these being computation of image differences vs. ratios. The theory suggests that the difference image method should be numerically more stable as well as more immune to noise. To test the theory, a Hoffman brain phantom was repeatedly scanned in one position and images of variable statistical quality and spatial frequency content were prepared. These data were then submitted for realignment according to either the difference or the ratio image method. The difference image error function yielded consistently better precision in all but the most blurred data, in which case the two methods performed comparably. The precision advantage of the difference image method was attributable mainly to better determination of angular registration error as a consequence of reduced sensitivity to noise and therefore greater tolerance of increased spatial frequency bandwidth. These results indicate that a modest improvement in realignment precision can be achieved by the use of error functions based on image differences as opposed to ratios.

I. INTRODUCTION AND THEORY

Interscan head movement causes an artifact in the difference images acquired in functional mapping experiments based on subtractive methodology. Several automated procedures for minimizing this artifact have been described (Andersson, 1995; Eberl *et al.*, 1993; Hoh *et al.*, 1993; Mintun and Lee, 1990; Woods *et al.*,

1992). All work by resampling one member of an image pair while searching for that rigid body coordinate transformation that minimizes the registration error. The various algorithms differ primarily in the functional form used to compute this error. In the method of ratio image variance minimization (Woods *et al.*, 1992), the registration error is computed as

$$\varepsilon_r^2 = \frac{1}{V} \iiint \left[\bar{r} - \frac{f_2(x', y', z')}{f_1(x, y, z)} \right]^2 dV$$

where $f_1(x, y, z)$ and $f_2(x', y', z')$ are the image activity profiles and $\bar{r}$ is the mean activity ratio. Alternatively, it is possible to directly minimize difference image variance. Registration error is then computed as

$$\varepsilon_d^2 = \frac{1}{V} \iiint [f_1(x, y, z) - cf_2(x', y', z')]^2 dV$$

where c is a scalar compensating for unequal global activity. If both images are scaled to a common whole brain mean, then $\bar{r} = c = 1$, as is assumed in what follows. It is evident that ε_r^2 is asymmetric with respect to f_1 and f_2 whereas in ε_d^2, f_1 and f_2 are equivalent. Numerical instability due to division by small numbers is a consideration in computing ε_r^2. Nevertheless, in the absence of noise, either functional form must lead to the correct result (assuming $f_1 \neq 0$ everywhere), because the unique coordinate transformation that brings the images into register corresponds to $\varepsilon_d^2 = \varepsilon_r^2 = 0$. It should be noted that ε_d^2 is closely related to the sum of absolute differences measure (SAD) (Hoh *et al.*, 1993; Eberl *et al.*, 1993).

To examine the question of precision in the presence of noise, suppose that both images represent the same

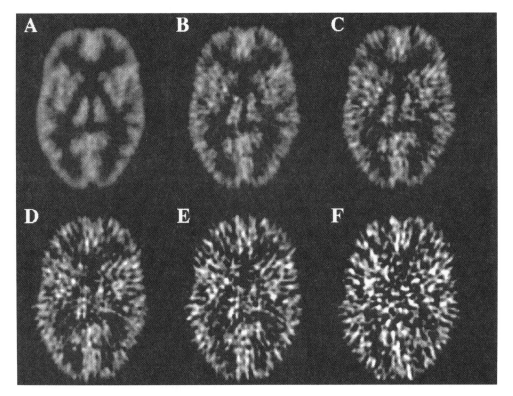

FIGURE 1 One slice from Hoffman phantom images of varying statistical quality A, 110×10^6 counts; B, 16×10^6 counts; C, 8×10^6 counts; D, 4×10^6 counts; E, 2×10^6 counts; F, 1×10^6 counts. All images are scaled to the same whole brain activity mean. The precision measures shown in Figures 2, 3, and 4 have been averaged over multiple scan pairs numbering as follows: B, 42; C, D, E, 90; F, 120.

underlying activity profile and that they are in register. That is,

$$f_1(x, y, z) = f(x, y, z) + z_1(x, y, z)$$
$$f_2(x', y', z') = f(x, y, z) + z_2(x', y', z')$$
$$[x', y', z'] = [x, y, z]$$

where z_1 and z_2 represent image noise. Now suppose $[x', y', z']$ is in error by some displacement (a) in x. Then

$$f_1 - f_2 = f(x, y, z) - f(x - a, y, z) + z_1(x, y, z)$$
$$- z_2(x - a, y, z) \simeq aD_x f + z_{\text{dif}}$$

where $aD_x f$ represents the first term in the Taylor series expansion of $f(x, y, z) - f(x - a, y, z)$. Inserting this approximation into the definition of ε_d^2 yields

$$\varepsilon_d^2 = \frac{1}{V} \iiint [f_1 - f_2]^2 \, dV$$
$$\simeq \frac{a^2}{V} \iiint [D_x f]^2 \, dV + \frac{2a}{V} \iiint [D_x f] [z_{\text{dif}}] \, dV$$
$$+ \frac{1}{V} \iiint [z_{\text{dif}}]^2 \, dV$$

where ε_d^2 is quadratic in a. The constant term corresponds purely to noise and depends in no systematic way on image registration, assuming z_1 and z_2 are uncorrelated. The quadratic term is entirely deterministic; more generally it is proportional to the volume average of $|\nabla f|^2$. Now minimizing ε_d^2 with respect to a gives

$$a = \delta x' = \frac{\iiint [D_x f] [z_{\text{dif}}] \, dV}{\iiint [D_x f]^2 \, dV}$$

whereas the correct answer is $a = 0$. It is thus demonstrated that realignment precision depends on a sort of "gradient-to-noise" ratio. It is reasonable to expect no systematic errors, assuming $D_x f$ and z_{dif} are uncorrelated.

Applying the previous example to the analysis of ε_r^2, we have

$$\varepsilon_r^2 = \frac{1}{V} \iiint \left[\frac{f(x, y, z) + z_1 - f(x - a, y, z) - z_2}{f(x, y, z) + z_1} \right]^2 dV$$

Inserting $f(x, y, z) - f(x - a, y, z) \simeq aD_x f$ gives

$$\varepsilon_r^2 \simeq \frac{1}{V} \iiint \left[\frac{aD_x f + z_{\text{dif}}}{f + z_1} \right]^2 dV$$

$$\simeq \frac{a^2}{V} \iiint [D_x \ln f]^2 \, dV + \frac{2a}{V} \iiint [D_x \ln f] \, [z_{\text{dif}}] \, dV$$

$$+ \frac{1}{V} \iiint \left[\frac{z_{\text{dif}}}{f} \right]^2 dV$$

The last approximation is valid when $z_1 \ll f$. As before, registration error is quadratic in a. Now, however, precision depends on a ratio in which the underlying activity distribution (but not difference image noise) enters as its logarithm.

$$a = \delta x' = \frac{\iiint [D_x \ln f] \, [z_{\text{dif}}] \, dV}{\iiint [D_x \ln f]^2 \, dV}$$

When $z_1 \simeq f$ or $z_1 > f$, ε_r^2 tends to behave more like ε_d^2. But this means that the noise dominated parts of the data contribute disproportionately to the realignment computations.

The preceding arguments are somewhat more tedious but essentially the same when f_1 and f_2 are related by an arbitrary rigid body transformation. The theory was tested as described next.

II. METHODS

A Hoffman brain phantom filled with 75 MBq ^{18}F was scanned in stationary mode (Siemens ECAT 953B) with the septa extended. Then, 120 runs with 1.0×10^6 net true counts each, all at the same phantom position, were acquired and conventionally 2D reconstructed. Four additional groups of scans with graded statistical quality were created by summing together 2, 4, 8, or 16 of the 10^6 count images (Fig. 1). Afterward, 21–60 independent scan pairs from each statistical quality group were submitted for realignment according to either ε_r^2 or ε_d^2. The computations were run in both directions; that is, with f_1 and f_2 exchanging roles. Early and late scans were paired to minimize within-group inhomogeneity of rate dependent statistics (randoms fraction 0.03 to 0.08). The volume of evaluation was consistently restricted to the region for which both f_1 and f_2 fell within the interior of a mask prepared from a high (110×10^6) count image by filtering (2.2 cm FWHM Gaussian) and thresholding at 20% maximum.

Before being submitted for realignment the images were low-pass filtered (fifth-order Butterworth) with the cutoff frequency systematically varied between 0.2 cm^{-1} and 1.1 cm^{-1}. Realignment precision was evaluated separately for each statistical quality group, prefilter, and error function. For each realignment, the obtained translation $(\delta x, \delta y, \delta z)$ and rotation $(\delta \alpha, \delta \beta, \delta \gamma)$ parameters were combined into total root mean squares (rms) linear and angular precision measures:

$$\delta r = \sqrt{(\delta x)^2 + (\delta y)^2 + (\delta z)^2}$$
$$\delta \eta = \sqrt{(\delta \alpha)^2 + (\delta \beta)^2 + (\delta \gamma)^2}$$

Movement due to angular motion was computed as an intensity weighted average by analogy with rigid body angular momentum:

$$(\delta r_{\text{ang}})^2 = \frac{\iiint f(x, y, z) \, |\delta \omega \times \mathbf{u}|^2 \, dV}{\iiint f(x, y, z) \, dV}$$
$$\text{where } \delta \omega = [\delta \alpha \, \delta \beta \, \delta \gamma]^t$$
$$\mathbf{u} = [x \, y \, z]^t$$

The total translation and rotation movement was computed as $\delta r_{\text{tot}} = \sqrt{(\delta r)^2 + (\delta r_{\text{ang}})^2}$. Finally, for each statistical quality group, prefilter and error functional form and arithmetic averages of the measures δr, $\delta \eta$, and δr_{tot} were obtained over all scan pairs.

III. RESULTS AND DISCUSSION

The main results are shown in Figures 2 and 3. Several features consistent with the present theory are evident. In particular, the data show that realignment precision generally scales with difference image noise as

$$\delta r_{\text{tot}} \propto \langle [\nabla f] \, [z_{\text{dif}}] \rangle \propto \frac{1}{\sqrt{N}}$$

using the well-known relationship between noise and the square root of net true counts (N). The ratio and difference image error functions performed comparably when the images were prefiltered to exclude frequencies greater than 0.3 cm^{-1}. However, the ratio image method precision deteriorated monotonically as progressively more high spatial frequencies were admitted (Fig. 2), whereas the difference image method characteristically performed nearly optimally over a broad range of filters (Fig. 3). It is noted that the ratio image method results shows a consistent optimum at 0.25 cm^{-1}, but this feature occurs very close to a precipitous fall in performance. It would, therefore, seem prudent, if ratio image uniformity is used for realignment, to blur images well before presentation to the algorithm, as recommended by the original authors (Woods *et al.*, 1992).

Figure 4 shows the total movement measures (δr_{tot}) corresponding to Figures 2 and 3. Table 1 lists, for

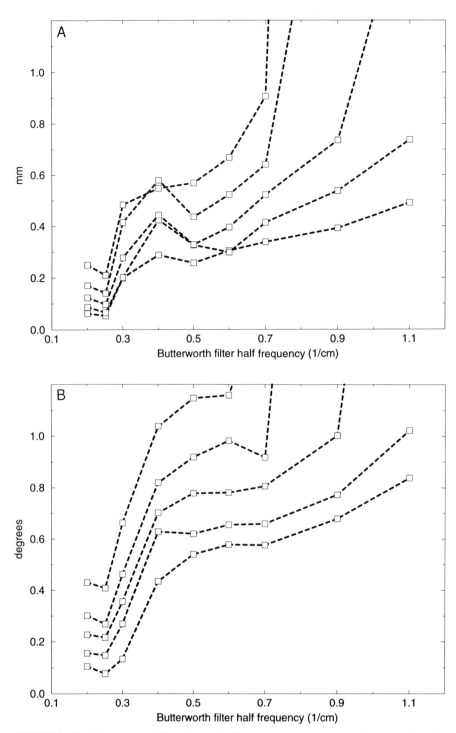

FIGURE 2 Realignment precision obtained with the ratio image registration error function ε_r^2. The five curves correspond, from bottom to top, to the statistical qualities B, C, D, E, and F shown in Figure 1; (A) translation (δr); (B) rotation ($\delta \eta$).

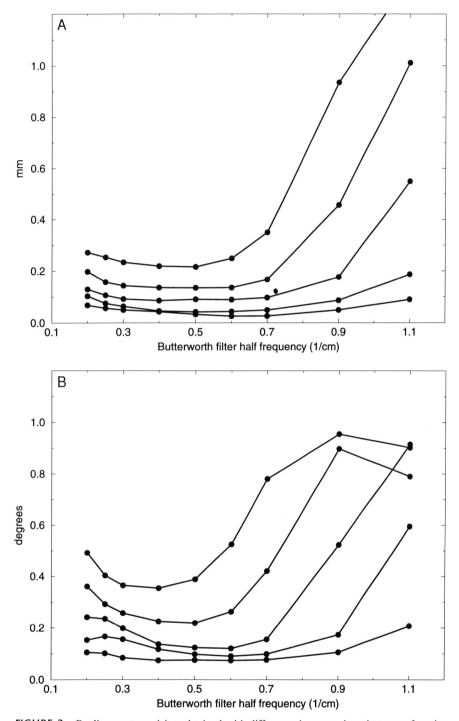

FIGURE 3 Realignment precision obtained with difference image registration error function ε_d^2; all else as in Figure 2.

each statistical quality group, the best precision (least measured total movement) achieved by both realignment methods. The difference image method yielded consistently better precision. It is, however, unclear that the gain of reducing image registration uncertainty from, say, 0.20 to 0.13 mm is of particularly great practical importance. Perhaps more of a practical advantage would result from the fact that the ratio image method tends to numerical instability unless the error function is evaluated on a fairly dense three-dimensional grid,

TABLE 1   Best Achieved Precision

Net trues per image	Ratio image method		Difference image method	
	Best prefilter (cm⁻¹)	Precision (rms mm)	Best prefilter (cm⁻¹)	Precision (rms mm)
16×10^6	0.25	0.082	0.6	0.067
8×10^6	0.25	0.135	0.6	0.088
4×10^6	0.25	0.206	0.6	0.131
2×10^6	0.25	0.266	0.5	0.224
1×10^6	0.25	0.396	0.4	0.361

Note. The prefilter (low-pass fifth-order Butterworth) yielding the best precision is identified by its half-amplitude (cutoff) frequency.

such as one sample every 4 mm³. The difference image method tolerates considerably more coarse sampling, such as one sample every 8 mm³, and so executes much faster.

Angular uncertainty (δr_{ang}) contributes more to total imprecision than translational uncertainty (δr) in most of the data. Figure 4 therefore resembles Figure 2(B) and 3(B) more than Figures 2(A) and 3(A). It may not be generally recognized that the translational part of

the realignment problem can be solved even with very blurred images, assuming that the brain edges are within the field of view, simply by aligning the centers of mass. Note the relative flatness of the curves in Figure 3(A) at cutoff frequencies less than 0.6 cm⁻¹. The angular part of the problem, on the other hand, depends on resolution of brain structure. Note the presence of clear minima in Figure 3(B). Excessive blurring is, therefore, counterproductive when realigning on the

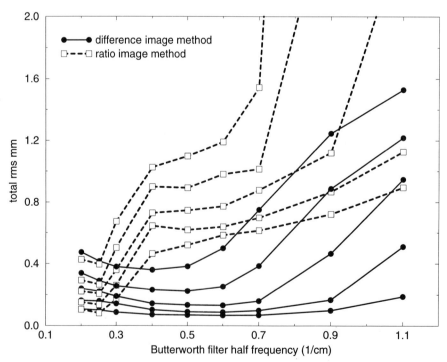

FIGURE 4   Whole brain realignment uncertainty (δr_{tot}) corresponding to the results shown in Figures 2 and 3. Please note a change in ordinate scale in comparison to Figures 2(A) and 3(A).

basis of ε_d^2. However, ε_d^2 can be understood as a more robust measure in comparison to ε_r^2 because it makes better use of the available "gradient-to-noise" ratio (defined previously) and consequently is more tolerant of broad spatial frequency bandwidth. The increased bandwidth can then be used to determine the angular component of image realignment. A very blurred PET image of the human brain begins to approximate a spherical shell for which, because of symmetry, the angular part of the realignment problem is completely unconstrained.

Acknowledgments

Supported by National Institute of Neurological and Communicative Disorders and Stroke Grant NS06833 and the Charles A. Dana Foundation.

References

Andersson, J. L. R. (1995). A rapid and accurate method to realign PET scans using image edge information. *J. Nucl. Med.* **36:** 657–669.

Eberl, S., Kanno, I., Fulton, R. R., *et al.* (1993). Automatic 3D spatial alignment for correcting interstudy patient motion in serial PET studies. *In:* "Quantification of Brain Function: Tracer Kinetics and Image Analysis in Brain PET" (K. Uemura, N. A. Lassen, T. Jones, and I. Kanno, Eds.), pp. 419–426. Elsevier Science Publishers B. V., Amsterdam.

Hoh, C. K., Dahlbom, M., Harris, G., *et al.* (1993). Automated iterative three-dimensional registration of positron emission tomography images. *J. Nucl. Med.* **34:** 2009–2018.

Mintun, M. A., and Lee, K. S. (1990). Mathematical realignment of paired PET images to enable pixel-by-pixel subtraction. *J. Nucl. Med.* **31**(Suppl.), 816.

Woods, R. P., Cherry, S. R., and Mazziotta, J. C. (1992). Rapid automated algorithm for aligning and reslicing PET images. *J. Comput. Assist. Tomogr.* **16:** 620–633.

27

Tailored Coregistration of Striata for Dopaminergic PET

W. D. BROWN,[1] R. PYZALSKI,[1] M. CROSSNOE,[1] S. J. SWERDLOFF,[2] and J. E. HOLDEN[2]

[1]*Department of Radiology*
[2]*Department of Medical Physics*
University of Wisconsin Medical School
Madison, Wisconsin 53792

Although several intrasubject and intersubject brain image coregistration methods show great elegance and have been used very successfully in countless experiments, this chapter begins with the assertion that no coregistration method is perfect. In fact, the assumptions and weaknesses of each method usually are most apparent in the anatomical "outlier," who is in some cases the patient whose anatomy is distorted by the very disease being studied with PET. The authors, therefore, make the assertions that a method for intersubject coregistration is only as "good" as its success in handling outlier and pathologic anatomy and that the optimal methods for handling the data will be heavily dependent on the nature of the subject or patient population and on the portion of the brain of particular interest. In particular, coregistration methods that are explicitly or implicitly weighted toward fitting the cerebral cortex may not be optimal when the organs of primary interest are the deep nuclei. The specific example developed in this chapter is, therefore, one piece of evidence in a larger argument: that the anatomical intersubject coregistration used for a particular task can and should be tailored to the specific anatomy and pathology being currently studied. The specific example used is the neostriatum, of particular interest in dopaminergic and other ligand studies; a description of its particular biological variability and corollary coregistration requirements are presented.

I. INTRODUCTION

There is infinite variety in the gross anatomy of the human brain. Initially for reasons of safer stereotaxic surgery (see Talairach and Tournoux, 1988, as a recent example) and later for reasons of combination and reporting of physiologic image data (Fox *et al.*, 1985; Friston *et al.*, 1989; Pelizzari *et al.*, 1989; Alpert *et al.*, 1990; Pietrzyk *et al.*, 1990; Greitz *et al.*, 1991; and Woods *et al.*, 1993), both manual and automated methods have been developed for the (co)registration of brain images into a standard coordinate system, or "stereotaxic space." As with many numerical methods applied to data with a high degree of variance, the accuracy, precision, and usefulness of any such method is necessarily dependent on specific sets of data as well as on the measure(s) used to determine "goodness of fit." As is also generally the case, *a priori* knowledge of the nature of the data will assist in optimizing the result. This chapter uses the example of the variation in position of the striatal nuclei with respect to overall brain size, as evaluated using high-resolution brain MRI scans, to demonstrate the need for context-specific optimization of coregistration methods.

II. MATERIALS AND METHODS

The data for this study are 3D MRI data sets, obtained using a gradient-recalled echo with a spoiler gradient (SPGR, for the earlier studies; fast, FSPGR, for the later studies) sequences reconstructed into 1.0 mm axial slices. All data were acquired on a clinical MRI scanner (GE Signa Advantage, 1.5 T). Image display, determination of landmark coordinates, and creation of volumes of interest (VOIs) were performed

---

using the program Pinnacle, originally developed at the University of Wisconsin for use in planning of stereotaxic radiosurgery.

Though the applicability of these results are not dependent on the choice of anatomic standard and are not strictly dependent on the choice of affine vs. plastic transformation method, for reasons of common use and simplicity of demonstration, the following assumptions are represented in the various data identified as "normalized": (1) The Talairach atlas (Talairach and Tournoux, 1988) was used as the registration "goal"; and (2) affine transformations would be performed such that lateral scaling would be performed based on whole brain width.

The initial measurements consisted of simply finding suitably reliable "landmark" points that provided indices of the size and position of the caudate nuclei and putamina bilaterally, with their distances from the anatomical midplane of the brain. These were functionally defined as follows:

1. The cortical points (in the posterior part of the superior temporal gyri) that were farthest from the midplane to the left and right;
2. The greatest distance each putamen reaches from the midplane at the coronal level of the anterior commissure (AC);
3. The nearest distance each caudate head reaches with respect to the midplane at the coronal level of the AC;
4. The (distance from midplane of the) most superior point of the body of each caudate nucleus.

From these were derived the following direct indices of striatal size and location:

1. Whole brain width (W);
2. Whole striatal width for each hemisphere (S)—the distance along the axis normal to the midplane from medial caudate to lateral putamen in each hemisphere;
3. Lateral putaminal separation (P)—from right to left lateral putaminal excursions;
4. Superior caudate separation (C)— from right to left superior-most caudate points;
5. Medial caudate separation—from right to left most medial caudate points.

Because of the very small absolute value of this last parameter with respect to the uncertainty of measurement, no reproducible results could be obtained, and so these numerical data will not be presented here. Index 1 will be expressed as a normalized value, divided by the value from Talairach. Indices 2–4 will be presented as ratios of the measurement to the total

TABLE 1   Discrete-Point-Derived Indices of Striatal Size and Position

Index	Normalized mean	Std. dev.	Coeff. of var.	Outliers (divided by mean)
W	.98	.03	3%	.94 (= −2.1 s.d.)
S	1.09	.05	5%	.88 (= −2.3 s.d.)
P	1.08	.03	3%	1.06 (= +2.1 s.d.)
C	1.07	.16	15%	.74 (< 1 s.d.)
				.89 (< 1 s.d.)
				1.42 (= +2.8 s.d.)

Note. For definition of indices and description of normalization, see the text.

width of the brain, normalized to the corresponding ratio from the Talairach atlas.

Because the method described previously, based on determination of single points, may be subject to errors in landmark localization, additional indices of putaminal and caudate location were obtained as follows: The anatomic boundaries of the caudate nuclei and putamina were outlined manually, yielding a volume of interests for each nucleus; each VOI was converted into a synthetic "image set" in which all voxels internal to the VOI were given the same positive value and all external voxels were set to 0; and the anatomic "center of mass" (all voxels given equal weight) was calculated for each nucleus. Since standard centers of mass of the striatal nuclei could not be derived precisely from the Talairach atlas, these data will be presented in terms of variation from the mean of each index.

The preceding measures were compared to visual interpretation of ventricular size. An "outlier" was functionally defined as any measure that exceeded two standard deviations from the mean for that measure or any measure that deviated from the mean for that measure by more than 10%. This boundary is somewhat arbitrary but reflects a level of error that would be visible as "misregistration" in an affine coregistration as described previously and is described for that reason.

III. RESULTS AND DISCUSSION

The results of the discrete-point measures are given in Table 1. The results of the center-of-mass measures are given in Table 2. From these tables it is clear that whole brain width, striatal width, and putaminal localization are fairly well-behaved; that is, they are clustered fairly tightly around the mean. In sharp contrast,

TABLE 2   Center-of-Mass Derived Indices of
Striatal Position

Index	Coeff. of var.	Outliers (divided by mean)
Interputaminal distance	4%	1.10
Intercaudate distance	12%	.78
		.86
		1.31

Note. For definition of indices and description of normalization, see the text.

the locations of the caudate nuclei is far more variable. This largely reflects the sizes of the lateral ventricles and is a particularly prominent effect when the ventricles are truly enlarged. It should also be pointed out that this error effectively results in a rotation of the striatum around an axis roughly parallel to the anterior–posterior axis of the brain.

Several points should be emphasized, in particular with respect to this emphasis on the extreme cases, the so-called outliers. In general, PET scanning of diseased persons does not permit casting off "anatomic outliers," as may sometimes be done in studies of young healthy volunteers. In the particular example of dopaminergic studies in Parkinson's disease, patients are often elderly, increasing the probability that "anatomic outliers" will be found. For striatal coregistration, this can perhaps best be performed by individual coregistration of the two striata from each scan, rather than whole brain coregistration intact, to handle the problem of size mismatching location.

The coregistration method used in any study must handle extreme cases adequately. In general, the tracer used, age, and pathology all affect the potential accuracy of a given coregistration algorithm. We believe these statements justify the assertions that (1) a coregistration method is only "as good" as its handling of extreme cases and, therefore, (2) coregistration meth-

ods should be tailored to the anatomy, pathology, and patient population of interest in a particular study. With such variety, it seems that a given PET facility should have available a "toolbox" of different coregistration methods unless it wishes to create new software for each coregistration problem. This chapter has demonstrated the use of high-resolution MRI anatomical scanning for delineation of the special needs for coregistration of corresponding structures in physiologic PET scans.

Acknowledgments

The authors gratefully acknowledge the financial support of the National Institute for Neurological Disorders and Stroke (grant NS31612) and the University of Wisconsin Departments of Radiology and Medical Physics. The authors also thank Kevin Dabbs for his programming work related to this chapter.

References

Alpert, N. M., Bradshaw, J. F., Kennedy, D., and Correia, J. A. (1990). The principal axes transformation—A method for image registration. *J. Nucl. Med.* **31:** 1717–1722.

Fox, P. T., Perlmutter, J. S., and Raichle, M. E. (1985). A stereotactic method of anatomical localization for positron emission tomography. *J. Comput. Assist. Tomogr.* **9:** 141–153.

Friston, K. J., Passingham, R. E., Nutt, J. G., Heather, J. D., Sawle, G. V., and Frackowiak, R. S. (1989). Localisation in PET images: Direct fitting of the intercommissural (AC-PC) line. *J. Cereb. Blood Flow Metab.* **9:** 690–695.

Greitz, T., Bohm, C., Holte, S., and Eriksson, L. (1991). A computerized brain atlas: Construction, anatomical content, and some applications. *J. Comput. Assist. Tomogr.* **15:** 26–38.

Pelizzari, C. A., Chen, G. T., Spelbring, D. R., Weichselbaum, R. R., and Chen, C. T. (1989). Accurate three-dimensional registration of CT, PET and/or MR images of the brain. *J. Comput. Assist. Tomogr.* **13:** 20–26.

Pietrzyk, U., Herholz, K., and Heiss, W.-D. (1990). Three-dimensional alignment of functional and morphological tomograms. *J. Comput. Assist. Tomogr.* **14:** 51–59.

Talairach, J., and Tournoux, P. (1988). "Co-Planar Stereotaxic Atlas of the Human Brain." Thieme, New York.

Woods, W. P., Mazziotta, J. C., and Cherry, S. R. (1993). MRI-PET registration with automated algorithm. *J. Comput. Assist. Tomogr.* **17:** 536–546.

28

Optimization of PET–MRI Image Registration

D. BERDICHEVSKY, Z. LEVIN, E. D. MORRIS, and N. M. ALPERT

PET Imaging Laboratory
Massachusetts General Hospital
Boston, Massachusetts 02114

We report a system that optimizes PET–MRI registration. The optimization is at three levels: (1) automatic segmentation replaces manual drawing operations, (2) visual assessment of registration quality is enhanced by composite imaging methods, and (3) the entire procedure is embedded in a commercially available scientific visualization package, thereby providing a consistent graphical user interface. The segmentation procedure removes confounding extracranial structures from magnetic resonance images using a sequence of morphological operations and connected components analysis. Composite fusion in the 2D slice-by-slice mode and in 3D ray-traced volume renderings allows the operator to vary the fusion of PET and MRI in real time. The scientific visualization system provides a consistent user interface. The segmentation algorithm was tested on more than 30 MRI data sets and was successful in all cases. The composite imaging techniques provide a convenient, robust method for assessing the registration. These results are important because this procedure can be performed by technicians with no anatomic knowledge and reduces the required time from hours to about 5 min on a modern computer workstation.

I. INTRODUCTION

Several different methods for the registration of PET and MRI images have been described and validated (Pelizzari *et al.*, 1989; Woods *et al.*, 1993; Strother *et al.*, 1994; Turkington *et al.*, 1995). Although the registration is usually computed automatically, a sequence of manual steps is required to prepare the PET and MRI data. These manual steps often require hours of work and some knowledge of neuroanatomy. Generally, an operator must segment the MRI images, slice by slice, to remove extracranial structures, usually by manually drawing the brain surface. MRI data sets typically have between 64 and 124 slices, so this procedure is tedious and limits the application of these methods to research studies.

Another important component in the optimization of registration techniques is the visualization of the result, used to confirm the adequacy of the registration or for further analysis. The fusion of overlayed images is appealing for these purposes, provided it can be completely automated and controlled in a convenient fashion.

The goal of our work was to provide software that automates and systematizes this procedure.

II. METHODS

Software was written in ANSI C code to extend the capabilities of a commercial scientific visualization package, AVS (Advanced Visual Systems, Waltham, Massachusetts). PET data were ^{15}O-CBF studies, gathered with a GE-4096 PET camera with 15 slices, 6.5 mm axial thickness, and 8 mm transverse resolution. MRI data were acquired on GE-SIGNA scanners. Pulse sequences were either T_1-weighted or SPGR, with slice thickness ranging from 1.5 to 5 mm.

The registration procedure has four basic steps: (1) prepare the PET data, (2) prepare the MRI data, (3) perform the registration, and (4) use visualization techniques to confirm the registration. These will be detailed.

A. Preparation of PET Data

The PET data are thresholded to eliminate noise outside the brain volume. Cropping is used to restrict the field of view to the cerebrum and cerebellum.

B. Preparation of MRI Data

The image volume is resampled to cubic voxels. Cropping is used to restrict the volume to cerebral hemispheres and cerebellum. The volume histogram of gray levels is computed. Upper and lower thresholds are applied according to the histogram of gray levels. Binary erosion separates the image volume into clusters of voxels representing brain and extracranial tissues (Morris *et al.*, 1993). Connected components analysis is employed to find the largest cluster; that is, the brain. Binary dilation, performed on the brain cluster, restores the brain surface.

Several features of the process merit further comment. Resampling to cubic voxels is accomplished by trilinear interpolation, according to the known physical dimensions of the original MRI voxels. The two-dimensional connected components algorithm of Haralick (1981) was extended to three dimensions by altering the kernel and applying it in top-down and bottom-up passes in *x*, *y*, and *z*. Three-dimensional binary erosion and dilation were accelerated by implementation at the bit level using volume-shifting operations and logical operators as described by Haralick and Shapiro (1992) rather than voxel-by-voxel application of the erosion–dilation kernel through the volume.

The segmentation can be controlled by varying several parameters. The lower threshold is set to eliminate background noise from the image, whereas the upper threshold is set to contrast voxels whose intensity values are distinct from those in the brain tissue. This thresholding creates a wider space between intra- and extracranial structures. Remaining islands connecting intra- and extracranial structures are broken by binary erosion, which can be controlled by choice of kernel size, shape, and the number of erosion passes. The computational elements of this procedure on volumes of $256 \times 256 \times 180$ voxels require less than 1 min on a 100 MHz workstation. Accordingly, adjustment of the segmentation parameters can be based on visualization of the resulting segmentation and thus allows fine control of the segmentation process. However, it should be noted, for a given pulse sequence and im-

aging protocol, all erosion–dilation parameters can be fixed, only the lower threshold need be adjusted.

C. Image Registration

Image registration was performed using the Woods algorithm (Woods *et al.*, 1993) on PET images of blood flow and MRI images of structural–anatomic data.

D. Visualization

Visualization is accomplished using standard composite image and volume rendering modules from the AVS library along with custom extensions that synchronize the independent processes. In general, PET and MRI are handled separately until the compositing step. In the 2D mode, three views are provided: transverse, coronal, and sagittal. Widgets control slice selection, image contrast, color mapping, and the proportion of PET and MRI in the fusion. Alternatively, with the computer mouse, the operator can select three orthogonal views passing through a chosen point.

In the 3D mode the user constructs a fused ray-traced volume rendering. The volume can be excavated to reveal internal structures of interest. The procedure employs a ''pilot view'' in which the operator uses the mouse to point at structures to be excavated and sees the result as a monochrome ray-traced image of the MRI data. When satisfied with the orientation and excavation of the volume, the user selects fusion to initiate the computation of the final image. Rendering of the monochrome image for the pilot view is fast, near real time. The composite rendering employs more rays and interpolation to give a higher quality image.

III. RESULTS AND DISCUSSION

The key steps in the registration procedure are illustrated in Figures 1–3. Figure 1 shows the volume histogram of an SPGR image set with pixel size $0.937 \times 0.937 \times 1.5$ mm^3. The histogram is characterized by three features: low-level noise, a peak corresponding (mostly) to gray matter pixels, and a lower height, broad peak that corresponds to white matter and extracranial structures. The low-level threshold is set to eliminate the low-level noise. Figure 2 shows 3D renderings of segmented MR data from several brains, visually confirming the quality of the segmentation.

Figure 3 shows an example of the color fusion of a PET CBF and MRI SPGR volume. In this case, the PET data are resliced to the MRI data (about

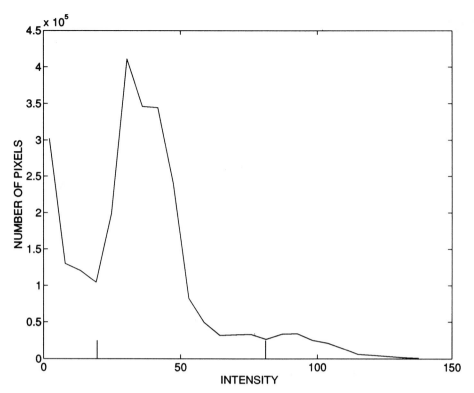

FIGURE 1   Volume histogram of MRI (SPGR) intensity levels before surface segmentation. The solid vertical lines indicate the thresholds used in the segmentation processing. Voxels to the left of the first vertical line usually represent noise outside the brain volume. Voxels to the right of the second vertical line correspond to (mostly) extracranial tissues.

180 slices). Shown are transverse, coronal, and sagittal slices along with a volume rendering that was excavated to remove about one-quarter of a hemisphere.

Our procedure has been tested on more than 30 PET–MRI data sets. The segmentation procedure was successful in all cases. Volume rendering and visual slice-by-slice comparison of slices before and after segmentation were performed to evaluate the quality of the segmentation.

The performance of registration algorithms depends on accurate location of brain surface and/or removal of confounding extracranial structures (surface segmentation). Segmentation of extracranial structures in MRI images of the human brain is often required in the processing or visualization of anatomic data. For example, removal of extracranial structures, such as scalp and meninges, is essential for computing a three-dimensional rendering of the brain surface and for accurate functioning of image-registration algorithms (Pelizzari et al., 1989; Woods et al., 1993; Morris et al., 1993). With the increasing resolution of volumetric MRI image data, often consisting of more than 100 slices, manual segmentation techniques become impractical for routine clinical and research applications and automated techniques become more appealing, even necessary.

It should be obvious that the quality of the MR data influences the quality of the brain surface segmentation. Neither manual nor our automatic segmentation can be perfect because the MRI gray levels do not always unambiguously identify intracranial and extracranial structures. The contrast between white and gray matter is also important, both for our algorithm and for manual segmentation. Despite these caveats, we found we were always able to get adequate surface segmentation. During the development and assessment of the segmentation procedure, we found that the result was most sensitive to the low-level threshold, whereas the setting of the upper threshold was not critical. Controlling the number of erosion-dilation iterations and the size and shape of the erosion–dilation kernel was essential for high-quality segmentation. But, for a given pulse sequence and slice thickness, all parameters except the low-level threshold could be fixed.

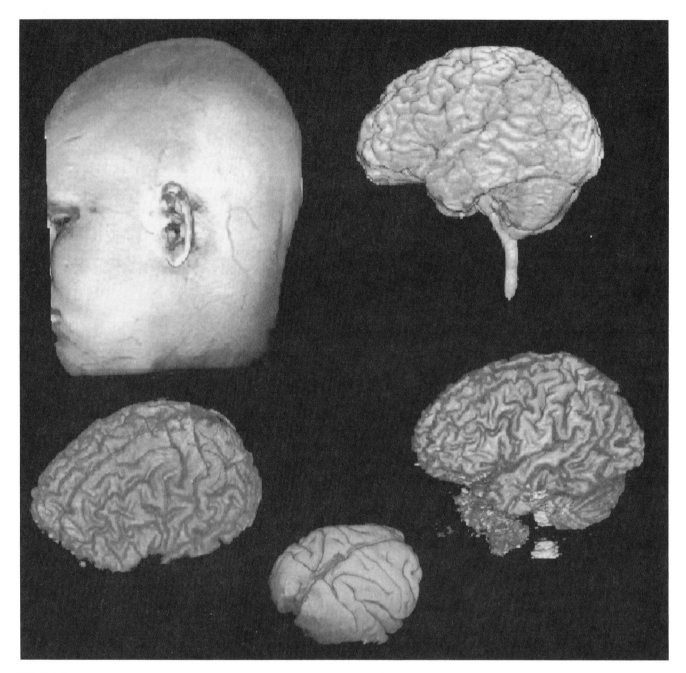

FIGURE 2   Ray-traced renderings of the surface segmentation produced with the procedure described in the text. Clockwise from the upper left corner, we show a ray-traced volume rendering of the human skull, the corresponding surface segmentation, two additional examples of surface segmentations of the human brain, with the surface segmentation of a monkey brain between them. The original data were acquired using an SPGR pulse sequence in 124 coronal sections with 256 × 256 pixels per plane.

In our work, the visualization of the registration is systematized with a consistent graphical user interface. This assists in training technicians and researchers in the use of the system. The ability to manipulate the fusion in real time has proven to be a desirable feature, both for assessing the quality of registration and for subsequent analysis.

We conclude that the techniques described here provide an automated procedure for performing PET–MRI image registration. The results are important because this procedure can be performed routinely by technicians with no anatomic knowledge and the time required is reduced from hours to about 5 min on a modern computer workstation.

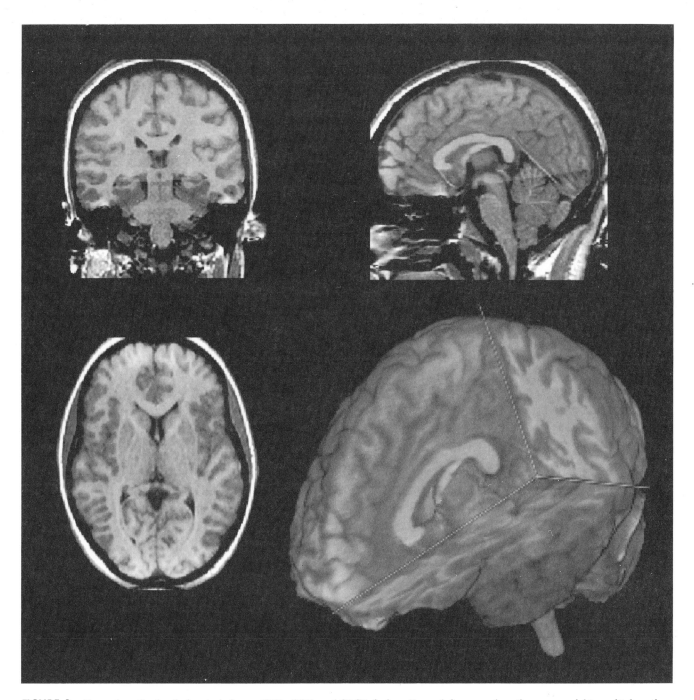

FIGURE 3 Examples of color fusion techniques, PET rCBF, and SPGR fusion: Upper left, coronal section; upper right, sagittal section; lower left, transverse section; lower right, ray-traced volume rendering with excavation. In this case, the PET data are resliced to the MRI data (about 180 slices). Inspection of data such as these provide direct confirmation of registration quality.

Acknowledgments

This work was supported in part by a grant from the Charles A. Dana Foundation Consortium on Memory Loss and Aging. Dr. Morris's contributions were supported, in part, by a PHS postdoctoral training grant, 2T32CA09362.

References

Haralick, R. M. (1981). Some neighborhood operators. *In:* "Real-Time Parallel Computing Image Analysis." (M. Onoe, K. Preston, Jr., and A. Rosenfeld, Eds.). Plenum, New York.

Haralick, R. M., and Shapiro, L. G. (1992). "Computer and Robot

Vision," Vol. 1. Chaps. 2 and 5. Addison–Wesley, Reading, Mass.

Morris, E. D., Muswick, G. J., Ellert, E. S., Steagall, R. N., Goyer, P. F., and Semple, W. E. (1993). Computer-aided techniques for aligning interleaved sets of non-identical medical images. Proceedings of the SPIE, Image Processing, Vol. 1898, pp. 146–157.

Pelizzari, C. A., Chen, G. T. Y., Spelbring, D. R., and Weichslebaum, R. R. (1989). Accurate three-dimensional registration of CT, PET and/or MR images of the brain. *J. Comput. Assist. Tomogr.* **13:** 20–26.

Strother, S. C., Anderson, J. R., Xu, X. L., Liow, J. S., Bonar, D. C., and Rottenberg, D. A. (1994). Quantitative comparisons of image registration techniques based on high-resolution MRI of the brain. *J. Comput. Assist. Tomogr.* **18,** 954–962.

Turkington, T. G., Hoffman, J. M., Jaszczak, R. J., MacFall, J. R., Harris, C. C., Kilts, C. D., Pelizzari, C. A., and Coleman, R. E. (1995). Accuracy of surface fit registration for PET and MR brain images using full and incomplete brain surfaces. *J. Comput. Assist. Tomogr.* **19:** 117–124.

Woods, R. P., Mazziotta, J. C., and Cherry S. R. (1993). MRI-PET registration with automated algorithm. *J. Comput. Assist. Tomogr.* **17:** 536–546.

Feature-Matching Axial Averaging Method for Enhancing Signal-to-Noise Ratio of Images Generated by New Generation PET Scanners

S. C. HUANG, J. YANG, M. DAHLBOM, C. HOH, J. CZERNIN, Y. ZHOU, and D. C. YU

Division of Nuclear Medicine and Biophysics
Department of Molecular and Medical Pharmacology
UCLA School of Medicine, Los Angeles, California 90095

Reduced per-plane detection efficiency of the new generation PET scanners increases the noise level of the reconstructed tomographic images. Axial smoothing of image values across planes can compensate for the efficiency reduction, but the image spatial resolution is usually degraded. A new axial averaging method that can reduce noise level with minimal resolution loss is therefore developed and evaluated in this study. The new method uses elastic image mapping to track the image features across planes. Following the path along matched features, the image values can be filtered to reduce noise without causing much loss in image resolution. The new method was evaluated with computer simulated images of brain FDG studies. The simulated images were generated from realistic 3D digital phantoms. As compared to the conventional method that uses the same filter to smooth the image values along the direction parallel to the z-axis, the new method is shown to have lower spatial resolution loss but with comparable noise reduction. Alternatively, using the new method, one can obtain images of comparable spatial resolution as those by the conventional method but of lower noise levels. The new method was also applied to real PET images from a new generation PET scanner to show the signal-to-noise ratio improvement.

I. INTRODUCTION

As the detector size of new generation PET scanners is decreased to give smaller intrinsic resolution and better axial sampling, the detection sensitivity per plane is markedly reduced (Wienhard *et al.*, 1994). This resulted in a large increase in the noise level of the reconstructed images. Although the use of 3D acquisition in these scanners can partly make up for the sensitivity loss, the full potential of these new scanners for delivering very high spatial resolutions is not achievable without additional efforts to address the issue of high image noise. A conventional method of smoothing images across different planes can reduce the noise, but the spatial resolution of the image is degraded. In this study, we have developed a novel processing method to reduce the image noise without causing much loss in spatial resolution.

II. THEORY AND METHODS

Figure 1 illustrates the general concept of the new method, which uses elastic mapping to find the spatial mapping vectors that track the locations of local features of the images from plane to plane. Thus, instead of smoothing along the z-axis direction by the conventional method, the averaging can be performed along the mapping vectors between the planes. The noise component in the images is expected to be reduced by the same amount as for the conventional axial smoothing (if the same filter is used). However, the image resolution is not seriously degraded, because the mapping vectors are obtained by matching the same image features across planes.

A neural network algorithm for elastic image mapping (Lin and Huang, 1993; Lin *et al.*, 1994; Kosugi *et al.*, 1993) was used to track the image features from

---

plane # i-3 i-2 i-1   i   i+1 i+2 i+3 i+4

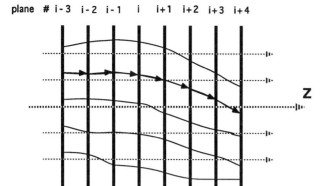

Z

FIGURE 1   Illustration of the concept of the new axial averaging method. The vertical lines denote the side view of different planes. Different curves in the figure represent the paths, along which various image features move across different planes. Mapping vectors along the image features are obtained by elastic mapping of images between planes. Averaging or smoothing along the curve (path) formed by the mapping vectors effectively reduces image noise with minimal loss of image resolution. Conventional axial averaging method smooths along the lines (dashed lines) parallel to the axial (z) axis.

plane to plane by mapping each image to those of its adjacent planes. Based on the resulting mapping vectors between adjacent planes, the image values along a path through any particular pixel across planes were obtained. The image values were then filtered to give a lower noise image value for that pixel. After going through this process for each pixel of each image plane, the images would have improved noise level without much degradation in the spatial resolution of the images.

To test the performance of this new method, computer simulated brain FDG images based on realistic 3D digital phantoms were generated. The true image was known and was used as the reference image to evaluate systematically the performance of the method as compared to that of the conventional method. The method was also applied to real brain FDG PET images to demonstrate the ability of the new method to increase the signal-to-noise ratio of real images.

A. Computer Simulations

A 3D voxel-based digital brain phantom obtained by segmenting a set of MRI images of a normal subject was used to simulate the brain FDG images. Relative radioactivity levels in gray matter, white matter, CSF, and muscle were 4, 1, 0, 0, respectively. Sinograms were generated with the following configuration parameters that approximated those of a Siemens/CTI EXACT HR scanner: transverse sampling distance = 0.165 cm, number of transverse samples = 336, number

of angular projections = 196, intrinsic spatial resolution = 0.4 cm FWHM in the transverse direction and 0.5 cm FWHM in the axial direction. Interplane distance was 0.3125 cm. Poisson noise was added to the sinograms to simulate images of various noise levels. The noise-added sinograms were then reconstructed using a filtered back-projection algorithm with various reconstruction filters to give tomographic images of various spatial resolutions.

The simulated images were then axial averaged separately by the conventional method and the new method. The filters used were to achieve the same axial spatial resolution as the in-plane resolution for the conventional method.

The effective in-plane resolution loss after the axial averaging is measured by the "effective global Gaussian resolution" (EGGR) (Chinn and Huang, 1993; Liow and Strother, 1993) using the noise-free image without axial averaging as the reference standard.

B. Real PET Images

Tomographic images obtained from brain FDG studies in human subjects using a Siemens/CTI EXACT HR scanner at UCLA were used to test the new axial averaging method. The images corresponded to about 200K counts per plane.

III. RESULTS AND DISCUSSION

Figure 2 shows the images before and after axial averaging. Images processed by the new method are shown along with those processed by the conventional method. The images were reconstructed with a Hanning filter of cutoff = 0.6 times the Nyquist frequency. The images by the conventional method are shown to have lower spatial resolution compared to the ones by the new method and the unprocessed ones. The difference images for the conventional method contains more the structural pattern of the original images, indicating a larger loss of spatial resolution. The total sum of squares of the pixel values in the difference image of the conventional method is about twice as large as for the difference image of the new method. Since the same axial filters were used in both cases, the images by the two methods have comparable noise levels.

Figure 3 shows the image pixel values along the axial direction at a fixed x, y location as compared to that along the feature-matched path of the same x, y location. The data were from a pixel near the parietal cor-

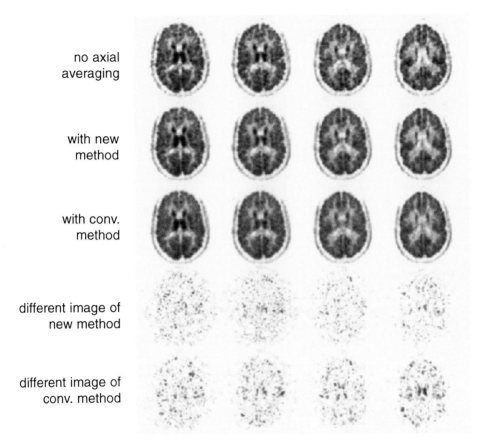

no axial
averaging

with new
method

with conv.
method

different image of
new method

different image of
conv. method

FIGURE 2 Computer simulated brain FDG PET images. Top row, original noisy images; second row, images processed by the new method; third row, images processed by the conventional method; fourth row, difference image between the images in the second row and the noise-free true images; fifth row, difference image between the images in the third row and the true images. The images of the first three rows were scaled according to the same gray level scale. The difference images were scaled up by a factor of 3 to reveal more clearly the differences (i.e., the darkness level is increased by a factor of 3).

tex. The variation along the feature-matched path is shown to be much lower than those along the axial (z-axis) direction. Therefore, the smoothed value along the feature-matched path was closer to the "true" value (noise free and without axial averaging) than the value smoothed along the z-axis direction. The variation along the z-axis consists of not only variation due to noise but also variation of the radioactivity distribution along the axial direction. Therefore, the conventional method of axial averaging reduces the noise as well as the effective in-plane spatial resolution.

The amount of effective in-plane spatial resolution loss as quantified by EGGR is shown in Figure 4. The new method is shown to cause smaller resolution loss at various image resolutions compared to the conventional method. In other words, using the conventional method to achieve the same effective in-plane spatial

resolution would require the original images to be reconstructed to a higher resolution and allow less smoothing in the axial averaging step. Therefore, for the same effective resolution, the conventional method would give images of higher noise level than with the new method. Based on the results in Figure 4, the amount of noise reduction by the new method as compared to the conventional method that gives the same effective in-plane resolution was estimated theoretically to be at least 30%.

Figure 5 shows the real brain FDG PET images after being processed by the new method. No noticeable image artifacts and little spatial resolution loss were seen in the real PET images processed by the new method. As compared to those processed by the conventional method, images by the new method are shown to have a larger reduction in image noise than by the conventional method.

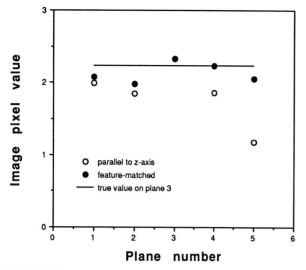

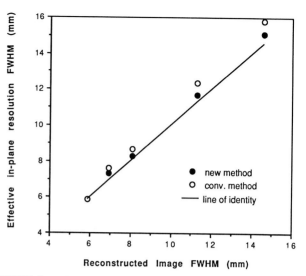

FIGURE 3   Image pixel values along the feature-matched path (filled circles) at a fixed *x, y* location compared to image pixel value along the axial direction (open circles) of the same *x, y* location.

FIGURE 4   Effective in-plane resolutions of the images processed by the new method (closed circles) compared to those by the conventional method (open circles).

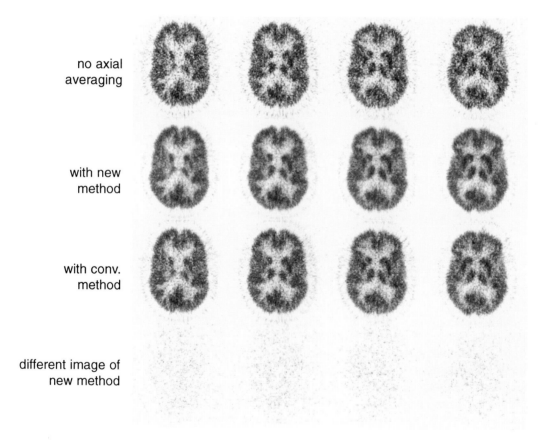

FIGURE 5   Brain FDG images obtained by Siemens/CTI EXACT HR scanner. Top row, original images; second row, images processed by the new method; third row, images processed by the conventional method; fourth row, difference image between the images of the new method (second row) and the original images (top row). All images in this figure were scaled according to the same gray level scale.

Results in this study indicate that the new method can provide noise reduction comparable to the conventional method but with less resolution reduction or more noise reduction with comparable spatial resolution. Although the method still needs to be more fully developed and characterized, the performance is expected to be better for images from scanners of finer axial sampling (e.g., Siemens/CTI Exact HR+ PET scanner). The method is also expected to be applicable to images from direct 3D acquisition.

Acknowledgment

We want to thank David Truong and Kent Gardner for computer system support, Ron Sumida and the PET technical staff for acquiring the real PET images. This work was partially supported by DOE contract DE-FC03–87ER60615 and NIH grants CA56655 and HL29845.

References

Chinn, G., and Huang, S. C. (1993). Noise and resolution of Bayesian reconstruction for multiple image configurations. *IEEE Trans. Nucl. Sci.* **40:** 2059–2063.

Kosugi, Y., Sase, M., Kuwatani, H., Kinoshita, N., Momose, T., Nishikawa, J., and Watanabe, T. (1993). Neural network mapping for nonlinear stereostactic normalization of brain MR images. *J. Compt. Assist. Tomog.* **17:** 455–460.

Lin, K. P., and Huang, S. C. (1993). An elastic mapping algorithm for tomographic images. Proceedings of Annual Conference of Biomedical Engineering. **1:** 40–41.

Lin, K., Huang, S., Baxter, L., and Phelps, M. (1994). An elastic image transformation method for 3-dimensional inter-subject medical image registration. *J. Nucl. Med.* **35** (Suppl.): 186P.

Liow, J., and Strother, S. (1993). The convergence of object dependent resolution in maximum likelihood based tomographic image reconstruction. *Phys. Med. Biol.* **38:** 55–70.

Wienhard, K., Dahlbom, M., Eriksson, L., Michel, C., Bruckbauer, T., Pietrzyk, U., and Heiss, W.-D. (1994). The ECAT EXACT HR: Performance of a new high resolution positron scanner. *J. Compt. Assist. Tomogr.* **18:** 110–118.

MR-Based Correction of Partial Volume Effects in Brain PET Imaging

J. JAMES FROST[2,3,4], CAROLYN CIDIS MELTZER[1,2], JON KAR ZUBIETA[2],
JONATHAN M. LINKS[2,3], PAUL BRAKEMAN[4], MARTIN J. STUMPF[2], and MARK KRUGER[2]

Department of Radiology
[1]Divisions of Neuroradiology and
[2]Nuclear Medicine
[3]Department of Environmental Health Sciences
[4]Department of Neuroscience
The Johns Hopkins Medical Institutions
Baltimore, Maryland 21205

Partial volume and mixed tissue sampling errors can cause significant inaccuracy in quantitative positron emission tomographic (PET) measurements. We previously described a method of correcting PET data for the effects of partial volume averaging on gray matter quantitation; however, this method may incompletely correct gray matter structures when local tissue concentrations are highly heterogeneous. We have extended this three-compartment algorithm to include a fourth compartment: a gray matter (GM) volume of interest (VOI) that can be delineated on magnetic resonance imaging (MR).

I. INTRODUCTION

Functional brain imaging using positron emission tomography permits quantitative *in vivo* measurement of regional cerebral metabolism, blood flow, and neuroreceptor concentration. The accuracy of quantitation of PET data is affected by its finite spatial resolution, which causes significant underestimation of the true isotope concentration in structures smaller than about 2.5 times the full-width at half-maximum (Hoffman *et al.*, 1979; Kessler *et al.*, 1984). Much of the prior work demonstrating this effect of underestimation of tracer concentration in small structures was performed using geometric phantoms consisting of hot spheres in a cold

background (Mazziotta *et al.*, 1981), a situation that does not accurately reflect a PET study of the human brain. The accuracy of quantitative measurements of radioactivity in small volumes is further affected by the structure's shape, background, and z-axis sampling (Hoffman *et al.*, 1979; Mazziotta *et al.*, 1981; Kessler *et al.*, 1984). Although the substantial effect of background radiation on the measurement of a hot spot was recognized by Kessler *et al.* (1984), the issue of heterogeneity of background was not addressed by these early experiments.

We previously developed an MR-based two-compartment technique for partial volume correction of PET data, based on that described by Videen *et al.* (1988), which addressed the underestimation of quantitative cortical tracer measurements in the presence of dilated sulci (Meltzer *et al.*, 1990b). A modification of this approach using a spoiled gradient recall (SPGR) MR pulse sequence to obtain high-contrast differences among gray matter (GM), white matter (WM), and cerebrospinal fluid (CSF) permitted the determination of cortical GM tracer concentration (Mueller-Gaertner *et al.*, 1992). Limitations of this latter approach include the assumption of homogeneous cortical GM activity and the undercorrection of small GM structures, such as the amygdala, where spill-in of activity from surrounding structures greatly influences the apparent tracer concentration. We describe our recent developments on an extension to this method that improves partial volume correction of heterogeneous GM radioactivity when structures of interest can be delineated by MR. We also describe implementation of this new algorithm using Application Visualization Software (AVS).

II. METHODS AND MATERIALS

A. Theory

The first steps in the algorithm are identical to that previously published. We modeled the PET image as a sum of three compartments: gray matter (GM), white matter (WM) and cerebral spinal fluid (CSF). The corrected GM compartment was given by (Mueller-Gaertner et al., 1992):

$$\tilde{I}_{gray} = (I_{obs} - \tilde{I}_{white} X_{white} \otimes h)/X_{gray} \otimes h \qquad (1)$$

where $\tilde{I}_{gray}$ is the three compartment corrected image, $\tilde{I}_{white}$ is the WM intensity image, X_{gray} and X_{white} are the GM and WM tissue maps derived from the MR, and h is the system point spread function of the PET scanner.

Equation (1) is valid only when (1) $\tilde{I}_{gray}$ is constant (i.e., spatially homogeneous) or (2) h is a delta function (i.e., the imaging system has perfect resolution). In practice, neither of these conditions is perfectly met, and thus the general approach is unable to completely recover $\tilde{I}_{gray}$. Our previous work (Mueller-Gaertner et al., 1992) indicated that the method was least successful for subcortical GM or small cortical GM "hot spots" (focal areas of increased activity). To account for heterogeneous $\tilde{I}_{gray}$, we have extended this three-compartment algorithm by including a fourth compartment: a GM volume of interest (VOI) such that $I_{VOI} \neq I_{gray}$ (Meltzer et al., 1996). Equation (1), therefore, takes the following form:

$$\tilde{I}_{VOI} = (I_{obs} - \tilde{I}_{gray} X_{gray} \otimes h \\ - \tilde{I}_{white} X_{white} \otimes h)/X_{VOI} \otimes h \qquad (2)$$

where $\tilde{I}_{gray}$ is defined by the three-compartment correction, that is, as the result of equation (1), and X_{gray} is defined as the tissue map of GM excluding the VOI.

B. MR Acquisition

MR data were acquired on a Signa 1.5 T scanner (General Electric, Milwaukee, Wisconsin). SPGR MR (TE = 5, TR = 65, flip angle = 45°, NEX = 2) images were acquired coplanar to the PET imaging planes (for phantom and human study), using an individually fitted thermoplastic face mask (Polysplint, Poly-Med Manufacturing Co., Baltimore, Maryland) and an MR-visible

fiducial marker for plane localization (Meltzer et al., 1990a). Each MR data set consisted of 60 1.5 mm thick contiguous images (24 cm field of view, image matrix = 256 × 256 pixels, pixel size = 0.94 mm). The high-resolution, high-contrast SPGR MR data permitted accurate segmentation of GM, WM, and CSF and delineation of subcortical structures of interest.

C. PET Acquisition

PET studies were performed on a G.E. 4096 plus whole body scanner (General Electric, Milwaukee, Wisconsin). Each PET data set consisted of 15 images (in a 128 × 128 matrix with a 2 mm pixel size) with a slice separation of 6.5 mm. Transmission scans were utilized to correct PET data for attenuation. The data were corrected for decay and scatter and smoothed using a 2D low-pass Hann filter ("6 mm width," corresponding to a cutoff frequency = 0.33 Nyquist) to a final resolution of FWHM = 8.0 mm in the z-axis and 7.0 mm in-plane. Scanner resolution was measured empirically from point sources positioned in the center of the field of view (FOV).

D. Image Processing

The MR data segmentation, convolution, and image manipulation steps necessary for partial volume correction in simulated PET images were initially performed using Macintosh-based image analysis software (Digital Image Processing Station, Hayden Image Processing Group, Cleveland, Ohio). These steps were subsequently implemented on data from human subjects using the AVS environment (Advanced Visual Systems Inc., Waltham, Massachusetts).

E. Computer Simulations

SPGR MR image data acquired on two male subjects (ages 64 and 77) were segmented into GM, WM, and CSF elements by histogram analysis of the pixel intensities, as previously described (Mueller-Gaertner et al., 1992). The midpoints between adjacent pixel intensity peaks, as fit by Gaussians, were used as cutoff values for defining pixels as GM, WM, or CSF. Simulated PET images were created by arbitrarily assigning GM, WM, and CSF pixels values as follows: CSF = 0, WM = 40, and GM = 120, and convolving the MR data with the PET point-spread functions (z-axis FWHM = 8.0 mm, in-plane FWHM = 7.0 mm). Subcortical VOIs were defined by cylinders (oriented longitudinally in the z-axis) and ellipsoids in the anatomic position of the amygdala and were coded over a range of contrast values from equal to WM to 4 × GM and a range of sizes (at constant contrast of 2 × GM) (152, 429, 518, and 725 mm³; i.e., representative values from MR measurements of the amygdala in 10 patients with Alzheimer disease and 10 elderly controls). Additional subcortical VOIs were defined by the boundaries of the caudate and thalamus in the MR data set and these structures coded as 480 (i.e., 4 × GM). The center image in the MR data set used to create a simulated PET image corresponded to the z-axis midpoint of the subcortical VOI. A 6 mm z-axis shift between the center of the MR data set and the center of the caudate simulated z-axis undersampling of a structure of interest with PET.

Four-compartment correction of quantitative measurements for subcortical VOIs was performed on the simulated PET data. Data sampling was performed using 8 × 8 mm square regions of interest (ROI) on both the simulated and corrected PET data. Our previously published three-compartment technique of partial volume correction (Mueller-Gaertner *et al.*, 1992) was also used to correct simulated PET measurements of the amygdala over a range of contrast values and sizes.

F. Human Study

The four-compartment correction was performed using AVS on [¹¹C]carfentanil (CFN) PET data acquired on a 69-year-old healthy man (Frost *et al.*, 1985, 1988). For opiate receptor imaging, scans were acquired over 90 min following intravenous injection of 740 MBq CFN and summed over the interval 35–70 min postinjection (Frost *et al.*, 1988). Paired 8 × 8 mm (2 mm/pixel) ROI were used to sample the cortex and amygdalae before and after correction.

G. Implementation of Partial Volume Correction in AVS

The most recent refinements in the implementation of partial volume correction (PVC) were performed using AVS. This program served as a base to automate the preceding algorithms and reduce operator dependence. This would be of importance in routine PVC of human studies with large data sets. The practical application of PVC using AVS is now described. To perform a four-compartment partial volume correction, it is first necessary to determine the average CSF, WM, and GM values and the spatial distributions of the brain tissues. Since WM and CSF are assumed to be homogeneous and not significantly affected by partial volume averaging, their mean values can be taken from the original PET scan in areas that are far from tissue boundaries. The heterogeneous GM values must be

corrected for partial volume averaging with WM and CSF before a GM average can be calculated.

H. Brain or Nonbrain Segmentation

The partial volume correction algorithm assumes that only pixels inside the skull cavity are significant. Therefore, the first step was to remove the nonbrain pixels on both the PET and the MR data sets. This was done by first using a thresholding operation to identify brain pixels and creating a binarized volume, where a value of 1 is *potentially* brain tissue. Then, a series of 3D morphologic operators was used to separate the brain pixels from the surrounding nonbrain pixels. Erosion was used to break any artifactual connections between brain and nonbrain, and connected component analysis was used to identify the largest object in the data set, which was assumed to be the brain. Finally, dilation was used to recover pixels lost in the previous erosion, and the holes in the volume were filled.

I. Registration

Although MR and PET data were acquired coplanar by the use of an individually fitted thermoplastic mask, exact coregistration is an essential part of PVC as described. To correct for small misalignments or minor head motion within the mask, a MR-PET coregistration algorithm was added to the AVS routines. The transformation matrix that makes the MR volume exactly registered with the PET volume was determined by an AVS based volumetric registration package called *Image-Match* (Focus Graphics Inc., San Mateo, California). This method models the PET and MR brains as solid objects in a potential energy field and finds the transform that minimizes the energy between them. This method is insensitive to local minima and the problem of missing data, which is of importance when a limited field of view and a stack of 2D PET data constructions are utilized.

J. Tissue Classification and Segmentation

The tissue maps X_{gray}, X_{white}, and X_{CSF} were determined by an automated statistical process. The MR data set was modeled as a finite normal mixture of the three tissue classes whose parameters were determined by the expectation maximization (EM) algorithm on a slice-by-slice basis. These parameters were then used in conjunction with a Bayesian hypothesis testing algorithm to discretely classify each pixel as one of the three classes (Lei and Sewchand, 1992). The VOI tissue map X_{VOI} was defined by manually tracing the boundaries of the volume on consecutive MR slices. Improvements to the VOI definition could include tracing on multiple orthogonal slices and shape-based nonlinear warping of geometric shapes to match the contours of the structures.

K. Mathematical Computations

All smoothing was performed by a 3D frequency convolution of the data with the system function of the PET scanner. The PVC equations 1 and 2 were implemented on a pixel-by-pixel basis.

III. RESULTS

A. Computer Simulations

Comparison was made among simulated PET data in the uncorrected state, after application of the previously published three-compartment correction (Mueller-Gaertner *et al.*, 1992) and following four-compartment correction of VOIs of varying contrasts and sizes. Over a variety of contrasts, ranging from 0.3 to 2.0 times GM concentration, errors in the recovery of assigned values in cylindrical VOIs observed in the uncorrected simulated PET data were as follows: 120, 15, 24, 32, 37, 48, and 65% at contrasts ratios of 0.3, 1.0, 1.2, 1.3, 1.5, 2.0, and 4.0 (contrast ratio = assigned value/GM value), respectively. Three-compartment correction of GM activity resulted in errors of 145, 0.8, 11, 19, 26, 38.3, and 57.7% at the same contrast ratios. In both the uncorrected and three-compartment corrected data, the largest errors occurred when activity in the VOI differed most from surrounding GM activity. Underestimation of assigned tracer concentration was observed when the VOI value was greater than neighboring tissue, and overestimation occurred when the VOI was colder than the surroundings. Four-compartment correction recovered the assigned VOI value with a maximum error of 1.9% (mean error = 1.3 ± 0.6% s.d.) for all contrast ratios.

The effect of size of the GM VOI was demonstrated with ellipsoid amygdalae ranging in size from 152 to 725 mm^3. ROI sampling of VOI tracer concentration in the simulated PET data resulted in errors ranging from 39.1 to 49.7%. This error decreased to 27.7–41.9% following three-compartment correction and to 0–0.4% with four-compartment correction.

Four-compartment correction of the thalamus and caudate in a simulated PET resulted in complete recovery of the coded value, as compared with 14.8 and 50% underestimation in the uncorrected data, respectively. Full recovery was also achieved by four-compartment correction of a caudate that was positioned at a 6 mm

offset from the *z*-axis center of the simulated PET slice, whereas underestimation of 64.4% was demonstrated in the uncorrected simulated PET (i.e., an additional underestimation of true caudate value by 14.4% over that obtained with the caudate aligned with the *z*-axis center of the PET slice).

B. Application to Human PET Data

Figure 1 demonstrates partial volume correction of single slice CFN PET data in an elderly human subject. Cortical GM activity increased 55% in the CFN data after three-compartment correction. Four-compartment correction of CFN amygdala activity resulted in an uncorrected to corrected ratio of 1.2.

IV. DISCUSSION

Partial volume and mixed tissue sampling errors can significantly influence the quantitative accuracy of PET. We and others have previously described approaches that attempt to account for some or all of these errors. We previously reported the implementation of a two-compartment correction method of partial volume correction of PET data (Meltzer *et al.*, 1990b), which uses MR data to correct PET measurements for the partial volume effects caused by metabolically inactive CSF spaces. The two-compartment correction method does not take into consideration partial volume averaging of gray and white matter activity, which is inherent given the typical differences in activity in GM and WM. Since the proportion of gray and white matter may be altered in disease states and normal aging, simply correcting for brain–CSF partial volume effects may confound the comparison of such subjects with young healthy individuals (Miller *et al.*, 1980; Prohovnik *et al.*, 1989; Rusinek *et al.*, 1991; Lim *et al.*, 1992). A three-compartment modification additionally corrected for potential differences in the gray–white matter proportions between groups by determining the tracer concentration of cortical GM (Mueller-Gaertner *et al.*, 1992). The major advantage of the new procedure for partial volume correction of PET images over the two- and three-compartment approaches is the accurate correction of small subcortical structures and irregular objects such as small cortical VOIs that can be defined by MR. Application of the four-compartment extension permits valid comparison of radioactivity concentration in selected brain regions between healthy control subjects and patients in whom the structure of interest may be morphologically reduced in size. This method would also allow partial volume correction of specific

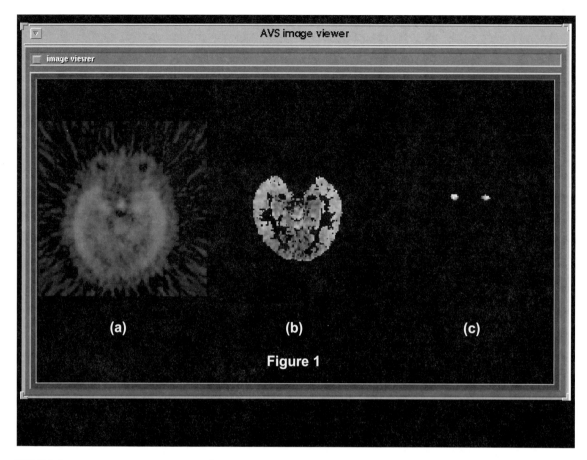

FIGURE 1   Partial volume correction of [^{11}C]carfentanil PET image in elderly man: (a) uncorrected CFN image, (b) three-compartment corrected image masked with the GM (excluding VOI) tissue map, (c) four-compartment corrected image masked with the VOI tissue map.

small cortical regions that exhibit abnormal signal on MR and may be expected to differ in metabolic activity or receptor concentration from surrounding tissue. Delineation of the structure of interest by MR is a requisite parameter for the algorithm. The actual gray matter PET radioactivity concentration of GM regions identified by functional MR techniques may also be potentially derived by this method.

The accurate determination of the true tracer concentrations in heterogeneous GM achieved with this partial volume correction technique represents a significant advantage over the previously published three-compartment method (Mueller-Gaertner *et al.*, 1992). Validation of the four-compartment correction in simulated PET images created from human brain MR data demonstrated an error of less than 2% in the determination of a wide range of assigned activity values in GM VOIs such as the amygdala, caudate, and thalamus. Under correction of small structures such as the amygdala with the three-compartment approach is due to

partial volume averaging between areas of relatively high radioactivity and surrounding structures with lower tracer concentrations. The four-compartment model removes this source of error by defining a VOI as having a different tracer concentration from neighboring structures. Full correction of cortical VOIs with the three-compartment approach is achieved when such areas are large in size relative to scanner resolution. Small cortical VOIs that do not span the full z-axis thickness of the PET slice would behave like subcortical structures, and in this case, full correction would be expected only with the four-compartment modification.

In the human PET studies, four-compartment correction of CFN PET data resulted in a mean decrease of 10% in amygdala activity. A larger increase in surrounding GM activity after correction resulted in very similar corrected values for the amygdala and temporal lobe GM, both known areas of high binding (Frost *et al.*, 1985, 1988).

In summary, we present a four-compartment approach to partial volume correction of PET data that represents a substantial improvement in accuracy over previous methods. This method permits the determination of the true radioactivity concentration in heterogeneous gray matter when specific regions of potentially different tracer concentration from neighboring structures can be defined by MR. The accuracy of this approach has been demonstrated in computer simulations of brain PET images derived from human MR data. The four-compartment correction method eliminates the substantial error caused by partial volume effects, permitting greater accuracy of quantitative PET measurements in selected brain regions of healthy control subjects and patients with cortical or subcortical atrophy.

Acknowledgments

We would like to thank Jerry L. Prince for helpful discussions. This work was supported by U.S.P.H.S. grants AG08740 and AG10624.

References

Frost, J. J., Mayberg, H. S., Fisher R. S., Douglass K. H., Dannals, R. F., Links, J. M., Wilson, A. A., and Ravert, H. T. (1988). Mu-opiate receptors measured by positron emission tomography are increased in temporal lobe epilepsy. *J. Comput. Assist. Tomogr.* **9:** 231–236.

Frost, J. J., Wagner, H. N., Dannals, R. F., Ravert, H. T., Wilson, A. A., Burns, H. D., Wong, D. F., McPherson, R. W., Rosenbaum, A. E., Kuhar M. J., and Snyder, S. H. (1985). Imaging opiate receptors in the human brain by positron emission tomography. *J. Comput. Assist. Tomogr.* **9:** 231–236.

Hoffman, E. J., Huang, S. C., and Phelps, M. E. (1979). Quantitation in positron emission computed tomography: 1. Effect of object size. *J. Comput. Assist. Tomogr.* **3:** 299–308.

Kessler, R. M., Ellis, J. R., and Eden, M. (1984). Analysis of emission tomographic scan data: Limitations imposed by resolution and background. *J. Comput. Assist. Tomogr.* **8:** 514–522.

Lei, T., and Sewchand, W. (1992). A new stochastic model-based image segmentation technique for X-ray CT imaging. *IEEE Trans. Med. Imag.* **11:** 53–61.

Lim, K. O., Zipursky, R. B., Watts, M. C., and Pfefferbaum, A. (1992). Decreased gray matter in normal aging: An in vivo magnetic resonance study. *J. Gerontol.* **47:** B26–30.

Mazziotta, J. C., Phelps, M. E., Plummer, D., and Kuhl, D. E. (1981). Quantitation in positron emission tomography: 5. Physical-anatomical effects. *J. Comput. Assist. Tomogr.* **5:** 734–743.

Meltzer, C. C., Bryan, R. N., Holcomb H. H., Mayberg, H. S., Sadzot, B., Leal, J. P., Wagner, H. N., and Frost J. J. (1990a). A method of anatomical localization for positron emission tomography using magnetic resonance imaging. *J. Comput. Assist. Tomogr.* **14:** 418–426.

Meltzer, C. C., Leal, J. P., Mayberg, H. S., Wagner, H. J., and Frost, J. J. (1990b). Correction of PET data for partial volume effects in human cerebral cortex by MR imaging. *J. Comput. Assist. Tomogr.* **14**(4): 561–570.

Meltzer, C. C., Zubieta, J. K., Links, J. M., Brakeman, P., Stumpf, M. J., and Frost, J. J. (1996). MR-based correction of brain PET measurements for heterogeneous gray matter radioactivity distribution. *J. Cereb. Blood Flow Metab.*, in press.

Miller, A. K. H., Alston, R. L., and Corsellis, J. A. N. (1980). Variation with age in the volumes of grey and white matter in the cerebral hemispheres of man: Measurements with an image analyzer. *Neuropathol. Appl. Neurobiol.* **6:** 119–132.

Mueller-Gaertner, H. W., Links, J. M., Prince, J. L., Bryan, R. N., McVeigh, E., Leal, J. P., Davatzikos, C., and Frost, J. J. (1992). Measurement of radiotracer concentration in brain gray matter using positron emission tomography: MRI-based correction for partial volume effects. *J. Cereb. Blood Flow Metab.* **12**(4): 571–583.

Prohovnik, I., Smith, G., Sackeim, H. A., Mayeux, R., and Stern, Y. (1989). Gray-matter degeneration in presenile Alzheimer's disease. *Ann. Neurol.* **25:** 117–124.

Rusinek, H., de Leon M. J., George, A. E., Stylopoulos, L. A., Chandra, R., Smith, G., Rand, T., Mourino, M., and Kowalski, H. (1991). Alzheimer disease: Measuring loss of cerebral gray matter with MR imaging. *Radiology* **178:** 109–114.

Videen, T. O., Perlmutter, J. S., Mintun, M. A., and Raichle, M. E. (1988). Regional correction of positron emission tomography data for the effects of cerebral atrophy. *J. Cereb. Blood Flow Metab.* **8:** 662–670.

In Vivo Correction Method for Partial Volume Effects in Positron Emission Tomography
Accuracy and Precision

OLIVIER G. ROUSSET[1], YILONG MA[1], STEFANO MARENCO[2], DEAN F. WONG[2], and ALAN C. EVANS[1]

[1]Positron Imaging Laboratories, McConnell Brain Imaging Centre
Montreal Neurological Institute, McGill University
Montreal, Quebec H3A-2B4, Canada
[2]Johns Hopkins Medical Institution
Department of Radiology, Baltimore, Maryland 21205

Previous methods to compensate for partial volume effects (PVE) in PET have accounted for dilution of gray matter activity by nonactive tissues like CSF (Meltzer et al., 1990) or for contamination of activity from white matter for which PVE are considered negligible (Müller-Gärtner et al., 1992). We have previously described a general 3D method for measuring the fractional regional recovery and interregional contamination independent of tracer activity levels (Rousset et al., 1993b). The method requires the identification of the tissue components from high-resolution MR images registered with the PET data. Simulation of PET physics (Ma et al., 1993) allows for calculating regional blurring factors that represent the contribution of each tissue component to any selected set of ROIs (Rousset et al., 1993b).

In the present study, the accuracy and precision of the correction method were assessed using a multicavity basal ganglia (BG) brain phantom (Wong et al., 1984). Corrected activity was within 2% of the true activity for a BG to background ratio of 3.5 : 1 and with over 300 kcounts/slice. The intraregional noise amplification factor is <1.3 for BG over the range of total counts studied. A dual-isotope experiment showed <4% inaccuracy in the half-life of each tracer derived from the PVE-corrected TACs. Also, the ability of this method to recover tissue time–activity curve (TAC) in PET-like noise conditions was investigated by simulations of typical tracer course in a normal human brain and demonstrated the ability of the method to provide accurate estimates, while offering the opportunity of estimating the precision of corrected regional activity for various brain regions.

I. INTRODUCTION

With varying contrast, as it is the case with dynamic tracer uptake studies, the bias introduced by limited spatial resolution of PET becomes nonlinear (Rousset et al., 1993a), and time-varying cross-contamination between functional tissues lead to distortions in the time–activity curve (TAC) shape (Rousset et al., 1993b). In vivo correction approaches using high-resolution MRI or transmission computerized tomography (CT) images were first developed to correct for PVE due to cerebrospinal fluid in 2D (Videen et al., 1988) and 3D (Meltzer et al., 1990). In 1992, Müller-Gärtner et al. proposed an MRI-based method for PVE correction in gray matter structures (Müller-Gärtner et al., 1992). Their method assumes that white matter activity is homogeneous throughout the brain, and can be accurately measured within the real PET image, in order to subtract its contribution to gray matter activity. However, this method does not account for activity spilled over from regions themselves suffering from PVE.

In our present approach, also based on MRI data, we assess the magnitude of cross-contamination between tissue components, independent of tissue activity levels. For computational efficiency, and because of the poor statistics of PET images, the method was first developed to correct regional measurements, that is, using ROIs, as it is generally the case with PET data. The accuracy of the correction method was examined using a multicavity brain phantom aimed to assess quantitation losses due to PVE in realistic conditions (Wong et al., 1984). Simulations of tracer uptake in a normal human brain were also performed in an effort to investigate the contrast recovery capability of the method in the presence of PET-like noise, and that of the precision of corrected estimates for various structures of the brain.

II. MATERIALS AND METHODS

A. Anatomical Information

To build up a model of the brain that can provide the structural information necessary for partial volume correction, volumetric high-resolution MRI data are registered with the corresponding PET data (Evans et al., 1991a). Semiautomatic as well as manual procedures are used for the segmentation of the coregistered MRI volume into its various components believed to have different kinetics for the tracer used (Rousset et al., 1993a). The resulting coded MRI volume can be assigned with tracer concentrations representing true activity distributions, assuming that the PET tracer is uniformly distributed over each identified tissue component.

B. Generation of Simulated PET Data

To characterize the PET response to the particular object under study, the coded MRI volume is sampled according to the geometry of our GE-2048 PET scanner (Ma et al., 1993; Rousset et al., 1993a, 1993b). As a first approximation, the 3D point-spread function (PSF) of the tomograph was taken as a spatially invariant Gaussian function ($6 \times 6 \times 6$ mm FWHM) (Evans et al., 1991b). The coded MRI volume is first convolved with a 1D Gaussian function to simulate the axial aperture function of the scanner. Sinogram projections are then computed from each axially weighted slice using an algorithm developed at University of Pennsylvania (Herman et al., 1989). The resulting projection profiles with adequate radial and angular sampling rates are then convolved with a 1D Gaussian function (6 mm FWHM) simulating the in-plane detector intrinsic re-

sponse. Beyond resolution, other physical factors inherent in PET data acquisition, such as photon attenuation and scatter counts, can be included according to the method described in Ma et al. (1993). For instance, noisy data were simulated by incorporation of Poisson noise at the projection stage, after attenuation simulation, based on estimated count density profiles, global efficiency of the scanner, duration of scan, and tracer's half-life. This approach, in contrast to techniques that add noise directly to the image, properly models the noise introduced by a count-limited data acquisition process at the scanner detectors.

C. Principle of the Correction Method

Since the point-spread function of the system is assumed to be a spatially invariant function, the PET image $I(\mathbf{r})$ is then equivalent to a 3D convolution of the PSF with the activity distribution $O(\mathbf{r})$:

$$I(\mathbf{r}) = \int_{FOV} O(\mathbf{r}')\mathrm{PSF}(\mathbf{r} - \mathbf{r}')\, d\mathbf{r}' = O(\mathbf{r}) * \mathrm{PSF}(\mathbf{r}) \quad (1)$$

If we consider that the activity distribution $O(\mathbf{r})$ is composed of N functional tissue components of true activity concentration T_i, each distributed over a spatial domain D_i, the image $I(\mathbf{r})$ can be derived using the linear character of the scanner, as expressed by

$$I(\mathbf{r}) = \sum_{j=1}^{N} \int_{D_j} T_j(\mathbf{r}')\mathrm{PSF}(\mathbf{r}, \mathbf{r}')\, d\mathbf{r}' \quad (2)$$

Since $T_j(\mathbf{r})$ is considered to be constant (i.e., homogeneous activity distribution within each tissue component), equation (2) can be written as

$$I(\mathbf{r}) = \sum_{j=1}^{N} T_j \int_{D_j} \mathrm{PSF}(\mathbf{r} - \mathbf{r}')\, d\mathbf{r}' \quad (3)$$

Since we want to correct regional values as generally obtained with PET, we can restrain the domain of calculation of the geometric transfer function (GTF) expressed by equation (3) to a limited area that constitutes a ROI. Then t_i, the mean value observed within ROI_i is given by

$$t_i = \frac{1}{n_{\mathrm{pix}}} \sum_{j=1}^{N} T_j \int_{\mathrm{ROI}_i} \int_{D_j} \mathrm{PSF}(\mathbf{r}, \mathbf{r}')\, d\mathbf{r}'\, d\mathbf{r} \quad (4)$$

where n_{pix} is the number of pixels in ROI_i.

Equation (4) can be re-expressed as

$$t_i = \sum_{j=1}^{N} \omega_{ij} T_j \quad (5)$$

where

$$\omega_{ij} = \frac{1}{n_{\text{pix}}} \int_{\text{ROI}_i} \int_{D_j} \text{PSF}(\mathbf{r}, \mathbf{r}') \, d\mathbf{r}' \, d\mathbf{r} \qquad (6)$$

The weighting factors ω_{ij} of the GTF represent the fractions of activity from each component in the observed measurement for any ROI, assuming unit activity in each structure. Therefore, voxels GTFs within each component of nonzero activity are integrated to generate a matrix of regional GTFs; that is, the contribution of each tissue to any region (ROI) of the image. This transfer matrix is thereafter referred to as the *geometric transfer matrix* (GTM), as in

$$\begin{bmatrix} t_1 \\ t_2 \\ \vdots \\ t_N \end{bmatrix} = \begin{bmatrix} \omega_{11} & \omega_{12} & \cdots & \omega_{1N} \\ \omega_{21} & \omega_{22} & & \\ \vdots & & \ddots & \vdots \\ \omega_{N1} & \omega_{N2} & \cdots & \omega_{NN} \end{bmatrix} \times \begin{bmatrix} T_1 \\ T_2 \\ \vdots \\ T_N \end{bmatrix} \qquad (7)$$

The diagonal terms of this matrix represent tissue self-interaction, or *recovery coefficient* (RC); that is, measured to true activity ratio in the absence of surrounding activity (Hoffman *et al.*, 1979). The other terms ω_{ij} ($j \neq i$) refer to the spillover fraction; that is, the fraction of true activity (T_j) of tissue j integrated in ROI$_i$. The regional values actually observed with PET and these known regional GTFs then represent a system of linear equations that can be solved for the true regional values. The GTFs are dependent on geometrical relationships between the structures of interest and on the ROIs and image resolution used but are independent of tracer activity distribution.

D. Accuracy vs. Precision

The implication of equation (5) is that the corrected value of tissue i is given by equation (8), where w'_{ij} represent the elements of the inverse of the GTM given in equation (7); that is, the matrix of correction factors to apply to the observed measurements:

$$T_i = \sum_{j=1}^{N} \omega'_{ij} t_j \qquad (8)$$

Apart from being dependent on geometrical interactions between the structures and the PET detection system, the recovery factors constituting the GTM, as well as the observed measurements and their precision, are dependent on the location and dimensions of the ROIs used and on the image resolution. Their covariance therefore would have been necessary to assess for a rigorous estimation of the degradation of data precision. However, the error attached to the corrected value, in terms of its standard deviation dT_i, cannot

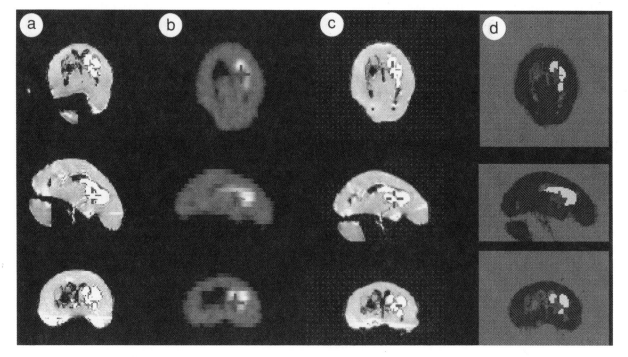

FIGURE 1   A 3D physical brain phantom after anatomical segmentation of the MRI volume registered with the PET data: (a) original MRI, (b) original PET, (c) realigned MRI volume in PET native space (2-mm thickness), (d) coded MRI after segmentation into various components.

exceed that obtained in the case of independent variables:

$$dT_i^2 \le \sum_{j=1}^{N} \left(\frac{\partial T_i}{\partial t_j} dt_j\right)^2 = \sum_{j=1}^{N} (\omega_{ij}' dt_j)^2 \qquad (9)$$

Where dt_j represents the standard deviation of the mean pixel value in ROI_i. The initial estimate of the noise enhancement phenomenon introduced by the N-fold correction process therefore was computed from the precision of the corrected values in terms of standard deviation derived from equation (9), which represents the worst case.

E. Accuracy and Limits of the Method

1. Experiment I: Physical Brain Phantom

We used a plastic model of the brain consisting of separately fillable compartments in the shapes of the caudate, putamen, globus pallidus, and ventricle, located in a main chamber (BKG) simulating the rest of the brain, all surrounded by a real skull. The design was based on digitized brain slices (Wong *et al.*, 1984). Structures located in the left hemisphere tended to leak; therefore, only the right caudate nucleus (CN), putamen (PU), and globus pallidus (GP) were considered in the present experiments.

To study static tracer distribution, the physical brain phantom was filled with a solution of [^{18}F]FDG at two different concentrations: one for the basal ganglia and

one for the main chamber, in the ratio of 3.5 to 1. The phantom was scanned for 2 hr to provide 27 images with frame lengths ranging from 30 sec to 10 min. Subsequently, a T_1-weighted sequence of the phantom was acquired with an MRI unit (GE, 1.5 T). The MRI volume was registered with the 15-slice PET volume (Evans *et al.*, 1991a) and then resampled to 2-mm thick images that were segmented into its various components (Fig. 1). Regional concentrations within the phantom were measured using anatomical (i.e., irregular) user-defined ROIs for each compartment with nonzero activity. Simulated images of each component were generated, and the GTM for the particular ROI template chosen was extracted. The observed regional values were then corrected according to the estimated GTM, considering a four-tissue system: CN, PU, GP, and BKG.

To test the ability of PVE-correction method to recover the activity with varying contrast conditions, the deep cavities were filled with a solution of fluorine-18 and the main chamber was filled with a radioactive solution containing carbon-11. Starting concentrations were 74 kBq·ml^{-1}, and 51.8 kBq.ml^{-1}, respectively, for ^{11}C and ^{18}F. The phantom was scanned for 85 min, and time–activity curves were derived by applying the ROI template defined from MRI on the corresponding PET slice from a total of 100 reconstructed images that were not corrected for radioisotope decay. The same procedures of simulation described earlier were applied to provide a GTM characteristic of the geometric conditions of the experiment. Both observed and corrected TACs were fitted with monoexponential functions to derive tracer half-life.

2. Experiment II: Simulation of Dynamic Tracer Uptake

This set of experiments was designed to investigate the PVE occurring in the normal human brain and the ability of the proposed method to provide accurate corrected estimates of regional radioactivity concentrations in PET-like noise conditions. Arbitrary shaped time–activity curves were assigned to various identified components of a normal brain (i.e., white matter, cortical gray matter, basal ganglia, thalamus), to simulate the time course of a hypothetical tracer within this brain. These curves were derived from functions in the form of $a \times \ln(t + 1) \times \exp(-b \times t)$, where t represents the time expressed in minutes, and a and b are constants chosen so as to provide TACs covering a wide range of image contrast range and activity levels (Fig. 2). The time-sampling scheme, typical for [^{18}F]fluorodopa studies in human subjects, consisted of 27 frames of 30 sec, 1 min, 2 min, 5 min, and 10 min lengths (Kuwabara *et al.*, 1993). The mean regional activity of

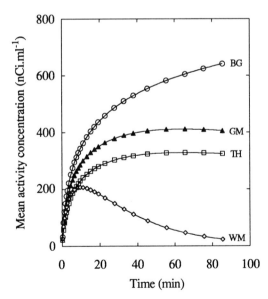

FIGURE 2 Arbitrary TACs used to simulate tracer uptake in the basal ganglia (BG), gray matter (GM), thalamus (TH), and white matter (WM).

TABLE 1   Recovery of Half-Life Characteristics of the Tracers[a]

Structure	FWHM (mm)	Observed			Corrected		
		$T_{1/2}$ (min)	Recovery (%)	rms[b] (%)	$T_{1/2}$ (min)	Recovery (%)	rms[b] (%)
CN	6	89.4	81.3	6.2	112.3	102.5	7.0
[18]F	12	74.1	67.4	4.3	113.2	103.3	5.4
PU	6	76.8	69.8	4.1	109.6	100.0	4.2
[18]F	12	61.5	55.9	3.6	113.7	103.7	3.5
BKG	6	20.1	98.5	1.1	20.1	98.5	1.2
[11]C	12	20.2	99.0	0.6	20.1	98.5	0.5

[a]True half-life periods $T_{1/2}$ were taken as 109.6 min for ^{18}F and 20.4 min for [11]C.
[b]Mean root mean square error between data points and fitting curve.

interest was taken as the average value of the right and left sides, and the ROI template was therefore selected as a set of pairs of anatomical ROIs placed on each five components: caudate (CN), putamen (PU), gray matter (GM), thalamus (TH), and white matter (WM). Poisson noise was added to each projection element according to the number of recorded counts, after simulation of photon attenuation in matter, along with ran-

dom and scatter counts according to the method proposed in Ma *et al.* (1993).

Each observed tissue TAC was corrected according to the 5 × 5 GTM extracted from ROI sampling of the simulated PET images of each identified component.

III.   RESULTS AND DISCUSSION

A.   Experiment I: Physical Brain Phantom

1.   Static Tracer

The apparent recovery coefficient (ARC), defined as the ratio of observed to true activity, is plotted as a function of accumulated counts in the slice analyzed, for both observed and corrected data range 68k to 1 million, (Fig. 3). The PVE correction allows signal recovery of nearly 100% of the true activity present in the various compartments. The accuracy of the observed data proved to be of the order of 70% at a resolution of 6 mm, and corrected data were within 2% of the true value for CN and 4% for PU for a number of accumulated counts >300k. The precision was found to be moderately affected by the correction. For instance, the degradation of data precision was estimated by comparing the coefficient of variation (COV = SD/mean) before and after correction. The noise magnification factor (NMF), ratio of the COVs after/before correction, was computed against the number of accumulated counts and found not to exceed 1.2 for the caudate and 1.4 for the putamen, with the expected tendency to decrease with increasing accumulated counts. Such figures can be derived for various contrasts, ROI sizes, or resolutions. In the last case, we noted that both accuracy and precision were degraded

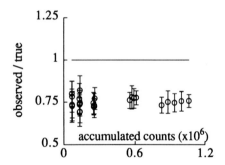

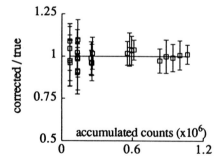

FIGURE 3   The apparent recovery coefficients, defined as the ratio of observed to true tracer concentration—ideally 1—and their relative precision in terms of Standard Deviation of the Mean Pixel Valve (SDMPV), plotted as a function of the number of accumulated counts, before (top) and after correction (bottom).

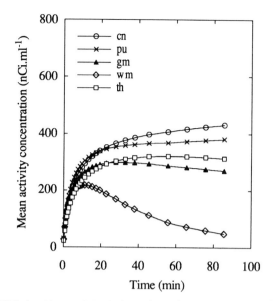

FIGURE 4 Observed TACs in various tissue components of the human brain when no other effects but resolution are simulated. They were extracted from the noise-free simulated PET images reconstructed with a 6 mm FWHM Hanning filter.

when increasing the width of the reconstruction filter.

2. Dynamic Tracer

The original TACs extracted for the deep nuclei filled with ^{18}F showed an underestimation of half-life due to contaminating activity from the faster kinetic component of the main compartment filled with ^{11}C (Table 1). Although the corrected activity level for CN was found to be underestimated by more than 10% (data not shown), the shape of its decay curve was accurately restored. The least squares fitting of the corrected TAC provided half-life values within 3% of the true value for the isotope used. The putamen gave the best results,

TABLE 2 Percentage rms Distance between Corrected Estimates and True Activity Concentrations

Structure	Noiseless		Noisy	
	Mean	**SD**	**Mean**	**SD**
CN	0.94	0.37	9.26	10.78
PU	1.11	0.51	8.97	9.70
GM	1.05	0.43	4.21	4.05
WM	1.66	1.60	6.85	7.10
TH	1.40	0.63	6.42	8.32

with only 1% underestimation of the activity at the beginning of the scan (not shown) and a 100% half-life recovery at a resolution of 6 mm FWHM. The underestimation encountered with CN is believed to be due to the presence of bubbles in this cavity, leading to "partial volume averaging" of a hot region with nonradioactive voids. For instance, the recovery of tracer's half-life to within 3% (Table 1), despite the underestimation of absolute regional tracer concentration, could prove to involve a time-invariant factor. Indeed, an overestimation of caudate's RC would produce an underestimation mainly in the recovery factor applied to the observed activity within CN and would therefore lead to a systematic underestimation of absolute tracer concentration. We found that a 14% depression of RC would provide accurate corrected estimates and would correspond to the presence of a bubble of less than 2 mm in diameter according to the calculation proposed by Kessler *et al.* (1984), assuming that CN can be locally assimilated to a sphere of roughly twice the resolution (6 mm FWHM) in diameter.

B. Experiment II: Contrast Recovery, Simulations

The TACs presented in Figure 4 are regional values observed with the user-defined ROI templates and from the simulated dynamic PET images obtained in noiseless conditions. They are differentially distorted, with greater loss for small structures, due to relatively larger PVE. For instance, CN and PU were originally as-

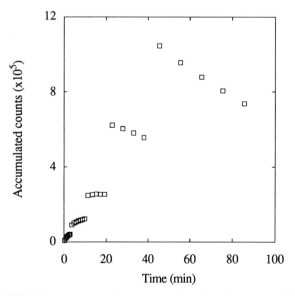

FIGURE 5 Accumulated counts as a function of time providing various statistics for the simulated images produced.

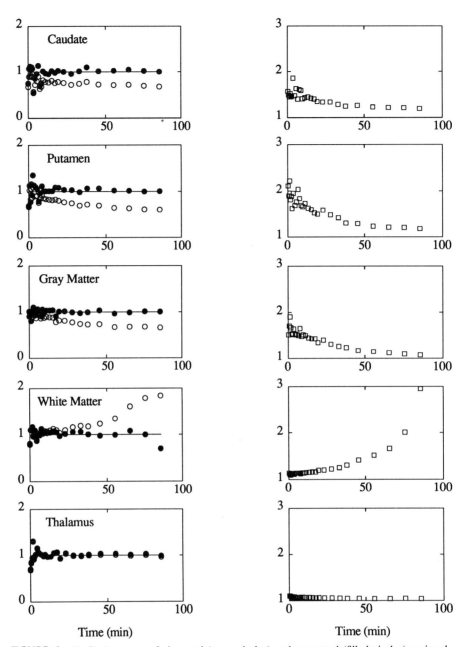

FIGURE 6 (Left) Accuracy of observed (open circles) and corrected (filled circles) regional activity as a function of time, when Poisson noise is incorporated in the simulation. Values are given as the recovery factor, defined as the ratio of observed (resp. corrected) to true activity initially assigned to the coded brain (Fig. 2). Images were reconstructed with a 6 mm FWHM Hanning filter. (Right) Degradation of precision of the corrected estimates computed as the noise magnification factor, defined as $(SD/mean)_{corr}/(SD/mean)_{obs}$.

signed the same tracer kinetics, represented by the basal ganglia (BG) curve shown in Figure 2, but they exhibit a different PET response due to different geometrical conditions; that is, different regional GTFs (equation (7)). After application of the inverse GTM, the shape of each TAC was fully restored. The corrected regional values were found to almost perfectly match the arbitrary tissue TACs chosen for simulating

dynamic tracer uptake, with a mean coefficient of variation with respect to the true value of smaller than 2% when analyzing noise-free images (Table 2). For the results presented, using anatomical ROIs of size ranging from 44 pixels to 269 pixels (2 × 2 mm) and at a resolution of 6 mm FWHM, RC was of 58% for CN and that of 52% for PU. The fraction of GM true activity contaminating the measurement (spillover fraction) was slightly greater for CN (14%) than for PU (9%), which was found to be more sensitive to white matter activity (39%) compared to CN (17%). Whereas cortical gray matter exhibited a 65% RC in ROIs over 200 pixels, 32% of white matter activity was integrated in its measurement. White matter (WM) regions as well as thalamus (TH) were affected far less by resolution, thanks to their ≈90% RC. These reported values do not constitute an absolute reference, because differences in ROI size, shape, and placement, as well as image resolution, may slightly modify these patterns.

TACs extracted from the noisy simulated images were corrected with an average rms error of corrected versus true values varying from 4.2% for GM to 9.3% for CN (Table 2) over the range of counts presented in Figure 5. The recovery factors of observed activity compared to corrected estimates for each tissue component are presented in Figure 6(left). The deterioration of the precision of the corrected estimates is presented in Figure 6(right) as the ratio of regional coefficients of variation before and after correction, or noise magnification factor. The sensitivity of the measurements to the various levels of noise is depicted by the behavior of the NMF curves, which are relatively high at the beginning when the statistics are low and then tend to decrease mono-exponentially as the number of accumulated counts increases. The poor recovery of activity within WM for the last time frame comes from the very low uptake value assigned (Fig. 2). Despite limited partial volume losses due to its relatively large dimension, WM activity can be overestimated due to the significant contribution of GM activity with increasing contrast. The few percent integrated from GM (≈6% in the present case) can then participate significantly in the observed low measurement within WM, which sees its activity overestimated by almost a factor of 2 for the last frame (Fig. 6(left)). In this case, even though the SD of the corrected estimate is similar to the SD of the measurement, the NMF goes off as the result of a concomitant overestimation of observed activity, which lowers the corresponding COV, and an underestimation of the corrected estimate.

In conclusion, apart from being independent of tracer activity levels allowing us to account for activity spilled over from regions suffering from PVE, the method provides simple estimate of degradation of precision that proved to be reasonable. The method is believed to be less sensitive to noise than a pixel-by-pixel deconvolution, although the present method could be extendable to one. Finally, assuming that we are capable of reproducing realistic imaging conditions, we can estimate the accuracy and precision of tissue curve, allowing us to optimize the imaging protocol or data sampling strategy to adopt for getting the most

suitable results. It would be interesting to compute the covariance factors to optimize the image analysis strategy, especially when analyzing dynamic data that need to be obtained at a rather low resolution.

Acknowledgments

Supported in part by USPHS grants HD24061, HD24448, and MH42821.

References

Evans, A. C., Marrett, S., and Collins, L. (1991a). MRI-PET correlation in three dimensions using a volume-of-interest (VOI) atlas. *J. Cereb. Blood Flow Metab.* **11, 2:** A69–A78.

Evans, A. C., Thomson, C. J., Marrett, S., Meyer, E., and Mazza, M. (1991b). Performance evaluation of the PC-2048: A new 15-slice encoded-crystal PET scanner for neurological studies. *IEEE Trans. Med. Imag.* vol. 10, no. 1.

Herman, G. T., Lewitt, R. M., Odhner, D., and Rowland, S. W. (1989). Snark 89, a programming system for image reconstruction from projections. no. MIPG160.

Hoffman, E. J., Huang, S. C., and Phelps, E. (1979). Quantitation in positron emission tomography: 1. Effect of object size. *J. Comput. Assist. Tomogr.* **3:** 299–308.

Kessler, R. M., Ellis, J., and Eden, M. (1984). Analysis of emission tomographic scan data: Limitations imposed by resolution and background. *J. Comput. Assist. Tomogr.* **8, 3:** 514–522.

Kuwabara, H., Cumming, P., Reith, J., Léger, G., Diksic, M., Evans, A. C., and Gjedde, A. (1993). Human striatal L-DOPA decarboxylase activity estimated in vivo using 6-[18F]fluoro-DOPA and positron emission tomography: Error analysis and application to normal subjects. *J. Cereb. Blood Flow Metab.* **13:** 43–56.

Ma, Y., Kamber, M., and Evans, A. C. (1993). 3-D simulation of PET brain images using segmented MRI and positron tomograph characteristics. *Comput. Med. Imaging Graphics* **11, 4/5:** 365–371.

Meltzer, C. C., Leal, J. P., Mayberg, H. S., Wagner, H. N., and Frost, J. J. (1990). Correction of PET data for partial volume effects in human cerebral cortex by MR imaging. *J. Comput. Assist. Tomogr.* **14:** 561–570.

Müller-Gärtner, H. W., Links, J. M., Leprince, J. L., Bryan, R. N., McVeigh, E., Leal, J. P., Davatzikos, C., and Frost, J. J. (1992). Measurement of radiotracer concentration in brain gray matter using positron emission tomography: MRI-based correction for partial volume effects. *J. Cereb. Blood Flow Metab.* **12:** 571–583.

Rousset, O., Ma, Y., Kamber, M., and Evans, A. C. (1993a). 3-D simulations of radio tracer uptake in deep nuclei of human brain. *Comput. Med. Imaging Graphics* **11, 4/5:** 373–379.

Rousset, O. G., Ma, Y., Léger, G. C., Gjedde, A. H., and Evans, A. C. (1993b). Correction for partial volume effects in PET using MRI-based 3D simulations of individual human brain metabolism. *In:* "Quantification of Brain Function. Tracer Kinetics and Image Analysis in Brain PET." (K. Uemura, N. A. Lassen, T. Jones, and I. Kanno, Eds.), pp. 113–125. Elsevier Science, Amsterdam.

Videen, T. O., Perlmutter, J. S., Mintun, M. A., and Raichle, M. E. (1988). Regional correction of positron emission tomography data for the effects of cerebral atrophy. *J. Cereb. Blood Flow Metab.* **8:** 662–670.

Wong, D. F., Links, J. M., Molliver, M. E., Hengst, T. C., Clifford, C. M., Buhle, L., Bryan, M., Stumpf, M., and Wagner, H. M. (1984). An anatomically realistic brain phantom for quantification with positron tomography. *J. Nucl. Med.* **25:** P108.

Dissolution of Partial Volume Effect in PET by an Inversion Technique with the MR-Embedded Neural Network Model

YUKIO KOSUGI[1], MIKIYA SASE[2], YUSUKE SUGANAMI[1], TOSHIMITSU MOMOSE[2], and JUNICHI NISHIKAWA[2]

[1]*Tokyo Institute of Technology*
Yokohama 226, Japan
[2]*University of Tokyo, School of Medicine*
Bunkyoku, Tokyo 113, Japan

Conventional deconvolution of PET images alone will not provide sufficient information for a precise study of localized brain function. In the deconvolution process, which is a type of inverse problem, it is important to confine the solution space by incorporating such a priori knowledge as the tissue distribution given by MR images. In this chapter, we propose an MR-embedded neural-network model to reduce the partial volume effect in the restoration of blood flow profiles from PET images. In the model, the hypothesized blood flow profile was iteratively modified to reduce the error between the synthesized and the observed PET images. This process, based on the network-inversion technique, is equivalent to realizing a deconvolution process. We tested our method on brain PET images from three normal subjects, as well as on a three-compartment phantom. After 10 updating iterations, clear activity profiles appeared in the hidden layer of the network. The activities were attributed mostly to those physiologically anticipated cortical areas: Activities miscellaneously assigned to the ventricles, to the bone, even to areas outside the head were restored to be in the appropriate cortical areas. We also tested the validity of the network model, by changing the weighting ratio w(gray matter)/w(white matter) to find that the error between the synthesized image and the actual PET image was minimum when the ratio was set at 1:4.

I. INTRODUCTION

In neuroactivation and neuroimaging with positron emission tomography (PET) or single photon emission tomography (SPECT), due to a limited number of detectors, as well as the random process involved in the positron recombination, spatial resolution is sometimes poorer than the physiological needs (George *et al.*, 1991). Deconvolution or conventional filtering of the reconstructed image will not provide sufficient information for a precise study of the localized brain function. In the deconvolution process, which is a type of inverse problem, it is important to confine the solution space by incorporating such *a priori* knowledge as the tissue distribution given by MR images. In this chapter, we propose an MR-embedded neural-network model to reduce the partial volume effect in the restoration of blood flow profiles from PET images.

II. METHOD

A. Conventional Deconvolution

If we have an infinite resolution of observed images in two-dimensional space (x, y), the observed image $s(x, y)$ might be obtained by the convolution of the true

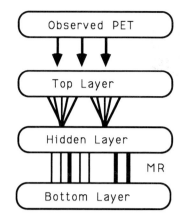

FIGURE 1   Neural network architecture.

distribution $f(x, z)$ with the spread function $g(\xi, \zeta)$ as

$$s(x, y) = \iint g(\xi, \zeta) f(x - \xi, y - \zeta)\, d\xi d\zeta$$
$$= g(x, y) * f(x, y) \qquad (1)$$

where $*$ denotes the convolution operator. If we have an ideal technique to observe the true distribution without ambiguity, $g(x, y)$ in (1) is the delta function, that is, $s(x, y) = f(x, y)$, but in actual systems $g(x, y)$ will have a distribution of a finite range describing the spatial resolution of the system.

When we apply the Fourier transform, the image profile in the space–frequency domain can be expressed simply as the product of F and G:

$$S(\omega_x, \omega_y) = G(\omega_x, \omega_y) \times F(\omega_x, \omega_y) \qquad (2)$$

where G and F are Fourier transforms of $g(x, y)$ and $f(x, y)$, respectively. This means, if we have the complete information about $s(x, y)$ and $g(x, y)$, we may be able to get the true distribution $f(x, y)$ as

$$f(x, y) = F^{-1}[S/G] \qquad (3)$$

where $F^{-1}[\ ]$ is the inverse Fourier transform. However, in practice, we cannot realize the spatial frequency range required for calculation of (3) in its ideal form. With the data insufficiently given, the deconvolution process, that is an inverse problem, turns out to be *ill-posed*; that is, we cannot determine the unique solution. To solve the problem, we should confine the solution space by giving *a priori* knowledge obtained from other observations, preferably based on image-generation processes including physiological and anatomical *a priori* knowledge.

B. The Neural Network Model

We modeled the PET image generation process based on a layered neural network consisting of linear neural elements as shown in Figure 1. Units in the bottom layer indicate a normalized physiological activity of the tissue, whereas the hidden layer units describe the positron generation profile attributed to the blood flow. The top layer describes the synthesized PET image, to be compared with the actual PET. Divergent connections from the hidden layer units to the top layer describe the diffusing process that causes the partial volume effect, which is equivalent to the convolution process of equation (1), in a discrete form.

That is, the top layer jth unit activity can be described as

$$s_j = \sum_i f_i g_{ji} \qquad (4)$$

where f_i is the hidden layer ith unit's activity, g_{ji} is the connection weight between the ith hidden unit and the jth top layer unit.

The one-to-one connection between the bottom layer and the hidden layer of the MR embedded network are prewired according to the gray matter and the white matter distribution given by the corresponding MR of 256×256 pixel resolution. We gave a weight of 4 to the gray matter, 1 to the white matter, and 0 to the CSF and other parts as

$$f_i = w_i a_i \qquad (5)$$

with the weight values $w_i = 1$ for white matter, 4 for gray matter, and 0 for the CSF and other parts; where a_i is the bottom layer ith unit's activity. The rationale for this ratio will be explained in the discussion. To classify these cerebral tissues, we used another three-layered back-propagation neural network system.

C. Network Inversion for Fitting the Model

In the model fitting procedure, the blood flow profile hypothesized in the model will be modified to reduce the error between the synthesized and the observed PET images. In updating the activity profile of the hidden and bottom layers, we modify the network inversion technique proposed by (Linden *et al.*, 1989). This process is equivalent to realizing a deconvolution process under the condition given by an MR image, which is a special case of an inverse process to the diffusion process modeled in the network (Sase *et al.*, 1994).

In short, this model fitting process is done by modifying the bottom layer activity with the iterative use of the following equation:

$$a_i(t + 1) = a_i(t) - \eta[\partial E/\partial a_i] \qquad (6)$$

where $a_i(t)$ is the activity of the ith unit in the previous step, $a_i(t + 1)$ is the new activity, η is the learning coefficient, E is the squared error between the synthe-

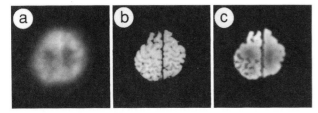

FIGURE 2   Dissolution result: (a) brain PET image without processing, (b) brain MR image, (c) PET image after neural-net processing.

sized PET image and the actually observed PET image, defined as

$$E = (1/2)\sum_j (t_j - s_j)^2 \qquad (7)$$

where t_j is the jth tutorial signal given by the actual PET.

Substitution of (4), (5), and (7) into (6) yields the explicit update formula

$$a_i(t + 1) = a_i(t) - \eta \sum_j (s_j - t_j)\, g_{ji} w_i \qquad (6')$$

During the blood flow update process, *a priori* knowledge regarding the tissue profile given by the MR helps to dissolve the partial volume effect; for example, blood flow in the gray matter is four times that of the white matter (Ingvar *et al.*, 1965). Connection weights from the bottom layer to the hidden layer describe this intensity profile. Absence of connection from the CSF prevents misinterpretation of the activity from the inactive region.

III. RESULTS

We tested our method on brain PET images from three normal subjects, as well as on a three-compartment phantom. The artificial PET image synthesized in the network was compared with the actual PET image obtained by $H_2^{15}O$ bolus injection and HeadTome IV. Each PET image, with a resolution of 128×128, was given to the MR-embedded network.

After 10 updating iterations using equation (6') with $\eta = 0.003$, starting with all the initial values of the bottom layer activities set to 0, clear activity profiles appeared in the hidden layer of the network. An example of the results is shown in Figure 2, with respect to a volunteer normal subject reading sentences aloud. Figure 2(a) shows the original PET image with the filtering or the conventional deconvolutional process off, Figure 2(b) is the MR image of the corresponding slice level, Figure 2(c) is the resultant image that ap-

peared in the hidden layer of the MR embedded network, after 10 fitting iterations under the supervision of actual image Figure 2(a). The activities were attributed mostly to those cortical areas where physiological activity was expected during the examination: Activities miscellaneously assigned to the ventricles, to the bone, even to areas outside the head were restored to be in the appropriate cortical areas.

In the model fitting process we imposed a restriction on the bottom layer activity profile that the activity of each unit a_j should be within a level zone $[a_{j(av)} - \theta < a_j < a_{j(av)} + \theta]$, where $a_{j(av)}$ is the averaged activity of the neighboring units, θ is the threshold level. This restriction was imposed only on the units within the white matter area, because the excessive restrictions may prevent the activity of a meaningful fine area within the gray matter to grow. This restriction should confine the solution space; however, there was no significant change in the resultant images, except when the original image was contaminated with high-frequency noise.

As shown in Table 1, we also tested the validity of the network model, by changing the weighting ratio w(gray matter)/w(white matter) from 1 : 1 to 1 : 10 and found that the error between the synthesized image and the actual PET image was minimum when the ratio was set at 1 : 4. This ratio agreed with the estimated regional cerebral blood flow for human brain (Ingvar *et al.*, 1965). In our current model, connection weights between the top and the hidden layers are all fixed at the one calculated based on point-source measurements. However, the convolution parameters can be treated as trainable variables, to be trained with the ordinary back-propagation algorithm with respect to some standard phantom sources to compensate for the nonuniform sensitivity as well as the aging effect of the γ-ray detectors. This flexibility is one of the significant advantages when compared with the similar MR-based model (Müller-Gärtner *et al.*, 1992).

TABLE 1   Model Fitting Error as the Function of the Weight Ratio

w(gray)/w(white)	Squared error
1.0	31.77
2.0	17.21
3.0	17.96
4.0	14.29
5.0	15.82
6.0	18.28
10.0	19.80

References

George, M. S., Ring, H. A., Costa, D. C., *et al.* (1991). "Neuroactivation and Neuroimaging with SPECT." Springer-Verlag, London.

Ingvar, D. H., Cronovist, S., Ekberg, R., *et al.* (1965). Normal values of regional cerebral blood flow in man, including flow and weight estimates of gray and white matter. *Acta Neurol. Scand.* **41** (suppl. 14): 72–78.

Linden, A., and Kindermann, J. (1989). Inversion of Multilayer Nets. Proc. Int. Joint Conf. on Neural Networks. pp. 425–432.

Müller-Gärtner, H. W., Links, J. M., Prince, J. L., *et al.* (1992). Measurement of radiotracer concentration in brain gray matter using positron emission tomography: MRI-based correction for partial volume effects. *J. Cereb. Blood Flow Metab.* **12,** 571–583.

Sase, M., Kinoshita, N., and Kosugi, Y. (1994). A neural network for fusing the MR information into PET images to improve spatial resolution. *Proc. IEEE Int. Conf. Image Processing.* pp. 908–911.

The Effect of Spatial Correlation on the Quantification in Positron Emission Tomography

G. BLOMQVIST, L. ERIKSSON, and G. ROSENQVIST

Department of Clinical Neuroscience
Experimental Alcohol and Drug Addiction Research Section
and Section of Clinical Neurophysiology
Karolinska Hospital
S-17176 Stockholm, Sweden

In positron emission tomography the values in adjacent parts of reconstructed images of radioactivity distributions are correlated. These correlations were examined by phantom measurements. The corresponding correlations in the parametric maps, derived from a time series of radioactivity maps, were investigated analytically and by simulation. As expected, the correlation was found to depend strongly on the distance between the pixels and on the cutoff frequency of the filter function used in the image reconstruction. With 3D data acquisition, there is also a considerable axial correlation, which was found to be largest between the outer planes and to increase with distance from the camera axis. The effect of correlation on the SEM of the pixel values in a region was found to be considerable and depend on both the size and shape of the region. For kinetic models, linear in the parameters, it was shown that the correlation coefficient between parameter values in two pixels is equal to or smaller than the correlation coefficient between the corresponding radioactivity values. Equality holds only when the ratio between the errors in two pixels are the same in all time intervals. The simulations showed that parameters entering nonlinearly in the model equation tend to have smaller correlation coefficient than parameters entering linearly, which have almost the same correlation coefficient as the underlying radioactivity data.

I. INTRODUCTION

In positron emission tomography (PET), the results of the measurements are often presented in the form of parametric maps with local values of CBF, CMR_{glc}, and so forth in each picture element (pixel). Normally the arithmetic mean of the individual pixel values in a region of such a map is used as a measure of the average parameter value in that region. The corresponding standard error of the mean (SEM) depends both on the standard errors of the individual pixel values in the region and on the correlation between the pixel values. These correlations, which depend on the camera geometry and the image reconstruction algorithm, are transferred from the reconstructed images of the radioactivity distribution to the parametric images derived from the time–activity data.

Normally, a PET study includes data from a number of subjects (or from repeated measurements on the same subject). From each subject and from each region, one parameter value is obtained: the arithmetic mean of the pixels in the region. From these values, the arithmetic mean and the SEM of the sample are calculated, and the effects of correlations between pixel values need not be known. However, an important question that requires knowledge about correlations is this: How much of the SEM in a region depends on the measurement error and how much depends on the true variation of the parameter value between the subjects? Knowledge of the measurement errors and the correlations is also required when only one measurement has been made (e.g., on one patient or on one special state), and one wishes to know whether or not the parameter value in some region deviates significantly from some (normal) value.

The aim of this study was threefold. First, the correlations in the reconstructed maps of the radioactivity concentration were investigated. The influence of the pixel positions and the filtering in the reconstruction algorithm was studied. Second, the effect of the correlations on the SEM in a region was investigated. Regions of different sizes and shapes were examined. Third, the correlation in the parametric maps, derived from the time sequence of the images of the radioactivity concentration, was studied.

II. MATERIALS AND METHODS

A. Measurement of Correlations in Activity Maps

The random errors in PET measurements originate in the fluctuations of the radioactive decay. These fluctuations imply that the projection data obey Poisson statistics, at least for moderate count rates, when dead time corrections are small. Using explicit expressions of the reconstruction algorithm, these fluctuations can provide errors and correlations in the maps of the radioactivity concentrations. However, the function connecting the projection data with the pixel data is complex, and therefore, we have chosen to estimate the errors by measurements on phantoms. Two types of phantoms were studied, a cylindrical, homogeneous phantom (radius 10 cm) filled with Ge-68 in a solid matrix and a Ge-68 line source. Each phantom was measured repeatedly, 10 times during 10 min in an ECAT EXACT HR positron camera (47 reconstructed image slices, 4 mm spatial resolution, and 4.5 mm transaxial resolution in the center of the plane). Due to the long half-life (275 days), the radioactivity was regarded as constant during the measuring time. Both 2D and 3D data acquisitions were applied. The images of the radioactivity distribution were reconstructed using a Hanning filter with the cutoff frequencies 0.3 and 0.5. The pixel size in the resulting images of the radioactivity concentration was 2×2 mm. The correlation coefficient between the data in two pixels was estimated from the 10 independent pairs of measurements. Pairs of pixels evenly distributed in the phantom image (4 mm apart in the x- and y-directions, respectively) were selected and averages of the corresponding correlation coefficients were calculated.

B. The Effect of Correlations on the SEM in a Region

With correlations present, the SEM of the pixel values X_i ($i = 1, n_p$) in a region is

$$\sigma[X] = \frac{1}{n_p} \sqrt{\sum_i \sigma_{X_i}^2 + 2 \sum \sum_{i<j} \sigma_{X_i} \sigma_{X_j} \rho_{ij}} \qquad (1)$$

where n_p is the number of pixels in the region, σ_{X_i} is the standard deviation in pixel i, and ρ_{ij} is the correlation coefficient between the values in pixels i and j. With equal standard deviations σ in all pixels, equation (1) simplifies to

$$\sigma[X] = \frac{\sigma}{\sqrt{n_p}} \sqrt{1 + \frac{2}{n_p} \sum \sum_{i<j} \rho_{ij}} \qquad (2)$$

Without correlations $\sigma[X]$ becomes $\sigma/\sqrt{n_p}$. Therefore, when the error is the same in all pixels of a region, the correlation effects enter as a correction factor to the usual expression for SEM, valid for independent and identically distributed random variables.

C. Estimation of Correlation Effects in Parametric Maps

1. Analytical

The algorithm for parameter estimation, including stopping rules for iterations and so on, is the same in all pixels of the parametric map, and therefore, the estimate of a certain parameter is related to the observed time sequence of radioactivities by the same function in all pixels. This function depends on auxiliary variables, in particular the input function (e.g., the time course of the tracer concentration in the plasma), assumed to be common for all pixels. As a rule, the input function is much more precisely determined than the radioactivity concentration in individual pixels, and accordingly, the measurements of this function are treated as nonrandom.

Because observations in different time frames are independent, the following relations between the time sequences of measurements $X_1, \ldots, X_{nt}$ and $Y_1, \ldots, Y_{nt}$ in two pixels are valid:

$$\begin{aligned} \text{cov}[X_i, X_j] &= 0 & \text{if } i \neq j, \quad i,j = 1, \ldots, n_t & \quad (3a) \\ \text{cov}[Y_i, Y_j] &= 0 & \text{if } i \neq j, \quad i,j = 1, \ldots, n_t & \quad (3b) \\ \text{cov}[X_i, Y_j] &= 0 & \text{if } i \neq j, \quad i,j = 1, \ldots, n_t & \quad (3c) \end{aligned}$$

The origin of the correlations, the camera geometry and the reconstruction algorithm, is the same for all time frames. As will be shown later, the correlation coefficient is nearly independent of the radioactivity distribution in the object. This motivates the assumption that the correlation coefficient, ρ_{XY}, between the observations in two pixels is common to all time frames; that is,

$$\text{cov}[X_i, Y_i] = \sigma_{X_i} \sigma_{Y_i} \rho_{XY}, \qquad i = 1, \ldots, n_t \qquad (4)$$

Only exceptionally is the explicit form of the function relating the time–activity data to the parameter estimate known. An example is the frequently utilized linear approximation, which is valid at late times in many situations (Patlak et al., 1983). Linear models have an important property: The (linear least squares) estimates of the parameters are, in turn, linearly related to the measurements (see, e.g., Beck and Arnold, 1977). Thus, in two pixels, the estimates P and Q of a parameter are related to the corresponding time series $X_1, \ldots, X_{nt}$ and $Y_1, \ldots, Y_{nt}$ by the same linear expression:

$$P = \Sigma \, b_i X_i \quad\quad\quad (5a)$$
$$Q = \Sigma \, b_i Y_i \quad\quad\quad (5b)$$

How is the correlation coefficient ρ_{PQ} between the parameter values P and Q in two pixels related to the correlation coefficient ρ_{XY} between the corresponding time–activity data X_i and Y_i ($i = 1, \ldots, n_t$)? Using equations (3a) to (3c), (4), (5a), and (5b), and common rules for the variance and covariance of linear functions, the following result is obtained:

$$\rho_{PQ} = \frac{\mathrm{cov}[P, Q]}{\sigma_P \sigma_Q} = \frac{\sum b_i^2 \, \sigma_{X_i} \sigma_{Y_i}}{\sqrt{\sum b_i^2 \, \sigma_{X_i}^2} \sqrt{\sum b_i^2 \, \sigma_{Y_i}^2}} \rho_{XY} \quad (6)$$

Applying the Cauchy–Schwarz inequality, $|\mathbf{u} \cdot \mathbf{v}| \leq |\mathbf{u}||\mathbf{v}|$, on the vectors $\mathbf{u} = (b_1 \sigma_{X_1}, b_2 \sigma_{X_2}, \ldots, b_{nt} \sigma_{X_{nt}})^T$ and $\mathbf{v} = (b_1 \sigma_{Y_1}, b_2 \sigma_{Y_2}, \ldots, b_{n_t} \sigma_{Y_{nt}})^T$, one obtains

$$|\rho_{PQ}| \leq |\rho_{XY}| \quad\quad\quad (7)$$

The equality sign is valid if and only if the vectors $\mathbf{u}$ and $\mathbf{v}$ are proportional; that is, if

$$\frac{\sigma_{X_i}}{\sigma_{Y_i}} = \text{constant, independent of } i \quad\quad (8)$$

Thus, when kinetic models that are linear in the parameters are applied, the absolute values of ρ in the parametric maps are no larger than the absolute value of ρ in the underlying maps of the radioactivity distribution. Further, if the ratio between the errors of the measurements in the two pixels are the same in all time intervals, the absolute values of ρ in the radioactivity and parametric maps are the same.

2. Simulations

Two more important questions remain: First, when there is strict inequality in equation (7), how much smaller is ρ in the parametric maps than in the radioactivity maps; and second, what happens when, as is often the case, the tracer model is nonlinear in the parameters? These questions were addressed using simulations. A large number of uptake curves, that is, the integrated radioactivity concentration in prescribed time intervals, were generated. The common three-parameter model,

$$C_{\text{tiss}}(T) = k_1 \int_0^T e^{[-(k_2 + k_3)(T-t)]} C_{\text{pl}}(t)dt + \frac{k_1 k_3}{k_2 + k_3} \int_0^T \{1 - e^{[-(k_2 + k_3)(T-t)]}\} C_{\text{pl}}(t) \, dt \quad (9)$$

was used. Here $C_{\text{pl}}(t)$ is the fixed input function and $C_{\text{tiss}}(T)$ is the theoretical radioactivity concentration at time T. For each generated pair of uptake curves, correlated random errors were superimposed on the data. In each time interval, the two correlated errors were assumed to follow a normal bivariate distribution with the expectation values equal to 0, with the variances equal to the radioactivity concentration divided by the time interval, and with the correlation coefficient, ρ_{act}, equal to a preset value between 0 and 1. In addition, the variance could be scaled by a factor. The errors were generated with the aid of routines in the IMSL program library. The errors in different time intervals and for different pairs of uptake curves were uncorrelated. The components of each correlated pair of time–activity curves could be generated with equal or unequal sets of rate constants, k_1, k_2, and k_3.

The model expression was fitted to the generated time–activity data using a fast algorithm, suitable for construction of parametric maps (Blomqvist, 1984). In this way 1,000 correlated pairs of the rate constants and the macro parameters $K_{\text{MR}} = k_1 k_3/(k_2 + k_3)$, the "metabolic rate constant," and DV = $k_1/(k_2 + k_3)$, the volume of distribution, were created. Finally, the correlation coefficients of these pairs of parameters were calculated. Using Fishers's z-transformation the corresponding 95% confidence intervals were also calculated.

III. RESULTS AND DISCUSSION

A. Measured Correlations

1. Transaxial Correlations

For the homogeneous cylinder phantom, the transaxial ρ was examined as function of the distance between (the central points) of the pixels. The pixels were oriented in two ways: in the "x-direction," that is, with the azimuthal angle equal to 0, and in the radial direction. For both orientations, the correlation between adjacent pixels was found to be considerable ($\rho = 0.75$ at cutoff frequency 0.3), but ρ decreased rapidly with increasing distance between the pixels.

The correlations in the radial and x-directions were almost the same at short distances but, in contrast to the negative values found in the x-direction at larger distances, ρ in the radial direction was nonnegative at all pixel distances. The correlation did not vary significantly between different slices. The correlation between pixels oriented in the radial direction and separated with a fixed distance increased monotonously with increasing distance of the pixel pair from the camera axis (z-axis). The dependence of ρ on the radial distance was much smaller for pixels oriented parallel to the x-axis. The correlation was found to decrease with increasing cutoff frequency.

The correlation was found to be almost the same for the homogeneous phantom and the line source. Further, the ρ values between pixels outside the cylindrical phantom were close to the ρ values between pixels within the phantom. Thus, ρ was found to be almost independent of the shape and magnitude of the radioactivity distribution in the object. These results justify the assumption behind equation (4). With 2D data acquisition, ρ between adjacent pixels was almost the same as with 3D data acquisition, but became more negative at larger distances. Our results for the transaxial correlation using 2D data acquisition are in accordance with previous findings (Tanaka and Murayama, 1982; Huesman, 1984; Carson et al., 1992).

2. Axial Correlations

In this case, only 3D data acquisition was considered, because with 2D acquisition a coincidence detection contributes in only one transaxial plane, whereas with 3D acquisition a coincidence contributes in all transaxial planes intersected by the line of response. Averaged over all slices and distances from the camera axis, the axial correlation between pixels oriented parallel to the camera (z-)axis was found to be weaker than the transaxial correlation. With cutoff frequency 0.3 and for pixels with the same transaxial position (same distance from the axis and same azimuthal angle in a transaxial plane), the ρ value was found to be 0.19 between pixels in adjacent slices, 0.02 between pixels two slices apart, and 0.01 between pixels three slices apart. The axial ρ was found to vary appreciably with the distance of the pixels from the camera axis. Averaged over all slices, ρ between pixels in adjacent slices and with the same transaxial position was only 0.09 in a central circular region (radius = 1 cm) but increased to a maximum 0.25 in an annulus between 4 and 5 cm from the center.

The axial correlation was found to be larger in the peripheral slices than in the central ones. Pixel values in different slices and different transaxial position were also correlated. If the x-coordinate differed by one

pixel, ρ was 0.16 between pixels in adjacent slices. The correlation between pixels oriented in the axial direction was found to be almost unaffected by changes in the cutoff frequency, whereas the correlation between pixels oriented at an angle with the camera axis decreased when the cutoff frequency increased.

In summary, in addition to a strong dependence of ρ on the distance between the pixels, ρ depends on the cutoff frequency used in the reconstruction, on the position of the pixel pair, and also on the orientation of the pixel pair in space. The dependence on the radioactivity distribution in the measured object is small.

B. The Effect of Correlations on the SEM in a Region

The correlations in the phantom images were approximated to be a function of the distance between the pixels only, which made it possible to use a simple lookup table with the experimentally determined ρ tabulated as a function of the distance between the pixels. This distance was calculated for each pixel pair in a region within the cylindrical phantom and the corresponding ρ-value was estimated by linear interpolation in the lookup table. As the errors in the pixels of the phantom image can be assumed to be the same, the effect of correlation was estimated using equation (2). Results obtained with the cutoff frequency 0.3 were utilized for generating the lookup table. For each distance the tabulated ρ value was an average of the ρ values measured in the radial and x-directions.

Two extreme shapes of regions were investigated: circular discs and straight lines. Different sizes of the regions were investigated. With a circular region, the correlation correction factor was found to increase from 2.4 at radius = 4 mm to 2.9 at radius = 20 mm and thereafter to stay quite constant. With pixels on a straight line, the correction factor was found to be 1.6 for 5 pixels (10 mm) and 1.8 for 50 pixels (100 mm). Thus, not only the number of pixels but also the shape of a region is important. The origin of this dependence is topological: The correlation between two pixels is preferentially positive and decreases with the distance between the pixels. For a fixed number of pixels forming a region, the average distance between the pixels is minimum when the region is circular, whereas this distance is maximum when the region is pixels on a straight line. Clearly, the SEM increases considerably when the correlation effects are taken into account.

C. Correlations in Parametric Maps

Both identical sets ($k_1 = 0.1$, $k_2 = 0.2$, $k_3 = 0.3$) and unequal sets of rate constants ($k_1 = 0.1$, $k_2 = 0.2$,

TABLE 1   Correlation Coefficient ρ_{param} of Parameters Fitted to 1000 Correlated Pairs of Simulated Time–Activity Curves with ρ_{act} Equal to 0.8

Parameter	Equal rate constants			Unequal rate constants		
	ρ_{param}	95% Confidence interval	% Difference from ρ_{act}	ρ_{param}	95% Confidence interval	% Difference from ρ_{act}
K_{MR}	0.81	0.79–0.83	+1.3	0.80	0.78–0.82	±0.0
DV	0.81	0.78–0.83	±0.0	0.77	0.74–0.80	−3.6
k_1	0.79	0.77–0.82	−1.0	0.78	0.75–0.80	−2.5
k_2	0.78	0.76–0.81	−2.0	0.76	0.73–0.78	−5.6
k_3	0.80	0.78–0.82	±0.0	0.76	0.73–0.78	−5.1

Note. Parameter settings in the simulation are given in the text.

$k_3 = 0.3$, and $k_1 = 0.2$, $k_2 = 0.4$, and $k_3 = 0.4$, respectively) were used for generating the pairs of correlated time–activity curves. A total measuring time of 30 min divided into 18 intervals was assumed. Two values of ρ_{act}, 0.4 and 0.8, were examined. The results for $\rho_{act} = 0.8$ are summarized in Table 1. The results indicate that, within the experimental uncertainty, the ρ_{param} values become the same as ρ_{act} when equal sets of rate constants are used. Analogous results were obtained with $\rho_{act} = 0.4$. This result should be compared with the corresponding result obtained analytically for linear models (equal rate constants imply equal errors).

When two unequal sets of rate constants were used, the displayed data showed that also in this case $\rho_{K_{MR}}$ and ρ_{k_1} were equal to ρ_{act} within the experimental uncertainty, whereas ρ_{k_2}, ρ_{k_3}, and ρ_{DV} were significantly smaller ($p <= 0.05$). Analogous results were found for $\rho_{act} = 0.4$, but in this case ρ_{k_2}, ρ_{k_3}, and ρ_{DV} were considerably (40–80%) smaller than ρ_{act}. Therefore, the results indicate that ρ_{param} is practically the same as ρ_{act} for parameters that, like K_{MR} and k_1, enter linearly in the operational equation, whereas ρ_{param} is smaller than ρ_{act} for parameters that enter nonlinearly into the operational equation. In no case was a ρ_{param} value found to be significantly higher than the corresponding ρ_{act} value.

D. Calculation of SEMs in Parametric Maps

The correlation coefficient is found to be mainly a function of the distance between the pixels, and for parameters that enter linearly in the model equation,

the correlation coefficients are approximately the same in the parametric maps as in the maps of the radioactivity concentrations. Accordingly, for such maps, the effect of correlation can be estimated using a common lookup table, providing the correlation coefficient as a function of the distance between the pixels. The software used for constructing parametric maps should also provide "error maps," presenting the SDs of the parameter estimates in each pixel. Error maps together with a lookup table for ρ should be the most flexible method for estimating SEMs in arbitrary regions of parametric maps. In conclusion, with knowledge of the spatial correlations better estimates of the errors in radioactivity and parameter data can be achieved.

References

Beck, J. V., and Arnold, K. J. (1977). "Parameter Estimation in Engineering and Science." Wiley, New York.

Blomqvist, G. (1984). On the construction of functional maps in positron emission tomography. *J. Cereb. Blood Flow Metab.* **4:** 629–632.

Carson, R. E., Yan, Y., Daube-Witerspoon, M. E., Freedman, N., Bacharach, S. L., and Herscovitch, P. (1992). An approximation formula for the variance of PET region-of-interest values. *IEEE Trans. Med. Imag.* **4:** 240–250.

Huesman, R. H. (1984). A new fast algorithm for the evaluation of regions of interest and statistical uncertainty in computed tomography. *Phys. Med. Biol.* **29:** 543–552.

Patlak, C. S., Blasberg, R. G., and Fenstermacher, J. D. (1983). Graphical evaluation of blood-to-brain transfer constants from multiple-time uptake data. *J. Cereb. Blood Flow Metab.* **3:** 1–7.

Tanaka, E., and Murayama, H. (1982). Properties of statistical noise in positron emission tomography. *In:* Proc. Int. Workshop Phys. Eng. Med. Imaging. New York: IEEE. pp. 158–164.

34

Integrated Quantitative Analysis of Functional and Morphological 3D Data by Volumes of Interest

K. HERHOLZ, S. DICKHOVEN, H. KARBE, M. HALBER, U. PIETRZYK, and W.-D. HEISS

Max Planck Institute for Neurological Research and
University Hospital
Department of Neurology, D-50931
Cologne, Germany

In this chapter, we describe tools for 3D data analysis based on volumes of interest (VOIs). Although these tools can be used for PET data alone, their full potential to demonstrate individual functional anatomy and pathology can be used best in connection with coregistered high-resolution MRI. They include tools for VOI generation (manually, by geometric primitives, or by thresholding), for VOI processing (by Boolean operations, shift, rotation, dilation, and erosion), and VOI display (as orthogonal cuts, as projections onto orthogonal image cuts, or as 3D renderings of multiple VOI objects). Quantitative and statistical data analysis can be done on VOI contents. Thus, tools for 3D image segmentation and for quantitative VOI analysis are brought together in a unified concept. This is illustrated by application examples from functional activation studies in normal subjects and patients with focal brain lesions (e.g., brain tumors).

I. INTRODUCTION

Current PET scanners provide 3D data acquisition of the whole brain in nearly isotropic voxels, and techniques for coregistration with high-resolution MRI images are well established. Traditional 2D plane-by-plane quantitative analysis of reconstructed data is no longer adequate in view of these technical developments and the complex 3D topography of brain structures. Although averaging over functional tomograms from different subjects after image smoothing and stereotactic normalization is still being used in cognitive activation studies in normal subjects, this technique

has obvious limitations with regard to accurate anatomical localization of activated brain structures. We therefore developed a strategy and the necessary software to quantify and visualize PET data in volumes of interest, which are defined with reference to the individual anatomy, as suggested by Mazoyer *et al.* (1993). This strategy is particularly well suited to study the individual variability of the relation between brain function and anatomy in normal subjects and to study pathological changes in patients.

II. METHODS

As outlined schematically in Figure 1, data analysis starts with registration of MRI data (typically T_1-weighted FLASH images, $256 \times 256 \times 64$ voxels of $0.98 \times 0.98 \times 2.5$ mm size) in standard position, as defined by the AC–PC line. All PET images (typically $128 \times 128 \times 47$ voxels of $2.17 \times 2.17 \times 3.125$ mm voxel size) are then coregistered with the MRI data. PET images often represent results of functional activation studies, that is, images of metabolic or CBF changes during activation, generated with routines similar to those described previously (Herholz *et al.*, 1994). Data sets representing the same rectangular volume (comprising the entire brain) are resampled using trilinear interpolation and saved on disk with typical voxel sizes of $1 \times 1 \times 1$ mm for MRI, and $2 \times 2 \times 2$ mm for PET data. For these steps, a recent modification of the multipurpose matching routine described by Pietrzyk *et al.* (1990, 1994) is used (MultiPurpose Imaging, or MPI-Tool, coded in C for SUN workstations under Solaris 2).

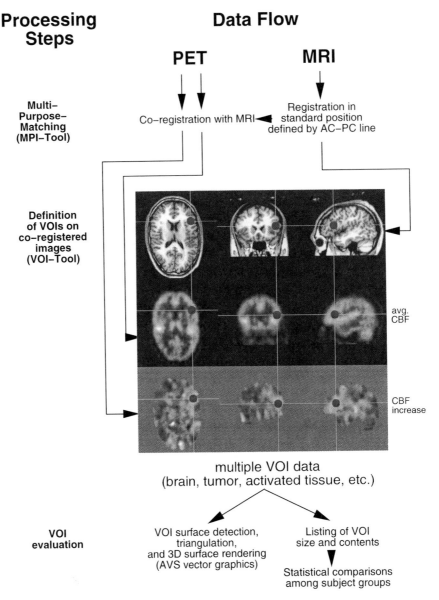

Processing Steps

Multi–Purpose–Matching (MPI-Tool)

Definition of VOIs on co-registered images (VOI-Tool)

VOI evaluation

Data Flow

PET   **MRI**

Co–registration with MRI ◄ Registration in standard position defined by AC–PC line

avg. CBF

CBF increase

multiple VOI data
(brain, tumor, activated tissue, etc.)

VOI surface detection, triangulation, and 3D surface rendering (AVS vector graphics)

Listing of VOI size and contents

Statistical comparisons among subject groups

FIGURE 1   Scheme of 3D VOI processing.

Next, definition of volumes of interest (VOIs) is done using a menu-driven program (VOI-Tool) written in IDL (Interactive Data Language, Version 4.0, Research Systems Inc., Boulder, Colorado), running on SUN and Silicon Graphics workstations. It features simultaneous display of up to three data sets as transaxial, coronal, and sagittal cuts, similar to the main display mode of the MPI-Tool. The position of these cuts is selected by cursor click or by specification of stereotactic coordinates. It provides routines for VOI generation that include

- Sequential manual drawing on multiple adjacent slices (transaxial, coronal, or sagittal),

- Geometric primitives (sphere, box, etc.), set optionally at predefined stereotactic coordinates for simple standardized PET quantification,
- Thresholding (globally, within predefined template VOI, or growing three-dimensionally or within a selected plane from a seed point) for delineation of specific brain areas or tissue.

In current applications, sequential manual drawing is usually preferred for VOIs of high anatomical accuracy, guided by MRI (Szelies *et al.*, 1995; Karbe *et al.*, 1995). Geometric primitives are currently used mainly for analysis of functional activation data. The primitives are often used as stereotactically placed target

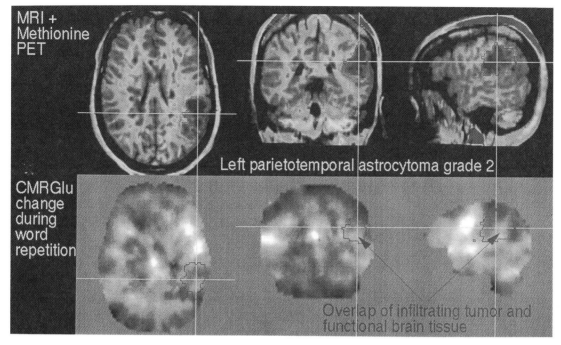

FIGURE 2   VOI delineating increased uptake of C-11-methionine in an astrocytoma of WHO grade 2. It was defined by the following steps: (1) draw crude tumor VOI; (2) mirror that to contralateral brain; (3) determine the average and SD of normal methionine uptake; (4) grow final VOI within crude tumor VOI by including all contiguous voxels with higher uptake than normal average + 2 SD. In the lower row, this tumor VOI is superimposed onto an image of functional activation by word repetition, demonstrating overlap of infiltrating tumor and functional brain tissue.

areas, in which focal activations are expected for a particular activation paradigm, and local activation maxima are then determined within these target VOIs (e.g., Fink *et al.*, Chapter 79 in this volume). The 3D VOI growing is used mainly to determine the extent of activation foci (Herholz *et al.*, 1994, 1995) or abnormal PET findings (e.g., abnormal methionine accumulation in a brain tumor, see Fig. 2). In some instances, the 3D VOI growing may be difficult to control, because unexpected bridges to other structures (e.g., eye muscles or major vessels at the skull base) may produce erratic results. Then, limiting growth within the currently displayed plane or by a predefined crude target VOI is a useful option.

Options for VOI processing include Boolean operations (e.g., VOI junction to determine overlap of invasive tumor and functionally activated areas), shift and rotation (which is most useful for adjustment of geometric primitives to individual anatomy), and 3D morphologic operators dilation and erosion (mainly used to smooth VOI shapes or to break erratic connections between the different tissue volumes that can occur with thresholding). A combination of thresholding, manual drawing, and Boolean and morphologic operators permits segmentation of brain on MRI rather com-

fortably. It extends the 3D segmentation concept described by Höhne and Hanson (1992) to VOI generation. Standard display shows the borders of a selected VOI (or of all VOIs simultaneously) as they are cut by the selected orthogonal planes. Alternatively the projections of the complete VOI onto these planes can be shown. These projections provide a better overview over the full extent of a VOI, but the cuts are needed to examine topographical details (see Fig. 3).

VOI data are stored within a $1 \times 1 \times 1$ mm voxel matrix. Voxels common to an old and a newly generated VOI can be assigned either to the old or the new VOI or stored as a separate, third VOI. Thus, each voxel is assigned uniquely to no more than one VOI. VOIs can be used as templates for subsequent analyses of data from the same or other individuals (optionally, linear stereotactic scaling of coordinate axes for adaption to individual brain size is also provided). Listings of VOI size and contents (average, standard deviation, median, minimum and maximum of voxel values from all three data sets) provide quantitative VOI data. Images can be masked by VOIs. These data can then be analyzed by standard statistical procedures (e.g., comparison of magnitude and location of activation maxima between patients and controls; Herholz *et al.*,

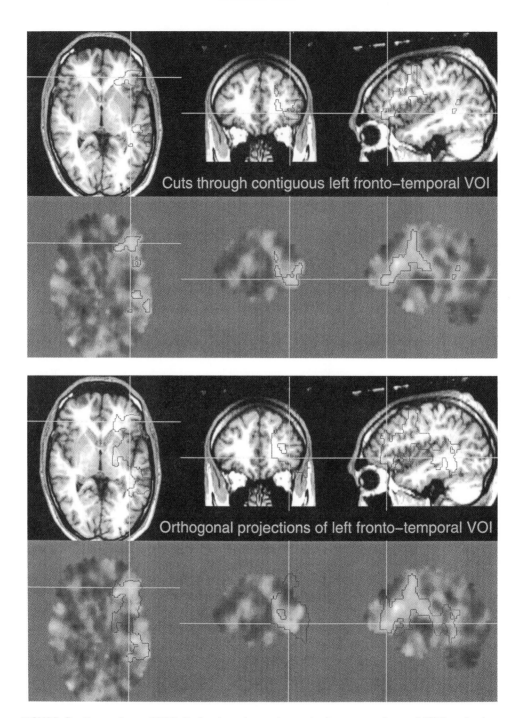

FIGURE 3   Comparison of VOI display in orthogonal cuts (top) versus orthogonal VOI projections (bottom). The projections give a better impression of the full extent of a contiguous region activated by silent verb generation (defined by CBF increase ≥7%), but the cuts are needed to recognize details (e.g., the sparing of basal ganglia from activation).

1995). Image and VOI output for further processing by vector graphics routines is also provided.

For a surface-rendered display, masked images and VOI data are loaded into a program package for vector graphics (AVS, Advanced Visual Systems, Waltham, Massachusetts), running on a 24-bit-color SGI workstation. Surfaces are detected by isocontouring with appropriate thresholds, triangulated and displayed from

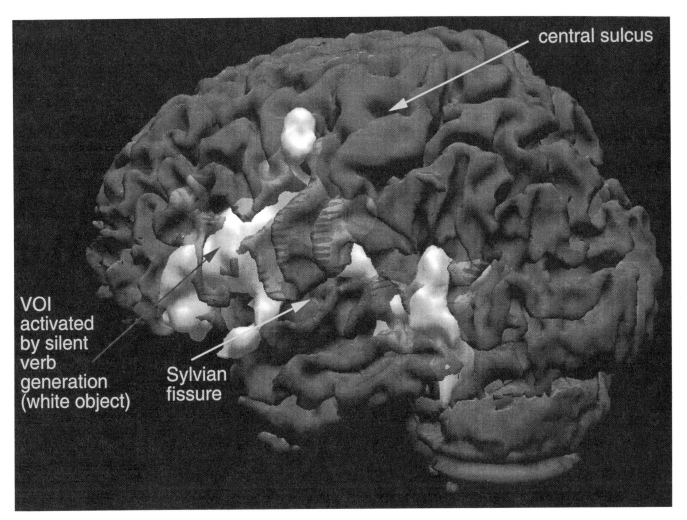

FIGURE 4 Transparent rendering of brain surface (using a high threshold to widen the sulci) and the same VOI as in Figure 3, demonstrating some topographic anatomical details.

appropriate viewpoints, with color, transparency, and lighting adjusted to demonstrate their topographic anatomic relations.

III. COMMENT

Our strategy employs 3D morphological tools not only for image segmentation and 3D visualization but also for quantitative PET data analysis by VOIs. In the literature (see Thatcher *et al.*, 1994, for a recent overview) and also by commercially available image analysis software, such as Analyze (Biomedical Imaging Resource, Mayo Foundation), image segmentation and quantitative analysis of VOI content are usually treated separately. By the examples (see Figs. 2–4) described in this chapter, we seek to demonstrate how analysis of quantitative PET data can be enhanced con-

siderably by use of morphological tools for VOI definition and subsequent 3D MRI–PET fusion display. The combination of segmentation and 3D visualization tools also facilitates definition of anatomical VOIs on MRI for quantitative analysis of coregistered PET data.

References

Herholz, K., Pietrzyk, U., Karbe, H., Würker, M., Wienhard, K., and Heiss, W. D. (1994). Individual metabolic anatomy of repeating words demonstrated by MRI-guided positron emission tomography. *Neurosci. Lett.* **182:** 47–50.

Herholz, K., Karbe, H., Ghaemi, M., Pietrzyk, U., Kessler, J., Würker, M., and Wienhard, K. (1995). Compensatory activations of frontal and thalamic regions in subacute aphasia during word repetition. *J. Cereb. Blood Flow Metab.* **15**(Suppl. 1), S186.

Höhne, K. H., and Hanson, W. A. (1992). Interactive 3D segmentation of MRI and CT volumes using morphological operations. *J. Comput. Assist. Tomogr.* **16:** 285–294.

Karbe, H., Würker, M., Herholz, K., Ghaemi, M., Pietrzyk, U., Kessler, J., and Heiss, W. D. (1995). Planum temporale and Brodmann's area 22: MRI and high-resolution PET demonstrate functional left-right asymmetry. *Arch. Neurol.,* **52:** 869–874.

Mazoyer, B. M., Tzourio, N., Frak, V., Syrota, A., Murayama, N., Levrier, O., Salamon, G., Dehaene, S., Cohen, L., and Mehler, J. (1993). The cortical representation of speech. *J. Cogn. Neurosci.* **5:** 467–479.

Pietrzyk, U., Herholz, K., and Heiss, W.-D. (1990). Three-dimensional alignment of functional and morphological tomograms. *J. Comput. Assist. Tomogr.* **14:** 51–59.

Pietrzyk, U., Herholz, K., Fink, G., Jacobs, A., Mielke, R., Slansky, I., Würker, M., and Heiss, W. D. (1994). An interactive technique for three-dimensional image registration: Validation for PET, SPECT, MRI and CT brain studies. *J. Nucl. Med.* **35:** 2011–2018.

Szelies, B., Weber-Luxenburger, G., Pawlik, G., Pietrzyk, U., Kessler, J., Holthoff, V., Mielke, R., Herholz, K., Wagner, R., and Heiss, W. D. (1995). Improved focus localization in temporal lobe epilepsy by MRI guided flumazenil and FDG PET. *J. Cereb. Blood Flow Metab.* **15**(Suppl.1), S779.

Thatcher, R. W., Hallett, M., Zeffiro, T., John, R. E., and Huerta, M. (Eds.) (1994). "Functional Neuroimaging. Technical Foundations." Academic Press, San Diego.

Data Processing Summary

S. C. STROTHER

PET Imaging Section (11P), VA Medical Center, Minneapolis, Minnesota 55417
Radiology Department, University of Minnesota, Minneapolis, 55455

The majority of the data processing papers presented at Brain PET 95 were concerned with improving signal or noise levels. This is a research endeavor with a long and successful history in PET (e.g., Hoffman *et al.*, 1991). Nevertheless, I believe the time has come to reassess the way in which we plan and perform such studies. Rarely is a new algorithm for improving signal quantification, or reducing image noise, presented along with a careful study of the variance and bias trade-offs for a specific research task. This failure to demonstrate improvements in specific tasks results in great difficulty in evaluating the significance of much of the PET data processing literature.

I believe the impact of data processing developments on our colleagues and in our day-to-day practice can be improved by routinely adopting a different view of data processing research. Figure 1 schematically depicts two approaches to PET data processing research, from the perspective of the "PET data processing chain" previously discussed by Strother *et al.* (1991).

Much data processing research is based on current methodological and technological practices and the assumptions associated with a single modeling stage in the "PET chain." This is represented by the technology and methodology driven development arrow at the top of Figure 1. For example, as demonstrated by a number of the data processing papers, an appropriate research goal is considered to be improving the signal-to-noise (S/N) ratio of the reconstructed images of radioactive tracer concentration. However, this is typically pursued in isolation from the bias–variance trade-offs associated with specific physiological and/or data analysis models.

The PET research community needs to balance such work on generic S/N ratio improvement with a concentrated effort in the clinical research and diagnostic question driven direction, depicted by the arrow at the bottom of Figure 1. This research is motivated by identifying and studying specific diagnostic and research tasks, and their associated data analysis models. It seeks to establish what constitutes task-specific signal and noise, and what, for example, is the optimal resolution for a particular task. We should adjust the reconstruction and physiological models to optimize the bias variance trade-offs for a specific task only after we understand the methodological and physiological signal and noise sources for that task. This still constitutes data processing research but *the motivation for developing a new processing technique and a metric for evaluating its importance is tightly coupled to, as opposed to loosely motivated by, a real-world problem.* One consequence of adopting real-world, task-driven approaches to data processing is that methodology will become very task specific. Such task-driven research is difficult to perform because it is often highly interdisciplinary, time consuming, and includes all the uncontrolled factors that attend real data. Sometimes this makes the problem of obtaining a definite result for the significance of a new data processing method difficult; however, we should bear in mind the statistician John Tukey's comment: "It is often better to get an approximate solution to a real problem than an exact solution to an oversimplified one."

An example of such clinical research-driven development is the study of Kippenham *et al.* (1994) of the classification of normal and Alzheimer's disease subjects as a function of high- and low-resolution PET cameras. They support the earlier finding of Strother

Technology/Methodology Driven Development

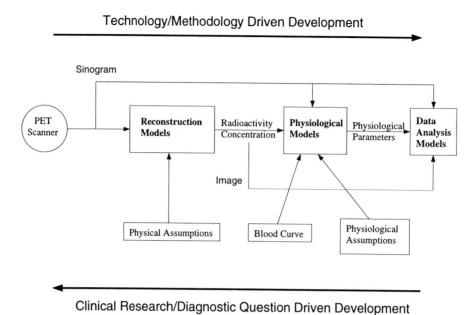

Clinical Research/Diagnostic Question Driven Development

FIGURE 1   A schematic representation of the flow of PET data from collection in the PET scanner as raw data sinograms through a "chain" of complex model transformations. The "models" are designed to create images of radioactive tracer concentration, convert these concentrations into physiological parameters and analyze the quantitative results over many scans to, for example, track disease progression. Alternate processing paths bypassing the various modeling stages are shown for sinograms and images.

et al. (1991) that optimal detection of disease is not necessarily dependent on absolute quantification of metabolism. By focusing on several specific clinical research tasks we find that improving absolute quantification of the physiological modeling stage does not necessarily improve the task of disease discrimination.

Most of the data processing papers that did not address methodologically driven signal or noise improvement dealt with various aspects of the image registration problem. This research may be viewed as a response to the experimental observation that anatomical and functional misregistration—a form of "anatomical and functional noise"—dominate the bias–variance trade-offs in the data analysis of groups. This noise source has emerged because of the change from analyses using volumes of interest (VOI) to the higher resolution promised by voxel based data analysis. In addition to the desire for higher resolution results, goals of image registration research are automated data processing, and anatomic segmentation and labeling. As with reconstruction techniques that promise higher resolution early in the PET processing chain, we will need to be watchful that these image registration goals do not become methodological ends in their own right. For example, comparisons of voxel versus VOI based analyses of clinical research problems have been performed (e.g., Rottenberg *et al.*, 1995) but it is far from clear that other tasks should adopt the voxel-based data

processing developments emerging from [^{15}O]-water activation studies.

The reasons for developing a particular data processing technique must be carefully considered. Ideally these reasons will emerge from an understanding of the bias–variance trade-offs for a specific diagnostic or research task. Researchers should identify a task and an associated data analysis model that together provide a metric with which to evaluate the significance of a new processing technique.

References

Hoffman, E. J., Cutler, P. D., Guerrero, T. M., Digby, W. M., and Mazziotta, J. C. (1991). Assessment of accuracy of PET utilizing a 3-D phantom to simulate the activity distribution of [^{18}F]Fluorodeoxyglucose uptake in the human brain. *J. Cereb. Blood Flow Metab.* **11:** A17–A25.

Kippenham, J. S., Barker, W. W., Nagel, J., Grady, C., and Duara, R. (1994). Neural-network classification of normal and Alzheimer's disease subjects using high-resolution and low-resolution PET cameras. *J. Nucl. Med.* **35:** 7–15.

Rottenberg, D. A., Sidtis, J. J., Strother, S. C., Schaper, K. A., Anferson, J. R., Nelson, M. J., and Price, R. W. (1995). Abnormal cerebral glucose metabolism in HIV-1 seropositives with and without dementia. *J. Nucl. Med.,* in press.

Strother, S. C., Liow, J.-S., Moeller, J. R., Sidtis, J. J., Dhawan, V., and Rottenberg, D. A. (1991). Absolute quantitation in neurological PET: Do we need it? *J. Cereb. Blood Flow Metab.* **11:** A3–A16.

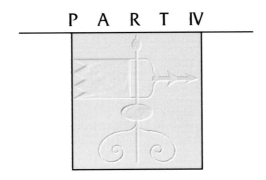

PART IV

KINETIC ANALYSIS

Absolute Cerebral Blood Flow with [^{15}O]Water and PET

Determination Without a Measured Input Function

RICHARD E. CARSON,[1] YUCHEN YAN,[1] and RICHARD SHRAGER[2]

[1]PET Department
[2]Division of Computer Research and Technology
National Institutes of Health
Bethesda, Maryland 20892

PET cerebral blood flow (CBF) methods require tissue and arterial blood radioactivity measurements to yield absolute values. We have developed a method to estimate CBF without a measured input function. For N pixels and M scan frames, we estimate N + M parameters (N flow values and M input function integrals) from N × M measurements with weighted least squares using the iterative Gauss–Newton (GN) algorithm. Tracer distribution volume V is assumed to be known. This method was tested with simulated and human image data. Simulation GN errors in whole brain CBF were −3 ± 2%, with uniform percentage errors for all flow values. GN image quality was comparable to that obtained from algorithms that require the measured input function. Results with actual scan data (eight subjects, four studies each) showed good correlation with global flow values using measured input functions but had errors in global flow of −77 ± 3% due to violations of the model assumptions, particularly tissue heterogeneity. Use of two modified algorithms that included either (1) an empirical formula for V as a function of CBF or (2) interpixel variations in V to account for heterogeneity reduced the bias but produced poor correlation with measured global flow values. Although this method theoretically can provide absolute CBF, it will be useful in practice only if its large sensitivity to model inaccuracies can be controlled.

I. INTRODUCTION

There are many methods to measure cerebral blood flow (CBF) with PET and diffusible tracers (Frackowiak *et al.*, 1980; Holden *et al.*, 1981; Huang *et al.*, 1982; Herscovitch *et al.*, 1983; Koeppe *et al.*, 1985a). These techniques, particularly those using bolus injections, require accurate measurement of the arterial input function. Some authors have presented noninvasive methods that use external measurements to estimate the input function without arterial sampling (Koeppe *et al.*, 1985b; Nelson *et al.*, 1993). Alternatively, input function measurements are avoided and qualitative flow measurements are made from the PET tissue data alone using the first 40–90 sec of scanning (Fox *et al.*, 1984; Mazziotta *et al.*, 1985). However, measurement of absolute CBF would be useful for many of these studies to distinguish between changes in global and regional flow. Therefore, a reliable method to measure absolute CBF without a measured input function would be widely applied.

We present a method to measure absolute CBF following a bolus injection using only dynamic tissue radioactivity values derived from reconstructed image data. As in all CBF methods, the input function is assumed to be common to all brain pixels. Each pixel's time–activity curve therefore has information about the local blood flow and the input function. By analyzing all pixels simultaneously, the input function can be estimated. Then CBF can be determined by any method of choice. We describe the theory and implementation of the new method and present results from simulated data and human studies.

II. MATERIALS AND METHODS

A. Estimation Problem

The one-compartment model for a diffusible tracer follows the differential equation

$$\frac{dC_i}{dt} = F_i C_a(t) - \frac{F_i}{V_i} C_i(t) \tag{1}$$

where $C_a(t)$ is the input function, and F_i, V_i, and $C_i(t)$ are the flow, distribution volume, and activity in pixel i. All radioactivity values are corrected for decay. Following a bolus injection, M scans are acquired, consecutive in time, of duration $\Delta t_j, j = 1, \ldots, M$. Integrating equation (1) from 0 to t_j, the mid-time of scan j, yields M equations for each pixel:

$$C_i(t_j) = F_i \int_0^{t_j} C_a(t)\, dt - \frac{F_i}{V_i} \int_0^{t_j} C_i(t)\, dt \tag{2}$$

We approximate $C_i(t_j)$, the instantaneous activity at mid-scan time, with the reconstructed pixel value c_{ij} (pixel i, scan j), which is integrated over each scan interval. The rightmost integral term is calculated by summing the scan values:

$$\int_0^{t_j} C_i(t)\, dt \cong \left(\sum_{k=1}^{j-1} c_{ik} \Delta t_k \right) + \frac{c_{ij} \Delta t_j}{2} \tag{3}$$

where the integral over the first half of scan j is approximated by half of its full integral. Equation (2) then becomes

$$\mathbf{c}_i = F_i \mathbf{x} - \frac{F_i}{V_i} U \mathbf{c}_i \tag{4}$$

where $\mathbf{c}_i$ is the M-vector of c_{ij} values, $\mathbf{x}$ is the M-vector of input function integrals, $x_j = (\int_0^{t_j} C_a(t)\, dt)$, and U is the matrix

$$U = \begin{pmatrix} \dfrac{\Delta t_1}{2} & 0 & 0 & \cdots & 0 \\[2mm] \Delta t_1 & \dfrac{\Delta t_2}{2} & 0 & \cdots & 0 \\[2mm] \Delta t_1 & \Delta t_2 & \dfrac{\Delta t_2}{2} & \cdots & 0 \\[2mm] \vdots & \vdots & \vdots & \ddots & \vdots \\[2mm] \Delta t_1 & \Delta t_2 & \Delta t_3 & \cdots & \dfrac{\Delta t_M}{2} \end{pmatrix} \tag{5}$$

Solving equation (4) for $\mathbf{c}_i$ yields

$$\mathbf{c}_i = F_i \left(I + \frac{F_i}{V_i} U \right)^{-1} \mathbf{x} = V_i k_i (I + k_i U)^{-1} \mathbf{x} \tag{6}$$

where $k_i = F_i/V_i$ and I is the $M \times M$ identity matrix. Equation (6) is the model describing the $N \times M$ tissue radioactivity values c_{ij}. In its initial implementation, we assume that all distribution volume values V_i are known and constant. The goal then is to estimate the $N + M$ unknowns $\beta = (k_1, k_2, \ldots, k_N, x_1, x_2, \ldots, x_M)$ from the $N \times M$ measurements.

B. Iterative Solution

Equation (6) is nonlinear in k_i and linear in x_j. Estimates of the parameter vector β will be determined by iterative weighted least squares (Beck and Arnold, 1977) by minimizing the optimization criterion:

$$\Psi = \sum_{i=1}^{N} \sum_{j=1}^{M} w_{ij} (c_{ij} - \hat{c}_{ij})^2 \tag{7}$$

where $\hat{c}_{ij}$ is the model estimate of c_{ij} (equation (6)) and w_{ij} is the corresponding data weight. We used a single weight for each image because filtered back-projection noise is relatively homogeneous (Alpert et al., 1982). Average pixel variance is computed using an approximation formula that includes the effects of reconstruction and all the corrections (Carson et al., 1993).

The algorithm steps are as follows: (1) Define brain pixels. This is performed with whole brain ROIs defined by an edge-finding algorithm applied to images summed over the first 60 sec post injection. (2) Calculate the noise of each brain pixel at each time point with the approximation formula. (3) Provide an initial guess for the parameter vector β (see later) and define the distribution volume. (4) Calculate the increment in β at iteration i ($\Delta \beta^{(i)}$) from the solution of the normal equations:

$$(X^T W X) \Delta \beta^{(i)} = X^T W \Delta c \tag{8}$$

where Δc is the residual vector ($c_{ij} - \hat{c}_{ij}$, an $N \times M$ vector), X is the sensitivity matrix ($\partial c/\partial \beta$, $N \times M$ by $N + M$ matrix), and W is the diagonal weighting matrix ($N \times M$ by $N \times M$). The matrix ($X^T W X$) is called the *information matrix* and has dimension $N + M$ by $N + M$. Using Gaussian elimination, equation (8) can be reduced to a set of M linear equations, which can be easily solved (see later). (5) Update the parameter vector β, calculate the new value of Ψ, and determine if it has been reduced from the previous iteration. If not, halve the size of the parameter vector step and repeat step 5. (6) Check for convergence.

C. Implementation of the GN Algorithm

Equation (8) uses extremely large matrices. For example, in a 15-slice scanner, reconstructing 128×128 2-mm pixels, there are $\sim 50,000$ (N) brain pixels. We routinely collect 16 (M) sequential scans for quantitative CBF studies. So Equation (8) is a set of 50,016 equations. Here, we reduce Equation (8) to a computable form. Define $Q(k_i) = k_i(I + k_i U)^{-1}$, an $M \times M$ matrix. Therefore, $\mathbf{c}_i = V_i Q(k_i)\mathbf{x}$. The sensitivity matrix X can be written in partitioned form as

$$X = \begin{pmatrix} \mathbf{y}_1 & 0 & \cdots & 0 & \bigm| & V_1 Q(k_1) \\ 0 & \mathbf{y}_2 & \cdots & 0 & \bigm| & V_2 Q(k_2) \\ \vdots & \vdots & \ddots & 0 & \bigm| & \vdots \\ 0 & 0 & \cdots & \mathbf{y}_N & \bigm| & V_N Q(k_N) \end{pmatrix} \quad (9)$$

where $\mathbf{y}_i = V_i Q'(k_i)\mathbf{x}$. For computational speed, a table of matrices Q and $Q'(\partial Q / \partial k)$ are precomputed for the physiological range of k values. Actual values of this matrix for any k_i value are determined by interpolation from this table.

Equation (8) can then be written in partitioned form as follows:

$$\begin{pmatrix} A & D \\ D^T & B \end{pmatrix} \begin{pmatrix} \Delta k \\ \Delta x \end{pmatrix} = \begin{pmatrix} g \\ h \end{pmatrix} \quad (10)$$

Here Δk (an N-vector) and Δx (an M-vector) make up $\Delta \beta$, the change in the parameter vector to be determined. The matrices A, D, and B are $N \times N$, $N \times M$, and $M \times M$, respectively; and A is diagonal. Then, by Gaussian elimination,

$$(B - D^T A^{-1} D) \Delta x = h - D^T A^{-1} g \quad (11)$$

Equation (11), a system of M linear equations, can be readily solved. Then, instead of solving for Δk from equation (10), the best k_i value for each pixel is determined independently by a least squares search procedure keeping $\mathbf{x}$ fixed. Each iteration requires ~ 2 min on a VAX 4000 computer and convergence is reached in 10–20 iterations.

An initial guess for F_i values was chosen by assuming that activity is linear in flow for the first 60 sec of scanning (Herscovitch et al., 1983; Fox et al., 1984; Mazziotta et al., 1985). Those scans were averaged and normalized to a mean of 40 ml/min/100 gm. The k_i values were computed from F_i/V_i. An initial guess for $\mathbf{x}$ is determined by a linear least squares solution for x_j given the k_i values. This is analogous to the iteration equations, but without the Gaussian elimination step.

D. Simulation Study 1

For CBF methods using a measured blood curve, simulation studies can be performed by considering

each pixel individually because the data from each pixel are analyzed independently. For the GN method, data from all pixels are used simultaneously to estimate $\mathbf{x}$. Therefore, a whole brain simulation is required. Quantitative human CBF images from multiple [^{15}O]water studies acquired on the Scanditronix PC2048-15B scanner were averaged creating a set of 15 "true" flow slices. Flow values for all pixels outside the brain were set to 0. Measured arterial curves from these studies (see later) were also averaged. Time–activity curves ($M = 16$ scans; 12×10 sec, 4×30 sec) were calculated for each pixel using that pixel's "true" flow, a volume of distribution (V) of 85 ml/100 gm, and the convolution solution to equation (1). These curves were reformatted into dynamic images, and sinogram data were simulated. The projection model included detector efficiencies and the subject's attenuation, randoms, scatter, and dead time (Carson et al., 1994). No resolution loss was applied to this projection data because the "true" CBF images were based on 7-mm FWHM reconstructions. Four independent realizations of Poisson noise, consistent with the actual total counts per scan, were added and new images were reconstructed by filtered back projection. The GN method was applied to these simulated images using the "correct" V value. The resulting CBF images were compared to the "true" images.

CBF was also determined with the autoradiographic (AR) method (Herscovitch et al., 1983) using the first six scans (60 sec). Two least squares methods (Holden et al., 1981; Koeppe et al., 1985a) were also applied. One method estimates both F and V values (LS2) and the other assumes a fixed value for V and estimates only one parameter (LS1).

E. Human Study

Data from 32 [^{15}O]water studies (four each from eight subjects, 1100–1500 MBq) were analyzed (Berman et al., 1995). Acquisition of dynamic scans began automatically following a step increase in the scanner count rate. Images were reconstructed with a Hanning filter resulting in a transverse resolution of 7 mm. Corrections included measured attenuation, normalization, random counts, scatter, and dead time. A postreconstruction Gaussian smoothing (FWHM 4 mm) was also applied.

Input functions were measured with an automated blood counting system. Blood was withdrawn at 3.8 ml/min and coincident events were counted at 1-sec intervals by paired NaI(T_1) detectors. These data were corrected for random counts, dead time, and sensitivity. Dispersion correction was performed by deconvolution of the measured dispersion function, a sum of two exponentials (Daube-Witherspoon *et al.*, 1992). Time shifts between blood and brain data were determined by aligning scanner count rate data (measured once per second) to the blood data in a manner similar to that described by Iida *et al.* (1988).

To apply the GN method, an assumed value for *V* is required. To determine the most appropriate value, the LS1 method was applied to the 32 data sets to determine the value of *V* that produced the minimum total Ψ (equation (7)). Across the 32 studies, the best *V* value was 74.4 ± 4.8 ml/100 gm. The GN method was then applied with *V* = 74 ml/100 gm. For the human studies, we did not directly compare the GN flow images to LS2 and AR. This comparison was not made because these methods apply different assumptions concerning *V* and have different sensitivity to errors in *V*. Instead, we used only the estimates of the blood activity produced by the GN method. Thus, CBF images were produced by the AR and LS2 methods using (1) the measured blood curve and (2) the GN-estimated input function, and these images were compared.

III. RESULTS AND DISCUSSION

A. Simulation Study 1

Image quality of the CBF images from the GN method was indistinguishable from the LS1 method (which also uses an assumed value for *V*) and was slightly superior to that of the AR and LS2 methods. However, errors in the estimation of the input function produce biases that affect every pixel. Therefore, the important measure for this algorithm is the percentage error, particularly in global flow. In four noisy realizations, the global flow error was −2.8 ± 2.2%. These percentage errors were very similar across all flow values. For pixels with CBF values in the ranges 20–25, 40–45, and 60–65 ml/min/100 gm, the errors were −0.8 ± 1.2%, −3.0 ± 2.2%, and −3.1 ± 2.4%, respectively. Therefore, when the scan data are consistent with the one-compartment model, the GN method can estimate both the input function and the global flow with good accuracy and reliability. The small variability in the global flow values was due to random errors in the estimation of the input function. This magnitude of error is smaller than that introduced by actual measurement of an input function (Carson, 1991).

B. Human Study

Unlike the simulation, the GN-estimated input function produced huge negative biases in human CBF data.

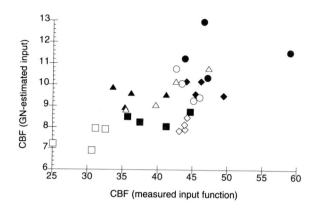

FIGURE 1 Relationship of global CBF values determined by the LS2 method using measured and GN-estimated input function. Four studies were performed with eight subjects. Each subject has a unique symbol.

The error in global flow was −77.2 ± 3.1% for LS2 and −76.7 ± 3.3% for AR. As in the simulations, the percentage errors were very similar across different flow values. The correlation of global CBF values between GN-estimated and measured input functions was 0.62 for LS2 and 0.58 for AR (Fig. 1). Although the positive correlation is encouraging, the large bias indicates that the GN method is extremely sensitive to violations of the assumptions of the model present in human data.

C. Simulation Study 2

Tissue heterogeneity was believed to be the most likely cause of the GN bias. Therefore, the simulation study described earlier was repeated with the sinogram simulation modified to include detector resolution in the projection model. After addition of Poisson noise (10 realizations), sinograms were reconstructed and the GN method was applied to these images to estimate the input function. For each image set, CBF images were then calculated with the AR and LS2 methods using the "true" and the GN-estimated input functions, and these images were compared.

The increased heterogeneity introduced by the detector model produced a negative bias in flow. The global errors were −16.8 ± 1.9% for both LS2 and AR methods. Even though this bias is smaller than that found in the human data, the amount of heterogeneity in this simulation is also smaller. Here, the "true" CBF distribution was obtained from images with 7-mm resolution, so the amount of heterogeneity introduced by the projection model is less than that found in real data.

A possible explanation for the large GN biases is as

follows. When the one-compartment model is applied to data from pixels in heterogeneous regions, V values are substantially underestimated (Iida *et al.*, 1989). Therefore, a single uniform value for V is inappropriate for many pixels. The V value influences the model prediction most heavily at later times, particularly for high-flow pixels, as tissue–blood equilibrium nears. If the presumed value of V is incorrect for some pixels due to heterogeneity, there will be a large difference between the late data points and the best fit. Because the GN algorithm estimates both flow values and the input function, it has substantial flexibility in adjusting these parameters to minimize the weighted sum of squares, Ψ. By dramatically underestimating the flow values, the late data become less sensitive to V and more sensitive to F, allowing a better fit. In order to compensate for the resulting error at early times, the algorithm significantly overestimates the input function, $\mathbf{x}$.

D. Modified Method 1

Clearly, a more sophisticated model is required to suppress GN bias. A number of strategies were evaluated including (1) a Bayesian prior applied to $\mathbf{x}$ and (2) operating only on pixels considered to be in homogeneous regions. Another approach to extend the GN method is to develop a model for V. To determine an appropriate formulation, estimates of V produced by the LS2 method were analyzed. Pixels with low flow were found to have lower V values than pixels with higher flows. This is not surprising because of the lower partition coefficient in white matter than gray matter and because of heterogeneity effects. An empirical formula to describe the mean V as a function of flow was specified:

$$V(F) = V_0 + V_1 \operatorname{erf}[(F - F_0)/F_1)] \qquad (12)$$

where erf is the error function. This formula was structured so that V is constrained between the values V_0 and $(V_0 + V_1)$.

Best fit values for V_0, V_1, F_0, and F_1 were determined using the LS1 method with measured input functions applied to the 32 bolus studies. Figure 2 shows the fitted $V(F)$ functions. The mean of these curves was then fit to equation (12) and the best fit parameters were $V_0 = 51.9$, $V_1 = 41.2$, $F_0 = 47.0$, and $F_1 = 13.3$. This $V(F)$ function was incorporated into the GN model, and the revised method was applied to the original 32 studies (used to determine $V(F)$) and to a new group of studies (also eight subjects, four runs each). As before, x_j was estimated and used to calculate LS2 flow and compared to results using the measured input function. The percent error in global flow was $3.1 \pm$

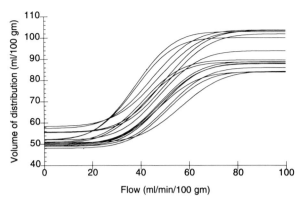

FIGURE 2 Best fit values for $V(F)$ from two runs each in eight subjects.

22.0% and -0.9 ± 17.7 for the two groups. However, the correlation of GN CBF values with the measured input values was negative: -0.62 and -0.45 for the two groups. Although the mean errors in global flow were virtually eliminated, there were large errors in global flow for some subjects. The magnitude of error in global flow correlated with the difference between the average $V(F)$ used in the GN model and each individual's best $V(F)$.

E. Modified Method 2

Another possible modification of the GN method is to allow V_i to float along with k_i and x_j. As can be seen from equation (6), V_i and $\mathbf{x}$ are both linear terms in the model equation, so their values cannot be separately identified. Therefore, a Bayesian term was added to the optimization criterion:

$$\Psi' = \Psi + \sum_{i=1}^{N} \frac{(V_i - \overline{V})^2}{\sigma^2(\overline{V})} \qquad (13)$$

where $\overline{V}$ is the presumed mean V value (74 ml/100 gm) and $\sigma(V)$ is the assumed standard deviation of V_i values across all pixels. This new algorithm was applied to the original 32 [^{15}O]water studies. For 10% $\sigma(\overline{V})$, the error in global flow was reduced to $-42 \pm 8\%$ and the correlation with the measured CBF values was 0.67. For 15% variability, the global flow bias became $+31 \pm 30\%$ and the correlation dropped to 0.15. Thus, the negative bias is reduced by inclusion of variability in V_i, but the variability in global flow error increases. For 20% $\sigma(\overline{V})$, global flow is significantly overestimated ($+111\%$) and the correlation with measured CBF is negative ($-.42$). This revised method is overly sensitive to the value of $\sigma(\overline{V})$.

F. Summary

The GN method can produce accurate CBF measurements only when the measurements follow the assumed model. Tissue heterogeneity and other factors produce large bias in the GN flow values. These model errors produce much smaller biases in other algorithms that use a measured input function. By estimating both flow and the input function, the GN algorithm has more flexibility in minimizing Ψ and, therefore, is more sensitive to model errors. Two modified methods presented here reduced the global flow bias, but eliminated the positive correlation of GN results with those using the measured input functions. Therefore, a better model for the distribution volume is required for the GN approach to produce accurate and reliable human CBF data.

Acknowledgments

The authors acknowledge Kim Robles and Gerard Jacobs for data processing assistance and Drs. Stephen Bacharach, Margaret Daube-Witherspoon, Peter Herscovitch, and Julie Price for helpful discussions.

References

Alpert, N. M., Chesler, D. A., Correia, J. A., Ackerman, R. H., Chang, J. Y., Finklestein, S., Davis, S. M., Brownell, G. L., and Taveras, J. M. (1982). Estimation of the local statistical noise in emission computed tomography. *IEEE Trans. Med. Imaging* **1:** 142–146.

Beck, J. V., and Arnold, K. J. (1977). "Parameter Estimation in Engineering and Science." Wiley, New York.

Berman, K. F., Ostrem, K. A., Randolph, C., Gold, J., Goldberg, T. E., Coppola, R., Carson, R. E., Herscovitch, P., and Weinberger, D. R. (1995). Physiological activation of a cortical network during performance of the Wisconsin card sorting test: A positron emission tomography study. *Neuropsychologia,* **33:** 1027–1046.

Carson, R. E. (1991). Precision and accuracy considerations of physiological quantitation in PET. *J. Cereb. Blood Flow Metab.* **11:** A45–50.

Carson, R. E., Yan, Y., Chodkowski, B., Yap, T. K., and Daube-Witherspoon, M. E. (1994). Precision and accuracy of regional radioactivity quantitation using the maximum likelihood EM reconstruction algorithm. *IEEE Trans. Med. Imaging* **13:** 526–537.

Carson, R. E., Yan, Y., Daube-Witherspoon, M. E., Freedman, N., Bacharach, S. L., and Herscovitch, P. (1993). An approximation formula for the variance of PET region-of-interest values. *IEEE Trans. Med. Imaging* **12:** 240–250.

Daube-Witherspoon, M. E., Chon, K. S., Green, S. L., Carson, R. E., and Herscovitch, P. (1992). Factors affecting dispersion correction for continuous blood withdrawal and counting systems. *J. Nucl. Med.* **33:** 1010.

Fox, P. T., Mintun, M. A., Raichle, M. E., and Herscovitch, P. (1984). A noninvasive approach to quantitative functional brain mapping with H$_2$^{15}O and positron emission tomography. *J. Cereb. Blood Flow Metab.* **4:** 329–333.

Frackowiak, R. S. J., Lenzi, G.-L., Jones, T., and Heather, J. D. (1980). Quantitative measurement of regional cerebral blood flow and oxygen metabolism in man using ^{15}O and positron emission tomography: Theory, procedure and normal values. *J. Comput. Assist. Tomogr.* **4:** 727–736.

Herscovitch, P., Markham, J., and Raichle, M. E. (1983). Brain blood flow measured with intravenous H$_2$^{15}O. I. Theory and error analysis. *J. Nucl. Med.* **24:** 782–789.

Holden, J. E., Gatley, S. J., Hichwa, R. D., Ip, W. R., Shaughnessy, W. J., Nickles, R. J., and Polcyn, R. E. (1981). Cerebral blood flow using PET measurements of fluoromethane kinetics. *J. Nucl. Med.* **22:** 1084–1088.

Huang, S., Carson, R., and Phelps, M. (1982). Measurement of local blood flow and distribution volume with short-lived isotopes: A general input technique. *J. Cereb. Blood Flow Metab.* **2:** 99–108.

Iida, H., Kanno, I., Miura, S., Murakami, M., Takahashi, K., and Uemura, K. (1988). Evaluation of regional differences of tracer appearance time in cerebral tissues using [^{15}O]water and dynamic positron emission tomography. *J. Cereb. Blood Flow Metab.* **8:** 285–288.

Iida, H., Kanno, I., Miura, S., Murakami, M., Takahashi, K., and Uemura, K. (1989). A determination of regional brain/blood partition of coefficient of water using dynamic positron emission tomography. *J. Cereb. Blood Flow Metab.* **9:** 874–885.

Koeppe, R. A., Holden, J. E., and Ip, W. R. (1985a). Performance comparison of parameter estimation techniques for the quantitation of local cerebral blood flow by dynamic positron computed tomography. *J. Cereb. Blood Flow Metab.* **5:** 224–234.

Koeppe, R. A., Holden, J. E., Polcyn, R. E., Nickles, R. J., Hutchins, G. D., and Weese, J. L. (1985b). Quantitation of local cerebral blood flow and partition coefficient without arterial sampling: Theory and validation. *J. Cereb. Blood Flow Metab.* **5:** 214–223.

Mazziotta, J. C., Huang, S. C., Phelps, M. E., Carson, R. E., MacDonald, N. S., and Mahoney, K. (1985). A noninvasive positron computed tomography technique using oxygen-15-labeled water for the evaluation of neurobehavioral task batteries. *J. Cereb. Blood Flow Metab.* **5:** 70–78.

Nelson, A. D., Miraldi, F., Muzic, R. F., Leisure, G. P., and Semple, W. E. (1993). Noninvasive arterial monitor for quantitative oxygen-15 water blood flow studies. *J. Nucl. Med.* **34:** 1000–1006.

Noninvasive Quantification of rCBF Using Positron Emission Tomography

H. WATABE,[1] M. ITOH,[2] V. J. CUNNINGHAM,[3] A. A. LAMMERTSMA,[3] P. M. BLOOMFIELD,[3] M. MEJIA,[2] T. FUJIWARA,[2] A. K. P. JONES,[4] T. JONES,[3] and T. NAKAMURA[2]

[1]National Cardiovascular Center Research Institute
Osaka, Japan
[2]Cyclotron and Radioisotope Center, Tohoku University
Sendai 980-77, Japan
[3]MRC Cyclotron Unit, Hammersmith Hospital
London W12 ONN, United Kingdom
[4]Rheumatic Diseases Centre, Hope Hospital
Manchester, United Kingdom

A new analysis for the pixel-by-pixel quantification of rCBF with PET and $H_2^{15}O$ is presented. It involves a reference region approach based on the simultaneous analysis of regions with different flows and the algebraic elimination of the arterial input function term. The method, therefore, requires no arterial blood sampling. Simulation studies were carried out to evaluate the method. The rCBF images of 17 subjects were calculated by the present method and the dynamic–integral method, and comparisons of the two methods were performed. The CBF images calculated by the present method correlated with those obtained by the dynamic–integral method. The method may prove a useful adjunct to those protocols, such as are often used in activation studies, which do not routinely involve arterial blood sampling.

I. INTRODUCTION

Techniques to calculate regional cerebral blood flow using positron emission tomography (PET) and water (or inhaled carbon dioxide) radiolabeled with the positron emitter, O-15, have been developed by several investigators. These include the steady state technique (Frackowiak *et al.*, 1980) and the autoradiographic, weighted integral, and dynamic–integral methods (Raichle *et al.*, 1983; Kanno *et al.*, 1984; Huang *et al.*,

1983; Lammertsma *et al.*, 1990). All these techniques require the sampling and assay of radioactivity in arterial blood.

We now propose a new numerical solution for the calculation of rCBF that involves the elimination of the arterial input function term. Thus, no arterial cannulation is needed in the protocol. Furthermore, corrections for dispersion and time delay in the model associated with the collection and assay of radioactivity in blood are avoided. The method can produce pixel-by-pixel functional images of rCBF with short calculation times.

II. THEORY

The model is based on the single tissue compartment model originally developed by Kety (1951), in which the differential equation relating the concentration of radioactivity in the tissue at time t, $C_t(t)$, and the arterial input function, $C_a(t)$, is given by

$$\frac{dC_t(t)}{dt} = fC_a(t) - \frac{f}{V_d}C_t(t) \qquad (1)$$

where f and V_d are the regional blood flow and the volume of distribution for water, respectively.

Now we consider any two distinct regions, Region 1 and Region 2, in the brain. Equation (1) can then be applied to both regions as follows:

$$\frac{dC_{t1}(t)}{dt} = f_1 C_a(t) - \frac{f_1}{V_{d1}} C_{t1}(t) \qquad (2)$$

$$\frac{dC_{t2}(t)}{dt} = f_2 C_a(t) - \frac{f_2}{V_{d2}} C_{t2}(t) \qquad (3)$$

where it is assumed that the input function, $C_a(t)$, is the same for the two regions. Integration of equations (2) and (3) twice from time 0 to T, gives the following derived equations:

$$\int_0^T C_{t1}(t)\,dt = f_1 \int_0^T dt \int_0^t C_a(s)\,ds$$
$$- \frac{f_1}{V_{d1}} \int_0^T dt \int_0^t C_{t1}(s)\,ds \qquad (4)$$

$$\int_0^T C_{t2}(t)\,dt = f_2 \int_0^T dt \int_0^t C_a(s)\,ds$$
$$- \frac{f_2}{V_{d2}} \int_0^T dt \int_0^t C_{t2}(s)\,ds \qquad (5)$$

where T represents the time of the last frame for PET scan.

From equations (4) and (5), the arterial input function $C_a(t)$ can be eliminated to give

$$\int_0^T C_{t1}(t)\,dt = \frac{f_1}{f_2} \int_0^T C_{t2}(t)\,dt + \frac{f_2}{V_{d2}} \int_0^T dt \int_0^t C_{t2}(s)\,ds$$
$$- \frac{f_1}{V_{d1}} \int_0^T dt \int_0^t C_{t1}(s)\,ds \qquad (6)$$

For a PET scan with n frames, n data sets for equation (6) are obtained as

$$\left\{ \int_0^T C_{t1}(t)\,dt \right\}_{i=1,\dots n} = \left\{ \frac{f_1}{f_2} \int_0^T C_{t2}(t)\,dt \right.$$
$$\left. + \frac{f_2}{V_{d2}} \int_0^T dt \int_0^t C_{t2}(s)\,ds - \frac{f_1}{V_{d1}} \int_0^T dt \int_0^t C_{t1}(s)\,ds \right\}_{i=1,\dots n} \qquad (7)$$

To calculate rCBF on a pixel-by-pixel basis, we first define the whole brain as Region 1 and all pixels within 10% of the maximum counts (i.e., gray matter) as Region 2. Data for Region 1 were obtained by applying elliptical ROIs just surrounding the brain on the middle five planes of the scans. By means of equation (7), whole brain CBF, f_1, and distribution volume of water, V_{d1}, together with f_2 for Region 2 were fitted using nonlinear regression techniques. The distribution volume for Region 2 was fixed to 0.86 ml/ml. Because of correlated errors in f_1 and f_2 it also proved necessary at this stage to include a penalty term biasing estimates of f_1 toward a predetermined mean value. Hence, another fitting condition with $f_1 = 50$ with a variance of 50 was added to the data represented by equation (7).

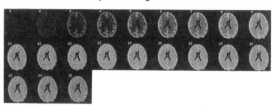

FIGURE 1   Simulation of data corresponding to a quantitative PET cerebral blood flow study.

The flow of each pixel, f_p, was then calculated from equation (8), which is derived from equation (6),

$$f_p =$$
$$\frac{\int_0^T c_{tp}(t)\,dt}{\frac{1}{f_1} \int_0^T C_{t1}(t)\,dt + \frac{1}{V_{d1}} \int_0^T dt \int_0^t C_{t1}(s)\,ds - \frac{1}{V_{dp}} \int_0^T dt \int_0^t C_{tp}(s)\,ds} \qquad (8)$$

where the fitted values for f_1 and V_{d1} were obtained as previously.

III. RESULTS AND DISCUSSION

A. Simulation

To validate the present method, we carried out the following simulation studies. First, simulated CBF images were generated. A plane of an MRI image was divided into two regions, white matter and gray matter. The values of pixels within the white matter region were determined as the flow values for white matter by a Gaussian random number generator with mean value of 30 ml/dl/min and standard deviation of 5. The rCBF values for the gray matter were also determined as the mean value CBF_g and standard deviation of 10. The values of CBF_g were varied from 70 to 90 ml/dl/min.

According to the typical PET protocol, the sequential images of dynamic study were generated using the typical input curve and the simulated rCBF image as shown in Figure 1. Using these dynamic images, the

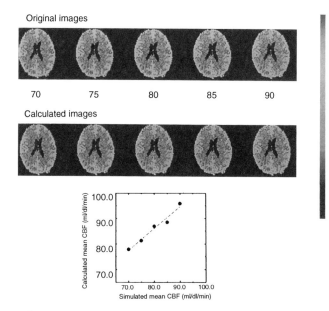

Original images

70   75   80   85   90

Calculated images

FIGURE 2   Analysis of the simulated data. A comparison of the calculated images with the original images.

calculated rCBF image was produced by the present method. Simulated rCBF images and calculated rCBF images were compared.

Figure 2 shows the results of simulation studies. The first row shows the simulated CBF images. Mean CBF values of gray matter are 70, 75, 80, 85, and 90, respectively. The second row shows the results of flow calculation by the present method.

The graph in Figure 2 represents the plots of mean blood flow for gray matter between simulated and calculated images. As shown in the figure, the calculated CBF were overestimated by about 8% from the simulated CBF. However significant correlation was found between simulated and calculated CBF values, as shown in the graph. The correlation coefficient was 0.984. One reason of the overestimation may be numerical errors involved in the numerical integration of equations (4) and (5).

B. Experiment

Actual PET data were utilized also for validation of the present method. Experiments were carried out using an ECAT 931-08/12 positron emission tomograph. Data was taken from PET studies with CO_2 inhalation from 17 normal volunteers aged 20–59 years, mean 40.8 ± 14. The experimental protocol was 30 sec of background scan, 4×5 sec scans and 16×10 sec scans. The subjects inhaled $C^{15}O_2$ gas for 2 min.

Before each scan a transmission scan was carried

out using external $[^{67}Ge]/[^{68}Ga]$ ring sources for tissue attenuation correction. Arterial blood was withdrawn continuously through a radial artery at a speed of 5 ml/min using polyethene tubing, and the counts of arterial blood were measured by the scintillation detector placed on the tube.

Reconstructed images were transferred to workstations, and the CBF images were calculated by the present method and the dynamic integral technique developed by Lammertsma *et al.* (1990).

Table 1 shows the results of comparison between the dynamic–integral method and the present method for 17 volunteers. The second column represents the mean CBF values calculated by the dynamic–integral method, and the third column represents the mean CBF values calculated by the present method. (Note that these mean values were extracted from the parametric images using the transmission image as a mask, and hence the mean values are low.) As shown in the fourth column, the correlation coefficients between two methods were unity for every case. This high intrasubject correlation is to be expected, however, as the data are common and both analyses are derived from the same model.

Figure 3 shows the regression curve between mean whole brain CBF values for the dynamic–integral

TABLE 1   Comparison of Two Methods

Run no.	Mean[a]	Mean[b]	Correlation coefficient	Slope	Intercept
p1414	26.8	27.7	1.00	1.04	−0.119
p1474	28.7	26.3	1.00	0.909	0.167
p1597	24.9	24.8	1.00	0.985	0.0061
p1634	29.3	28.3	1.00	0.958	0.275
p1639	25.7	26.7	1.00	1.05	−0.128
p1644	36.7	28.0	1.00	0.745	0.659
p1657	33.1	27.2	1.00	0.808	0.470
p1672	26.9	30.9	1.00	1.16	−0.384
p1770	23.4	25.2	1.00	1.08	−0.172
p1803	22.5	22.8	1.00	1.01	−0.0867
p1831	37.8	33.0	1.00	0.861	0.449
p1852	24.5	25.8	1.00	1.06	−0.108
p1865	25.2	25.0	1.00	0.990	0.0144
p1949	27.7	26.9	1.00	0.969	0.0308
p2018	35.3	35.4	1.00	1.00	−0.0098
p2037	33.1	34.8	1.00	1.06	−0.159
p2122	33.4	29.5	1.00	0.875	0.319
Average	29.1	28.1	1.00	0.974	0.0720
SD	4.8	3.6		0.107	0.277

[a] Mean CBF value (ml/dl/min) of whole brain image by the dynamic–integral method.

[b] Mean CBF value (ml/dl/min) of whole brain image by the present method.

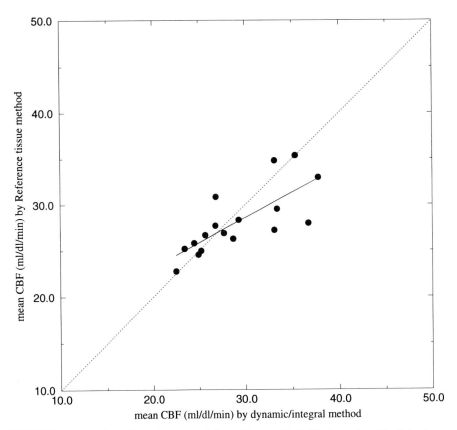

FIGURE 3   Comparison of results obtained from 17 normal individuals analyzed both by the present reference tissue method and the dynamic–integral method.

method and for the present method between the different subjects. The correlation coefficient was 0.749, with a significant correlation between two methods (paired *t* test, $p < 0.0005$). However, some data found disagreement between two methods. Several reasons for these disagreements can be considered. One reason is, as described in the simulation study, the numerical calculations such as integration or decay correlation produce the errors of calculation.

The main problem of the present method is that the solution of equation (7) is very near to singular, so sometimes the solution depended on the starting point of the fitting routine. To avoid the fitting routine falling into the abnormal solution, the constrained condition of 50 ml/dl/min was set, which means the flow of Region 1 will never be far away from 50 ml/dl/min. Further optimization of the scanning procedure and constraint conditions are probably necessary.

IV. SUMMARY

A new solution for the calculation of rCBF with positron emission tomography is proposed. The

method requires no arterial cannulation for the input function and can produce pixel-by-pixel functional images of rCBF with short calculation times. The principal problem with the method is the instability of the solution, which necessitates the introduction of a penalty function in the fitting procedure. Despite this shortcoming, the method may prove a useful adjunct to those protocols, such as are often used in activation studies, that do not routinely involve arterial blood sampling.

References

Frackowiak, R. S. J., Lenzi, G. L., Jones, T., and Heather, J. D. (1980). Quantitative measurement of regional cerebral blood flow and oxygen metabolism in man using ^{15}O and positron emission tomography: Theory, procedure, and normal values. *J. Comput. Assist. Tomogr.* **4**: 727–736.

Huang, S. C., Carson, R. E., Hoffman, E. J., Carson, J., MacDonald, N., Barrio, J. R., and Phelps, M. E. (1983). Quantitative measurement of local cerebral blood flow in humans by positron computed tomography and ^{15}O-water. *J. Cereb. Blood Flow Metab.* **3**: 141–153.

Kanno, I., Lammertsma, A. A., Heather, J. D., Gibbs, J. M., Rhodes, C. G., Clark, J. C., and Jones, T. (1984). Measurement of cerebral blood flow using bolus inhalation of C15 O2 and positron emission tomography: Description of the method and its comparison with the $C^{15}O_2$ continuous inhalation method. *J. Cereb. Blood Flow Metab.* **4:** 224–234.

Kety, S. S. (1951). The theory and applications of the exchange of inert gas at the lungs and tissues. *Pharmacol. Rev.* **3:** 1–41.

Lammertsma, A. A., Cunningham, V. J., Deiber, M. P., Heather, J. D., Bloomfield, P. M., Nutt, J., Frackowiak, R. S. J., and Jones, T. (1990). Combination of Dynamic and Integral Methods for Generating Reproducible Functional CBF Images. *J. Cereb. Blood Flow Metab.* **10:** 675–686.

Raichle, M. E., Martin, W. R. W., Herscovitch, P., Mintun, M. A., and Markham, J. (1983). Brain blood flow measured with intravenous H2150. II. Implementation and validation. *J. Nucl. Med.* **29:** 241–247.

38

A Sensitivity Analysis of Model Parameters in Dynamic Blood Flow Studies Using $H_2{}^{15}O$ and PET

P.-J. TOUSSAINT and E. MEYER

Positron Imaging Laboratories, McConnell Brain Imaging Centre, and
Montreal Neurological Institute, McGill University
Montreal, Quebec, Canada H3A 2B4

Cerebral blood flow (CBF) can be estimated from dynamic positron emission tomographic (PET) data using $H_2{}^{15}O$ and multiparameter nonlinear least squares fitting. This requires the simultaneous determination of additional model parameters, which include the partition coefficient of water, p, the initial tracer distribution volume, V_o, as well as the arterial blood radioactivity correction factors tracer delay, Δt, and dispersion time constant, τ. The fitting approach therefore is successful only if the parameters involved are sufficiently uncorrelated. We have qualitatively studied this question by means of computer simulations and a sensitivity analysis, which indicated that Δt, τ, and V_o were significantly correlated. By lumping the latter two parameters into Δt and performing a three-parameter fit for CBF, p and Δt_{lumped} (one-compartment model), we found that CBF could be estimated with a less than 3% error for brain regions with average vascularity (V_o ~2 ml/100 g). For more vascular regions, ignoring the nonextracted vascular radioactivity, that is, V_o, rapidly leads to an overestimation of CBF by over 50%, particularly for areas with low CBF. Inclusion of V_o in the analysis (two-compartment model) yielded excellent estimates of CBF and p over a wide range of V_o values, provided that Δt and τ were known. Our results indirectly demonstrate that CBF is overestimated with the conventional one-compartment analysis that ignores unextracted vascular radioactivity.

I. INTRODUCTION

Estimation of physiological parameters such as cerebral blood flow (CBF), oxygen metabolic rate (CMR_{O_2}), water partition coefficient (p), and initial tracer distribution volume (V_o) from dynamic positron emission tomography (PET) data requires accuracy and precision as well as knowledge of the correction parameters tracer delay (Δt) and dispersion time constant (τ) of the continuously sampled arterial blood data. Frequently, nonlinear least squares multiparameter fitting is used to determine the parameters of interest for a given model (Meyer, 1989). The question that arises is this: How many of the parameters may be simultaneously determined by this approach? The procedure is successful only if the parameters are sufficiently uncorrelated. This may be qualitatively assessed by means of a sensitivity analysis (Huang *et al.*, 1986).

Using as an example the two-compartment model of Ohta, Meyer, and Gjedde (1990) (Fig. 1, bottom), which, unlike Kety's (1951) one-compartment model (Fig. 1, top), accounts for nonextracted intravascular radioactivity, we have performed simulations and calculated sensitivity functions (SFs) to evaluate the accuracy and precision with which various sets of parameters may be determined. In addition, we have investigated the importance of including V_o in the CBF analysis by comparing the simulation results for the two models.

II. METHODS

The arterial blood activity curve from a dynamic PET $H_2{}^{15}O$ study was used to generate a bolus-type input function by approximation to a sum of four

ONE – COMPARTMENT

CBF′·C$_a$

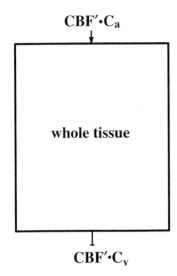

whole tissue

CBF′·C$_v$

TWO – COMPARTMENT

CBF·C$_a$

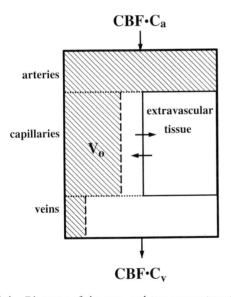

arteries

extravascular tissue

capillaries   V$_0$

veins

CBF·C$_v$

FIGURE 1 Diagrams of the one- and two-compartment cerebral blood flow models.

gamma variates: $C_a(t) = \sum_{i=1}^{4} a_i \cdot t^{n_i} \cdot \exp(-t/b_i)$. This ideal input function was delayed by Δt sec and dispersed by means of convolution with a mono-exponential dispersion function to yield the measured input function $g(t + \Delta t) = C_a(t) * (1/\tau) \exp(-t/\tau)$ (Iida *et al.*, 1986).

By deconvolution of the above expression, $C_a(t)$ can

be obtained from the measured delayed and dispersed input function, $g(t + \Delta t)$, as follows:

$$C_a(t) = g(t + \Delta t) + \tau \frac{dg}{dt}(t + \Delta t) \qquad (1)$$

The tissue time activity curve for the two-compartment model (Fig. 1, bottom) is given by

$$C(t) = CBF \int_0^t C_a(u)e^{-\frac{CBF}{p}(t-u)} du + V_o \cdot C_a(t) \quad (2)$$

Inserting $C_a(t)$ from equation (1), we obtain

$$
\begin{aligned}
C(t) = {} & \tau \cdot CBF \cdot g(t + \Delta t) \\
& + \left(1 - \tau \frac{CBF}{p}\right) e^{-\frac{CBF}{p}(t+\Delta t)} \int_{\Delta t}^{t+\Delta t} g(u)e^{\frac{CBF}{p}u} du \quad (3) \\
& + V_o \cdot \left[g(t + \Delta t) + \tau \frac{dg}{dt}(t + \Delta t) \right]
\end{aligned}
$$

By setting $V_o = 0$, equation (3) describes the tissue activity for Kety's one-compartment model (Kety, 1951), which does not distinguish between tissue- and blood-borne radioactivity (Fig. 1, top).

Equation (3) was used to generate tissue data with the addition of 5% random Gaussian noise. For the simulations, the input values of p, Δt, and τ were fixed to 0.9 ml/g, at 10 sec and 5 sec, respectively. For V_o, two values were used: 2 ml/100 g (average vascularity) and 10 ml/100 g (high vascularity). Four values were used for CBF: 25, 50, 75, and 100 ml/100 g/min.

From these tissue data, together with $g(t + \Delta t)$, we tried to determine how many and which of the five parameters could be determined reliably and simultaneously by multiparameter fitting, using equation (3). To

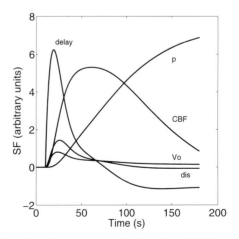

FIGURE 2 Sensitivity functions for blood flow (CBF), water partition coefficient (p), tracer delay (Δt), dispersion (τ), and initial distribution volume (V_o) where CBF = 50 ml/100 g/min, p = 0.9 ml/g, Δt = 10 sec, τ = 5 sec.

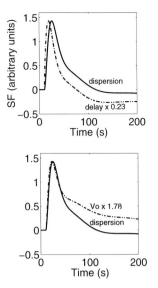

facilitate this task, a sensitivity analysis was performed to qualitatively ascertain the degree of accuracy with which the model parameters could be recovered from the simultaneous fits. Sensitivity functions (SFs) were calculated as

$$SF(t, p_i) = \frac{C(t, p_i + \Delta p_i) - C(t, p_i)}{\Delta p_i} \qquad (4)$$

where p_i represents any of the five parameters CBF, p, Δt, τ, or V_o (Huang et al., 1986). They are a measure of the change in $C(t)$ brought upon by a small variation in any one of the parameters of the function (e.g., $\Delta p_i / p_i = 0.01$). The more similar are the shapes of the SFs, the greater is the degree of correlation between the respective parameters, and vice versa.

In a subset of simulations we assumed that Δt and τ were known from other sources such as [11C]- or [15O]carbon monoxide studies (Kuwabara et al., 1993; Murase et al., 1995). The values of Δt and τ were, therefore, fixed to their input values (10 sec and 5 sec) and a three-parameter fit for CBF, p, and V_o performed using equation (3) (two-compartment model). To assess

FIGURE 3 Sensitivity functions for Δt and τ (top) and for V_o and τ (bottom), scaled to equal peak height.

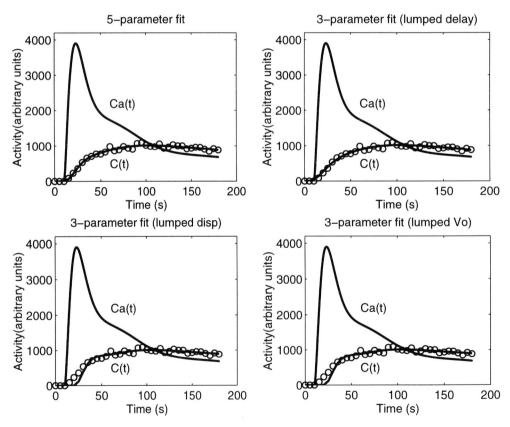

FIGURE 4 Simulated input function and tissue time activity curve with 5% Gaussian random noise (○) and its fit (−) for a five-parameter fit of CBF, p, Δt, τ, V_o (top left), and three-parameter fits of CBF, p, Δt_{lumped} (top right), CBF, p, τ_{lumped} (bottom left), and CBF, p, $V_{o_{lumped}}$ (bottom right).

the importance of including V_o in the analysis, the fit was repeated with V_o set to 0 (two-parameter fit, one-compartment model) and the estimates of CBF and p were compared with their input values.

III. RESULTS AND DISCUSSION

The SFs for τ, Δt, and V_o look very similar (Fig. 2), suggesting that these three parameters might not be recovered with accuracy and precision from a multiparameter fit. Scaling of the SFs of these parameters to the same peak height accentuates this finding (Fig. 3). On the other hand, relatively accurate estimates of CBF and p may be expected.

Fitting of all five parameters, as expected, gave an excellent fit (Fig. 4, top left); however, the estimates of τ, Δt, and V_o were meaningless whereas those of CBF and p were within 10% of their true values. Similar results for CBF and p were obtained by fitting only for CBF, p, and either τ, Δt, or V_o, setting the remaining two parameters to 0 (three-parameter fits). In fact, when τ and V_o were "lumped" into Δt_{lumped}, the estimates for CBF and p were significantly better than with the five-parameter fit (deviation of <3% from true value at V_o = 2 ml/100 g and <14% for V_o = 10 ml/100 g; Fig. 5, top). In fact, the two fits were practically indistinguishable (Fig. 4, top right). When τ and V_o were "lumped" in turn (Fig. 4, bottom left and right), the estimates for CBF and p became progressively worse (Fig. 5, center and bottom). The estimate of the "lumped" parameter, of course, substantially exceeded its true value in all instances because it was compensating for the absence of the other two parameters, as predicted by the sensitivity analysis.

When Δt and τ were fixed to their input values, CBF and p were accurately estimated (error <2%) from a three-parameter fit (two-compartment analysis) for all conditions tested and V_o was somewhat underestimated (up to 12%). When V_o was set to 0 in the fit (one-compartment analysis), CBF and p were still within 8% of their true values for a low V_o (2 ml/100 g), with the error decreasing as CBF increased. For a high V_o, CBF was significantly overestimated, with the error ranging from +60% at a low CBF to +24% at a high CBF.

Our simulation results suggest that, as long as V_o does not exceed 10 ml/100 g, CBF may be estimated with less than 10% error from a three-parameter fit of CBF, p, and a *lumped* Δt, which is achieved by setting τ and V_o to 0 in the fitting equation. This finding does not suggest, however, that V_o should be neglected when estimating CBF. On the contrary, it indirectly demonstrates that CBF is overestimated, particularly for large

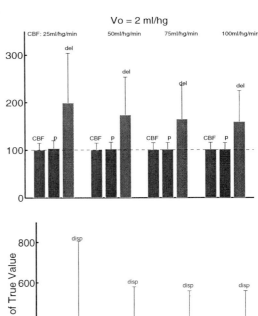
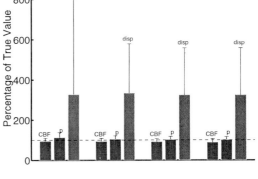
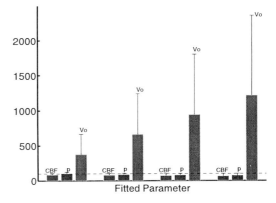

FIGURE 5 Mean values (±rms) of CBF, p, Δt (delay), τ (dispersion), and V_o, in terms of their percentage of the true values, obtained from three-parameter fits for the three cases where (1) τ and V_o are lumped into Δt_{lumped} (top), (2) Δt and V_o are lumped into τ_{lumped} (center), and (3) Δt and τ are lumped into $V_{o_{lumped}}$ (bottom). Results from n = 50 simulations; hg = 100 g.

values of V_o, by the one-compartment analysis, because (1) the "lumped" value of Δt obtained from the three-parameter fit, which represents a weighted mixture of corrections for true delay, dispersion, and vascular radioactivity (V_o), is significantly larger than its true value (i.e., Δt determined by accepted methods applying to the one-compartment model; Iida *et al.*, 1988) and (2) the larger is Δt in the one-compartment analysis, the smaller is the calculated value of CBF. For a small V_o (~2 ml/100 g), the one-compartment model overestimates CBF by approximately 10%, with the error rapidly rising, reaching 60% at a large V_o (~10 ml/100 g). The largest errors were found for the smallest CBF values and vice versa.

It goes without saying that, by ignoring V_o in the analysis, one deprives oneself of the potentially useful information contained in this exclusively vascular parameter that may be obtained from the same CBF study.

The two-compartment CBF model with inclusion of V_o yields excellent estimates of CBF and p over a wide range of V_o values, provided that Δt and τ are known. However, estimation of V_o itself is a challenge as this parameter seems to be the most fragile of all.

In conclusion, we have demonstrated the usefulness of SFs for the qualitative assessment of correlations between model parameters. Such an analysis assists in the initial evaluation of multiparameter fitting problems, indicating which parameters may or may not be estimated accurately and reliably. It also helps to develop the appropriate fitting strategies to recover the major parameter(s) of interest.

We found that CBF by the $H_2^{15}O$ bolus method can be safely estimated for brain regions with average vascularity from a three-parameter fit of CBF, p, and a *lumped* Δt that compensates for the ignored parameters τ and V_o. This result indirectly demonstrates that CBF is overestimated with the conventional one-compartment analysis that ignores unextracted vascular radioactivity (V_o).

Acknowledgments

This work was supported by MRC (Canada) grant SP-30, the Isaac Walton Killam Fellowship Fund of the Montreal Neurological Institute and by the McDonnell-Pew Program in Cognitive Neuroscience.

References

Huang, S. C., Feng, D. G., and Phelps, M. E. (1986). Model dependency and estimation reliability in measurement of cerebral oxygen utilization rate with oxygen-15 and dynamic positron tomography. *J. Cereb. Blood Flow Metab.* **6:** 105–119.

Iida, H., Kanno, I., Miura, S., Murakami, M., Takahashi, K., and Uemura, K. (1986). Error analysis of a quantitative cerebral blood flow measurement using O-15 H2O autoradiography and positron emission tomography, with respect to the dispersion of the input function. *J. Cereb. Blood Flow Metab.* **6:** 536–545.

Iida, H., Higano, S., Tomura, N., *et al.* (1988). Evaluation of regional differences of tracer appearance time in cerebral tissues using [^{15}O] water and dynamic positron emission tomography. *J. Cereb. Blood Flow Metab.* **8:** 285–288.

Kety, S. S. (1951). The theory and application of the exchange of inert gas at the lungs and tissues. *Pharmacol. Rev.* **3:** 1–41.

Kuwabara, H., Fujita, H., Vafaee, M., Yasuhara, Y., Gjedde, A., and Meyer, E. (1993). Measurement of tracer arrival delay and dispersion using positron emission tomography and tracer [^{15}O] carbon monoxide. *In* "Tracer Kinetics and Image Analysis in Brain PET" (K. Uemura *et al.*, Eds.), pp. 61–67. Elsevier Science Publishers, BV.

Meyer, E. (1989). Simultaneous correction for tracer arrival delay and dispersion in CBF measurements by the $H_2^{15}O$ autoradiographic method and dynamic PET. *J. Nucl. Med.* **30:** 1069–1078.

Murase, K., Kuwabara, H., Vafaee, M., Toussaint, P.-J., Gjedde, A., Evans, A. C., and Meyer, E. (1995). Generation of maps of dispersion time constant and tracer arrival delay using [O-15]carbonmonoxide. Abstract presented at PET95.

Ohta, S., Meyer, E., and Gjedde, A. (1990). Weighted integration method with CBV correction to estimate rCBF by PET. *Eur. J. Nucl. Med.* **16**(Suppl): S178.

Generation of Maps of Dispersion Time Constant and Tracer Arrival Delay Using [^{15}O]Carbon Monoxide

K. MURASE, H. KUWABARA, M. VAFAEE, P.-J. TOUSSAINT, A. GJEDDE, A. C. EVANS, and E. MEYER

Positron Imaging Laboratories, McConnell Brain Imaging Centre
Montreal Neurological Institute McGill University,
Montreal, Quebec, Canada H3A 2B4

We proposed a method for generating the averaged maps of dispersion time constant (τ) and tracer arrival delay (δ) using [^{15}O]carbon monoxide and dynamic PET data. Although there is some room for improvement, especially in determination of the τ image, our preliminary results suggest that this method is useful for estimating regional τ and δ values, which may be applicable for routine dispersion and delay correction of PET data on a pixel-by-pixel basis.

I. INTRODUCTION

Because the time course of radioactivity measured in the periphery ($C_a^M(t)$) is usually modulated in terms of dispersion and tracer arrival delay (Iida *et al.*, 1986; Meyer, 1989), $C_a^M(t)$ does not represent the time course of radioactivity at the site of tracer exchange between the circulation and the organ of interest ($C_a^*(t)$). Kuwabara *et al.* (1993) previously developed a method for determining the dispersion time constant and tracer arrival delay simultaneously, using [^{15}O]carbon monoxide (CO), which is retained in red blood cells and does not enter the brain. In this chapter, we extended this method to the estimation of dispersion time constant and tracer arrival delay pixel by pixel, to generate averaged maps for the investigation of regional differences in these parameters.

II. MATERIALS AND METHODS

A. Theory

When $C_a^*(t)$ is related to $C_a^M(t)$ as

$$C_a^*(t) = C_a^M(u) + \tau \frac{dC_a^M(u)}{du} \qquad (1)$$

where $u = t + \delta$, τ is the dispersion time constant, and δ is the tracer arrival delay of $C_a^M(t)$ relative to $C_a^*(t)$ (Iida *et al.*, 1986; Meyer, 1989), then the radioactivity at pixel (x, y) in the brain measured during the *i*th scan ($A_i^{x,y}$) can be expressed by the following multilinear regression equation:

$$[A_i^{x,y}] = V_b[B_i] + V_b\tau[C_i] \qquad i = 1,2,3, \ldots \quad (2)$$

In Equation (2), B_i and C_i are given by

$$B_i = \int_{T_{i-1}}^{T_i} C_a^M(t + \delta)\, dt$$
$$C_i = C_a^M(T_i + \delta) - C_a^M(T_{i-1} + \delta)$$

where T_{i-1} and T_i are the start and end times of the *i*th scan, respectively, and V_b, the cerebral blood volume (Kuwabara *et al.*, 1993). Equation (2) allows simple and fast determination of V_b and τ for various values of δ. In this study, we changed δ from -5 to 10 sec in 0.5 sec increments and chose values of δ, τ, and V_b that minimized $\sum \omega_i (A_i^{x,y} - \hat{A}_i^{x,y})^2$, where $\omega_i = (A_i^{x,y})^2$ and $\hat{A}_i^{x,y}$ is the value for $A_i^{x,y}$ calculated using equation (2).

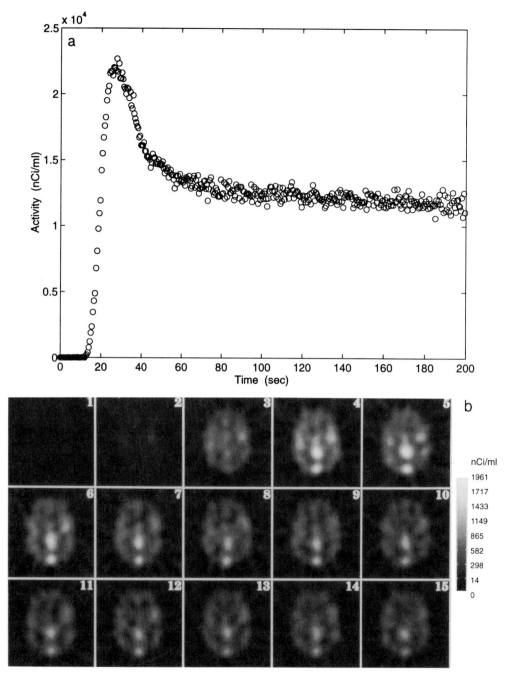

FIGURE 1   Typical example of arterial blood curve (a) and dynamic image (b). Figure 1(b) shows 15 of 21 frames of the sixth slice.

B. PET Studies

We studied seven healthy, neurologically normal subjects (age 23.0 ± 3.7 years old). Permission to conduct the study was granted by the Ethics and Research Review Committee of Montreal Neurological Institute and Hospital and signed consent forms were obtained from the subjects before the study. The tracer was prepared with a medical cyclotron (IBA cyclone 18/9), and the PET studies were performed with a Scanditronix PC-2048 15B eight-ring, 15-slice BGO head tomograph with a spatial resolution of about 6 mm FWHM in all three dimensions (Evans *et al.*, 1991a). After correction of tissue attenuation, dead time, scatter, and coincident counts, each PET image was reconstructed in a 128 × 128 matrix of 2 × 2 mm pixels (25.6 mm³ in volume) using the filtered back-projection method with a 20 mm FWHM

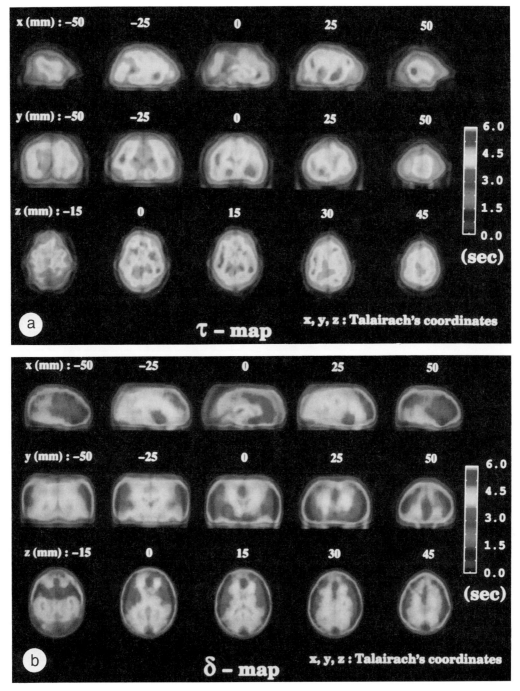

FIGURE 2   Averaged images of τ (a), δ (b), and V_b (c), which were generated using the present method.

Hanning filter. The subjects were positioned in the tomograph with their heads immobilized by means of a customized self-inflating foam headrest. A short indwelling catheter was placed into the left brachial artery for arterial blood sampling. During a 3 min period following a bolus inhalation of ~1480 MBq of CO, we acquired 21 frames with Scanditronix PC-

2048 15B (12×5 sec, 6×10 sec, and 3×20 sec). Arterial blood was drawn at 7.5 ml/min through an 18G catheter in the brachial artery and through a polyethylene tube connected to the Scanditronix automated blood sampling device. Whole blood radioactivity was reported continuously as the mean of half-second acquisitions.

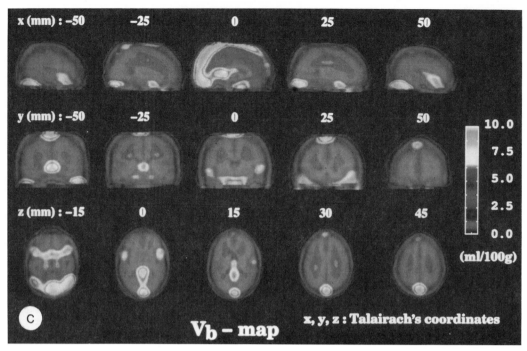

FIGURE 2 *(continued)*.

C. Superimposition of PET and MRI Images

All subjects also underwent a magnetic resonance imaging (MRI) examination on a Philips Gyroscan, 1.5 T superconducting magnet system. The MRI data volume consisted of 64 contiguous slices of 2 mm thickness. Each PET image dataset was first coregistered with its corresponding MRI image volume using a three-dimensional landmark-matching algorithm (Evans *et al.*, 1988, 1991b). The images of τ, δ, and V_b, generated from the raw PET data, were projected into Talairach's stereotaxic coordinates (Talairach and Tournoux, 1988) using the MRI volume for identification of the bicommissural plane (Evans *et al.*, 1991b) and were averaged across subjects.

III. RESULTS AND DISCUSSION

Figure 1(a) shows a typical example of an arterial blood curve ($C_a^M(t)$), and Figure 1(b) shows typical dynamic images ($A_i^{x,y}$), with 15 of 21 frames of the sixth slice being displayed.

Figure 2 shows the averaged τ (a), δ (b), and V_b (c) images generated using the present method. It should be noted that τ value obtained here represents the net dispersion; that is, the dispersion between the heart and the sampling site relative to the dispersion between the heart and the brain. Therefore, the larger is the dispersion between the heart and the brain, the smaller is the τ value, and vice versa. Similarly, the δ value obtained here represents the net tracer arrival delay; that is, the delay between the heart and the sampling site minus the delay between the heart and the brain. Therefore, the larger the delay between the heart and the brain, the smaller is the δ value, and vice versa.

In the present study, we used a large image-reconstruction filter (20 mm FWHM) for image averaging. This has the effect of increasing the signal-to-noise ratio in the averaged image, but reduces the spatial resolution. Fox *et al.* (1985) introduced the stereotactic method for PET images, and they further developed an intersubject averaging technique to increase the signal-to-noise ratio, demonstrating the feasibility of stereotactic orientation (Fox *et al.*, 1988). In the present study, we used the same technique to get the averaged images of τ, δ, and V_b (Fig. 2). As shown in Figure 2, regional differences in δ and V_b were clearly observed, although the τ image was still noisy.

The regions with high δ values correspond to areas of major cerebral arteries, and the regions with low δ values correspond to areas of venous sinus (Fig. 2(b)). This finding can also be supported qualitatively by comparison with the V_b image (Fig. 2(c)).

$A_i^{x,y}$ in equation (2) represents the mean vascular radioactivity that contains the radioactivity in both the arteries and veins, rather than the radioactivity at the arterial end alone. Thus, the τ value may be underestimated when venous radioactivity with large dispersion (smaller τ) is predominant. Because $A_i^{x,y}$ in the brain close to the skull or venous sinus can be contaminated by the radioactivity from the veins due to partial volume effect, the τ values in these regions tend to be underestimated (Fig. 2(a)).

Iida *et al.* (1988) reported 8.2 sec as the mean of the tracer arrival delay to the radial artery relative to the brain input function for tracer [^{15}O]water with a regional range of 6.4–10.2 sec. They also recommended the use of 5 sec for the dispersion time constant to obtain the brain input function from the radial artery curve (Iida *et al.*, 1986). Meyer (1989) reported 7.0 sec for the tracer arrival delay, and 4.0 sec for the dispersion time constant, expressed as means of six normal subjects using [^{15}O]water. It is not reasonable to compare our data with their values, because they used the total coincidence count curve of a PET detector ring. However, our data show that the τ value is close to reported values, although the δ value is somewhat smaller than reported values (Fig. 2). The fact that we sampled from the brachial artery rather than the more distal radial artery explains the smaller δ value of the present study.

In conclusion, although there is some room for improvement, especially in determination of the τ image, our preliminary results suggest that this method is useful for estimating regional dispersion time constants and tracer arrival delays, which may be applicable for routine dispersion and delay correction of PET data on a pixel-by-pixel basis.

References

Evans, A. C., Beil, C., Marrett, S., Thompson, C. J., and Hakim, A. (1988). Anatomical functional correlation using an adjustable MRI-based region of interest atlas with positron emission tomography. *J. Cereb. Blood Flow Metab.* **8:** 513–530.

Evans, A. C., Thompson, C. J., Marrett, S., Meyer, E., and Mazza, M. (1991a). Performance evaluation of the PC-2048: A new 15-slice encoded-crystal PET scanner for neurological studies. *IEEE Trans. Med. Imag.* **10:** 89–98.

Evans, A. C., Marrett, S., Torrescorzo, J., Ku, S., and Collins, L. (1991b). MRI-PET correlation in three dimensions using volume-of-interest (VOI) atlas. *J. Cereb. Blood Flow Metab.* **11:** 69–78.

Fox, P. T., Perlmutter, J. S., and Raichle, M. E. (1985). A stereotactic method of anatomical localization for positron emission tomography. *J. Comput. Assist. Tomogr.* **9:** 141–153.

Fox, P. T., Mintun, M. A., Reiman, E. M., and Raichle, M. E. (1988). Enhanced detection of focal brain responses using intersubject averaging and chain-distribution analysis of subtracted PET images. *J. Cereb. Blood Flow Metab.* **8:** 642–653.

Iida, H., Kanno, I., Miura, S., Murakami, M., Takahashi, K., and Uemura, K. (1986). Error analysis of a quantitative cerebral blood flow measurement using O-15 H$_2$O autoradiography and positron emission tomography, with respect to the dispersion of the input function. *J. Cereb. Blood Flow Metab.* **6:** 536–545.

Iida, H., Higano, S., Tomura, N., Shishido, F., Kanno, I., Miura, S., Murakami, M., Takahashi, K., Sasaki, H., and Uemura, K. (1988). Evaluation of regional differences of tracer appearance time in cerebral tissues using [^{15}O] water and dynamic positron emission tomography. *J. Cereb. Blood Flow Metab.* **8:** 285–288.

Kuwabara, H., Fujita, H., Vafaee, M., Yasuhara, Y., Gjedde, A., and Meyer, E. (1993). Measurement of tracer arrival delay and dispersion using positron emission tomography and tracer [^{15}O] carbon monoxide. *In:* "Tracer Kinetics and Image Analysis in Brain PET" (K. Uemura *et al.*, Eds.), pp. 61–67. Elsevier Science Publishers, BV, Amsterdam.

Meyer, E. (1989). Simultaneous correction for tracer arrival delay and dispersion in CBF measurements by the H$_2$^{15}O autoradiographic method and dynamic PET. *J. Nucl. Med.* **30:** 1069–1078.

Talairach, J., and Tournoux, P. (1988). "Co-Planar Atlas of the Human Brain." Thieme, Stuttgart.

Quantitative Noninvasive Estimation of rCBF by Using [^{15}O]Water and PET

MARCO A. MEJIA,[1] MASATOSHI ITOH,[1] HIROSHI WATABE,[2] TAKEHIKO FUJIWARA,[1] and TAKASHI NAKAMURA[2]

[1]*Department of Nuclear Medicine*
[2]*Department of Radiation Protection*
Cyclotron Center, Tohoku University
Sendai 980, Japan

We propose a method to estimate rCBF by using [^{15}O]- water and positron emission tomography (PET). This method generates rCBF images on a pixel-by-pixel basis, and it is based on the acquisition of sequences of images with correction of nonlinearity of brain tissue counts. In this study, [^{15}O]water PET scans were performed on 13 normal human volunteers and continuous sampling from the radial artery was conducted to generate functional CBF images according to the invasive catheterization method. Also we evaluated the effect on distribution volume and compared the real and calculated flows. Although, there is a dependence in the whole brain and the assumption that the V_d is 1 for all regions, this method was demonstrated to provide accurate estimation of rCBF and may simplify the brain activation studies.

I. INTRODUCTION

Positron emission tomography (PET) is a unique tool, widely used for *in vivo* measurements of local brain function such as flow (Huang *et al.*, 1983; Raichle *et al.*, 1983). Most of the methods described to measure CBF used information derived from tissue counts and arterial blood samples with correction for delay and dispertion (Iida *et al.*, 1986). Also, measurement of the input function requires continuous arterial sampling with some discomfort for both patient and doctor. Recently, a noninvasive method, the double integration method (Mejia *et al.*, 1994), has been described to linearize brain activity without arterial blood sampling.

The method has the ability to produce pixel-by-pixel images of rCBF. The disadvantages of this method are the assumptions of the whole brain and distribution volume (Lammertsma, 1994). In the present study we investigate such effects and the error in calculated and true rCBF to evaluate the accuracy of this approach. In this study, both our method and the invasive method (Lammertsma *et al.*, 1989) were performed, and the results achieved by both procedures were correlated to assess the accuracy of our method.

II. THEORY

The theoretical basis of the method is based on the principle of inert gas exchange between capillary blood and tissue in a single compartment model for CBF measurement using [^{15}O]-labeled H_2O, developed by Kety. The tissue radiotracer concentration is expressed with the rate constant of K_1 (influx) and k_2 (efflux):

$$\frac{dC_i(t)}{dt} = fC_a(t) - k_2C_i(t) \tag{1}$$

where f is the rCBF, $k_2 = f/V_d$ (V_d = volume of distribution of water for brain tissue), $C_a(t)$ and $C_i(t)$ are decay-corrected arterial and tissue concentrations, respectively. After integrating equation (1) twice from time 0 to T and assuming whole brain as 50 ml/dl/min, regional blood flow can be expressed as

$$f = \frac{\int_0^T C_i(t)\,dt}{A - \frac{1}{V_d}\int_0^T dt \int_0^t C_i(u)\,du} \tag{2}$$

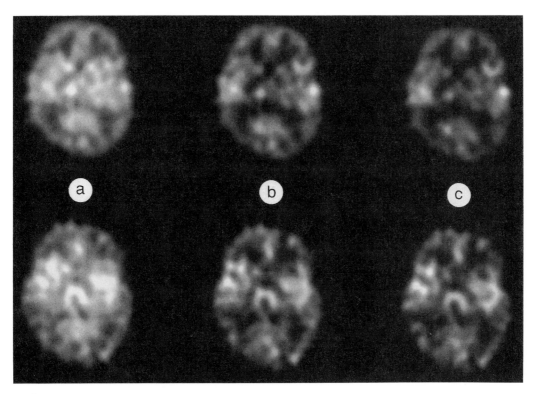

FIGURE 1   Raw images and quantitative images. The two original images were processed according to the invasive method and our method. This corresponds to one study.

where V_d was assumed to be unity. The $C_t(t)$ for each pixel was determined by dynamic data acquisition. In the application of this model, values of $\int_0^T C_w(t)$ were obtained by measuring the integral concentration of [^{15}O]water in the whole brain that is defined on the summated images. Instead of values of $C_a(t)$, we calculated A from the double integration function of $C_w(t)$. Hence, the rCBF for each pixel was estimated. The simulation algorithm has been described elsewhere (Mejia *et al.*, 1994).

III. MATERIALS AND METHODS

The study was performed on 13 normal volunteers (mean age $\pm$ SD, 27 $\pm$ 3). The CBF was measured using intravenous injection of 1480 MBq of [^{15}O]water and the ECAT 931 (CTI Inc., Knoxville, Tennessee). A transmission scan was performed for correction of tissue attenuation. The scanning protocol and the arterial monitoring system were identical to those described previously (Mejia *et al.*, 1994). In this study, only the first and last of these scans, collected during resting baseline conditions, were analyzed. After image

reconstruction, the images were transferred to a workstation for image processing.

With these images and the arterial radioactivity curve, CBF was calculated. Values of delay time were estimated from the least squares fitting between the initial slope of the total counts of the PET system and those of the estimated brain activity curve generated from the arterial curve using equation (5) with a dispersion time constant of 25 sec, according to Iida *et al.* Standard rCBF images were generated according to the autoradiographic technique using arterial input functions. On the other hand, we elaborated a program to calculate pixel-by-pixel rCBF images, according to our method just described.

Several elliptical ROIs were defined on the functional images generated by the autoradiographic method and projected with the same location on those by our method for comparison including the whole brain, the frontal cortex, and the frontal white matter.

IV. RESULTS AND DISCUSSION

It was observed that V_d values less than 1.0 produced a systematic underestimation in the calculated flow,

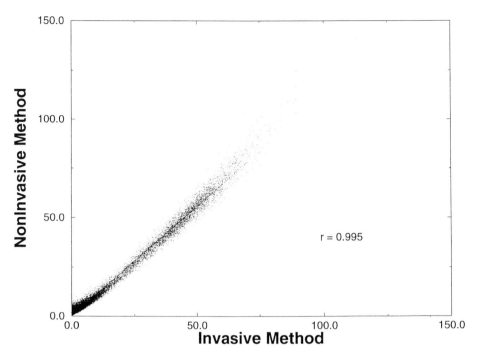

FIGURE 2 Comparison of rCBF values measured by our method and invasive method on a pixel-by-pixel basis, corresponding to a study. The solid line represents the linear regression line.

and a systematic overestimation accompanies V_d values more than 1.0, especially when flow was high. For example, more than 10% of error in CBF was resulted from 20% overestimation of V_d at a scan time of 100 sec.

Figure 1 shows the corresponding autoradiographic method images and our method images in a subject. CBF measurements were carried out on five normal volunteers with the PET dynamic approach using [¹⁵O]-water. Regional CBF images were generated using the invasive method and our method. Note that CBF values for whole brain in the invasive method are comparable with those in our method assumed at 50 ml/dl/min. Correlation between these images was examined by a pixel-by-pixel plot of all image pixel, as shown in Figure 2 for a typical case. A significant correlation was observed. The estimated CBF showed, for example, ~5% (underestimation) at 60 ml/dl/min.

The measurement of rCBF using [¹⁵O]water and positron emission tomography requires serial arterial blood samples to determine the input function. The double integration method is an attractive approach for estimating rCBF by using [¹⁵O]water.

It also assumes a fixed whole brain flow value normalized not only to flow but also to cancel out the arterial input function. There are several advantages in this approach. First, this method avoids the need for arterial blood sampling, a recognized drawback of quantitative PET (2). Second, it is not necessary to use the average standardized arterial curve or tissue counts

alone in the case of semiquantitative methods. Theoretically, it is possible that single scan data may be processed to solve count linearity. At least scan, protocols of 15 sec may be obtained to achieve this approach. In conclusion this method can be applicable to brain activation studies that require standardization of flow values without the least linearity distortion.

References

Huang, S. C., Carson, R. E., Hoffman, E. J., *et al.* (1983). Quantitative measurement of local cerebral blood flow in humans by positron computed tomography and ¹⁵O water. *J. Cereb. Blood Flow Metab.* **3:** 141–153.

Iida, H., Kanno, I., Miura, S., Muramaki, M., and Uemura, K. (1986). Error analysis of a quantitative cerebral blood flow measurement using H₂¹⁵O autoradiography and positron emission tomography, with respect to the dispersion of input function. *J. Cereb. Blood Flow Metab.* **6:** 536–545.

Lammertsma, A. A. (1989). Noninvasive estimation of cerebral blood. *J. Nucl. Med.* **35:** 1878–1879.

Lammertsma, A. A., Frackowiack, R. S. J., Hoffman, J. M., *et al.* (1989). The C¹⁵O₂ build-up technique to measure regional cerebral blood flow and volume of distribution of water. *J. Cereb. Blood Flow Metab.* **9:**461–470.

Mejia, M. A., Itoh, M., Watabe, H., Fujiwara, T., and Nakamura, T. (1994). Simplify nonlinearity correction of O-15 water CBF image without blood sampling. *J. Nucl. Med.* **35:** 1870–1877.

Raichle, M. E., Martin, W. R. W., Herscovitch, P., Mintun, M. A., and Markham, J. (1983). Brain blood flow measured with intravenous H₂¹⁵O. II. Implementation and validation. *J. Nucl. Med.* **24:** 790–798.

Correction for Global Metabolism in FDG PET Brain Images Using Linear Regression and Anatomic Standardization by Nonlinear Warping

M. HALBER,[1] **K. HERHOLZ,**[1] **S. MINOSHIMA,**[2] **and W.-D. HEISS**[1]

[1]*Max Planck Institute for Neurological Research*
Cologne D-50931, Germany
[2]*University of Michigan Medical School*
Cyclotron/PET Facility
Ann Arbor, Michigan

For intersubject comparison of FDG PET images of the brain, the influence of global effects on local metabolic rates was analyzed by a simple linear model: $P_i = a_i + b_i \cdot G$, in which every image voxel P_i is considered to be composed of a baseline value a_i and a proportionality factor b_i, representing the dependence on the global metabolic value G. This simple model was tested on high-resolution $rCMR_{glu}$ PET images of 18 healthy subjects without structural or functional brain damage, anatomically standardized using linear scaling and subsequent nonlinear warping, as described by Minoshima et al. (1994). For every image, global brain metabolism G was determined using the mean of the intracerebral voxels. The parameters a_i and b_i were determined using linear regression together with the corresponding squared correlation coefficient to estimate the regional validity of the approach for every voxel. The analysis of the spatial distribution of a_i and b_i showed uniform high b_i values in the cerebral cortex and even higher b_i values in thalamus and basal ganglia. The visual cortex showed only a small dependence on the total brain metabolism, suggesting a relative functional metabolic autonomy. This completely user-independent method can be used to correct a FDG PET image for the expected local metabolism at every single voxel location for the given individual global metabolism. Current analysis of patient data will show whether it improves sensitivity

and specificity for detection of areas with abnormal brain metabolism.

I. INTRODUCTION

Whenever metabolic PET images of the brain from different individuals are to be compared on a voxel-by-voxel basis, the confounding effect of global metabolic differences has to be taken into consideration. Usually, the global metabolic level, G, is estimated by the mean of all intracerebral voxels or all voxels above a certain threshold. Every voxel is then divided by G. Certainly, different areas of the brain contribute differently to the global metabolic value, so those simple proportional models are probably not adequate for intersubject, voxel-by-voxel comparison. Therefore, we considered the value of every single PET voxel P_i to be composed of a baseline value, a_i and another part representing the dependence on the global metabolic value G, quantified by a proportionality factor b_i. This very simple model, which is similar to that suggested by Friston *et al.* (1990) for activation studies, can be described by the following formula:

$$P_i = a_i + b_i \cdot G$$

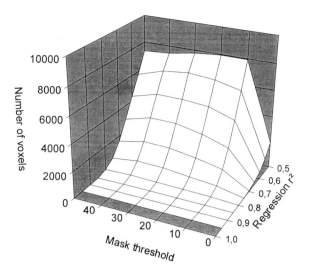

FIGURE 1   Frequency distribution of squared correlation coefficients (r^2) from linear regression with global metabolic level (G), giving an impression of the range of thresholds for which the number voxels with high r^2 values is maximal.

When a_i and b_i are determined voxel-by-voxel for coregistered PET scans from a sufficiently large population of normal subjects by voxelwise regression analysis, they can be used for normalizing a patient's PET scan by subtracting the expected P_i from every patient voxel p_i:

$$\Delta_i = p_i - P_i = p_i - (a_i + b_i \cdot G)$$

This approach produces normalized PET images (Δ images), in which every voxel represents the individual's deviation from the normal population's standard, depending on the individual global metabolic level. The squared correlation coefficient (r^2), as a measure of determination of the individual voxel level by the linear regression modeling, can be used to estimate the local validity of the approach. Finally, the normalized Δ images can be adjusted to the local variance by dividing through the regression residuals standard deviation (SD_{res}), resulting in z-score images:

$$z_i = \Delta_i / SD_{res} = [p_i - (a_i + b_i \cdot G)]/SD_{res}$$

The use of a population of normal subjects as reference makes further comparison comparatively robust against interindividual variance. Nevertheless, it should be kept in mind that there are many technical sources of error in metabolic images beyond the biological variation, as reviewed by Alavi, Smith, and Duncan (1994).

II. MATERIALS AND METHODS

For validation of this model, we used FDG PET images of 18 healthy subjects (16 male, 2 female) without structural or functional brain damage assessed by standard computed tomography or magnetic resonance imaging and clinical examination, including neurological examination and standard laboratory tests. The mean age ($\pm$ standard deviation) was 40.8 ± 11.6 years (range, 25 to 68 years). Four people were left-handed, one was ambidextrous, and the others were right-handed. None of the subjects had any history of chronic or brain diseases.

Images had been acquired with a high-resolution PET scanner (SIEMENS/CTI ECAT EXACT HR), giving 47 slices with an in-plane resolution of approximately 3.6 mm and an axial resolution of about 4.0 mm. The acquisition was performed in a darkened room at rest with eyes closed. Arterialized venous blood samples were used for quantification of $rCMR_{glu}$ applying the operational equation as described by Wienhard *et al.* (1985) with adjustment of K_1 to measured activity. Those images were anatomically standardized using linear scaling and subsequent nonlinear warping as described by Minoshima *et al.* (1994). This procedure gives consistent and reliable registration results superior to simple stereotactic transformation, because intersubject anatomic variability is greatly reduced. A mask image intended to define all intracerebral voxels was derived from the standard anatomic PET image taken from

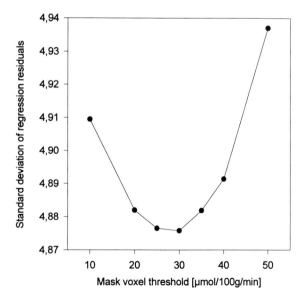

FIGURE 2   Optimum of standard deviation of regression residuals for different mask voxel thresholds.

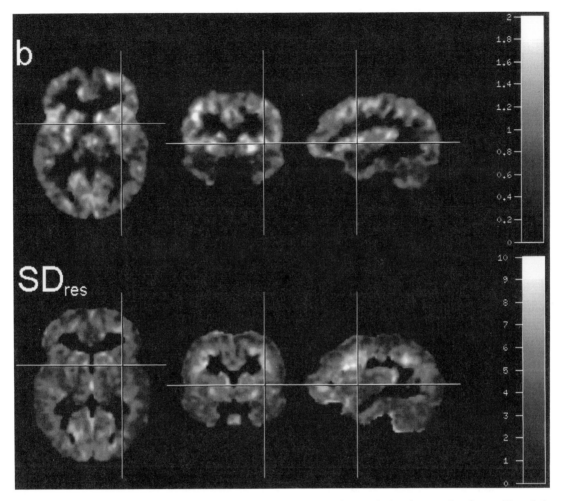

FIGURE 3   Transaxial, coronal, and sagittal tomographic aspects of the calculated regression factor (b) and the standard deviation of regression residuals (SD$_{res}$).

the work of Minoshima *et al.* (1994) by thresholding it at a certain level $T \in (0, 10, 20, 25, 30, 35, 40, 50)$.

Then, a mask-based global brain metabolism, G, was determined as the mean value of all subject's image voxels lying within the mask. Linear regression with G as the independent variable and P_i, the value of voxel i, as the dependent variable revealed approximation values for a_i and b_i. Additionally, the corresponding squared correlation coefficient r^2 was used to estimate the regional validity of the linear regression approach for every voxel, and the standard deviation of the residual voxel values were used to optimize the threshold for the global metabolic level calculation.

III. RESULTS AND DISCUSSION

Primary visual inspection of the resulting images revealed reasonable exclusion of ventricles and non-

brain areas at threshold levels of 20 μmol/100 g/min for T. Although the regression results, in particular the squared correlation coefficient, did not change very much with thresholds between 20 and 40 μmol/100 g/min (Fig. 1), the mean of the standard deviation of the regression residuals showed a minimum around 30 μmol/100 g/min (Fig. 2). The mask-based approach was chosen because it ensures inclusion of the same set of voxels every time, thus being robust against metabolic abnormalities in the image data set. Therefore, further analysis used the standard brain mask at a threshold of 30 μmol/100 g/min.

The analysis of the spatial distribution of a_i and b_i showed generally high b_i values in the cerebral cortex, as shown in Figure 3 (for a typical voxel in the frontal cortex: $a = -14.8$; $b = 1.85$; $r^2 = 0.66$), and even higher b_i values in thalamus and basal ganglia ($a = -23.2$; $b = 2.17$; $r^2 = 0.52$). The visual cortex, however, showed just marginal correlation with total brain metabolism.

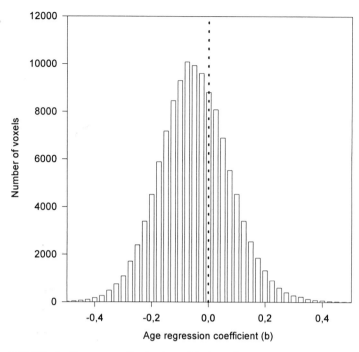

FIGURE 4 Frequency distribution of b_i from linear regression with the subject's age showing a shift of b_i toward the negative side, thus indicating voxels with negative correlation between glucose metabolism and age, mostly in the frontal and parietal association cortices.

The linear regression approach can easily be used for assessing the influence of other factors, such as the subject's age, to build hypotheses for further testing. The voxel-by-voxel regression with age as the independent variable and local cerebral glucose metabolism (in absolute units) as the dependent variable showed a tendency toward decreasing voxel values with increasing age, shown in the histogram as a shift of the resulting b_i values toward the negative side of the x-axis (Fig. 4). In comparison to previous findings by Wang *et al.* (1994), no marked side differences could be detected on the corresponding images. However, the spatial distribution of the age regression factor showed a prominent age-dependent decrease (negative b) in the prefrontal, temporal, parietal, and cingulate cortex.

The use of the normalized (z) images for examination of normal-to-pathological contrast is demonstrated here on a scan from a 54-year-old female patient with severe dementia of Alzheimer type (Fig. 5).

In conclusion, the model presented here can be used to correct an anatomically standardized PET image for the expected value at every single voxel location, depending on the individual global metabolism. The high regression coefficient values in the thalamus and in the basal ganglia correspond with the high contribution of gray matter areas to the global metabolic level and the multitude of thalamic projections. On the other hand, a relative functional metabolic autonomy of the visual cortex is suggested by its small correlation with the global metabolism. Effects of age appear most prominent in cortical structures. The visual cortex shows little dependence on age, similar to the regression on global metabolism, but basal ganglia and cerebellum also lack a prominent age dependence.

Note that the whole analysis, including linear scaling and nonlinear warping, is completely user independent. Current analysis of patient data will show whether it improves sensitivity and specificity for detection of areas with abnormal brain metabolism, such as in dementia of the Alzheimer type.

Acknowledgments

The authors thank Thomas Bruckbauer, Jan Löttgen, Alexander Thiel, and Gerald Weber-Luxenburger for helpful discussions and Gabi Bühler, Ursula Juchellek, Henning Schlüter, and Carmen Selbach for their skillful technical assistance.

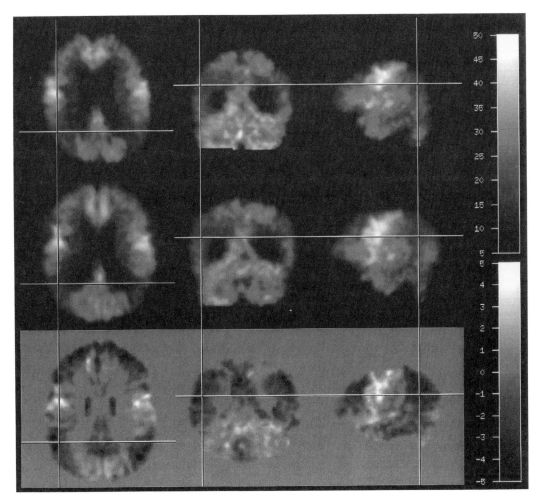

FIGURE 5 Transaxial, coronal, and sagittal aspects of a FDG scan from a 54-year-old female patient with severe dementia of Alzheimer type (top row) and its anatomic standardization by nonlinear warping (middle row), together with the corresponding normalized z-map image (bottom row), showing the prominent areas with negative z-values corresponding to brain areas affected by the disease.

References

Alavi, A., Smith, R., and Duncan, D. (1994). What are the sources of error in measuring and calculating cerebral metabolic rates with fluorine-18-fluorodeoxyglucose and PET? *J. Nucl. Med.* **35:** 1466–1470.

Friston, K. J., Frith, C. D., Liddle, P. F., Dolan, R. J., Lammertsma, A. A., and Frackowiak, R. S. J. (1990). The relationship between global and local changes in PET scans. *J. Cereb. Blood Flow Metab.* **10:** 458–466.

Minoshima, S., Koeppe, R. A., Frey, K. A., and Kuhl, D. E. (1994).

Anatomic standardization: Linear scaling and nonlinear warping of functional brain images. *J. Nucl. Med.* **35:** 1528–1537.

Wang, G. J., Volkow, N. D., Wolf, A. P., Brodie, J. D., and Hitzemann, R. J. (1994). Intersubject variability of brain glucose metabolic measurements in young normal males. *J. Nucl. Med.* **35:** 1457–1466.

Wienhard, K., Pawlik, G., Herholz, K., Wagner, R., and Heiss, W. D. (1985). Estimation of local cerebral utilization by positron emission tomography of (^{18}F)-2-fluoro-2-deoxy-D-glucose: A critical appraisal of optimization procedures. *J. Cereb. Blood Flow Metab.* **5:** 115–125.

A Kinetic Model for Double Injection ^{18}FDG Studies

DAVID C. REUTENS, SADAHIKO NISHIZAWA, ERNST MEYER, and HIROTO KUWABARA

Positron Imaging Laboratories
McConnell Brain Imaging Centre
Montreal Neurological Institute and McGill University
Montreal, Canada H3A 2B4

The use of two injections of [^{18}F]fluorodeoxyglucose in a single PET scanning session allows the examination of relationships between cerebral glucose metabolism and physiological alterations such as functional activation or changes in plasma glucose concentration. We present a kinetic model for the double injection method in which transfer coefficients are estimated independently for the second injection, allowing the second injection to be administered at a time when the steady state for the second physiological condition has been established. The method was tested using simulated noisy data and was then applied to real PET data in which the plasma glucose concentration was changed. It yielded physiologically meaningful values of transfer coefficients and the lumped constant in hyperglycemia.

I. INTRODUCTION

Sequential injections of [^{18}F]fluorodeoxyglucose (FDG) and positron emission tomography (PET) may be used to examine the relationships between cerebral glucose metabolism and physiological alterations such as functional activation or changes in plasma glucose concentration. There are advantages to a method that employs two FDG injections in a single PET scanning session, compared to two FDG PET scans performed on two separate days. Intrasubject variation in the regional cerebral metabolic rate for glucose (rCMR$_{glu}$) is greater for scans done on separate days (~25%; Duara *et al.*, 1987) than for scans performed 2 hr apart (7%;

Reivich *et al.*, 1982). In addition to reflecting true physiological changes in the subject's state, the variation in rCMR$_{glu}$ in two separate scans also includes variability due to errors in repositioning the subject in the scanner.

Any model of the double injection method must deal with the tracer remaining in brain tissue from the first injection. At the start of the second injection of FDG, it is not possible to measure separately ^{18}F activity due to FDG in tissue (M_e^*) and FDG-6-phosphate in tissue (M_m^*). This led Chang *et al.* (1987) to assume that the change in transfer coefficients between the first and second injections is instantaneous. The error incurred by this assumption is likely to be small when the rate constants change rapidly with respect to the duration of the second physiological state. However, considerable errors may result when the physiological change to be studied cannot be induced rapidly, and there is a substantial period between the first and second injections when the steady state assumption is violated. Such is the case when, for example, plasma glucose concentrations are altered.

We have devised a kinetic model of the double injection procedure that allows independent estimation of transfer coefficients for the second injection. The method was tested using simulated noisy data and was then applied to real PET data in which plasma glucose concentration was changed.

II. THEORY

We employed the deoxyglucose model with dephosphorylation of FDG-6-phosphate (k_4^* model) and incorporated biological constraints.

214

TABLE 1 Symbols, Definitions, and Units

Symbols	Definitions	Units
M_T^*	Brain ^{18}F content (^{18}FDG and ^{18}FDG-6-phosphate)	μmol g^{-1}
M_e^*	Brain ^{18}FDG content	μmol g^{-1}
M_m^*	Brain ^{18}FDG-6-phosphate content	μmol g^{-1}
K_1^*	Unidirectional plasma clearance of ^{18}FDG	ml g$^{-1}\cdot$min^{-1}
k_2^*	Fractional brain–blood clearance of ^{18}FDG	min^{-1}
k_3^*	Phosphorylation coefficient ^{18}FDG	min^{-1}
k_4^*	Dephosphorylation coefficient ^{18}FDG	min^{-1}
K^*	Net clearance ^{18}FDG	ml$\cdot$g^{-1}min^{-1}
V_0	Correction term for vascular volume	ml$\cdot$g^{-1}
V_d	Brain water volume	ml$\cdot$g^{-1}
K_t	Michaelis–Menten constant for transport between blood and brain	mM
Λ	Lumped constant	
J_{net}	Glucose metabolic rate	μmol/100 g^{-1}/min^{-1}

For the second injection, the differential equations

$$[M_e^*(t)]' =$$
$$K_1^* C_a^*(t) - (k_2^* + k_3^* + k_4^*)M_e^*(t) + k_4^* M_T^*(t) \quad (1)$$

$$[M_T^*(t) - M_e^*(t)]' = (k_3^* + k_4^*)M_e^*(t) - k_4^* M_T^*(t) \quad (2)$$

were solved in terms of measurable entities. Here M_m^* has been expressed in terms of M_e^* and M_T^* the total amount of activity in brain tissue:

$$M_m^*(t) = M_T^*(t) - M_e^*(t) \quad (3)$$

The asterisk indicates symbols that represent the tracer; symbols without an asterisk refer to native glucose (Table 1). The total ^{18}F activity at time t after the start of the second injection (when $t = 0$) is given by

$$\text{Act}^*(t) = A(t) \cdot [b_1 M_T^*(0) + K_1^* \int_0^t e^{q_1 u} C_a^*(u)\, du]$$
$$+ B(t) \cdot [b_2 M_T^*(0) + K_1^* \int_0^t e^{q_2 u} C_a^*(u)\, du]$$
$$- C(t) \cdot [M_T^*(0) + k_3^* \int_0^t e^{(k_3^* + k_4^*)u} M_T^*(u)\, du] \quad (4)$$
$$+ V_0 C_a^*(t)$$

where

$$b_{1,2} = \frac{k_2^* + k_3^* - k_4^* \pm \sqrt{(k_4^* - k_2^* - k_3^*)^2 + 4k_3^* k_4^*}}{2k_3^*} \quad (5)$$

$$q_{1,2} = \frac{k_4^*(b_{1,2} - 1)}{b_{1,2}} \quad (6)$$

$$B(t) = \frac{(1 - b_1) \cdot [e^{(k_3^* + k_4^*)t} - e^{q_1 t}]}{(1 - b_1) \cdot [e^{(k_3^* + k_4^*)t} - e^{q_1 t}] + e^{q_1 t}(1 - b_2) \cdot [e^{q_2 t} - e^{(k_3^* + k_4^*)t}]} \quad (7)$$

$$A(t) = \frac{1 - B(t)e^{q_1 t}}{e^{q_1 t}} \quad (8)$$

$$C(t) = \frac{A(t)e^{q_1 t}(b_1 - 1) + B(t)e^{q_2 t}(b_2 - 1)}{e^{(k_3^* + k_4^*)t}} \quad (9)$$

The amount of FDG in brain tissue at the start of the second injection can be expressed as

$$M_e^*(0) = \frac{M_T^*(t) - M_T^*(0) \cdot [A(t)b_1 + B(t)b_2] - A(t)K_1^* \int_0^t e^{q_1 u}C_a^*(u)\, du - B(t)K_1^* \int_0^t e^{q_2 u}C_a^*(u)\, du}{A(t)(1 - b_1) + B(t)(1 - b_2)} \quad (10)$$

Although $M_e^*(0)$ cannot be measured, with the correct transfer coefficients its value should remain constant and positive for all values of t.

The biological constraints employed were based on Michaelis–Menten kinetics; their validity was investigated in detail in a previous paper (Kuwabara *et al.*, 1990). The phosphorylation ratio ($\phi = k_3^*/k_3$) and the transport ratio ($\tau = K_1^*/K_1$) were assumed to be real constants, thus allowing k_2^* and k_1^* to be expressed in terms of K_1^* and K^*:

$$k_2^* = \frac{K_1^* + \mu K^*}{V_d} \qquad k_3^* = \frac{K^* \cdot k_2^*}{K_1^* - K^*} \quad (11)$$

where $\mu = \tau \cdot C_a / [\Lambda \cdot K_t]$. The lumped constant ($\Lambda$) is given by

$$\Lambda = \varphi + (\tau - \varphi) K^* / K_1^* \qquad (12)$$

We assumed that V_0, the correction term for cerebral vascular volume, remained constant for both injections and that its value could be accurately determined from the first injection. We fixed k_4^* using a value previously estimated with the constrained method (0.015 min^{-1}; Kuwabara and Gjedde, 1991). We chose $\tau = 1.1$, $\varphi = 0.33$, $K_t = 4.8$ mM, and $V_d = 0.77$ ml g^{-1} (Kuwabara *et al.*, 1990). The regional glucose phosphorylation rate (J_{net}) was calculated as

$$J_{net} = K^* \cdot Ca / \Lambda$$

III. METHODS

A. Simulated PET Studies

We simulated PET studies to assess the accuracy and precision of parameter estimates. "Noiseless" brain time–activity data were generated from sets of values of K_1^*, k_2^*, k_3^*, k_4^*, and V_0 and the plasma time–activity data from actual PET studies. Mean noise levels of 2 and 5% Gaussian noise were added to the noiseless data. The accuracy of the estimates was expressed as the coefficient of error [(root mean square error/input value) × 100%] for 100 sets of "noisy" brain time–activity data.

B. PET Studies

Dynamic FDG PET studies were performed in three healthy volunteers (age, 22–29 years) with a Scanditronix PC-2048 15B scanner; its performance characteristics have been described elsewhere (Evans *et al.*, 1992). Subjects fasted overnight prior to the scan. They were positioned in the scanner so that the uppermost slice was parallel to the orbitomeatal line and contained the high cerebral convexity.

Two slow (1 min) injections of FDG were used, the first being 3 mCi at the start of the study and the second being 2 mCi at 70 min. After each injection of FDG, a scan schedule of six 30 sec scans, seven 1 min scans, five 2 min scans, and six 5 min scans was employed. After the first 50 min, an intravenous infusion of 10% glucose was started and its rate adjusted so that a stable level of hyperglycemia was attained by 60 min and maintained throughout the remainder of the study.

Plasma radioactivity was measured in arterial blood sampled every 10 sec from 0–3 min, every 20 sec from 3–5 min, and every 1–5 min until 50 min after each injection of FDG. Arterial plasma glucose concentrations were measured at 10 min intervals throughout the study.

For the analysis of regional radioactivity, 202 MRI-based cortical regions of interest (ROIs) were drawn on a high-resolution MRI coregistered with the summed PET image. The average size of the ROIs was 2 cm^2. The ROIs were then applied to serial images obtained in the dynamic studies and the mean activity in each ROI at the midtime of each scan frame was used to form time–activity curves of brain radioactivity.

Estimation of K_1^*, K^*, and V_0 for the first injection was performed using nonlinear least squares regression and a previously described constrained method (Kuwabara *et al.*, 1990). For the second injection, the coefficients K_1^* and K^* were estimated using a commercial software package with sequential quadratic programming (MATLAB, The Mathworks Inc., Massachusetts). The fitting program incorporated a penalty function weighted against combinations of K_1^* and K^* that yielded negative or time-varying estimates of $M_e^*(0)$.

IV. RESULTS AND DISCUSSION

A. Simulation Studies

The coefficients of error for K_1^*, K^*, Λ, and glucose phosphorylation rate are shown in Table 2. The method yielded accurate estimates of these parameters with coefficients of error generally below 10% at realistic levels of noise. Parameter estimates were relatively insensitive to errors in k_4^* (Fig. 1).

B. PET Studies

The incorporation of biological constraints based on Michaelis–Menten kinetics reduces the number of parameters to be estimated. Kuwabara and Gjedde (1991) demonstrated that the use of these constraints interfered little with the appropriate description of the time course of tracer FDG and native glucose uptake into brain when the dephosphorylation coefficient (k_4^*) was included in the model. The biological constraints employed, the phosphorylation coefficient (τ) and the transport coefficient (φ), are likely to remain constant over a wide range of plasma glucose concentrations and metabolic rates and are assumed to have little regional or intersubject variation (Dienel *et al.*, 1991).

The mean arterial glucose concentrations for the first and second injections were 5.1 ± 0.6 mM (± standard deviation) and 15.8 ± 2.8 mM, respectively. We ob-

TABLE 2 Accuracy and Precision of Parameter Estimates for Simulated Data with 2 and 5% Noise

Noise	K^*			K_1^*			Λ			CMR_{glu}		
	True	Estimated[a]	COE[b]	True	Estimated	COE	True	Estimated	COE	True	Estimated	COE
2%	0.01	0.009 ± 0.002	18	0.04	0.041 ± 0.006	14	0.5	0.48 ± 0.04	8	0.3	28.4 ± 3.5	13
	0.02	0.019 ± 0.001	9	0.08	0.080 ± 0.009	11	0.5	0.49 ± 0.02	4	0.6	58.3 ± 4.8	9
	0.03	0.029 ± 0.001	6	0.12	0.117 ± 0.011	10	0.5	0.50 ± 0.02	3	0.9	87.1 ± 5.4	7
	0.04	0.039 ± 0.001	4	0.16	0.153 ± 0.014	10	0.5	0.50 ± 0.02	3	1.2	115.8 ± 5.9	6
5%	0.01	0.01 ± 0.002	23	0.04	0.040 ± 0.012	31	0.5	0.51 ± 0.09	19	0.3	27.8 ± 4.7	17
	0.02	0.019 ± 0.003	14	0.08	0.081 ± 0.017	21	0.5	0.49 ± 0.04	8	0.6	58.2 ± 7.4	13
	0.03	0.030 ± 0.003	9	0.12	0.120 ± 0.020	17	0.5	0.50 ± 0.04	7	0.9	88.4 ± 8.5	10
	0.04	0.039 ± 0.003	7	0.16	0.162 ± 0.024	15	0.5	0.50 ± 0.03	6	1.2	119.2 ± 9.2	8

[a]Mean ± standard deviation of parameter estimates.
[b]Coefficient of error: (root mean square error/input value) × 100%.

served a reduction in mean values of K_1^* and K^* with increased plasma glucose concentrations. This reflects competition between glucose and FDG for the carrier that mediates transport across the blood–brain barrier and for hexokinase (Table 3).

The constrained method does not require explicit knowledge of Λ, which is calculated in terms K^*, K_1^*, τ, and φ (equation (12)). The mean value of Λ for gray matter in normoglycemia was 0.63, similar to values previously obtained with this method (Kuwabara *et al.*, 1990). The value is higher than estimates of Λ based on direct measurements of the whole brain value (0.52; Reivich *et al.*, 1985) or calculated using an assumed gray/white matter ratio (0.50; Phelps *et al.*, 1979). However, the value is similar to one determined on the basis of the glucose/oxygen utilization ratio (0.61; Lammertsma *et al.*, 1987).

In keeping with previous observations in experimental animals (Mori *et al.*, 1989; Schuier *et al.*, 1990), Λ was significantly lower in hyperglycemia than in normoglycemia. The value of Λ is chiefly dependent upon and inversely related to brain glucose content, which increases as plasma glucose concentration increases (Crane *et al.*, 1981). Although the change in Λ is relatively small, accurate determination of $rCMR_{glu}$ in hyperglycemia requires the appropriate adjustment of Λ.

We observed a small but statistically significant increase in $rCMR_{glu}$ with hyperglycemia. A similar observation was made in rats by Gjedde and Diemer (1983) and Siemkowicz *et al.* (1982). However, others have found no increase in whole brain glucose utilization (Bachelard *et al.*, 1973) or significant increases in only a few discrete structures (Orzi *et al.*, 1988) in hyperglycemia.

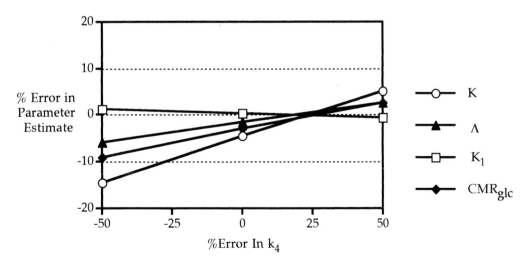

FIGURE 1 Accuracy of parameter estimates.

TABLE 3   Effect of Hyperglycemia on Transfer Coefficients, Λ and rCMR$_{glu}$

	Normoglycemia	Hyperglycemia	
K^*	0.037 ± 0.001	0.010 ± 0.0001	$p < 0.001$
K_1^*	0.095 ± 0.001	0.047 ± 0.001	$p < 0.001$
rCMR$_{glu}$	29.3 ± 0.3	32.3 ± 0.6	$p < 0.001$
Λ	0.63 ± 0.002	0.50 ± 0.004	$p < 0.001$

In conclusion, we present a kinetic model for the double injection method in which transfer coefficients are estimated independently for the second injection. It does not assume instantaneous changes in the transfer coefficients, hence allowing the second injection to be administered at a time when the steady state for the second physiological condition has been established. The method yielded physiologically meaningful values for K^*, K_1^*, Λ, and rCMR$_{glu}$ in hyperglycemia.

Acknowledgments

Dr. Reutens was supported by a Neil Hamilton Fairley Fellowship of the National Health and Medical Research Council of Australia.

References

Bachelard, H. S., Daniel, P. M., Love, E. R., *et al.* (1973). The transport of glucose into the brain of the rat in vivo. *Proc. R. Soc. London [Biol]* **183:** 71–82.

Chang, J. Y., Duara, R., Barker, W., Apicella, A., and Finn, R. (1987). Two behavioral states studied in a single FDG/PET procedure: Theory, method and preliminary results. *J. Nucl. Med.* **28:** 852–860.

Crane, P. D., Pardridge, W. M., Braun, L. D., *et al.* (1981). The interaction of transport and metabolism on brain glucose utilization: A reevaluation of the lumped constant. *J. Neurochem.* **36:** 1601–1604.

Dienel, G. A., Cruz, N. F., Mori, K., *et al.* (1991). Direct measurement of the λ of the lumped constant of the deoxyglucose method in rat brain: determination of λ and lumped constant from tissue glucose concentration or equilibrium brain/plasma distribution ratio for methylglucose. *J. Cereb. Blood Flow Metab.* **11:** 25–34.

Duara, R., Gross-Glen, K., and Barker, W. W. (1987). Behavioral activation and the variability of cerebral glucose metabolic measurements. *J. Cereb. Blood Flow Metab.* **7:** 266–271.

Evans, A. C., Marrett, S., Neelin, P., *et al.* (1992). Anatomical mapping of functional activation in stereotactic coordinate space. *Neuroimage* **1:** 43–53.

Gjedde, A., and Diemer, N. H. (1983). Autoradiographic determination of regional brain glucose content. *J. Cereb. Blood Flow Metab.* **3:** 303–310.

Kuwabara, H., Evans, A. C., and Gjedde, A. (1990). Michaelis-Menten constraints improved cerebral glucose metabolism and regional lumped constant measurements with [^{18}F]fluorodeoxyglucose. *J. Cereb. Blood Flow Metab.* **10:** 180–189.

Kuwabara, H., and Gjedde, A. (1991). Measurements of glucose phosphorylation with FDG and PET are not reduced by dephosphorylation of FDG-6-phosphate. *J. Nucl. Med.* **32:** 692–698.

Lammertsma, A. A., Brooks, D. J., Frackowiak, R. S. J., Beaney, R. P., Herold, S., Heather, J. D., Palmer, A. J., and Jones, T. (1987). Measurement of glucose utilization with [18F]2-fluoro-2-deoxy-D-glucose: A comparison of different analytical methods. *J. Cereb. Blood Flow Metab.* **7:** 161–172.

Mori, K., Cruz, N., Dienel, G., *et al.* (1989). Direct chemical measurement of the λ of the lumped constant of the [^{14}C]deoxyglucose method in rat brain: Effects of arterial plasma glucose level on the distribution spaces of [^{14}C]deoxyglucose and glucose and on λ. *J. Cereb. Blood Flow Metab.* **9:** 304–314.

Orzi, F., Lucignani, G., Dow-Edwards, D., *et al.* (1988). Local cerebral glucose utilization in controlled graded levels of hyperglycemia in the conscious rat. *J. Cereb. Blood Flow Metab.* **8:** 346–356.

Phelps, M. E., Huang, S. C., Hoffman, E. J., Selin, S., Sokoloff, L., and Kuhl, D. E. (1979). Tomographic measurement of local cerebral glucose metabolic rate in humans with (F-18) 2-fluoro-2-deoxy-D-glucose. Validation of method. *Ann. Neurol.* **6:** 371–388.

Reivich, M., Alavi, A., and Wolf, A. (1982). Use of 2-deoxyglucose-D-(1-11C) glucose for the determination of local cerebral glucose metabolism in humans: Variation within and between subjects. *J. Cereb. Blood Flow Metab.* **2:** 301–319.

Reivich, M., Alavi, A., Wolf, A., Fowler, J., Russell, J., Arnett, C., MacGregor, R. R., Shiue, C. Y., Atkins, H., Arnand, A., Dann, R., and Greenberg, J. H. (1985). Glucose metabolic rate kinetic model parameter determination in humans. The lumped constants and rate constants for [18F] fluorodeoxyglucose and [11C] deoxyglucose. *J. Cereb. Blood Flow Metab.* **5:** 179–192.

Schuier, F., Orzi, F., Suda, S., *et al.* (1990). Influence of plasma glucose concentration on lumped constant of the deoxyglucose method: Effects of hyperglycemia in the rat. *J. Cereb. Blood Flow Metab.* **10:** 765–773.

Siemkowicz, E., Hansen, A. J., and Gjedde A. (1982). Hyperglycemic ischemia of rat brain: The effect of post-ischemic insulin on metabolic rate. *Brain Res.* **243:** 386–390.

Combined FDOPA and 3-O-MFD PET Studies in Parkinson's Disease

Modeling Issues and Clinical Significance of Striatal Dopa Decarboxylase Activity

VIJAY DHAWAN,[1] TATSUYA ISHIKAWA,[1] CLIFFORD PATLAK,[2] THOMAS CHALY,[1] and DAVID EIDELBERG[1]

[1]*Departments of Neurology, Research, Medicine, and Biostatistics*
North Shore University Hospital/Cornell University Medical College
Manhasset, New York 11030
[2]*State University of New York at Stony Brook, New York*

Positron emission tomography (PET) has been used to quantify striatal 6-[^{18}F] fluoro-L-dopa (FDOPA) uptake as a measure of presynaptic dopaminergic function. It has been suggested that the estimation of dopa–decarboxylation (DDC) rate, k_3^D, using a compartmental approach to dynamic FDOPA/PET data, can provide a better objective marker of parkinsonism. However, this modeling process requires many assumptions to estimate DDC activity with acceptable errors.

We attempted to clarify these assumptions by performing combined FDOPA 3-O-methyl-fluorodopa PET studies on three normal subjects and five patients with Parkinson's disease (PD). In a separate group of 9 normal volunteers and 16 patients with PD, we also validated the use of population values of 3-O-MFD transport in simplifying the FDOPA model and correlated the estimated DDC activity with the quantitative disease severity ratings.

The modeling assumptions that are contradicted are (1) the rate constants across blood–brain barrier, K_1^D and k_2^D, for 3-O-MFD and FDOPA were in similar range (ratio $\cong$ 1), thus not equal to assumed values of K_1^M/K_1^D of 2.3 derived from rat studies and applied to human FDOPA studies; (2) the K_1^D/k_2^D ratio for frontal cortex was not equal to that for striatum (0.70 $\pm$ 0.15 vs. 1.07 $\pm$ 0.3; p < 0.002). Discriminant analyses indicate that simple estimates like the striatum-to-occipital ratio (SOR) or the graphically derived unidirectional transport rate constant (K_i^{FD}) separate normal subjects from PD patients at least as accurately as estimates of striatal DDC activity (k_3^D). K_i^{FD} and k_3^D both correlated significantly with disease severity ratings, with a similar degree of accuracy.

Direct measurements of 3-O-MFD rate constants facilitated the estimation of striatal DDC activity with dynamic FDOPA/PET without making some of the incorrect assumptions.

I. INTRODUCTION

FDOPA/PET studies must yield quantitative parameters that (1) correlate closely with independent disease severity measures and (2) discriminate reliably between patients with mild early disease, or with preclinical involvement, and normal control subjects.

A variety of compartmental models have been developed to quantitate FDOPA/PET images for these purposes. The differences in these model arise because of the different set of assumptions made in each case and the ultimate number of parameters estimated (Huang *et al.*, 1991; Kuwabara *et al.*, 1993; Wahl *et al.*, 1993a). We have analyzed the model shown in Figure 1. The metabolites FDA (fluorodopamine) and FMT (3-methoxy-6-[^{18}F]fluorotyramine) are considered to be nondiffusible metabolites, whereas FDOPAC (L-3,4-dihydroxy-6-[^{18}F]fluorophenylacetic acid) and FHVA

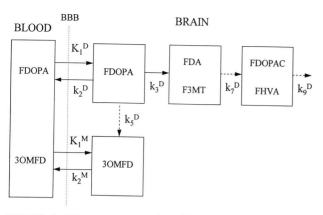

FIGURE 1 The compartmental model for the biodistribution of FDOPA. A similar model has been previously published by Kuwabara *et al.*, (1993) and the nomenclature has been kept the same for comparison purposes. The rate constants shown (dotted) are to emphasize the marginal contribution of these processes for a 100 min study (see text for details).

(6-[^{18}F]fluorohomovalinic) are considered to be diffusible metabolites. The rate constant k_7^D represents the conversion of FDA to FDOPAC and FHVA and k_9^D is the rate of loss of diffusible metabolites. A very small amount of O-methylation of FDOPA to O-MFD in the brain is shown by the rate constant k_5^D. The parameter of physiological significance in PD has been postulated to be the DOPA decarboxylase step in the metabolism of DOPA to dopamine (DA) (Gjedde *et al.*, 1991). This step is defined by the rate constant k_3^D and is thought to be more sensitive to presynaptic nigrostriatal dopaminergic process in PD than the unidirectional transfer

constant, K_i^{FD} estimated from the multiple time graphical approach (MTGA; Patlak *et al.*, 1983), which also includes the capillary exchange process. To address this issue, we used PET to study PD patients and normal subjects with FDOPA and with 3-O-MFD, a labeled metabolite of FDOPA that crosses the blood–brain barrier but is not significantly trapped in brain tissue.

II. MATERIALS AND METHODS

Five classical PD patients with mild or moderate clinical involvement and without dementia (two male, three female; age 63 ± 14 years) were studied with quantitative FDOPA and 3-O-MFD/PET. The control group consisted of three normal volunteer subjects (one male, two female; age 22 ± 4 years). This group will be referred to as *Group A*. An entirely separate group (B) consisting of 9 normal volunteers (3 male, 6 female; age 43 ± 20 years) and 16 patients (10 male, 6 female; age 60 ± 13 years) with PD were studied with FDOPA only.

A. Positron Emission Tomography

All subjects fasted overnight prior to PET scanning. All antiparkinsonian medications were discontinued at least 12 hr before PET investigations. PET studies were performed using the SuperPETT 3000 tomograph (Scanditronix; Essex, Massachussets). The performance characteristics of this instrument have been described elsewhere (Robeson *et al.*, 1993). Each slice is

TABLE 1 FDOPA Model M1 Estimated Parameters (K_1^D, k_2^D, k_3^D, and V_b) for Frontal, Occipital, and Striatum, with V_e^D a calculated parameter (K_1^D/k_2^D)

	K_1^D	k_2^D	k_3^D	V_b	V_e^D
Normal ($n = 3$)					
Frontal	0.039 ± 0.007	0.056 ± 0.004	0.005 ± 0.003	0.014 ± 0.005	0.696 ± 0.189
Occipital	0.050 ± 0.011	0.064 ± 0.007	0.004 ± 0.002	0.024 ± 0.009	0.791 ± 0.259
Striatum	0.042 ± 0.007	0.038 ± 0.008	0.024 ± 0.011*	0.019 ± 0.006	1.178 ± 0.414
PD ($n = 5$)					
Frontal	0.041 ± 0.005	0.060 ± 0.013	0.003 ± 0.005	0.030 ± 0.007	0.707 ± 0.149
Occipital	0.055 ± 0.013	0.070 ± 0.012	0.002 ± 0.003	0.025 ± 0.017	0.788 ± 0.190
L. striatum	0.045 ± 0.012	0.048 ± 0.013	0.007 ± 0.005*	0.035 ± 0.010	0.952 ± 0.196
R. striatum	0.044 ± 0.010	0.042 ± 0.010	0.006 ± 0.005*	0.036 ± 0.021	1.063 ± 0.239

Notes. All table entries are mean + SD.
PD = Parkinson's disease.
$V_e^D = K_1^D/k_2^D$
k_2^D and k_3^D are expressed as 1/min and K_1^D as ml/min/gm
M1 is the four-compartment FDOPA model described in the text
* indicates significant difference between normal and PD groups ($p < 0.015$)

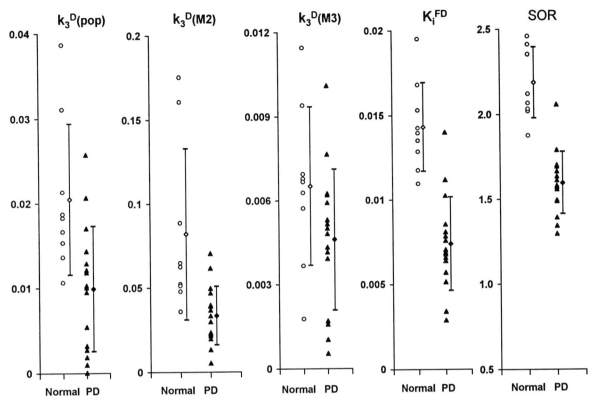

FIGURE 2   Discriminant analyses between PD patients and normal subjects for $k_3^D(\text{pop})$, $k_3^D(\text{M2})$, $k_3^D(\text{M3})$, K_i^{FD}, and SOR. K_i^{FD} and SOR separated PD patients from normal subjects more accurately than estimates of striatal DDC activities ($F[1,23]$ = 37.3, 54.2, 12.3, 10.2, and 3.0; p = 0.0001, 0.0001, 0.002, 0.004, and 0.09 for K_i^{FD}, SOR, $k_3^D(\text{M2})$, $k_3^D(\text{pop})$, and $k_3^D(\text{M3})$, respectively).

8 mm thick with in-plane resolution of 7.5 mm (full-width at half-maximum, FWHM).

All subjects received 200 mg carbidopa 1.5 hr before the study and 185–370 MBq of FDOPA was injected intravenously. Dynamic PET images acquired over 100 min were corrected for measured tissue attenuation, random coincidences, electronic dead time, and scatter effects. The time course of plasma ^{18}F radioactivity was determined by arterial blood sampling and HPLC. The procedure for 3-O-MFD/PET study was exactly the same as for FDOPA except no carbidopa was administered and 185–370 MBq 3-O-MFD was injected. Striatal and occipital ROIs were transferred to the 3-O-MFD images prealigned with the FDOPA images because the striatum was not clearly visualized in the 3-O-MFD scan. Kinetic measures of FDOPA uptake (k_i^{FD}) were calculated by MTGA (Patlak et al., 1983) using the time course of striatal radioactivity from 40 to 100 min post injection and the plasma FDOPA input function. We also calculated the ratio of striatal to occipital activity on the last 10 min scan (90–100 min post injection). The only parameters estimated from the 3-O-MFD kinetic data were K_1^M, k_2^M, and V_b.

Various models of increasing complexity (three to seven parameters) were tried with (1) K_1^M and k_2^M fixed to values obtained from the 3-O-MFD study or (2) allowed to be estimated as independent parameters. The models were evaluated for *bias*, using the residual plots, and *goodness-of-fit*, using weighted sum of squares (WSS). The models were compared using the F-test as well as AIC scores (Akaike information criteria, defined as AIC = $N \log(\text{WSS}) + 2p$, where N is the number of observations and p is the number of parameters; Akaike, 1978). A direct comparison of our proposed four-parameter model "M1" (fitted parameters are K_1^D, k_2^D, k_3^D, and V_b) in which K_1^M and k_2^M are fixed to the values obtained from 3-O-MFD studies was made with the Montreal Neurological Institute model "M2" (Kuwabara et al., 1993) and the McMaster University model "M3" (Wahl et al., 1993a). The parameter V_b refers to the blood volume in the region of interest. The model M2 estimates three parameters (K_1^D, k_3^D, and V_b) while fixing the value of striatal V_e^D to that obtained from a frontal region and assuming K_1^M/K_1^D = k_2^M/k_2^D = 2.3 based on data from rat experiments; the values of k_7^D and k_9^D were obtained empirically from

TABLE 2   Comparison of FDOPA Parameters from Compartmental Model M1 (k_3^D and K^D), Multiple Time Graphical Approach (K_i^{FD}) and Striato–Occipital ratio (SOR) Calculated from a 10-Min Scan Starting at 90 Min Postinjection

	k_3^D	K_i^{FD}	K^D	**SOR**
Normal ($n = 3$)				
L. striatum	0.019 ± 0.007*	0.015 ± 0.004†	0.016 ± 0.007‡	2.24 ± 0.24§
R. striatum	0.028 ± 0.014	0.016 ± 0.005	0.016 ± 0.005	2.37 ± 0.15
PD ($n = 5$)				
L. striatum	0.007 ± 0.005	0.007 ± 0.002	0.006 ± 0.004	1.51 ± 0.08
R. striatum	0.006 ± 0.005	0.007 ± 0.002	0.006 ± 0.005‡	1.58 ± 0.17

All table entries are mean ± SD.
PD = Parkinson's disease
SOR = Striato-Occipital ratio
$K^D = K_1^D k_3^D/(k_2^D + k_3^D)$
k_3^D and K^D are expressed as min^{-1} and K_i^{FD} as ml/min/gm
M1 is the 4 compartment FDOPA model described in the text
*, †, ‡, and § show significant differences between the mean striatal values for normal subjects and individual left and right striatal values for the PD group at $p < 0.015$, $p < 0.006$, $p < 0.039$, and $p < 0.0006$, respectively

the least normalized residual sum of squares criteria; and k_5^D was neglected. The model M3 estimates the least number of parameters (K_1, k_2, and k_3) that yield an optimum fit to the data. The UCLA model (M2') (Huang *et al.*, 1991) is a four-parameter model (K_1^D, k_2^D, k_3^D, and k_4^D are estimated, K_1^M/k_2^M is assumed to be 1.0 and K_1^M/K_1^D is fixed at 1.7) in which k_5^D and k_9^D are set to 0 and k_7^D is defined as k_4^D. The mathematical treatment of these models has been extensively reported and will not be duplicated here (Huang *et al.*, 1991; Kuwabara *et al.*, 1993; Patlak *et al.*, 1983, 1993).

For group A, striatal k_3^D values obtained from individually measured 3-O-MFD rate constants were compared with values of k_3^D (pop) obtained using the population mean values ($K_1^M = 0.04$ and $k_2^M = 0.042$). These estimates of k_3^D and k_3^D(pop) correlated significantly ($r = 0.98$, $p = 0.0001$). We, therefore, applied the mean population K_1^M and k_2^M values in the FDOPA model to estimate k_3^D for the Group B subjects.

III. RESULTS AND DISCUSSION

A. Plasma Analysis

Over the duration of the study, 3-O-MFD had negligible breakdown with < 5% of unknown metabolite. The breakdown function (FDOPA to total ^{18}F) could be modeled by a sum of two exponentials with rate constants of 0.71 ± 0.12 and 0.09 ± 0.02 min^{-1} for both groups, suggesting that the peripheral FDOPA breakdown is similar in normal subjects and PD patients.

B. 3-O-MFD

Good model fits were obtained with no bias and the standard error of estimate (s.e.e) of the parameters is < 15% for K_1^M and k_2^M and < 30% for V_b. For the normal group, there is no statistical difference between V_e^M for striatum (0.815 ± 0.139) and frontal (0.701 ± 0.038) ROIs ($p > 0.1$). The same was also true for the PD group. The striatal rate constants for normal subjects K_1^M (0.029 ± 0.003) and k_2^M (0.036 ± 0.006) from our 3-O-MFD study are similar to those measured by Doudet *et al.* (1991) for primates and by Wahl *et al.* (1993b) for humans. Normal subjects have a lower mean striatum K_1^M than the PD group (0.029 vs. 0.047; $p = 0.048$). Based on our previous data it is unlikely that, after a 12 hr fast, competition with plasma amino acid levels could have played a role in this observation (Eidelberg *et al.*, 1990).

C. FDOPA

1. Frontal and Occipital

The results from model M1 are presented in Tables 1 and 2. The DOPA decarboxylase rate constant, k_3^D, was found to be essential for obtaining a good fit (six out of eight subjects showed a significant decrease of bias and weighted sum of squares; $p < 0.01$ in each case). Mean k_3^D was 40% lower in the PD group than the normal one (Table 1) but was not statistically significant. The model M2 yields a higher k_3^D than our model, 0.0105 ± 0.0061 vs. 0.0035 ± 0.0043 ($N = 8$, $p < 0.002$). When experimentally derived 3-O-MFD values of K_1^M and k_2^M were used in our model, the estimated values of K_1^D and k_2^D were very similar to the corresponding 3-O-MFD parameters, yielding a q value of approximately 1.0.

2. Striatum

The lack of improvement in the model fits with and without k_5^D, k_7^D, and k_9^D (F-test on WSS; $p > 0.2$) suggests that unless these parameter values can be obtained independently (and then fixed to population averages in the model), there is no need to take into account the diffusible and nondiffusible metabolites of dopamine.

The simplest *mathematically justifiable* model (M3) (Wahl *et al.*, 1993a) did not yield the best AIC scores. The neglect of the known presence of 3-O-MFD in plasma and brain tissue makes the physiological interpretation of the micro-parameters difficult and the macro-parameter $K^D = K_1 k_3/(k_2 + k_3)$ does not provide more information than a simple influx constant obtained from the MTGA approach (K_i^{FD} vs K^D has a linear correlation, with $r = 0.77$, $p = 0.001$).

The parameter V_e^D for frontal cortex is 20–30% lower than for striatum ($p < 0.002$). The model fits for striatum obtained with V_e^D fixed to the frontal value did not improve the AIC scores. This suggests that K_1^D and k_2^D should be fitted as independent parameters.

The parameters K_1^D and k_2^D had a range similar to K_1^M and k_2^M with $K_1^M/k_2^M \cong 1.0$ for both normal and PD groups across all regions. Higher values of q (2.3 and 1.7) have been assumed in both the M2 and M2′ models. In the M2 model, q was determined in a separate rat study and the least sum-of-squares criteria for different ratios of K_1^M/K_1^D were used in M2′. Our data contradicts these assumed values for 3-O-MFD exchange across the blood–barrier.

For the larger group B, graphical influx constant K_i^{FD} separates the groups better than k_3^D and SOR distinguished PD patients from normal subjects more accurately than the other parameters (Fig. 2). Correlation analysis revealed a significant negative relationship between quantitative disease severity scores (UPDRS) and striatal K_i^{FD} ($r = -0.62$, $p < 0.01$), k_3^D(pop) ($r = -0.66$, $p < 0.006$), and k_3^D (M2) ($r = -0.63$, $p < 0.009$) in the PD group. These scores did not correlate with k_3^D(M3).

To summarize, the use of 3-O-MFD parameters in the FDOPA compartmental model allowed us to simplify the model without making assumptions that are otherwise required. The results show that striatal DDC activity estimated from a compartmental modeling approach is similar to the graphically derived unidirectional influx constant (K_i^{FD}) in discriminating normals

from PD patients. In addition, K_i^{FD} and various estimates of k_3^D have similar correlations with disease severity. This suggests that with present PET methods, clinically relevant information can be obtained from a simple graphical approach rather than a more computationally demanding compartmental technique.

Acknowledgment

This work was supported by grants from the Parkinson Disease Foundation and the Dystonia Medical Research Foundation. T. I. is a Veola S. Kerr fellow of the Parkinson Disease Foundation. D. E. is a faculty fellow of the Parkinson Disease Foundation and the United Parkinson Foundation.

References

Akaike, A. (1978). Posterior probabilities for choosing a regression model. *Ann. Inst. Math. Sci.* **30:** 9–14.

Doudet, D. J., McLellan, C. A., Carson, R., Adams, H. R., Miyake, H., Aigner, T. G., Finn, R. T., and Cohen, R. M. (1991). Distribution and kinetics of 3-O-methyl-6-[18F]fluoro-L-DOPA in the rhesus monkey brain. *J. Cereb. Blood Flow Metab.* **11:** 726–734.

Eidelberg, D., Moeller, J. R., Dhawan, V., Sidtis, J. J., Ginos, J. Z., Strother, S. C., Cedarbaum, J., Greene, P., Fahn, S., and Rottenberg, D. A. (1990). The metabolic anatomy of Parkinson's disease: Complementary [18F]Fluorodeoxyglucose and [18F]Fluorodopa positron emission tomographic studies. *Movement Disorders.* **5:** 203–213.

Gjedde, A., Reith, J., Dyve, S., Léger, G., Guttman, M., Diksic, M., Evans, A., and Kuwabara, H. (1991). DOPA decarboxylase activity of the living human brain. *Proc. Natl. Acad. Sci.* **88:** 2721–2725.

Huang, S. C., Yu, D. C., Barrio, J. R., Grafton, S., Melega, W. P., Hoffman, J. M., Satyamurthy, N., Mazziota, J. C., and Phelps, M. E. (1991). Kinetics and modeling of 6-[18F]fluoro-L-DOPA in human positron emission tomographic studies. *J. Cereb. Blood Flow Metab.* **11:** 898–913.

Kuwabara, H., Cumming, P., Reith, J., Leger, G., Diksic, M., Evans, A. C., and Gjedde, A. (1993). Human striatal L-DOPA decarboxylase activity estimated in vivo using 6-[18F]fluoro-Dopa and positron emission tomography: Error analysis and application to normal subjects. *J. Cereb. Blood Flow Metab.* **13:** 43–56.

Patlak, C. S., Blasberg, R. G., and Fenstermacher, J. D. (1983). Graphical evaluation of blood-to-brain transfer constants from multiple-time uptake data. *J. Cereb. Blood Flow Metab.* **3:** 1–7.

Patlak, C. S., Dhawan, V., Takikawa, S., Chaly, T., Robeson, W., and Eidelberg, D. (1993). Estimation of striatal uptake rate constant of FDOPA using PET: Methodological issues. *Ann. Nucl. Med.* **7**(Suppl): S46–S47.

Robeson, W., Dhawan, V., Takikawa, S., Babchyck, B., Zanzi, I., Margouleff, D., and Eidelberg, D. (1993). SuperPETT 3000 time-of-flight tomograph: Optimization of factors affecting quantification. *IEEE Trans. Nucl. Sci.* **40**(2): 135–142.

Wahl, L. M., Garnett, E. S., Chirakal, R., Firnau, G., and Nahmias, C. (1993a). Quantification of dopamine metabolism in man: What is the most justifiable approach? *J. Cereb. Blood Flow Metab.* **13**[Suppl. 1]: S722.

Wahl, L. M., Chirakal, R., Firnau, G., Garnett, S. E., and Nahmias, C. (1993b). The distribution and kinetics of [18F] 6-Fluoro-3-O methyl-L-dopa in the human brain. *J. Cereb. Blood Flow Metab.* **14:** 664–670.

Evaluation of Three Assumptions Regarding Blood–Brain Transport of 6-[18F]Fluoro-L-dopa and O-methyl-dopa in Healthy Volunteers

P. VONTOBEL, A. ANTONINI, M. PSYLLA, I. GÜNTHER, and K. L. LEENDERS

PET Department, Paul Scherrer Institute
CH5232 Villigen, Switzerland

Models for the simultaneous transport of FDOPA and OMFD (Hoshi et al., 1993) have to make assumptions about the ratios of forward transport rate constants (K_{1d} for FDOPA, K_{1m} for OMFD), to reverse transport rate constants (k_{2d}, k_{2m}); that is, $V_e = K_{1d}/k_{2d}$ and $V_m = K_{1m}/k_{2m}$ and the relative magnitude $q = K_{1m}/K_{1d}$ of the forward transport rate constants. Measurements of OMFD distribution and kinetics alone show a ratio q near unity and provide independent estimates for K_{1m} (Wahl et al., 1994). We evaluated three assumptions about the FDOPA and OMFD blood–brain transport to estimate the decarboxylase activity k_{3d} in 10 healthy volunteers. Fixing the V_e and V_m values from a nonspecific reference region instead of using a constant $q = 2.3$ and fixing V_e as proposed by Gjedde et al. (1991) resulted in values of K_{1m} too high for striatal regions. Alternatively, fixing q and V_m to values computed in the nonspecific region resulted in striatal K_{1m} values comparable with those found by Wahl et al. (1994). The value of k_{3d} for the putamen had about the same size as K_{1d} for fixed V_e and V_m, whereas for the latter assumption it was approximately half the size of K_{1d} in healthy volunteers. Assuming equal OMFD tissue activity in striatal regions as in the nonspecific region and the elimination of the FDOPA plasma input function by the nonspecific (reference) region's FDOPA time–activity curve in the third proposed method lead to k_{3d} values in the putamen with half the size of K_{1d}, too, but with a much lower percentage coefficient of variation for the group average.

I. INTRODUCTION

For the kinetic analysis of FDOPA PET data compartment models have been proposed by Gjedde *et*
al. (1991) and Huang *et al.* (1991). To estimate the decarboxylase activity rate constant k_{3d}, both groups had to assume a fixed value for the ratio q of the forward transport rate constants of OMFD and FDOPA. Gjedde *et al.* (1991) relied additionally on fixing $V_e = K_{1d}/k_{2d}$ for striatal regions to values calculated in the frontal cortex. The measurement of OMFD distribution and kinetics in human brain by Wahl *et al.* (1994) confirmed the assumption of a single reversible compartment for OMFD in tissue, but showed striatal OMFD forward transport rate constants of the same size as those published for FDOPA, leading to a value of q close to 1. The purpose of this communication is to assess the validity of three alternative hypotheses on combined FDOPA and OMFD blood–brain forward transport used to derive normal values for striatal decarboxylase activity rate constants k_{3d} in humans.

II. MATERIALS AND METHODS

We analyzed FDOPA data (2 hr scans) of 10 healthy subjects (age 52 ± 11 years). 2 mg/kg carbidopa was given 1 hr before tracer injection. FDOPA plasma metabolites were measured using HPLC and a γ-detector system. The generation and elimination of metabolites in plasma was calculated with a compartment model. The kinetics of FDOPA and OMFD in tissue (see Fig. 1) were calculated first in an average nonspecific region (ROI size averaged contributions from cerebellum, 50%; occipital lobe, 35%; frontal cortex, 15%) using a single reversible compartment for FDOPA and OMFD (see Fig. 2). Second for striatal regions we assumed negligible methylation of FDOPA in brain tissue and

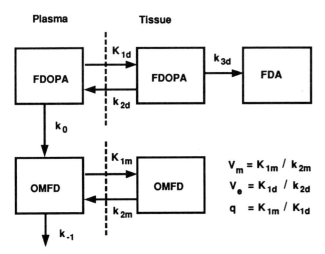

FIGURE 1   Compartment model for FDOPA and OMFD.

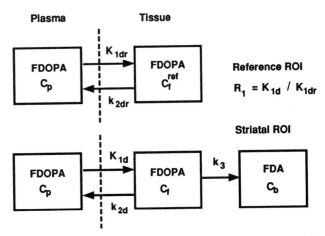

FIGURE 3   The k_3 reference tissue FDOPA compartment model.

no loss of FDA metabolites during the 2 hr scan. Additional assumptions used in the first method (1) were fixed values of V_e and V_m as calculated in the non-specific region: fit K_{1d}, K_{1m}, k_{3d}, and rcbv (regional cerebral blood volume). In method 2, we fixed the values of V_m and q as calculated in the nonspecific region: fit K_{1d}, k_{2d}, k_{3d} and rcbv. In method 3, we fixed the values for K_{1m} and V_m from the nonspecific region, subtracted the OMFD contribution in tissue as calculated in the nonspecific region both from the nonspecific region's and the striatal region's total activity, and used a reference tissue input model approach proposed for raclopride (Hume *et al.*, 1992) for the FDOPA kinetics alone (see Figs. 3 and 4): fit the ratio $R1 = K_{1d}/K_{1dr}$, k_{2d}, and k_3 ($k_4 = 0$). Elimination of the FDOPA plasma input with the reference tissue FDOPA activity with

$$\frac{dC_f^{\text{ref}}}{dt} = K_{1dr}C_p - k_{2dr}C_f^{\text{ref}} \therefore C_p = \frac{k_{2dr}}{K_{1dr}}C_f^{\text{ref}} + \frac{1}{K_{1dr}}\frac{dC_f^{\text{ref}}}{dt}$$

$$\frac{K_{1d}}{k_{2d}}C_p = \frac{K_{1d}}{k_{2d}}\frac{k_{2dr}}{K_{1dr}}C_f^{\text{ref}}$$

$$\approx 1$$

$$+ \frac{K_{1d}}{k_{2d}}\frac{1}{K_{1dr}}\frac{dC_f^{\text{ref}}}{dt}$$

$$K_{1d}C_p \approx k_{2d}C_f^{\text{ref}} + \frac{K_{1d}}{K_{1dr}}\frac{dC_f^{\text{ref}}}{dt}$$

$$= k_{2d}C_f^{\text{ref}} + R_1 \frac{dC_f^{\text{ref}}}{dt}$$

leads to the following set of differential equations for striatal FDOPA and FDA activity:

$$\frac{dC_f}{dt} = K_{1d}C_p \qquad\qquad \frac{dC_f}{dt} = k_{2d}C_f^{\text{ref}} + R1\frac{dC_f^{\text{ref}}}{dt}$$

$$- (k_{2d} + k_3)C_f \qquad\qquad - (k_{2d} + k_3)C_f$$

$$\Rightarrow$$

$$\frac{dC_b}{dt} = k_3C_f \qquad\qquad \frac{dC_b}{dt} = k_3C_f$$

III. RESULTS AND DISCUSSION

Average K_{1d} values for the putamen are the same for methods 1 and 2 (see Table 1). The average K_{1m} value for OMFD forward transport is high for method 1, whereas for method 2 it is in the same range as the FDOPA forward transport rate constant K_{1d}. The average k_{3d} value for the putamen is about the same size as K_{1d} for method 1. In methods 2 and 3, k_{3d} (or k_3) is approximately half the size of K_{1d}. Method 1

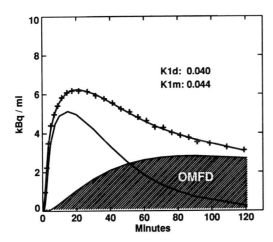

FIGURE 2   Fit in non-specific region.

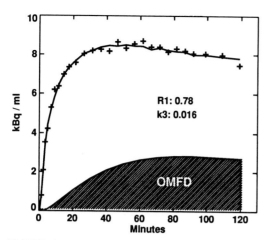

FIGURE 4 The k_3 reference input fit in the putamen.

FDOPA plasma input as described previously for method 3 results in decarboxylase activity rate constants with only 14.3% coefficient of variation and values comparable to those of method 2. The assumption of equal values for the distribution volume of OMFD V_m in striatal regions as in the average nonspecific region in the three methods tested was made for simplicity although it was shown by Wahl *et al.* (1994), that striatal V_m values are higher by about 10–15%. Because of the lowest variability of k_3 across the group in method 3, we conclude that this method gives a more reliable estimate of decarboxylase activity rate constants in healthy subjects than method 2. Method 1 is not suitable to estimate k_{3d}, because it leads to values of K_{1m}, that are more than a factor of 2 higher than those measured by Wahl *et al.* (1994).

(V_m and V_e fixed) overestimates the OMFD forward transport rate constant in the putamen (Wahl *et al.*, 1994: 0.044 [1/min]). Method 2 (V_m and q fixed) results in a higher variability of k_{3d} than method 1 or 3. Assuming equal OMFD tissue activity in the putamen as in a large average nonspecific region and replacing the

TABLE 1 Average Kinetic Parameters in the Putamen of Healthy Subjects

Method	K_{1d} (ml/g/min)	% COV	K_{1m}	% COV	k_{3d} (1/min)	% COV
1. V_e and V_m	0.036	20.0	0.113	37.7	0.0313	20.0
2. V_m and q	0.036	20.0	0.038	42	0.0156	27.2
3. Reference					0.0169	14.3

Note. Average ($n = 10$) kinetic parameters for the putamen of healthy subjects.

References

Gjedde, A., Reith, J., Dyve, S., Léger, G., Guttman, M., Diksic, M., Evans, A., and Kuwabara, H. (1991). Dopa decarboxylase activity of the living human brain. *Proc. Natl. Acad. Sci. USA.* **88:** 2721–2725.

Hoshi, H., Kuwabara, H., Léger, G., Cumming, P., Guttman, M., and Gjedde, A. (1993). 6-[^{18}F]fluoro-L-DOPA metabolism in living human brain: A comparison of six analytical methods. *J. Cereb. Blood Flow Metab.* **13:** 75–69.

Huang, S.-C., Yu, D., Barrio, J. D., Grafton, S., Melega, W. P., Hoffmann, J. M., Satyamurthy, N., Mazziotta, J. C., and Phelps, M. E. (1991). Kinetics and modeling of L-6-[^{18}F]Fluoro-DOPA in human positron emission tomographic studies. *J. Cereb. Blood Flow Metab.* **11:** 898–913.

Hume, S. P., Myers, R., Bloomfield, P. M., Opacka-Juffry, J., Cremer, J. E., Ahier, R. G., Luthra, S. K., Brooks, D. J., and Lammertsma, A. A. (1992). Quantitation of carbon-11 labeled raclopride in rat striatum using positron emission tomography. *Synapse* **12:** 47–54.

Wahl, L., Chirakal, L., Firnau, G., Garnett, E. S., and Nahmias, C. (1994). The distribution and kinetics of [^{18}F]6-fluoro-3-O-methyl-L-dopa in the human brain. *J. Cereb. Blood Flow Metab.* **14:** 664–670.

Links between 6-Fluorodopa and 6-Fluoro-3-O-methyldopa Kinetics
Prospects for Refined Graphical Analysis

J. E. HOLDEN, F. J. G. VINGERHOETS, B. J. SNOW, G. L-Y. CHAN, B. LEGG, S. MORRISON, M. ADAM, S. JIVAN, V. SOSSI, K. R. BUCKLEY, and T. J. RUTH

Neurodegenerative Disorders Centre and TRIUMF
University of British Columbia
Vancouver, British Columbia and
Department of Medical Physics
University of Wisconsin
Madison, Wisconsin 53706

The graphical analysis of 6-fluorodopa (6-FD) with the time course in cortex as the input function has been demonstrated to discriminate strongly between those with Parkinson's disease and normal subjects. However, this uptake measure is biased downward by the accumulation of the metabolite 6-fluoro-3-O-methyl-dopa (3-O-MFD) in the cortical input function. Methods to correct for this and other effects of the metabolite are limited by the large intersubject variability of 3-O-MFD kinetics and the large uncertainties of 3-O-MFD kinetics determined directly from 6-FD studies by compartmental analysis. Data from paired 6-FD and 3-O-MFD studies performed in 10 subjects were used to demonstrate that the required 3-O-MFD kinetic parameters may be derivable from graphical analysis of the 6-FD data. The same data were used to perform preliminary tests of particular correction schemes. Although the corrections yielded only marginal improvement in the discrimination of five parkinsonian subjects from five normal controls, results clearly indicated that the rank order of apparent disease severity can be influenced by extremes of metabolite distribution volume in brain.

I. INTRODUCTION

The graphical analysis of 6-fluorodopa (6-FD) with the time course in cortex as the input function has been demonstrated to discriminate strongly between those with Parkinson's disease (PD) and normal subjects (Hoshi *et al.*, 1993). However, the fitted slopes are biased downward by the accumulation of the metabolite 6-fluoro-3-O-methyldopa (3-O-MFD) in the cortical input function. Hybrid graphical methods that incorporate a correction for metabolites have been suggested (Patlak *et al.*, 1993), but have been provisionally rejected on the basis of the known intersubject variability of 3-O-MFD kinetics. Measures of 3-O-MFD kinetics determined directly from 6-FD studies have been thought to have unacceptably high uncertainties. However, the equilibrium distribution volumes (DV) of 6-FD and 3-O-MFD would be expected to be very similar; furthermore, the ratio of the graphical slope determined from the plasma input function to that determined from the cortical input function is predicted by compartmental theory to equal the 6-FD DV in striatum. We have determined in the present study that this ratio, despite 3-O-MFD contamination, may provide the required measure of 3-O-MFD DV in each subject.

The two major sources of error due to 3-O-MFD in the graphical analysis of 6-FD are (1) a residue of 3-O-MFD contribution to the specific striatal signal due to incomplete cancelation on subtraction of the cortical from the striatal time course and (2) a progressively increasing 3-O-MFD contribution to the cortical tissue input function that can reach 50% of the total by 2 hr post injection. This 3-O-MFD portion of the cortical

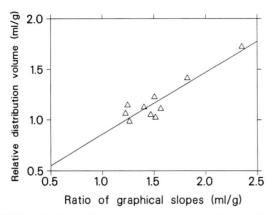

FIGURE 1 Relationship between two measures of tracer distribution volume determined in 10 subjects in two studies performed two weeks apart. Excursions of the 3-O-MFD distribution volume in two of the subjects are matched by corresponding excursions of a distribution volume measure derived from graphical analysis of 6-FD kinetics. The solid line is the result of linear regression.

signal cannot undergo trapping, and therefore the apparent 6-FD trapping rate is biased downward relative to its actual value.

Tracer 6-FD and 3-O-MFD are both transported by the same saturable neutral amino acid transport system, and their kinetics should therefore be linked in analogy with glucose and 3-O-methylglucose. Furthermore, graphical analysis can be shown on theoretical grounds to provide information on equilibrium DV. Let the compartmental parameter K_1 denote the clearance of 6-FD from plasma into striatum; k_2, the rate constant for backflow from brain to plasma; and k_3, the rate constant describing the trapping of brain 6-FD. The graphical slope derived from the plasma input function method is then expected to be

$$K_i = \left(\frac{K_1}{k_2 + k_3}\right)k_3$$

That is, a striatal precursor concentration proportional to the equilibrium DV is available to the trapping process k_3. The graphical slope derived from the cortical tissue input function is instead

$$K_o = \left(\frac{k_2}{k_2 + k_3}\right)k_3$$

If the true striatal precursor concentration could somehow be determined and used as the input function, the slope would be expected to equal k_3 itself. However, the concentration in the cortex is substituted in the method for that in striatum. The untrapped tracer in the striatum is expected to be smaller than that in the

cortex by the factor shown, and the expected value of the slope is reduced correspondingly. The ratio of these two graphical slopes is thus

$$\frac{K_i}{K_o} = \frac{K_1}{k_2}$$

that is, the equilibrium DV that 6-FD would have in the absence of the trapping process. We have performed paired 6-FD and 3-O-MFD studies in five normal control subjects and five subjects with PD. The results indicate that graphical analysis of 6-FD kinetics can provide quantitative information about the behavior of 3-O-MFD in individual subjects. The data from the paired studies were used to test particular schemes for correcting the graphical analysis of 6-FD for the effects of 3-O-MFD. Even though the corrections yielded only marginal improvement in the discrimination of disease, results clearly indicated that the rank order of apparent disease severity can be influenced by extremes of metabolite distribution volume in brain.

II. METHODS

A. PET Studies

Studies of [^{18}F]-6-FD and [^{18}F]-3-O-MFD were made at the TRIUMF-UBC Cyclotron facility using reported methods (Namavari *et al.*, 1992; Adam *et al.*, 1994). Five normal control subjects (three females) were age and gender matched to five subjects with PD. Each subject received both a 6-FD and a 3-O-MFD study

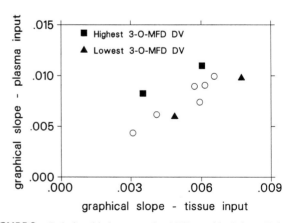

FIGURE 2 Relationship between the 6-FD graphical slope K_i determined from the plasma input function and the slope K_o determined from the cortical tissue input function. Mean striatal values are presented for five normal control subjects and five subjects with PD. The two subjects from each group having the highest and the two having the lowest 3-O-MFD DVs determined in separate studies in the same subjects are indicated by different plotting symbols.

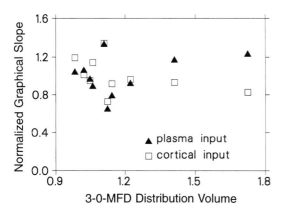

FIGURE 3 Graphical slopes from 6-FD studies plotted vs 3-O-MFD DV determined in separate studies in the same subjects. The plot is intended to show changes in the relative ordering of the values for each subject. See the main text for the normalization method.

within a two week period. Carbidopa pretreatment (200 mg 1 hr before injection) was used in all studies. Scans were performed in the Siemens/CTI 953B/31 tomograph at the Neurodegenerative Disorders Centre at the University of British Columbia. Tracer doses were 185 MBq. Arterial blood samples were drawn manually with continuous sampling in the first minute and with progressively decreasing frequency as the scans progressed. Plasma samples were counted for total radioactivity concentration and analyzed by HPLC to determine the percentage contributions of the injected compounds and their metabolites (Chan *et al.*, 1992). Purified plasma time courses of the injected compounds (6-FD, 3-O-MFD) were estimated by fitting the measured fractions to a smooth curve and multiplying the result against the total radioactivity at each time point. Time courses for 3-O-MFD in the 6-FD studies were generated using this same approach. An individually molded plastic mask was used to maintain anatomical registration between the two studies in the same subject. Visual inspection showed an adequate degree of identity in both position and orientation between the two scans in every case. The seven image planes in which striatal signal was clearly evident in the 6-FD study were summed axially to create a single slab of 20 mm thickness. Standardized regions of interest were placed corresponding to left and right total striatum and left and right occipital cortex. The same regions were then imported into the 3-O-MFD study. Region values were read out as radioactivity concentrations.

B. Graphical and Compartmental Analyses

The brain region time courses from the 3-O-MFD studies were fitted to a conventional one-tissue compartment model incorporating a clearance parameter,

K_1; a tissue–plasma backflow parameter, k_2, and an initial blood volume. The HPLC-purified 3-O-MFD time course was used in each case to fit the first 90 min of data post injection. The ratio of the fitted rate constants (K_1/k_2) was used as an estimator for the tissue–plasma equilibrium DV of 3-O-MFD in each region. Graphical analysis of the corresponding first 90 min of the 6-FD data was performed. Both the plasma input function (Martin *et al.*, 1989) and the cortical tissue input function (Brooks *et al.*, 1990) methods were applied. For both the DV values and the graphical slopes, left and right striatal values were averaged into a single value for each subject.

C. Corrections of 6-FD Graphical Analysis

Two model corrections of the graphical analysis with cortical tissue input function were implemented. In both, the cortical input function was corrected for the contribution of 3-O-MFD by subtracting a model estimate of the 3-O-MFD cortical time course. The plasma time course of 3-O-MFD in the 6-FD study was convolved with a single tissue compartment using kinetic parameters derived from fitting the 3-O-MFD bolus data in the same region. The specific striatal signal was estimated in the usual way by subtracting the occipital cortical time course from the striatal time course. In the second method, an additional correction was made to account for the possible failure of cancelation of 3-O-MFD in this subtraction step. The model estimate of the striatal 3-O-MFD time course was subtracted in place of the cortical time course.

III. RESULTS AND DISCUSSION

The striatal DVs measured in the 3-O-MFD studies were strongly correlated with the ratios of graphical

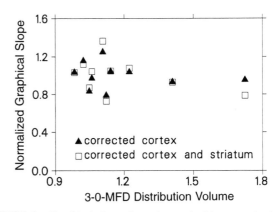

FIGURE 4 Graphical slopes from the cortical input method after the corrections described in the text.

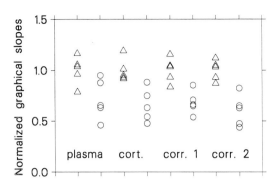

FIGURE 5 Discrimination between normal control subjects (triangles) and subjects with PD (circles) by the four graphical analysis approaches. Plasma: plasma input function; cort.: cortical input function method; Corr-1: correction of the cortical time course used as the input function; corr-2: correction of both the cortical time course and the specific striatal signal for incomplete cancellation of the 3-O-MFD signal.

slopes determined in the 6-FD studies ($r = 0.92$, Fig. 1). Regression of the nine subjects, excluding the subject with the highest values, was still significant ($r = 0.71$). In Figure 2, the slope with plasma input K_i is plotted vs. that from tissue input K_o, with the two subjects with the lowest and the two subjects with the highest measured values for the 3-O-MFD DV identified by alternative plotting symbols. The open circles denote the linear relationship between the two slopes when the DV is near its modal value. Subjects with high DV values are displaced from this curve upward, or to the left, or both. Those with small volumes are apparently displaced downward, to the right, or both.

Figure 3 presents the same results in yet a third way: Graphical slopes for each method and within each subgroup (normal and PD) were averaged and normalized values derived by dividing individual values by that average. The relationship between the DV and the slope ratio shown in Figure 1 now appears as a tendency of the values K_i to be larger when DV is large and smaller when DV is small, whereas the cortical input function values K_o are small when DV is large and large when DV is small. These data cannot be used to identify whether the change in the ratio is primarily a K_i or a K_o effect or a combination of the two. However, they do show that DV effects can cause the rank order of disease severity to differ in a systematic way for different analysis methods.

Figure 4 shows a similar plot for the two correction approaches. In the first approach the input function from cortex was corrected as described earlier. In the second, an additional correction to the specific striatal signal was made. Only subtle alterations appeared in the relative ordering of the 10 subjects. The primary

effect, exemplified by the simpler of the two correction methods, was a tightening of the distribution of values about their mean as the dependence of the values on DV is accounted for.

This last effect is apparent in Figure 5, which shows the discrimination between normal subjects and those with PD by the four graphical approaches applied to the data. The values for each method were normalized by setting the means of the normal controls to unity. The three cortical input function approaches apparently have very similar discriminant power. A trial with additional subjects would be required to determine whether there was a significant benefit from the correction process.

A. Conclusions

Indexes of tracer DV in brain derived from 3-O-MFD and from 6-FD analyzed by graphical methods identified similar large excursions from the modal values. The correlation between the two measures indicated that the implied DV excursions remained stable over the two week interval between the studies. The data suggest that, in the event of an extraordinarily high 3-O-MFD DV value in a given subject, the slopes K_i derived from plasma input functions may be biased upward, and the values K_i derived from the cortical tissue input may be biased downward, to a degree capable of changing the rank order of disease severity between the two methods. Corrections of the cortical input function method for 3-O-MFD effects showed only minimal improvement over the standard uncorrected approach in the overall discrimination between normal control subjects and those with PD. Further studies with additional subjects would be required to determine whether such corrections improved the correlation with clinical measures of disease severity.

Acknowledgments

This work was supported by the Medical Research Council of Canada and the National Institutes of Health, Grant R01-AG10217.

References

Adam, M. J., Lu, J., and Jivan, S. (1994). Stereoselective synthesis of 3-O-methyl-6-[18F]fluorodopa via fluoro destannylation. *J. Lab. Compd. Radiopharm.* **34:** 565–570.

Brooks, D. J., Ibanez, V., Sawle, G. V., Quinn, N., Lees, A. J., Mathias, C. J., Bannister, R., Marsden, C. D., and Frackowiak, R. S. J. (1990). Differing patterns of striatal [18F]-dopa uptake in Parkinson's disease, multiple system atrophy and progressive supranuclear palsy. *Ann. Neurol.* **28:** 547–555.

Chan, G. L. Y., Hewitt, K. A., Pate, B. D., Schofield, P., Adam, M. J., and Ruth, T. J. (1992). Routine determination of [18F]L-

6-fluorodopa and its metabolites in blood plasma is essential for accurate positron emission tomography studies. *Life Sci.* **50:** 309–318.

Hoshi, H., Kuwabara, H., Leger, G., Cumming, P., Guttman, M., and Gjedde, A. (1993). 6-[^{18}F]fluoro-L-DOPA metabolism in living human brain: A comparison of six analytical methods. *J. Cereb. Blood Flow Metab.* **13:** 57–69.

Martin, W. R. W., Palmer, M. R., Patlak, C. S., and Calne, D. B. (1989). Nigrostriatal function in humans studied with positron emission tomography. *Ann. Neurol.* **26:** 535–542.

Namavari, M., Bishop, A., Satyamurthy, N., Bida, G., and Barrio, J. (1992). Regioselective radiofluorodestannylation with [^{18}F]F$_2$ and [^{18}F]CH$_3$COOF: A high yield synthesis of 6-[^{18}F]fluoro-L-dopa. *Appl. Radiat. Isot.* **43:** 989–996.

Patlak, C., Dhawan, V., Takikawa, S., Chaly, T., Robeson, W., and Eidelberg, D. (1993). Estimation of striatal uptake rate constant of FDOPA using PET: Methodological issues. *In:* "Quantitation of Brain Function" (K. Uemura, N. A. Lassen, T. Jones, and I. Kanno, Eds.), pp. 263–268. Excerpta Medica, Amsterdam.

Fluorodopa Positron Emission Tomography with an Inhibitor of Catechol-O-methyltransferase

Effect of the Plasma 3-O-methyldopa Fraction on Data Analysis

TATSUYA ISHIKAWA,[1] VIJAY DHAWAN,[1] CLIFFORD PATLAK,[2] THOMAS CHALY,[1] and DAVID EIDELBERG[1]

[1]*Departments of Neurology, Research, Medicine, and Biostastistics*
North Shore University Hospital/Cornell University Medical College
Manhasset, New York 11030
[2]*State University of New York at Stony Brook, New York 11794*

Fluorodopa (FDOPA) is an analog of L-DOPA used to assess the nigrostriatal dopamine system in vivo with positron emission tomography (PET). However, FDOPA/PET quantitation is complicated by the presence of the 3-O-methyl-FDOPA (3-O-MFD) fraction in brain and plasma. Pretreatment with entacapone (OR-611), a peripheral catechol O-methyltransferase (COMT) inhibitor, greatly reduces the plasma 3-O-MFD fraction and provides an opportunity to evaluate the contribution of the plasma 3-O-MFD fraction in several kinetic models of FDOPA uptake.

We performed FDOPA/PET with and without the entacapone preadministration in six Parkinson's disease (PD) patients. We measured the time course of the plasma FDOPA and 3-O-MFD fractions using high pressure liquid chromatography (HPLC). We calculated striato–occipital ratios (SOR) and estimated the striatal FDOPA uptake rate constant graphically using the plasma FDOPA and occipital tissue time–activity curves (K_i^{FD} and K_i^{OCC}, respectively). We also estimated striatal DOPA decarboxylase (DDC) activity (k_3^D) using a model incorporating independent measurements of 3-O-MFD transport kinetic rate constants.

With the preadministration of entacapone, the pharmacological efficiency in plasma prolonged significantly (21.1 to 37.7%; $p < 0.01$). We also observed significant mean elevations in SOR and K_i^{OCC} by 21.8 and 53.5%, respectively ($p < 0.05$). K_i^{FD} and k_3^D showed no significant change.

We conclude that entacapone prolongs the circulation time of FDOPA in the plasma but does not alter rate constants for striatal FDOPA uptake or decarboxylation.

I. INTRODUCTION

Parkinson's disease (PD) is characterized by presynaptic nigrostriatal dopamine dysfunction. Therapy with L-DOPA (L-dihydroxyphenylalanine) remains the single most effective agent for the presynaptic treatment of PD. Methods for improving the bioavailability of L-DOPA may help to prolong its antiparkinsonian effect. In this regard, there has been much interest in several new catechol O-methyltransferase (COMT) inhibitors as an adjunct to L-DOPA therapy. Of these, entacapone (OR-611) appears to have utility in the treatment of L-DOPA related response fluctuations by blocking peripheral COMT activity (Linden *et al.*, 1990; Kaakkola *et al.*, 1994).

The agent 6-[^{18}F]fluoro-L-DOPA (FDOPA) is an analog of L-DOPA used to assess the presynaptic nigrostriatal dopamine system *in vivo* with positron emission tomography (PET). This method yields quantitative information on regional differences in FDOPA entry and metabolism in the brain. However, the kinetic analysis of FDOPA uptake is complicated by the presence of 3-O-methyl-FDOPA (3-O-MFD) fraction in the brain (Huang *et al.*, 1991; Kuwabara *et al.*, 1993). Peripheral inhibition of 3-O-MFD formation with COMT inhibitors provides an opportunity to assess the contribution of the plasma 3-O-MFD fraction in the kinetic models that have been developed to estimate striatal DDC activity. In this study, we performed FDOPA/PET to assess the effects of entacapone on the systemic metabolism and striatal uptake of FDOPA using a comprehensive kinetic model (Dhawan *et al.*, Chapter 43 in this book). These results were compared with those obtained through other proposed models to evaluate the sensitivity of each to the plasma 3-O-MFD fraction.

II. MATERIALS AND METHODS

We studied six patients (one woman and five men; mean ± SD age 57.7 ± 13.6 years) with mild to moderate parkinsonism (Hoehn and Yahr Stage I, four patients; Hoehn and Yahr Stages II and III, one patient each).

PET studies were performed using Superpett 3000 tomograph (Scanditronix; Essex, Massachusetts). Each patient underwent FDOPA/PET with and without preadministration of entacapone (400 mg) 60 min prior to the study. In each study, patients fasted overnight prior to PET scanning. All antiparkinsonian medications were discontinued at least 12 hr before PET investigations. All patients received 200 mg carbidopa 90 min before the study to inhibit decarboxylation. And 260–370 MBq (7–10 mCi) of FDOPA in 20–25 ml saline was injected intravenously. Emission scanning began simultaneously with the start of the FDOPA injection, and continuous scan data were acquired between 0 and 100 min post injection. The time course of plasma ^{18}F radioactivity was determined by radial arterial blood sampling followed by plasma centrifugation. In each of the paired FDOPA/PET studies, the specific time course of plasma activity for FDOPA and its metabolites was measured using high pressure liquid chromatography (HPLC).

We assessed the pharmacokinetics of FDOPA by calculating the pharmacokinetic circulation time, $\theta_T^{FD}(\theta_T^{FD} = \int_0^T Ca^{FD}(t)dt/Ca^{FD}(T))$, where $Ca^{FD}(t)$ is the radioactivity concentration of FDOPA in plasma as a function of time and $Ca^{FD}(T)$ is the concentration at specific time T (Gjedde, 1981). We also calculated an index of pharmacokinetic efficiency, E_p [$E_p = (T/\theta_T^{FD}) \times 100\%$], where θ_T^{FD} is the pharmacokinetic circulation time at specific time T (Guttman *et al.*, 1993).

Region of interest (ROI) analysis was performed on 256×256 PET reconstructions using a SUN microcomputer (490 SPARC Server) and Scan/VP software. Elliptical ROIs were placed to encompass the whole striatum (mean 90 pixels/striatum; pixel size, 4 mm^2). Background count rates were determined separately for an occipital ROI (mean size, 350 pixels). We estimated the striatal FDOPA uptake rate constant graphically by the multiple time graphical approach using the plasma FDOPA and occipital tissue time activity curves (K_i^{FD} and K_i^{OCC}, respectively; Takikawa *et al.*, 1994). We also calculated the striato–occipital ratio by dividing striatal count rates by occipital count rate measured on the last 10 min scan (90–100 min post injection).

We determined striatal DDC activity by the following two methods: (1) In our four-compartment model (Dhawan *et al.*, Chapter 43), we used population mean K_1^M and k_2^M values (0.0400 and 0.0420, respectively) obtained from independent 3-O-MFD/PET studies for the calculation of striatal k_3^D(pop). We set the values of k_5^D, k_7^D, and k_9^D all to 0 min^{-1} [k_5^D is the O-methylation coefficient of FDOPA, k_7^D is the lumped O-methylation and oxidation coefficient of FDA (fluorodopamine), and k_9^D is the fractional clearance from brain of the diffusible FDA metabolites], and estimated frontal and striatal K_1^D, k_2^D, k_3^D(pop), and V_b, the brain vascular volume. (2) In a second compartmental modeling approach, we used the constraints of a common value of the partition volume ($V_e = K_1/k_2$) for the frontal lobe and striatum, and a fixed K_1 ratio (q) for FDOPA and O-MFD (Model M2; Kuwabara *et al.*, 1993; Dhawan *et al.*, Chapter 43). We set the values of k_5^D, k_7^D, and k_9^D to 0, 0.02, and 0.005 min^{-1}, and estimated striatal K_1^D, k_3^D(M2), and V_b with several predetermined q values ($q = 0.5, 1.0, 1.7, 2.3,$ and 3.0). Based on the striatal kinetic rate constants (K_1^D, k_2^D, k_3^D(pop)) estimated from our model, we calculated composite rate constants of FDOPA uptake: K^D and $K^{D'}$ [$K^D = K_1^D \times k_3^D/(k_2^D + k_3^D)$; $K^{D'} = k_2^D \times k_3^D/(k_2^D + k_3^D)$] (Patlak and Blasberg, 1985).

The following statistical procedures were performed using SAS (SAS Institute, Cary, North Carolina): (1) The time course of plasma FDOPA metabolite fractions were compared with and without entacapone pretreatment using repeated measures ANOVA. The θ_T^{FD} and E_p values were also compared with and without entacapone using the paired Student's *t*-test. (2) The mean of left and right striatal K_i^{FD}, K_i^{OCC} and SOR values, estimates of striatal DDC activity (striatal k_3^D(pop) and striatal k_3^D(M2)) derived with different choices of q, and values for K^D and $K^{D'}$ were compared with and without the entacapone pretreatment using the paired Student's *t*-test.

TABLE 1 Estimated Parameters with and without Entacapone Pretreatment

		Placebo		Entacapone		
		Mean	S.D.	Mean	S.D.	p^b
θ_T^{FD} ($T = 55$ min)	min	271.0	(56.4)	147.6	(17.9)	$p < 0.001$
E_p^{FD} ($T = 55$ min)	%	21.2	(5.1)	37.7	(4.6)	$p < 0.001$
K_i^{FD}	ml/min/mg	0.0109	(0.0034)	0.0107	(0.0036)	N.S.
K_i^{OCC}	min^{-1}	0.0042	(0.0018)	0.0065	(0.0025)	$p < 0.05$
k_3^D(pop)	min^{-1}	0.0169	(0.0076)	0.0131	(0.0073)	N.S.
k_3^D(M2)	min^{-1} $q = 3.0$	0.0508	(0.0242)	0.0222	(0.0069)	$p < 0.05$
	$q = 2.3$	0.0470	(0.0204)	0.0218	(0.0068)	$p < 0.05$
	$q = 1.7$	0.0421	(0.0184)	0.0212	(0.0066)	$p < 0.05$
	$q = 1.0$	0.0315	(0.0138)	0.0203	(0.0068)	N.S.
	$q = 0.5$	0.0204	(0.0096)	0.0198	(0.0072)	N.S.
SOR (90–100 min)		1.72	(0.25)	2.09	(0.34)	$p < 0.01$
K^D	ml/min/mg	0.0139	(0.0046)	0.0136	(0.0040)	N.S.
$K^{D'}$	min^{-1}	0.0120	(0.0047)	0.0094	(0.0038)	N.S.

[a]See text for definition of θ^{FD}, E_p^{FD}, K_i^{FD}, K_i^{OCC}, k_3^D(pop), k_3^D(M2), SOR, K^D, and $K^{D'}$.

[b]See text for statistical tests and their significance.

III. RESULTS AND DISCUSSION

A. Plasma Analysis

Entacapone acts predominantly by inhibiting COMT at peripheral sites, such as liver, kidneys, gut, and red blood cells (Linden *et al.*, 1990). This compound was found to effectively increase the half-life of L-DOPA and reduced the formation of 3-O-MFD in cynomolgus monkeys (Guttman *et al.*, 1993). In our human study, the fraction of 3-O-MFD reached 70% and the fraction of FDOPA decreased to under 20% at 85 min after injection without COMT inhibition. With entacapone, the 3-O-MFD fraction was significantly inhibited to under 20% at the end of the study ($p < 0.001$). The FDOPA fraction, by contrast, increased significantly ($p < 0.01$), remaining above 50% throughout the study. The fraction of the unknown metabolite increased significantly to 30% after 30 min ($p < 0.05$). The precise identity of this metabolite is unresolved. However, the location of the peak in HPLC suggests that it may be assigned to 6-fluorodopamine sulfate (Firnau *et al.*, 1988). Mean θ_T^{FD} decreased significantly from 271.0 to 146.7 min ($p < 0.001$), and mean E_p increased significantly from 21.2 to 37.7% with the entacapone pretreatment ($p < 0.001$; Table 1), consistent with the corresponding values in the monkey study (Guttman *et al.*, 1993). Our results therefore demonstrate that entacapone is effective in prolonging the available time of L-DOPA in plasma in PD patients.

B. PET Analysis

Mean values and standard deviation for SOR, striatal K_i^{FD}, K_i^{OCC}, k_3^D(pop), k_3^D(M2) calculated for several q values, K^D and $K^{D'}$ are given in Table 1. Changes of individual values in striatal K_i^{FD}, K_i^{OCC}, SOR, and striatal DDC activity (k_3^D(pop) and k_3^D(M2)) with and without entacapone appear in Figure 1.

In their monkey study, Guttman *et al.* (1993) demonstrated 20% increase in the striatum–occipital cortex ratio with entacapone. Subsequently, Sawle *et al.* (1994) studied six normal subjects and four Parkinson's disease patients and found a mean increase in (striatum–cerebellum)/cerebellum ratio of approximately 38% by entacapone pretreatment. In our study, we noted a 21.8% SOR (calculated as striatum–occipital) increase with entacapone ($p < 0.05$), due to a combined 3% increase in the proportion of the injected dose within the striatum and a 13% decline in that proportion in occipital cortex. This decline in occipital cortex appears to have resulted from the approximately 20% increase of the unknown metabolite, probably 6-fluorodopamine sulfate, which does not cross the blood–brain barrier. Entacapone pretreatment thus gives rise to a net reduction in the combined FDOPA and 3-O-MFD plasma fraction and lowers the total activity in "neutral" brain regions such as the occipital cortex. This decrease in occipital cortex appears to play a greater role in raising the SOR than a concomitant increase in striatal FDOPA concentration.

Guttman *et al.* (1993) estimated striatal DDC activity by the method of Kuwabara *et al.* (1993), in which a fixed ratio (q) was assumed for the transport kinetic rate constants for FDOPA and 3-O-MFD (K_1^M/K_1^D). They selected $q = 2.3$ based on the data derived from rat experiments (Reith *et al.*, 1990). These investigators found that striatal k_3^D(M2) fell from 3.9 to 2.5 (hr^{-1})

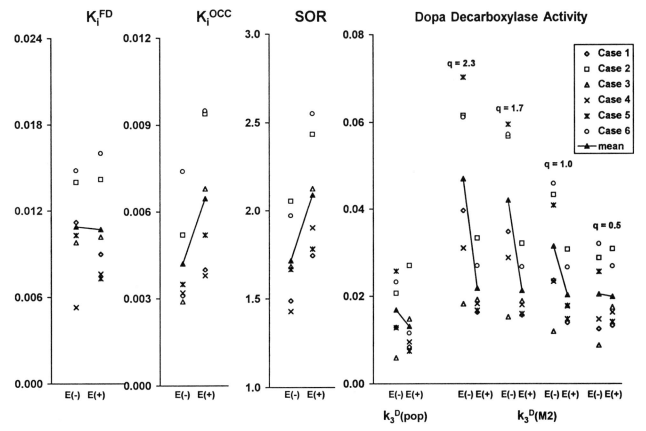

FIGURE 1 Changes in mean (left–right) striatal K_i^{FD}, K_i^{OCC}, SOR, and striatal DDC activity (k_3^D(pop), k_3^D(M2) sec for $q = 2.3$, 1.7, 1.0, and 0.5), with and without entacapone pretreatment ($E(+)$ and $E(-)$). With entacapone, (1) K_i^{FD} remained unchanged; (2) K_i^{OCC} increased significantly (mean change 60%, $p < 0.05$); (3) SOR increased significantly (mean change 20%, $p < 0.01$); (4) k_3^D(pop) did not significantly change; (5) k_3^D(M2) shows a significant decrease for all $q \geq 1.7$ ($p < 0.05$). In the ($E(+)$) studies, variation in the assumed values of q did not significantly alter k_3^D(M2) estimates.

following entacapone, although this decrease did not reach statistical significance. Similarly, Huang *et al.* (1991) found that the best fit of their constrained model occurred with q fixed at 1.7. To determine q explicitly, we performed combined PET studies with 3-O-MFD and FDOPA in humans and found limited intersubject variability in estimates of K_1^M and k_2^M (COV $<$ 30%) and that q approached unity (Dhawan *et al.*, Chapter 43). We also demonstrated that population values for K_1^M and k_2^M (0.0400 and 0.0420, respectively) can be applied in a comprehensive FDOPA kinetic model to estimate striatal DDC activity without adjunctive 3-O-MFD/PET scans (Dhawan *et al.*, Chapter 43). When we applied the model M2 with choices of q to our patient data, estimates of striatal k_3^D(M2) significantly decreased after entacapone pretreatment—but only when q values $\geq$1.7 were selected ($p < 0.05$). However, neither k_3^D(M2) values estimated with q values less than 1.0 nor did k_3^D(pop) values show significant change with COMT inhibition. We also note that in our study k_3^D

(M2) values were found to be sensitive to the choice of q, especially when 3-O-MFD is appreciably present in plasma. When the plasma 3-O-MFD fraction was reduced with entacapone pretreatment, k_3^D(M2) did not vary with q. Indeed, animal studies have demonstrated that entacapone does not cross the blood–brain barrier and does not effect central DDC activity (Mannisto *et al.*, 1992). For this reason, we conclude that M2 model may not be appropriate for DDC activity estimation in settings in which COMT is not effectively inhibited.

We found no change in K_i^{FD} with entacapone. On the other hand, we did find that K_i^{OCC} increased significantly by approximately 50% with the pretreatment of entacapone ($p < 0.01$). These findings are consistent with the animal experiments of Guttman *et al.* (1993) and with the human study of Sawle *et al.* (1994). These investigators speculated that the reason for the K_i^{OCC} increase was its sensitivity to the presence of 3-O-MFD in the periphery and suggested that the change in free brain FDOPA may be reflected in the magnitude of change in the value of K_i^{OCC}. We, however, did not find a change in the net uptake rate constants, K^D and $K^{D'}$, with entacapone treatment. Furthermore, mean K_i^{OCC} was elevated significantly with entacapone, but $K^{D'}$ was not significantly changed. These results suggest that the estimation of K_i^{OCC} is influenced greatly by the plasma fraction of the sulfated metabolite, which does not cross the blood–brain barrier. As mentioned earlier, our data suggest that the increase in the plasma concentration of this metabolite with entacapone pretreatment leads to a concomitant reduction in the combined FDOPA and 3-O-MFD plasma fraction. This in turn gives rise to a reduction in "neutral" region brain count rates. Such reductions in the occipital time–activity integral increase K_i^{OCC}, without necessarily affecting striatal FDOPA uptake.

In summary, our results suggest that entacapone has little effect on FDOPA kinetics in the striatum, and that the main pharmacologic effect of this agent is brought about by the prolongation of FDOPA circulation time in plasma.

References

Bernheimer, H., Birkmayer, W., Hornykiewicz, O., Jellinger, K., and Scitelberger, F. (1973). Brain dopamine and the syndromes of Parkinson and Huntington. *J. Neurol. Sci.* **20**: 415–455.

Eidelberg, D., Takikawa, S., Dhawan, V., Chaly, T., Robeson, W., Dahl, R., Margouleff D., Moeller, J. R., Patlak, C. S., and Fahn, S. (1993). Striatal 18F-DOPA uptake: Absence of an aging effect. *J. Cereb. Blood Flow Metab.* **13**: 881–888.

Fahn, S., Elton, R. L., and the UPDRS Development Committee (1987). Unified Parkinson disease rating scale. In: Fahn, S., Marsden, C. D., Calne, D., Goldstein, M., eds. "Recent Developments in Parkinson's Disease. vol. 2." Floral Park, New Jersey: Macmillan: 293–304.

Firnau, G., Sood, S., Chirakal, R., Nahmias, C., and Garnett, E. S. (1988). Metabolites of 6-[18F]fluoro-L-dopa in human blood. *J. Nucl. Med.* **29**: 363–369.

Gjedde A. (1981). High- and low-affinity transport of D-glucose from blood to brain. *J. Neurochem.* **36**: 1463–1471.

Gjedde, A., Reith, J., Dyve, S., Léger, G., Guttman, M., Diksic, M., Evans, A., and Kuwabara, H. (1991). DOPA decarboxylase activity of the living human brain. *Proc. Natl. Acad. Sci.* **88**: 2721–2725.

Guttman, M., Leger, G., Reches, A., Evans, A., Kuwabara, H., Cedarbaum, J. M., and Gjedde, A. (1993). Administration of the new COMT inhibitor OR-611 increases striatal uptake of fluorodopa. *Movement Disorders*, **8**: 298–304.

Hoehn, M. M., and Yahr, M. D. (1967). Parkinsonism: Onset, progression, and mortality. *Neurology* **17**: 21–25.

Huang, S. C., Yu, D. C., Barrio, J. R., Grafton, S., Melega, W. P., Hoffman, J. M., Satyamurthy, N., Mazziota J. C., and Phelps, M. E. (1991). Kinetics and modeling of 6-[18F]fluoro-L-DOPA in human positron emission tomographic studies. *J. Cereb. Blood Flow Metab.* **11**: 898–913.

Kaakkola, S., Teravainen, H., Athtila, S., Rita, H., and Gordin, A. (1994). Effect of entacapone, a COMT inhibitor, on clinical disability and levodopa metabolism in parkinsonian patients. *Neurology*, **44**: 77–80.

Kuwabara, H., Cumming, P., Reith, J., Leger G., Diksic, M., Evans, A. C., and Gjedde, A. (1993). Human striatal L-DOPA decarboxylase activity estimated in vivo using 6-[18F]fluoro-dopa and positron emission tomography: Error analysis and application to normal subjects. *J. Cereb. Blood Flow Metab.* **13**: 43–56.

Linden, I-B., Etemadzadeh, E., Schultz, E., and Pohto, P. (1990). Selective catechol-O-methyltransferase (COMT) inhibition as potential adjunctive treatment with L-DOPA in Parkinson's disease. [Abstract[. *Movement Disorders*, **5(Suppl. 1)**: 49.

Mannisto, P. T., Tuomanien, P., and Tuomanien, R. (1992). Different *in vivo* properties of three new inhibitors of catechol-O-methyltransferase in the rat. *Br. J. Pharmacol.* **105**: 569–574.

Patlak, C. S. and Blasberg, R. G. (1985). Grpahical evaluation of blood-to-brain transfer constants from multiple-time uptake data. *J. Cereb. Blood Flow Metab.*, **5**: 584–590.

Patlak, C. S., Blasberg, R. G., and Fenstermacher, J. D. (1983). Graphical evaluation of blood-to-brain transfer constants from multiple-time uptake data. *J. Cereb. Blood Flow Metab.* **3**: 1–7.

Reith, J., Dyve, S., Kuwabara, H., Guttman, M. Diksic, M., and Gjedde, A. (1990). Blood–brain transfer and metabolism of 6-[18F]fluoro-L-DOPA in rat. *J. Cereb. Blood Flow Metab.* **10**: 707–719.

Sawle, G. V., Burn, D. J., Morris, P. K., Lammertsma, A. A., Snow, B. J., Luthra, S.K., Osman, S., and Brooks, D. J. (1994). The effect of entacapone (OR-611) on brain [18F[-6-L-fluorodopa metabolism: Implications for levodopa therapy of Parkinson's disease. *Neurology*, **44**: 1292–1297.

Snow, B. J., Tooyama, I., McGeer, E. G., Yamada, T., Calne, D. B., Takahashi, H., and Kimura, H. (1993). Human positron emission tomographic [18F]fluorodopa studies correlate with dopamine cell counts and levels. *Ann. Neurol.* **34**: 324–330.

Takikawa, S., Dhawan, V., Chaly, T., Chaly, T., Robeson, W., Dahl, R., Zanzi, I., Mandel, F., Spetsieris, P., Eidelberg, D. (1994). Input functions for 6-[fluorine-18]fluorodopa quantitation in Parkinsonism: Comparative studies and clinical correlations. *J. Nucl. Med.* **35**: 955–963.

Wahl, L. M., Garnett, E. S., Chirakal, R., Firnau, G., and Nahmias, C. (1993). Quantification of dopamine metabolism in man: What is the most justifiable approach? *J. Cereb. Blood Flow Metab.* **13[Suppl. 1]**: S722.

47

Comparison of Ratio and Slope–Intercept Plot-Based Images of [18F]Fluoro-L-DOPA Uptake in Human Brain

MASAHIRO SHIRAISHI, HIROTO KUWABARA, PAUL CUMMING, MIRKO DIKSIC, and ALBERT GJEDDE

McConnell Brain Imaging Center
Montreal Neurological Institute and
Department of Neurology and Neurosurgery
McGill University Faculty of Medicine
Montreal, Quebec, Canada H3A 2B4

We constructed and compared functional 6-[18F]fluoro-L-DOPA (FDOPA) images of the pixel-to-occipital radioactivity ratio (ratio images) and of the graphical slope–intercept analysis, refering to the radioactivies in plasma (K^{pl} image) and in occipital cortex (k^r image). Striatal ratio values from ratio images increased as a function of study time from 40 to 90 min. The increase was more prominent in the head of caudate nucleus than in the putamen ($p < 0.05$). Individual putaminal K^{pl} and k^r values obtained directly from images correlated linearly to each other ($p < 0.001$ for both) and were practically identical to respective values obtained in the conventional way, in which regional rather than pixel radioactivies were used. Both methods discriminated subjects with PD from control subjects equally well. Averaged images following stereotactic transformation of these images of individual subjects of the two groups revealed relative sparing of the head of the caudate nucleus and severe involvement of the posterior part of the putamen in PD. These trends in PD were more apparent in K^{pl} and k^r images than ratio images. In conclusion, the images of slope–intercept plot methods are useful to visualize the net uptake of FDOPA in normal and PD subjects.

I. INTRODUCTION

The agent L-6-[18F]fluoro-L-DOPA (FDOPA) has been used to evaluate the striatal presynaptic dopamine metabolism in living humans with positron emission tomography (PET). Three major approaches have been used to quantify the uptake of FDOPA into striatum: the simple ratio of striatum to nonstriatal reference region (Martin *et al.*, 1986), the net FDOPA uptake constant using graphical slope–intercept analysis (Martin *et al.*, 1989; Brooks *et al.*, 1990b; Sawle *et al.*, 1990), and compartmental approaches that involve least squares optimization (Huang *et al.*, 1991; Kuwabara *et al.*, 1993). One of the great advantages of PET is to present physiological variables by means of tomographic images. Although the compartmental approach may be the most desirable in theory, the approach is not suitable for this purpose due to complexity of FDOPA kinetics and the intrinsic weakness of least squares optimization to noise. The simple ratio method is popular, but may be shown to be less sensitive to changes in diseases and less potent in discriminating between normal and PD subjects, and its relevance to the underlying physiology and biochemistry is not clear.

In this study, we introduce and compare two additional types of FDOPA images with a greater physiological relevance: images of the FDOPA uptake constant obtained as the slopes of pixel-by-pixel slope–intercept plots with a reference to the radioactivity in a reference brain region or the FDOPA activity in plasma. We applied recent intersubject stereotactic transformation and averaging to these functional images to visualize changes in the FDOPA uptake constant in Parkinson's disease.

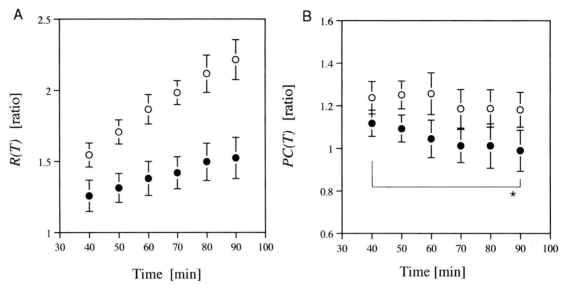

FIGURE 1 $R(T)$ (A) and putamen-to-caudate ratio ($PC(T)$) (B) in the putamen as a function of time. Open circles represent normal volunteers and filled circles, patients with Parkinson's disease: $*p < 0.05$.

II. METHODS

We studied six healthy, neurologically normal subjects (ages, 42–70 years) and six patients with Parkinson's disease (ages, 44–70 years).

A. PET Procedures

All subjects fasted overnight and received 150 mg carbidopa 90 min before the PET study. All medication to PD patients are interrupted at least 12 hr before the study. We used the Scanditronix PC-20481 15B PET scanner with 15 simultaneous planes at 6.5 mm intervals and a 12 mm effective reconstruction full-width at half-maximum. Tissue attenuation was determined with a 511 keV γ source (^{68}Ga). Twenty seven frames were taken in 90 min, including six 30 sec, seven 1 min, five 2 min, four 5 min, and five 10 min frames. Arterial blood was sampled through the brachial artery and separated for FDOPA and O-methyl-fluoro-DOPA with high-performance liquid chromatography (HPLC).

On a separate occasion, 64 axial magnetic resonance images (MRI) of 2 mm thickness were obtained. In each subject, the MRI volume was "resliced" along planes parallel to the PET planes following spatial alignment of MR and PET images using the three-dimensional landmark-matching method (Evans *et al.*, 1991). We identified and outlined the following cerebral structures as regions of interest (ROIs) on two adjacent "resliced" MRI planes; the head of the caudate nu-

cleus, putamen, and occipital cortex. The ROI templates were used to obtain ratio, K^{pl}, and k^r values from functional images and the time courses of radioactivity (TAC) in these structures.

B. Data Analysis

1. Simple-Ratio Method ($R(T)$)

We constructed ratio images by dividing radioactivity images by the radioactivity of the occipital cortex. We obtained ratio images for each PET frame between 40 and 90 min.

2. Plasma Slope–Intercept Plot (K^{pl}) and Tissue Slope–Intercept Plot (k^r)

The input function for the graphical method was either radioactivity in plasma (Gjedde, 1981; Patlak *et al.*, 1983; Martin *et al.*, 1989) or in a nonstriatal reference brain region (Patlak *et al.*, 1985; Brooks *et al.*, 1990b; Sawle *et al.*, 1990). In the plasma slope–intercept plot, we used the separated radioactivity of FDOPA in plasma ($C_a^D(T)$). In the tissue slope–intercept plot, we used TACs from the occipital ROI ($A^r(T)$) as the input function. In both methods, we calculate the uptake constants using data obtained between 40 and 90 min:

$$\frac{A^*(T) - A^r(T)}{C_a^D(T)} = K^{pl} \frac{\int_0^T C_a^D(t)\, dt}{C_a^D(T)} + V_q \qquad (1)$$

$$\frac{A^*(T) - A^r(T)}{A^r(T)} = k^r \frac{\int_0^T A^r(t)\, dt}{A^r(T)} + r_0 \qquad (2)$$

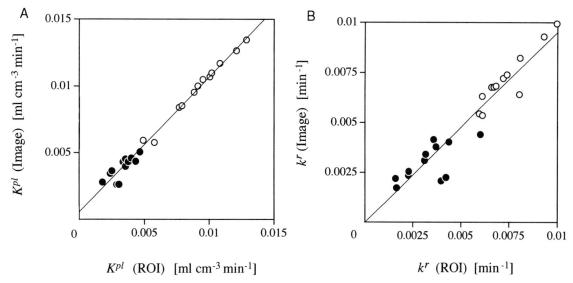

FIGURE 2   Plots of individual values of ROI analysis and image analysis for K^{pl} (A) and k^r (B) methods. Open circles represent normal volunteers and filled circles, patients with Parkinson's disease.

where, $A^*(T)$ is the total radioactivity in the target region at time T, V_q is a constant with the unit of volume, and r_0 is a constant with the unit of ratio.

We obtained striatal ratio, K^{pl}, and k^r values in two ways: directly from respective functional images (image analysis) and by applying equations (1) and (2) to regional TACs (ROI analysis) using the same template of regions of interest.

3. Averaged Images

The ratio K^{pl} and k^r images were transformed to a common Talairach's stereotactic space (Talairach et al., 1988), using a three-dimensional landmark-matching method and averaged across normal subjects or PD patients (Evans et al., 1992).

III. RESULTS AND DISCUSSION

Figure 1(A) shows changes of putaminal $R(T)$ as a function of time. The $R(T)$ values of both normal volunteers and PD patients increased with time. Therefore, it is better to select a later frame to obtain images of a better contrast between striatum and the rest of the brain. Usually, a frame starting 60 min or later is used (Martin et al., 1986; Leenders et al., 1986). We found that the putamen-to-caudate ratio of normal control subjects was stable over time, but that of PD patients decreased. There was a statistical difference between 40 (1.12 ± 0.061) and 90 (0.98 ± 0.096) min putamen-to-caudate ratio values in PD patients ($p <$

0.05) (Fig. 1(B)). Not only the striato–reference region ratio but also the putamen-to-caudate ratio was time dependent in PD. The difference between normal subjects and PD patients was greater in the putamen than in the caudate nucleus. We speculate that the difference may be explained by the spatially differential involvement of the striatum in PD (Brooks et al., 1990a; Kuwabara et al., 1995) and a reduced ability to retain dopamine in the putamen in PD (Kuwabara et al., 1992). In a primate model of parkinsonism induced with 1-methyl-4-phenyl-1,2,3,6-tetrahydropyridine (MPTP),

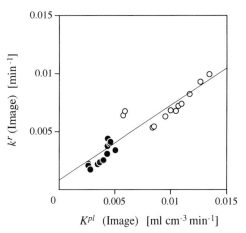

FIGURE 3   Plots of the k^r values from image analysis vs those of K^{pl} values. Open circles represent normal volunteers and filled circles, patients with Parkinson's disease.

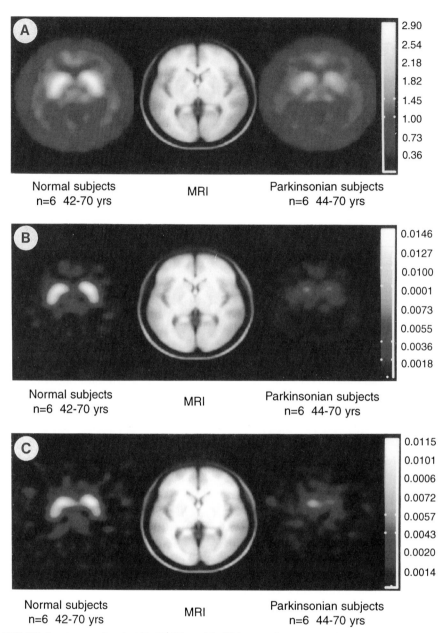

FIGURE 4 Averaged ratio (A), K^{pl} (B), and k^r (C) images for normal volunteers (left panel) and Parkinson's disease (right panel). The center image shows averaged MRI images of the same level as functional PET images.

the dopamine turnover increased dramatically in the putamen (Barrio *et al.*, 1990).

The graphical analyses for the FDOPA study are based on an assumption that the tracer is taken up and trapped irreversibly in striatum for the duration of a PET scan. If the assumption is correct, the plot of K^{pl} and k^r analyses will become linear some time after the tracer injection. The plot of k^r analysis never becomes strictly linear at least for 2 hr (data not shown). Because, for practical reasons, few patients can tolerate

more than 90 min of scanning and more data points produce better statistics, it may be a good compromise to include data obtained between 40 and 90 min.

Figure 2 shows the correlation between individual putaminal values of the image analysis and ROI analysis for the K^{pl} (A) and k^r (B) methods. We can expect the image analysis to be affected less by possible deviation due to heterogeneous FDOPA uptakes within a ROI, and the ROI analysis to be affected less by the noise. The regression lines were $y = 0.001 + 1.017x$

for the K^{pl} method (r = 0.99, p < 0.001) and y = 0.955x (r = 0.92, p < 0.001) for the k^r method, where x is values from ROI analysis and y, from image analysis. Therefore, we conclude that the image and ROI analyses are alternative to each other.

To obtain K^{pl} images requires serial samples of arterial blood from the beginning of tracer injection to the end of scan, and metabolites of FDOPA in plasma must be determined with HPLC. In contrast, the k^r analysis requires neither. Therefore, it is obvious that the k^r analysis is advantageous if the quality of images and values of the FDOPA uptake constant from the two analyses are equivalent. On viewing, k^r images are similar to K^{pl} images, although k^r images appeared slightly noisier. Quantitatively, individual k^r values from image analysis were linearly correlated with K^{pl} values (Fig. 3). The regression line was k^r = 0.645 K^{pl} + 0.001 (r = 0.94, p < 0.001). In addition, K^{pl} values were shown to be affected more by the presence of large neutral amino acids in plasma than k^r values (Leenders et al., 1986; Kuwabara et al., 1994).

Figure 4 shows the stereotactically averaged ratio, K^{pl}, and k^r images through a plane of middle striatum for control and PD subjects together with averaged MR images. In ratio images, the striatum of control subjects appeared as a homogeneous area of elevated ratio values (Fig. 4(A), left panel). In the striatum of PD subjects, the ratio was retained relatively more in the head of caudate nucleus but smoothly tapered toward the tail of the putamen (Fig. 4(A), right panel). Cortical ratio values remained unchanged in PD. The striatum of control subjects appeared less homogeneous in K^{pl} images than ratio images; K^{pl} values appeared higher in the head of caudate nucleus and the anterior putamen compared to the posterior putamen (Fig. 4(B), left panel). And, the K^{pl} images gave an impression that the right striatum had higher K^{pl} values than the left side. In PD, the reduction of K^{pl} values in the striatum were more apparent in K^{pl} images than in ratio images (Fig. 4(B), right panel). Again, K^{pl} values of the head of caudate nucleus were preserved relatively more than those of the putamen. In k^r images, the normal striatum appeared less homogeneous than in the previous two image modalities (Fig. 4(C), left panel). It was impossible to trace cerebral cortex in k^r images mainly due to a relatively large variance. In PD, we observed a marked side-to-side difference in the striatum in the k^r image (Fig. 4(C), right panel). The differences in the appearances of corresponding images of the three imaging modalities cannot be attributed to methodological errors associated with stereotactic transformation because we applied the same stereotactic transformation in all.

In conclusion, the slope–intercept plot methods, either plasma reference or tissue reference, are useful as functional images of the FDOPA/PET study and to visualize and detect changes in PD.

Acknowledgments

The present study was supported by grants from the Medical Research Council of Canada (SP-30).

References

Barrio, J. R., Huang, S. C., Melega, W. P., Yu, D. C., Hoffman, J. M., Schneider, J. S., Satyamurthy, N., Mazziotta, J. C., and Phelps, M. E. (1990). 6-[^{18}F]Fluoro-L-DOPA probes dopamine turnover rates in central dopaminergic structures. *J. Neurosci. Res.* **27:** 487–493.

Brooks, D. J., Ibanez, V., Sawle, G. V., Quinn, N., Lees, A. J., Mathias, C. J., Bannister, R., Marsden, C. D., and Frackowiak, R. S. J. (1990a). Differing patterns of striatal ^{18}F-Dopa uptake in Parkinson's disease, multiple system atrophy, and progressive supranuclear palsy. *Ann. Neurol.* **28:** 547–555.

Brooks, D. J., Salmon, E. P., Mathias, C. J., Quinn, N., Leenders, K. L., Bannister, R., Marsden, C. D., and Frackowiak, R. S. J. (1990b). The relationship between locomotor disability, autonomic dysfunction, and the integrity of the striatal dopaminergic system in patients with multiple system atrophy, pure autonomic failure, and Parkinson's disease, studied with PET. *Brain* **113:** 1539–1552.

Evans, A. C., Marrett, S., Torrescorzo, J., Ku, S., and Collins, L. (1991). MRI-PET correlation in three dimensions using a volume-of-interest (VOI) atlas. *J. Cereb. Blood Flow Metab.* **11:** A69–A78.

Evans, A. C., Marette, S., Neelin, P., Collins, L., Worsley, K., Dai, W., Milot, S., Meyer, E., and Bub, D. (1992). Anatomical mapping of functional activation in stereotactic coordinate space. *Neuroimage.* **1:** 43–53.

Gjedde, A. (1981). High- and low-affinity transport of D-glucose from blood to brain. *J. Neurochem.* **36:** 1463–1471.

Huang, S.-C., Yu, D.-C., Barrio, J. R., Grafton, F., Melega, W. P., Hoffman, J. M., Satyamurthy, N., Mazziotta, J. C., and Phelps, M. E. (1991). Kinetics and modeling of L-6-[^{18}F]fluoro-DOPA in human positron emission tomographic studies. *J. Cereb. Blood Flow Metab.* **11:** 898–913.

Kuwabara, H., Cumming, P., Léger, G., and Gjedde, A. (1992). Loss of 6-[^{18}F]fluoro-dihydroxyphenylalanine [FDOPA] metabolites from human striatum. *J. Nucl. Med.* **33:** 916.

Kuwabara, H., Cumming, P., Reith, J., Léger, G., Diksic, M., Evans, A. C., and Gjedde, A. (1993). Human striatal L-DOPA decarboxylase activity estimated in vivo using 6-[^{18}F]fluoro-DOPA and positron emission tomography: Error analysis and application to normal subjects. *J. Cereb. Blood Flow Metab.* **13:** 43–56.

Kuwabara, H., Cumming, P., Reutens, D., Diksic, M., Jolly, D., and Gjedde, A. (1994). Protein rich diet suppressed net and unidirectional clearances of 6-[F-18]fluoro-DOPA decarboxylase activity. *J. Nucl. Med.* **35:** 212P.

Kuwabara, H., Cumming, P., Yasuhara, Y., Léger, G. C., Guttman, M., Diksic, M., Evans, A. C., and Gjedde, A. (1995). Regional striatal DOPA transport and decarboxylase activity in Parkinson's disease. *J. Nucl. Med.*, **36:** 1226–1231.

Leenders, K. L., Poewe, W. H., Palmer, A. J., Brenton, D. P., and Frackowiak, R. S. J. (1986). Inhibition of L-[^{18}F]fluorodopa uptake into human brain by amino acids demonstrated by positron emission tomography. *Ann. Neurol.* **20:** 258–262.

Martin, W. R. W., Stoessl, A. J., Adam, M. J., Ammann, W., Bergstrom, M., Harrop, R., Laihienen, A., Rogers, J. G., Ruth, T. J., Sayre, C. I., Pate, B. D., and Calne, D. B. (1986). Positron emission tomography in Parkinson's disease: Glucose and DOPA metabolism. *Adv. Neurol.* **45:** 95–98.

Martin, W. R. W., Palmer, M. R., Patlak, C. S., and Calne, D. B. (1989). Nigrostriatal function in humans studied with positron emission tomography. *Ann. Neurol.* **26:** 535–542.

Patlak, C. S., Blasberg, R. C., and Fenstermacher, J. D. (1983). Graphical evaluation of blood-to-brain transfer constants from multiple-time uptake data. *J. Cereb. Blood Flow Metab.* **3:** 1–7.

Patlak, C. S., and Blasberg, R. G. (1985). Graphical evaluation of blood-to-brain transfer constants from multiple-time uptake data. Generalizations. *J. Cereb. Blood Flow Metab.* **5:** 584–590.

Sawle, G. V., Colebatch, J. G., Shah, A., Brooks, D. J., Marsden, C. D., and Frackowiak, R. S. (1990). Striatal function in normal aging: Implications for Parkinson's disease. *Ann. Neurol.* **28:** 799–804.

Talairach, J., and Tournoux, P. (1988). "Co-Plannar Stereotaxic Atlas of the Human Brain: 3-Dimensional Proportional System: An Approach to Cerebral Imaging." Thieme, Stuttgart.

Parametric Images of Benzodiazepine Receptor Concentration

J. DELFORGE,[1] L. SPELLE,[1] P. MILLET,[2] B. BENDRIEM,[1] Y. SAMSON,[1] and A. SYROTA[1]

[1]*C.E.A., Service Hospitalier F. Joliot, 91400 Orsay, France*
[2]*CERMEP, Lyon, France*

The in vivo *quantification of the benzodiazepine receptor concentration in the human brain using positron emission tomography and [^{11}C]flumazenil, is usually based on a three-compartment model and PET curves measured in large regions of interest. However, whereas experimental PET data are images, limiting the quantification of the receptor concentration to only some large brain regions is somehow a loss of information. Therefore, it should be interesting to obtain quantified images of the receptor concentration, whose main advantage is to allow visual screening of receptor site localization and quantitation over the entire brain.*

Two different methods allowing us to obtain parametric images of the benzodiazepine receptor concentration are proposed here: first, the multi-injection approach, which allows us to identify all the model parameters; second, the partial saturation approach, which leads to only receptor concentration and FMZ affinity estimates. The interests and the disadvantages of these two methods are discussed and compared to the previously proposed approaches. The multi-injection approach is difficult to use in human studies, but allows to obtain good images of all model parameters. The partial saturation approach can lead to some inaccurate values in receptor-poor regions, but it is the only method allowing us to obtain B_{max} and $K_d V_R$ images from a single 40 min experiment without blood sampling, an acceptable protocol for routine human examinations.

I. INTRODUCTION

The benzodiazepine receptors are usually studied in the human brain using [^{11}C]flumazenil (^{11}C-FMZ), an antagonist with a high affinity and selectivity for central benzodiazepine receptors. A quantification of these receptors is very useful for understanding the pharmacological properties of benzodiazepine receptor ligand and the role of the binding sites for benzodiazepine in pathological conditions. In particular, the study of changes in the density or affinity may be very useful in pathophysiology or neurology disorders. One of the challenges of the *in vivo* studies of ligand–receptor interactions is the quantification of these two parameters.

Many methods have been proposed to estimate all or part of the parameters of the ligand–receptor model from PET curves measured in regions of interest. However, whereas experimental PET data are images (of activity), limiting the quantification of the receptor concentrations to only some large brain regions is somehow a loss of information. Therefore, recent efforts have been devoted to the search for methods to obtain quantified images of the receptor concentration and affinity (Blomqvist *et al.*, 1990; Lassen *et al.*, 1995). The main advantage of such images is to allow visual screening of receptor site localization and quantitation in the entire brain. They could be very useful for the easy investigation of possible local changes in patients.

All the approaches allowing us to identify receptor concentration in large regions of interest are not adapted for parametric imaging, which requires model parameter estimation in very small brain regions to obtain images with good resolution. Indeed, due to the small number of counts in each voxel, some PET curves (corresponding mainly to regions with a low concentration of receptor sites) can be very noisy.

Thus, unadapted approaches can lead to badly identified parameters and unrealistic results (negative or too large values).

Two different methods to obtain parametric images of the benzodiazepine receptor concentration are proposed here, each having specific advantages compared to the previously proposed approaches. First, the multi-injection approach allows us to identify all the model parameters from a single PET experiment, including several injections of labeled or unlabeled ligand, but requires blood sampling and metabolite study. Second, the partial saturation approach allows us to estimate only the receptor concentration and the FMZ affinity, but its main interest is to avoid blood sampling.

II. METHODS

A. The Ligand–Receptor Model

The compartmental model used in this study is the usual nonequilibrium nonlinear model (Delforge *et al.*, 1993, 1995a). It includes three compartments (the unmetabolized free ligand in plasma, the free ligand, and the specifically bound ligand in the tissue) and four model parameters (the benzodiazepine receptor concentration, B'_{max}, and four kinetic parameters: the exchanges between plasma and tissue, k_1 and k_2, and the apparent association and dissociation rate constants, k_{on}/V_R and k_{off}). The apparent equilibrium dissociation rate constant $K_d V_R$ is deduced from the ratio of k_{off} to k_{on}/V_R. The vascular fraction is often assumed to be negligible. The parameter V_R is the reaction volume, which allows us to take into account the possibility for the free ligand concentration in the vicinity of the receptor sites to be different from the mean free ligand concentration in the tissue (which is the concentration used in the model). By definition, the reaction volume is the tissue volume in which the free ligand mass present in 1 ml of tissue would have been distributed with the same concentration as that in the receptor site vicinity. The reaction volume also allows us to take into account a possible nonspecific binding in an equilibrium state with the free ligand compartment (Delforge *et al.*, 1996).

B. The Multi-injection Approach

In previous papers, we proposed a kinetic approach, based on a multi-injection protocol and a global fitting procedure (Delforge *et al.*, 1993, 1995a). The typical protocol used to study the flumazenil kinetics in the human brain consisted of three injections. At the beginning of the experiment, about 555 MBq of ^{11}C-FMZ (about 5 μg) were injected intravenously over a time period of about 1 min. At 30 min, an intravenous injection of unlabeled ligand (about 10 μg per kg of body weight) was performed, followed at 60 min by a third injection, consisting of a mixture of labeled flumazenil (about 278 MBq at the injection time corresponding to about 20 μg) and unlabeled flumazenil (about 0.1 mg per kg of body weight) in the same syringe. The total experiment lasted 100 min. This method required blood sampling and metabolite analysis to estimate the input function.

For the parametric imaging, we have reduced the number of parameters by fixing one parameter, the dissociation rate constant k_{off} (the value of this parameter is estimated from a fitting procedure of the whole brain PET curve; see Millet *et al.*, 1995). Indeed, previous results showed that k_{off} could be considered as a constant for all regions (Delforge *et al.*, 1995a). Therefore, four quantified parameter images have been obtained: the receptor concentration, the FMZ affinity, and the k_1 and k_2 parameters (Millet *et al.*, 1995).

C. The Partial Saturation Approach

The partial saturation approach is a new method, based on a Scatchard analysis (which allows us to estimate the receptor concentration and the FMZ affinity), whose main interest is to avoid blood sampling. The protocol consists of a single coinjection of a tracer dose of ^{11}C-FMZ (about 740 MBq) and a partial saturation dose of FMZ (between a tracer dose and a saturation dose). The choice of the unlabeled FMZ amount is important, because it must be sufficiently large to occupy a significant percentage of receptor sites (at least 50%), but not too large, in order to observe a significant decrease of this percentage during the limited duration of the experiment (1 hr at most). We have used here 10 μg per kg of body weight. Data are analyzed using the Scatchard equation. The free ligand concentration F, assumed to be identical in all regions, is estimated from the pons, considered as a reference region. The bound ligand concentration B in any region is then obtained by subtracting the free ligand concentration F (estimated in the pons) from the PET-measured concentration.

The pons has often been assumed to be devoid of receptor sites and thus the PET concentration in the pons has often been used as an estimate of the free ligand concentration F. However, the multi-injection study has shown that the concentration of receptor sites in the pons is small, but not negligible: about 4.7 pmol/ml (Delforge *et al.*, 1995a). Because all the model parameters of the ligand kinetics in the pons have been identified using the multi-injection approach, it is possible to simulate the percentage of bound ligand in the pons as a function of time and of FMZ mass. This curve is used in each experiment to estimate the free ligand concentration F from the PET-measured pons concentration. The Scatchard analysis is performed using all the (F, B) pairs obtained at various times during the experiment. Except for the early data (where the equilibrium state may not have been yet reached), the points are aligned on a straight line, from which estimations of B'_{max} (the intercept of the straight line with the B-axis) and $K_d V_R$ (the inverse of the slope) are calculated. The Scatchard straight line is estimated using a minimization of a cost function.

III. REVIEW OF PREVIOUSLY PUBLISHED METHODS

A. Index Images (Distribution Volume and Delayed PET Activity Images)

Several methods have previously been proposed to obtain index images that are assumed to be correlated to the receptor concentration. The proof of this correlation requires validation studies, which are difficult without simulations studies (these simulations are now possible using the model parameters found with the multi-injection approach).

The easiest approach assumes that the regional ligand concentration images obtained about 20 min after tracer injection of [^{11}C]flumazenil reflect the benzodiazepine receptor density (Savic et al., 1988, Zilbovicius et al., 1993). The main advantage of this delayed image approach is its great simplicity (no blood sampling, no fitting procedure).

Koeppe et al., (1991) have suggested estimating the apparent distribution volume, which is considered an index of the receptor density. The two-compartment model used in the distribution volume approach is deduced from the usual three-compartment model by assuming that the free and bound ligand compartments can be lumped in a single tissue compartment. This assumes that the double equilibrium state is reached immediately after the tracer injection because the two-compartment model is applied to all points of the PET curve. With FMZ, this double equilibrium is reached only 5–15 min after a tracer injection, which leads to a small systematic bias. For example, a significant underestimation (from 5 to 15%) of K_1 using the two-compartment model, compared to the same parameter estimated with the three-compartement model, has been observed (Millet et al., 1995).

It can be easily shown that these two approaches are equivalent, because we have proven that the distribution volume images (V_d) are related to the PET activity images obtained at a delayed time t when the double equilibrium state is reached ($DA_{pet}(t)$). From this last hypothesis and using the model equations at the equilibrium state, the following relationship is immediately obtained:

$$DA_{pet}(t) = A_S V_d C_a(t) \qquad (1)$$

where A_s is the specific activity and $C_a(t)$ is the arterial concentration of the unmetabolized free ligand (Delforge et al., 1995c; Millet et al., 1995). This property has been tested on FMZ images obtained from human brain data and the correlation found between the delayed PET activity image and the distribution volume image was very strong ($r = 0.996$, $p < 0.005$, Millet et al., 1995). An advantage of the V_d images is to provide absolute values (because of the use of the input function) and thus to allow intersubject and intergroup comparisons. However, a single blood sample at the delayed time t is sufficient to estimate $C_a(t)$ and thus to deduce the distribution volume image from the delayed PET activity image by using equation (1).

These two index image methods are simple and need only a single injection of the tracer dose ligand. However, they can provide only indexes of receptor concentration, because the separate quantification of both the receptor density and the affinity requires different concentrations of bound ligand, usually obtained using at least two injections of the ligand with different specific radioactivities.

B. First Parametric Images of Receptor Concentration

The study of Blomqvist et al., (1990) was the first attempt to determine the quantified benzodiazepine receptor map. It used a method based on PET data obtained from two experiments on the same subject, but with high and low specific activity, respectively. The estimation of the three parameters (the receptor concentration and the association and dissociation rate constants) was obtained with a kinetic approach, the free radioligand concentration being estimated from a reference region (the pons) assumed to be free of receptor sites. The images of receptor concentration and affinity obtained by Blomqvist et al. are of good quality, in spite of some negative values and of biased values (due to the neglected concentration of receptor sites in the pons). The comparison between these two images shows, for the first time, a possible correlation between receptor concentration and affinity.

Recently, Lassen et al., (1995) proposed a new

method for the quantification of receptor concentration and the affinity, based on the steady-state principle and on the measurement of distribution volumes. The experimental protocol includes two experiments, consisting of a constant-infusion injection of ligand, with high and low specific activity, respectively. From the distribution volumes obtained from these two experiments, Lassen deduced the relations, giving the receptor concentration and the flumazenil affinity using many physiological considerations. A simple proof of these relations have been recently published (Delforge et al., 1995b). However, as the result of the equivalence between the distribution volume and the delayed PET activity images, the receptor concentration and the affinity can be deduced using the Lassen's equations directly from the delayed PET images. With this steady state approach, the receptor concentration images appear of good quality, but the affinity images are very noisy, with some negative values (Lassen et al., 1995; Lammertsma et al., 1993).

The main disadvantage of these two approaches is the need to perform two experiments with different specific activities. In particular, this can lead to uncertainties related to repositionning difficulties, whose effects can be very large in the receptor-poor regions.

IV. RESULTS AND DISCUSSION

A. The Multi-injection Approach

This multi-injection approach allows us to identify all model parameters from a single dynamic PET experiment. It has two main advantages. First, it relies on no particular hypothesis that can be difficult to justify entirely (such as equilibrium hypothesis or hypotheses needed for the use of a reference region); second, it allows various simulations (for example, to test and evaluate hypotheses or simplified quantitative methods) because all model parameters are identified. For example, the results of the flumazenil kinetics in baboon and human brains have shown that the double equilibrium hypothesis (kinetic equilibrium states between the three compartments) is valid for the FMZ kinetics 10 min after the injection (this property is due to the rapid and continuous exchanges between the compartments; see Delforge et al., 1993; 1995a).

With the multi-injection approach, four quantified parameter images are obtained: the receptor concentration, the FMZ affinity, and the K_1 and k_2 parameters (Millet et al., 1995). The B_{max} images reveal a relatively homogeneous pattern across major gray matter structures, with lower values observed in white matter. The k_2 map appears correlated with the K_1 map, which rep-resents the ^{11}C-FMZ transport rate. Large variations (ranging from 4 to 14 pmol/ml) are observed in the $K_d V_R$ map, and a correlation between the receptor concentration and the flumazenil affinity is clearly established ($K_d V_R = C_2 + C_3 B_{max}$; see Millet et al. 1995). Since this approach is based on a global fitting procedure (and not on a comparison between two similar and noisy curves), all the identified parameters have positive values even in the receptor-poor regions. A great advantage of this multi-injection protocol is a single experiment (no positioning problem) and its main disadvantage is the need for a blood sampling.

As a consequence of the correlation between the receptor concentration and the FMZ affinity, we deduce that the distribution volume is related to the distribution volume by a nonlinear relationship (Millet et al., 1995):

$$DA_{pet} = C_1(1 + B_{max}/K_d V_r) = C_1[1 + B_{max}/(C_2 + C_3 B_{max})] \quad (2)$$

where C_1, C_2, and C_3 are constants ($r = 0.72$ in the example given by Millet et al., 1995). However, due to the uncertainties, the linear correlation is not in contradiction with the experimental results in the usual range of benzodiazepine receptor concentrations ($r = 0.69$ in the example given by Millet et al., 1995).

B. The Partial Saturation Approach

The hypotheses of this partial saturation approach are the usual hypotheses of the Scatchard analysis and the reference region method. The Scatchard analysis assumes that an equilibrium state between the free and the bound ligand compartments is reached (which has been previously proven for FMZ; see Delforge et al., 1993). The estimation of the free ligand concentration from the PET-measured concentration in a reference region assumes that this reference region has no receptor site (or, as proposed here, can be corrected for the small concentration of ligand bound to pons receptor sites) and that the distribution volumes (defined by K_1/k_2) are identical in all regions, including the reference region (this hypothesis is supported by the distribution volume estimates obtained in human, although it seems slightly smaller in the pons; see Delforge et al., 1995a).

This method presents several advantages: It allows a separate estimation of B_{max} and $K_d V_R$ with a protocol including only a single injection without blood sampling and with a reduced scanning time (from 30 min to 1 hr). This single experiment is possible because we used, first, a reference region to estimate the free ligand concentration, and second, the natural decrease of the bound ligand concentration to obtain a large range of this value.

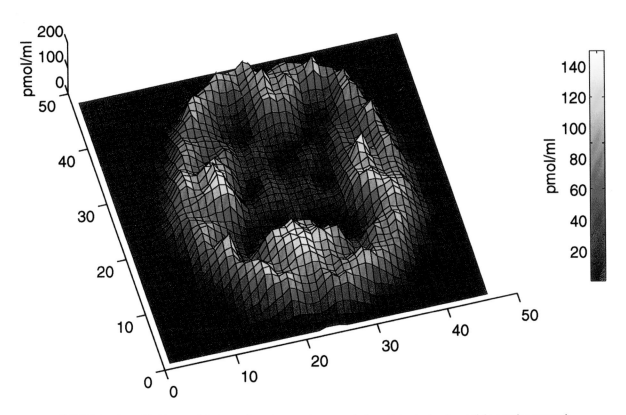

FIGURE 1   Quantified image of the benzodiazepine receptor concentration obtained using the partial saturation approach.

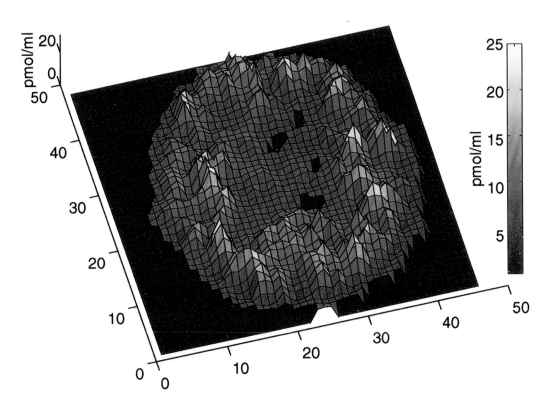

FIGURE 2   Quantified image of the *in vivo* flumazenil affinity (K_dV_r) obtained using the partial saturation approach.

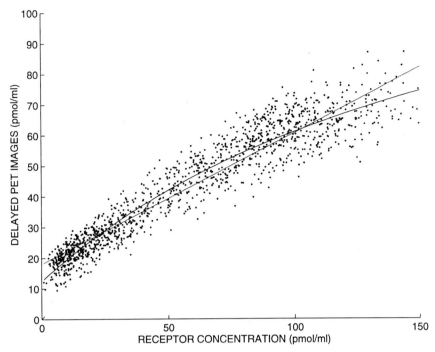

FIGURE 3 Correlation between the receptor density obtained using the partial saturation approach and the delayed PET images (30–60 min).

The partial saturation method is based on the comparison between two curves (the PET ligand concentrations in the interest and the reference regions), which can be very noisy and very close in the receptor-poor regions. If the difference between these two curves (which gives the bound ligand concentration) is too noisy and contains many with negative values, then the receptor concentration and the affinity are set to 0 [in the example given in Figs. 1 and 2, (Colorplates), there are about 1,200 small regions of interest and only 11 regions have not been usable]. Figures 1 and 2 (Colorplates) show the receptor concentration and flumazenil affinity images in a normal subject obtained from a PET slice parallel to the AC–PC plane and at the level +15 mm. Similarly, with the multi-injection approach results (Delforge *et al.* 1995a, Millet *et al.* 1995), these figures show clearly a correlation between the receptor concentration and the affinity.

Equation (1), relating the delayed PET images and the distribution volume, remains valid with the partial saturation protocol, because at the delayed times, the occupancy of the receptor sites becomes weak and the double equilibrium state is reached. Therefore, the distribution volume method can be tested using a delayed image obtained between 30 and 60 min. Figure 3 represents, pixel by pixel, the delayed PET concentrations as a function of the receptor concentrations

estimated by the partial saturation method. We found a significant linear correlation (solid straight line, $r = 0.94$, $p < 0.0005$). However, if we use the nonlinear equation (2), the result of the correlation between the receptor concentration and affinity, the correlation coefficient is better (solid line, $r = 0.96$).

V. CONCLUSION

The parametric imaging requires parameter estimation in very small brain regions to obtain images with good resolution. Moreover, some approaches are based on two experiments performed with different specific activities and thus on the comparison between two curves that are very close and very noisy in the receptor-poor regions. Such methods can lead to unrealistic results (negative or too large values). The same difficulty affects the partial saturation approach because the latter computes the difference between the interest and the reference region curves. However, such difficulties are not found in the multi-injection approach, which is well adapted to estimate the receptor concentration in receptor-poor regions.

In conclusion, the multi-injection approach is difficult to use in human studies, but the PET data obtained with multi-injection protocols allow us to obtain good images of four model parameters. This method is recommended for the study of receptor-poor regions, for preliminary studies of a new disease when the localizations of the receptor anomalies are not known, and as a reference method to test simplified approach. The partial saturation approach has the same disadvantage as the previously used methods (some unrealistic values can be obtained in receptor-poor regions), but it is the only method allowing us to obtain images of the B'_{max} map from a single 40 min experiment without blood sampling, an acceptable protocol for routine human examinations.

References

Blomqvist, G., Pauli, S., Farde, L., Eriksson, L., Persson, A., and Halldin, C. (1990). Maps of receptor binding parameters in the human brain—A kinetic analysis of PET measurements. *Eur. J. Nucl. Med.* **16**: 257–265.

Delforge, J., Syrota, A., Bottlaender, M., Varastet, M., Loch'h, C., Bendriem, B., Crouzel, C., Brouillet, E., and Mazière, M. (1993). Quantification of benzodiazepine receptor in human brain using PET, ^{11}C-flumazenil and a single-experiment protocol. *J. Cereb. Blood Flow Metab.* **15**: 284–300.

Delforge, J., Pappata, S., Millet, P., Samson, Y., Bendriem, B., Jobert, A., Crouzel, C., and Syrota, A. (1995a). Modeling analysis of ^{11}C-flumazenil kinetics studied by PET: application to a critical study of the equilibrium approaches. *J. Cereb. Blood Flow Metab.* **13**: 454–468.

Delforge, J., Bendriem, B., and Syrota, A. (1996). The concept of reaction volume in the in vivo ligand-receptor model. *J. Nucl. Med., in press.*

Delforge, J., Bendriem, B., and Syrota, A. (1995b). A direct proof of the Lassen equation relating to the steady-state approach of the receptor quantification (abstract). *J. Cereb. Blood Flow Metab.,* **15**: S639.

Delforge, J., Millet, P., Bendriem, B., Cinotti, L., Samson, Y., and Syrota, A. (1995c). Equivalence between the delayed PET activity and the distribution volume for the ligand verifying the double equilibrium property (abstract). *J. Cereb. Blood Flow Metab.,* **15**: S640.

Koeppe, R. A., Holthoff, A., Frey, K. A., Kilbourn, M. R., and Kuhl, D. E. (1991). Compartmental analysis of [11C]flumazenil kinetics for the estimation of ligand transport rate and receptor distribution using positron emission tomography. *J. Cereb. Blood Flow Metab.* **11**:735–744.

Lammertsma, A., Lassen, N., Prevett, M., Bartenstein, P., Turton, D., Luthra, S., Osman, S., Duncan, J., and Jones, T. (1993). Quantification of benzodiazepine receptors in vivo using ^{11}C-flumazenil: Application of the steady state principle. *In:* "Quantification of Brain Function (K. Uemura, N. A. Lassen, T. Jones, I. Kanno, Eds.), pp. 303–311. Excerpta Medica, Amsterdam.

Lassen, N., Bartenstein, P., Lammertsma, A., Prevett, M., Turton, D., Luthra, S., Osman, S., Bloomfield, P., Jones, T., Patsalos, P., O'Connell, M., Duncan, J., and Vanggaard Andersen J. (1995). Benzodiazepine receptor quantification in vivo in humans using ^{11}C-flumazenil and PET: Application of the steady-state principle. *J. Cereb. Blood Flow Metab.* **15**: 152–165.

Millet, P., Delforge, J., Mauguière, F., Pappata, S., Cinotti, L., Frouin, V., Samson, Y., Bendriem, B., and Syrota, A. (1995). Parametric images of benzodiazepine receptor concentration in human brain: Comparison with the distribution volume approach. *J. Nucl. Med.,* **36**: 1462–1471.

Savic, I., Persson, A., Roland, P., Pauli, S., Sedvall, G., and Widen, L. (1988). In vivo demonstration of reduced benzodiazepine receptor binding in human epileptic foci. *Lancet,* **2**: 863–866.

Zilbovicius, M., Rancurel, G., Leder, S., Raynaud, L., Loc'h, C., Wang, R., Crouzel, C., Cambier, J., and Samson, Y. (1993). PET study of benzodiazepine receptors with ^{11}C-flumazenil distinguishes cortical functional abnormalities from neuronal loss in frontal-type dementias. *Neurology* **43**, A213.

49

Analyzing PET Receptor Studies of Multiple Injections of Varying Specific Activities

Proper Modeling of the Unlabeled Ligand in Blood and Tissue

EVAN D. MORRIS, ALAN J. FISCHMAN, and NATHANIEL M. ALPERT

Radiology Department
Massachusetts General Hospital and Harvard Medical School
Boston, Massachusetts 02114

The goal of quantitative receptor-ligand PET studies is to estimate the receptor density B'_{max}, in vivo. An approach to this goal that is gaining wide acceptance is the use of multiple injections of radioligand of both high and low specific activity (SA). The information in the data produced by these studies is desirable in that it may allow the differentiation of B'_{max} from the association rate constant, k_{on}. However, if a significant amount of cold ligand is introduced by the low SA injection, the number of receptor sites will no longer be in excess compared with the total amount of injected ligand, and the saturable nature of the receptor binding must be taken into account by any kinetic model. Two different approaches have been taken in the literature toward modeling multiple injection data. The approach originally advanced by Huang et al. (1989) postulates compartments to represent only the labeled ligand species while the role of cold ligand is taken into account by use of the SA function. An alternative approach, introduced by Delforge, Syrota, and Mazoyer (1990) relies on explicit compartments for describing both hot and cold ligand species. In our simulation study, we compare and contrast these two approaches. We present results of simulations based on both models and examine their differences. We attempt to elucidate the behavior of the models by examining how each one represents the changes in receptor availability over time. Finally, we try to recover known values for B'_{max} from noisy and perfect test data generated with the latter model. In conclusion, we find that the more complicated modeling approach, which includes the cold species explicitly, is superior in its representation of receptor availability, and we attempt to explain the shortcomings of the former approach.

I. INTRODUCTION

One of the signature capabilities of positron emission tomography is the ability to image specific receptor systems *in vivo*. The quantification of these receptor-specific images, that is, the estimate of a receptor density, typically requires the comparison of the dynamic PET data to an appropriate nonlinear mathematical model. Even with an appropriate model, however, not be enough information may be available in the data to guarantee precise, uncorrelated parameter estimates. Accordingly, PET experiments to estimate receptor density have become more complicated, combining injections of high specific activity ligands with low specific activity displacement doses. In their latest incarnation, these experiments have included three or more injections of receptor ligand. We consider alternate ways to model the data from such multiple injection experiments.

A compartmental model including plasma, free, and receptor-bound species was first proposed by Mintun *et al.* (1984) to describe dynamic data from single injection PET studies with a labeled receptor ligand. Subsequently, Huang *et al.* (1989) introduced a double-injection technique with fluoroethyl-spiperone to estimate

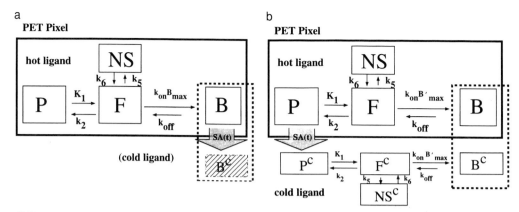

FIGURE 1 (a) Schematic of "Hot Only" model. Crosshatched compartment labeled B^c is not really a compartment but indicates that SA is used to account for cold ligand bound to receptor. (b) Schematic of "Hot and Cold" model. Large arrow labeled *SA* indicates that generalized SA function is used to create cold plasma input from hot plasma input.

the D2 receptor density, B'_{max}, as opposed to the compound parameter, binding potential (B'_{max}/K_D). This technique included the injection of a bolus of low SA ligand following an initial high SA injection. Huang *et al.* (1986) had previously proposed that the occupation of receptor sites by low a SA dose be modeled by a B/SA term in the nonlinear compartment model. Delforge *et al.* (1990) proposed a different model that included explicit compartments for labeled ("hot") and unlabeled ("cold") species to describe the dynamics of the muscarinic receptor ligand methyl quinuclidinyl-N-benzilate (MQNB) after multiple injections of varying specific activities. In that study, the authors found that two injections were inadequate to identify B'_{max} and the other model parameters. On the other hand, three injections were sufficient.

In this simulation study, we seek to elucidate the differences between these two established models and determine whether one is to be preferred in modeling PET data from three or more injections. We compare the predicted tissue activity curves from both models for a given set of test parameters and a test experimental protocol. The models can also be compared on the basis of their predicted receptor availability, which we believe is a revealing property of each model's inner workings. Finally, test data have been generated with and without noise. We report the ability of the two models to recover the original receptor density parameter from the various test data sets.

II. METHODS

A. Theory

The first of the models examined, based on the model proposed by Huang *et al.* (1989) is diagrammed in Fig-

ure 1(a). Because it contains compartments (i.e., balance equations) corresponding just to hot species, we refer to this model as the Hot Only (HO) model. The HO model follows:

$$\frac{dF}{dt} = K_1 C_p(t) - k_2 F - k_{on} F \left[B'_{max} - \frac{B}{SA(t)} \right]$$
$$+ k_{off} B - k_5 F + k_6 NS - \lambda F$$

$$\frac{dB}{dt} = k_{on} F \left[B'_{max} - \frac{B}{SA(t)} \right] - k_{off} B - \lambda B$$

$$\frac{dNS}{dt} = k_5 F - k_6 NS - \lambda NS$$

In the model, receptor availability is defined as $B'_{max} - B/SA(t)$. The second model, based on the work of Delforge *et al.* (1990) incorporates explicit mass balance equations for both the hot and cold species. Therefore, we refer to this model as the "Hot and Cold" (HC). The HC model is diagrammed in Figure 1(b). In the six HC model equations, superscript *c* refers to cold:

$$\frac{dF}{dt} = K_1 C_p(t) - k_2 F - k_{on} F [B'_{max} - B - B^c]$$
$$+ k_{off} B - k_5 F + k_6 NS - \lambda F$$

$$\frac{dB}{dt} = k_{on} F [B'_{max} - B - B^c] - k_{off} B - \lambda B$$

$$\frac{dNS}{dt} = k_5 F - k_6 NS - \lambda NS$$

$$\frac{dF^c}{dt} = K_1 C_p^c(t) - k_2 F^c - k_{on} F^c [B'_{max} - B - B^c]$$
$$- k_{off} B^c - k_5 F^c + k_6 NS^c$$

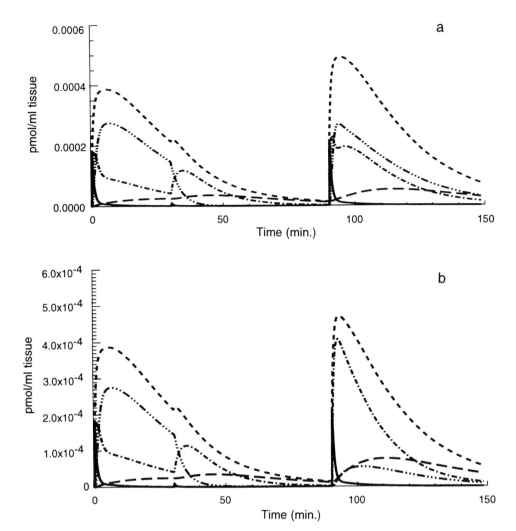

FIGURE 2   Simulation of concentrations of labeled ligand in plasma (————), free (–·–·–), bound (–···–), and nonspecific (————) compartments for both models: (a) HO model, (b) HC model. The total (——) is the weighted sum of all the compartments (i.e., its proportional to the PET activity).

$$\frac{dB^c}{dt} = k_{on}F^c\left[B'_{max} - B - B^c\right] - k_{off}B^c$$

$$\frac{dNS^c}{dt} = k_5 F^c - k_6 NS^c$$

In the HC model, receptor availability is defined as $B'_{max} - B - B^c$. Unlike the HO model, the HC model requires two input functions: one hot plasma function, one cold. They are related by SA:

$$C_p^c(t) = C_p(t)[1/SA(t) - 1]$$

Normally, the hot input function would be measured via arterial blood sampling. The cold input function is not measured directly. It is inferred from the hot input and knowledge of the specific activity of the ligand. Because of radioactive decay and mixing of various injectates in the plasma, the specific activity will vary

in time. We propose the generalized specific activity function that follows to account for these effects:

$$SA(t) = \frac{\sum_{i=1}^{n} MCP(t - t_i)U(t - t_i)e^{-\lambda(t-t_i)}}{\sum_{i=1}^{n} MCP(t - t_i)U(t - t_i)e^{-\lambda(t-t_i)}} + \sum_{i=1}^{n} MCP(t - t_i)U(t - t_i)$$

where MCP is a metabolite-corrected plasma activity pertaining to a single injection; U is a unit step function, λ is the decay constant of the isotope, t_i are the injection times. There are a total of n injections.

B. Simulation Protocol

All the simulations of both models that will be preed are based on one experimental protocol, a single set

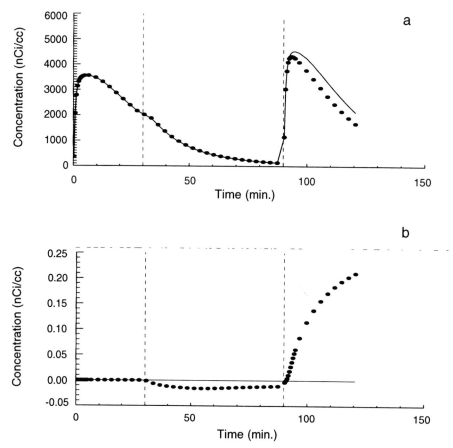

FIGURE 3 Simulation of PET activity for both models: (a) filled circles, HC model; solid line, HO model; (b) fractional residuals between the two curves in (a).

of model parameters. The protocol stipulated injections at 0, 30, and 90 min. The activity in these injections was 325.6, 17.02, and 410.7 MBq, respectively and the specific activities were 44.77, 0.0013, and 18.72 GBq/μmole. To assess how well B'_{max} could be recovered from data, test data was generated just with the HC model. For noisy test data, an error was added to tissue activity value according to $\sigma^2 = PET*f/\Delta T$, where σ^2 is the variance, f is the error level, and ΔT is the scan length. Data points were spaced every 30 sec near the time of injection and every 3 min for the remainder of the scans.

III. RESULTS AND DISCUSSION

A. Comparison of Model Outputs

Figure 2 displays the time-varying concentrations of total labeled ligand and ligand in each of the compartments as predicted by each of the models. Both simulations are based on the identical plasma input, injection protocol, and tissue parameters. Figure 2(a) displays the output of the HO model. Figure 2(b) displays the comparable output for the HC model. In both simulations, the concentrations in the various compartments (plasma, free, bound, nonspecific) are nearly identical until the third injection (at 90 min). Following the third injection, however, the HO model predicts that more than half of the total signal consists of receptor-bound species, whereas the HC model predicts that the majority of the signal following the third injection is due to labeled ligand in the free space. The time course of non-specifically bound ligand is quite similar although not identical in the two simulations. Despite the differences in the way each model apportions ligand between the compartments, the total ligand concentration (proportional to the PET activity) for the entire study is quite similar in the two simulations.

Figure 3(a) displays on the same axes the predicted PET activity curves (nCi/cc) for the two models. It is clear from Figure 3(a) that, for the same parameter, the HO model predicts higher PET activity following

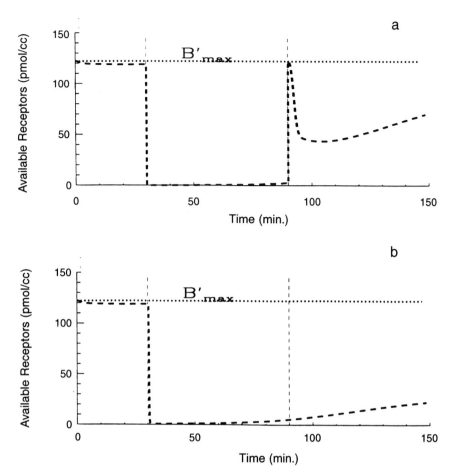

FIGURE 4   Simulation of receptor availability for both models: (a) HO model, (b) HC model. Vertical dashed lines mark injections. Horizontal dotted line marks B'_{max} value (i.e., maximum theoretical receptor availability).

the third injection. Based on Figure 2, we attribute this difference to higher predicted receptor binding by the HO model. Figure 3(b) shows the fractional residuals between the HO and HC model outputs in Figure 3(a). The residuals reveal that the two models predict identical PET curves only up to the second injection. Figure 3(b) shows that the HC model output is higher than the HO model output between the second and third injections and the HO model predicts higher activity than HC model after the third injection.

B. Receptor Availability

Let us consider the implications of the quite different amounts of receptor binding predicted by each of the models following a third injection. Figure 4 shows plots of the receptor availability, B_{avail}, as predicted by the HO and HC models. Plots (a) and (b) are identical between the first and second injections of high SA — B_{avail} is not affected appreciably. Both plots are similar but not identical in the period between the second and third injection. As expected, both models predict that the low SA injection causes an immediate and nearly complete obliteration of available receptor sites. Following the second injection the plots are still similar, although the freeing up of receptor sites proceeds slightly more quickly in the HC simulation prior to the third injection. However, the plots are very different following the third injection. According to the HO model (Fig. 4(a)), there is a sudden recovery of all the receptor sites previously blocked by the cold injection at 30 min. This sharp increase in B_{avail} after the injection of a tiny mass of ligand is reversed within 10 min of the injection (i.e., receptors become occupied again), then the gradual freeing up of sites resumes but at a pace faster than prior to the third injection. In contrast, the HC model indicates no effect whatsoever of the third injection (of high SA ligand) on the slow dissociation of ligand from receptor sites beginning after the low SA injection.

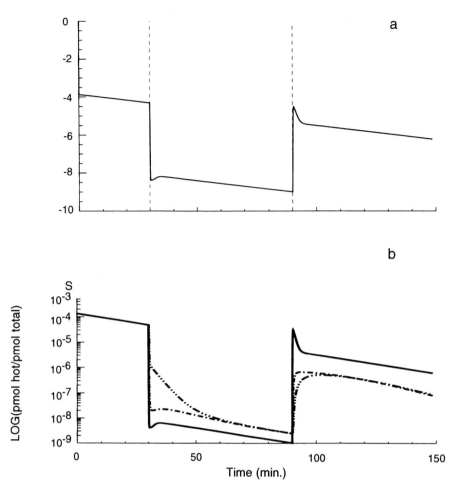

FIGURE 5   Specific activity: (a) Log SA vs time for HO model (generalized SA is defined for the plasma); (b) log SA vs time for HC model for plasma, free, and bound compartments. Plasma SA is same as function in (a), but functions for the free and bound compartments are calculated from state variables of HC model.

C. Specific Activity by Compartment

What might cause the HO model to make what seems an unphysiological prediction about the fraction of occupied binding sites? As discussed in Section II, B_{avail} for the HO model is explicitly dependent on SA, whereas SA does not appear explicitly in B_{avail} for the HC model. The time-varying function for SA, used in the HO model, is given as a log plot in Figure 5(a). Note that SA decreases with time even after a single injection because of radioactive decay. At each injection of ligand, the SA is changed to reflect the introduction of a new mixture of hot and cold ligand into the plasma, which differs significantly from the mixture already in the plasma. During these transitions, the SA overshoots and then settles down to a new (decaying) level. The overshoots are not artifactual. They result from modeling the plasma concentrations as sums of more than one exponential. The overshoot in SA at 90 min explains the overshoot in B_{avail} around the same time (see Fig. 4(a)). The SA function is not explicitly included in the state equations for the HC model. Rather, the SA function described in Section II applies only to the plasma compartment in the HC model and is necessary for generating a cold plasma function from a (measured) hot plasma function. The SA in the compartments can be calculated by the model because the concentrations of both hot and cold ligand in the different compartments are specified as state variables.

Figure 5(b) shows the SA for plasma (same as Fig. 5(a)), free and receptor binding compartments. Notice that the overshots in the plasma SA plot are absent from the free and bound SA functions. SA in the bound compartment, which is furthest from the plasma differs most from the plasma SA. In fact the bound SA appears to be a low-pass filtered version of SA in the plasma.

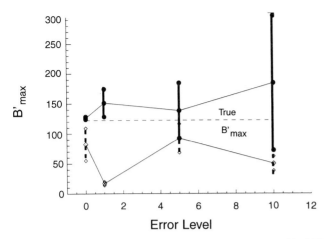

FIGURE 6 Error in B'_{max} estimated from test data generated by HC model with varying levels of additive noise. The error level corresponds to proportionally constant f defined in Section II. The true value of B'_{max} for the test data is indicated by horizontal dashed line (122 pmol/ml). The top curve shows estimates using the HC model. The error bars are ± 1 standard deviation, based on covariance matrix of the estimates. The bottom curve shows estimates using the HO model.

Notice also that, by 10 min following the third injection, the SA in the bound compartment is an order of magnitude smaller than that in the plasma. In other words, the HO model, in using the plasma SA function as an approximation of the bound SA, introduces a large error that then appears in the calculation of receptor availability as a severe underestimate of the B/SA term. This error leads to an overestimate of receptor availability. Because the model equations state that binding rate is proportional to receptor availability, the result of using the HO model to describe multiple injection data is to overestimate the amount of receptor binding that occurs following a blocking dose of cold ligand.

D. Magnitude of Errors in Estimates of B'_{max}

What size error might be committed by using the HO model to analyze three injection experiments? Figure 6 displays, for different error levels in the data, the B'_{max} values estimated by fitting both of the two models to test data generated by the HC model. The variance of each data point has been modeled as proportional to the PET signal and inversely proportional to the length of the scan (Mazoyer *et al.* 1986). Test data were generated with the HC model at four error levels, $f = [0, 1, 5, 10]$. Those data were then fit with both models and the resulting estimates of B'_{max} and its standard deviation are given in Figure 6. The true value of B'_{max} in the test data was 122 pmol/ml. The estimates

with the HO model were all lower than the true value and did not converge to the true value as the error in the data was reduced. The estimates with the HC model were all above the true value but they converged to the correct value as the test data was made less noisy. As the error in the data was reduced the estimated precision in the parameter estimates—as determined by the covariance matrix of the estimates—improved as well. In contrast, the precision of the estimates based on the HO model fits did not improve with better test data.

E. Conclusions

To this point, we have established that the HO and HC models are not identical for multiple injection studies. We have also shown that the HO model makes apparently unreasonable predictions about receptor availability following displacement doses of cold ligand. This unexpected behavior of the HO model can be traced to its application of the plasma SA function to the bound compartment as a means of accounting for competition between the hot and cold ligand for receptor sites. As simulations of the HC model indicate, the SA is not uniform across compartments once a second injection of a different SA from the first has been introduced. The error introduced into estimates of B'_{max} based on fits of the HO model to test data constructed with the HC model are significant. In the simulations examined, a 30% negative bias was introduced to estimates of B'_{max} even when the HO model was used to fit noiseless three-injection test data.

Finally we ask how easy would it be to identify a biased fit of the HO model to data in the literature, given that noise in actual PET data may make the fit look "good." Figure 7 displays the fits of each model to the test data at error level 10 shown in Figure 6. Figure 7(a) shows a fit of the HO model, and Figure 7(b) shows a fit of the HC. Although careful examination of the two plots reveals that the HO model undershoots the first peak at about 5 min, slightly overshoots most of the points in the displacement phase (30–90 min), and minimally overshoots the last peak following the third injection. Unfortunately, the corresponding estimate of B'_{max} (49 pmol/ml) is less than half the true value. Even though the covariance matrix of the estimates indicates that the estimate is precise, it is just not accurate. We conclude by pointing out that such a fit of the HO model to PET data as shown in Figure 7(a) might look pretty "good" but still be giving the wrong answers. Therefore, we recommend use of the HC model whenever describing data from multiple injection PET receptor ligand experiments.

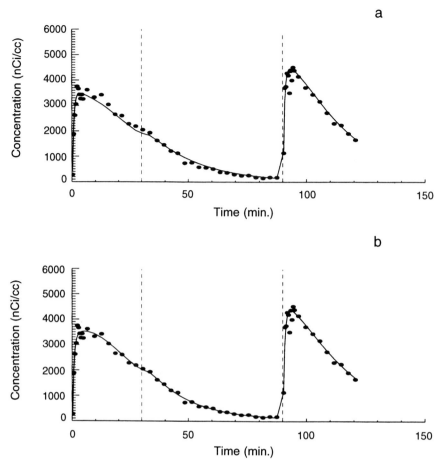

FIGURE 7 Fits of each model to test data (filled circles) generated at error level 10: (a) Fit (solid curve) of HO model; (b) fit (solid curve) of HC model.

Acknowledgments

Dr. Morris wishes to acknowledge support of PHS training grant T32 CA 09362.

References

Delforge, J., Syrota, A., and Mazoyer, B. M. (1990). Identifiability analysis and parameter identification of an in vivo ligand-receptor model from PET data. *IEEE Trans. Biomed. Eng.* **37:** 653–661.

Huang S-C., Barrio, J. R., and Phelps, M. E. (1986). Neuroreceptor assay with positron emission tomography: Equilibrium versus dynamic approaches. *J. Cereb. Blood Flow Metab.* **6:** 515–521.

Huang S.-C., Bahn, M. M., Barrio, J. R., Hoffman, J. M., Satyamurthy, N., Hawkins, R. A., Mazziotta, and J. C., and Phelps, M. E. (1989). A double-injection technique for the in vivo measurement of dopamine D2-receptor density in monkeys with 3-(2'-[18F] fluoroethyl)spiperone and dynamic positron emission tomography. *J. Cereb. Blood Flow Metab.* **9:** 850–858.

Mazoyer, B. M., Huesman, R. H., Budinger, T. F., and Knittel, B. L. (1986). Dynamic PET data analysis. *J. Comput. Assist. Tomogr.* **10:** 645–653.

Mintun, M. A., Raichle, M. E., Kilbourn, M. R., Wooten, G. F., and Welch, M. J. (1984). A quantitative model for the in vivo assessment of drug binding sites with positron emission tomography. *Ann. Neurol.* **15:** 217–227.

50

Kinetic Modeling of Serotonin-1A Binding in Monkeys Using [^{11}C]WAY 100635 and PET

J. C. PRICE, C. A. MATHIS, N. R. SIMPSON, K. MAHMOOD, and M. A. MINTUN

PET Facility, Department of Radiology
University of Pittsburgh
Pittsburgh, Pennsylvania 15213

[^{11}C]WAY 100635 localizes in primates in a manner consistent with the known distribution of 5-HT$_{1A}$ receptors. In this chapter, the usefulness of [^{11}C]WAY 100635 for the in vivo quantitation of 5-HT$_{1A}$ receptor binding was examined with tracer kinetic modeling. PET data were acquired in monkeys after high specific activity injections alone and after preinjection with either an agonist or antagonist (blocking studies). The cerebellar and blocking data (negligible receptor binding) were not well fit with a two-compartment model and significantly better fit (F-test) using three compartments (3C). For regions with specific binding, a 3C model was more suitable than constrained four compartment (4C) models (F-test) with distribution volume values that follow the rank order of 5-HT$_{1A}$ receptor density. A speculative model was proposed to address the apparent inconsistency of the suitability of a 3C model for all data. This model allowed for irreversible nonspecific binding. The Akaike information criteria indicated that this model was not superior to the 3C model for the cerebellar data, superior for the frontal cortex and temporal cortex (high specific binding), and equivalent for the striatum and thalamus (intermediate specific binding). An appropriate model that bridges the inconsistency between the nonspecific binding kinetics and the kinetics in specific-binding regions was not identified in this work, although adequate regional curve fits were obtained. The difficulty in applying conventional models may indicate that lipophilic metabolites of [^{11}C]WAY 100635 (labeled in the 2-methoxy position with ^{11}C) contribute to the observed PET signal.

I. INTRODUCTION

The serotonin (5-HT) receptor system has been linked to a variety of neuropsychiatric disorders and an area of active research interest is the identification of a suitable 5-HT radiotracer for use with positron emission tomography (PET) to permit the imaging and quantification of serotonin receptor function *in vivo*. Of particular interest is the 5-HT$_{1A}$ subtype because it plays a role in depression and anxiety disorders (Stahl *et al.*, 1992) and has been well characterized in animal and human brain (Pazos *et al.*, 1987).

The recent radiosynthesis of [^{11}C]WAY 100635 ([O-methyl-^{11}C]N-[2-[4-(2-methoxyphenyl)-1-piperazinyl]-ethyl]-N-(2-pyridinyl)cyclohexanecarboxamide) has provided a selective serotonin 5-HT$_{1A}$ antagonist that is currently being evaluated as a PET radiotracer.

Ex vivo rat biodistribution studies (Mathis *et al.*, 1994; Pike *et al.*, 1995) and PET imaging of monkeys (Mathis *et al.*, 1994) and rats (Pike *et al.*, 1995) have been performed with [^{11}C]WAY 100635. Frontal cortex : cerebellar ratios of 8 : 1 and of 4–6 : 1 were reported for the rat and monkey data, respectively. These studies also demonstrated that [^{11}C]WAY 100635 binding was decreased as a result of pretreatment with either the selective 5-HT$_{1A}$ agonist 8-OH-DPAT (Mathis *et al.*, 1994; Pike *et al.*, 1995) or WAY 100635 (Pike *et al.*, 1995).

Previously, kinetic modeling was applied to rat PET data, and these studies demonstrated that the cerebellar data could not be fit using a single tissue compartment (Hume *et al.*, 1994), although the application of a reference tissue model resulted in regional binding potential values that were correlated with the known distribution of 5-HT$_{1A}$ receptors.

In the present chapter, we further examine the binding of [^{11}C]WAY 100635 in monkeys to evaluate its usefulness for the *in vivo* quantitation of serotonin receptor binding in primates. This work was aimed at the following questions: (1) Can [^{11}C]WAY 100635 PET studies be used to quantify serotonin 5-HT$_{1A}$ receptor binding in primates? (2) Can we identify an appropriate tracer kinetic model?

II. MATERIALS AND METHODS

Eight rhesus monkeys were studied with [^{11}C]WAY 100635 at high specific activity (mean, 1.4 ± 0.3 Ci/μmole). Two monkeys had additional high specific activity (HSA) studies 15 min after pretreatment with 5 mg/kg of a selective 5-HT$_{1A}$ agonist (8-OH-DPAT) or antagonist (MPPI, 4-(2'-methoxyphenyl)-1-[2'-(N-2''-pyridinyl-p-iodobenzamido)ethyl]piperazine) (Zhuang *et al.*, 1994; Kung *et al.*, 1995).

Thirty-one imaging planes were simultaneously acquired using a Siemens-CTI 951R/31 PET scanner (in-plane resolution, 5.0 mm FWHM (ramp filter); axial slice width, 3.4 mm). Twenty frames (6 × 0.5 min, 1 × 1 min, 4 × 1.5 min, 2 × 5 min, and 7 × 10 min) were acquired over 90 min. Images were reconstructed with a Hanning filter (cutoff 0.4 Nyquist). Regions of interest were used to generate time–activity curves for

regions that are known to have specific 5-HT$_{1A}$ receptor binding: high, the frontal cortex (Frt) and temporal cortex (Temp); intermediate, the striatum (Str) and thalamus (Thal); and negligible, the cerebellum (Cer).

The plasma time–activity curve was determined from 34 arterial blood samples obtained throughout the study with about 20 samples collected during the initial 2 min. The kinetics of unchanged and metabolized [^{11}C]WAY 100635 in plasma were determined using thin layer chromatography at five times: 2, 10, 30, 60, and 90 min.

A. Kinetic Methods

The data were analyzed using linear compartment models. The general configuration is a conventional four-compartment (4C) model. In this model, C_1 contains the unmetabolized drug in plasma and C_2, C_3, and C_4, respectively, contain the free, specifically bound, and nonspecifically bound drug in the brain. The bidirectional transport of drug across the blood–brain barrier is described by K_1 (ml/min/ml) and k_2 (min^{-1}). The association and dissociation rates for specific binding are reflected in k_3 (min^{-1}) and k_4 (min^{-1}), and those for nonspecific binding in k_5 (min^{-1}) and k_6 (min^{-1}). The model equations are

$$\frac{dC_2}{dt} = K_1 C_1 - (k_2 + k_3 + k_5) C_2 + k_4 C_3 + k_6 C_4 \quad (1)$$

$$\frac{dC_3}{dt} = k_3 C_2 - k_4 C_3 \quad (2)$$

$$\frac{dC_4}{dt} = k_5 C_2 - k_6 C_4 \quad (3)$$

$$C_{\text{MOD}} = C_2 + C_3 + C_4 + (\text{BV})C_P \quad (4)$$

The model solution (C_{MOD}) of equation (4) includes an additional parameter for the tissue blood volume (BV) that corresponds to a fractional amount of the total plasma concentration (C_p).

TABLE 1 Compartmental Model Configurations, [^{11}C]WAY 100635 Monkey Data

Region	Model compartments	Method	Parameters floated	Parameters fixed
Nonspecific	2 (1 Tissue)	A_{NS}	K_1, k_2, BV	$k_3 = k_4 = k_5 = k_6 = 0$
	3 (2 Tissue)	B_{NS}	K_1–k_4, BV	$k_5 = k_6 = 0$
Specific	4 (3 Tissue)	A_{SP}	K_1–k_4, BV	$k_5 = k_{3\text{Cer}}$, $k_6 = k_{4\text{Cer}}$
	4 (3 Tissue)	B_{SP}	K_1, k_3, k_4, BV	$K_1/k_2 = K_1/k_{2\text{Cer}}$
				$k_5 = k_{3\text{Cer}}$, $k_6 = k_{4\text{Cer}}$
	3 (2 Tissue)	C_{SP}	K_1–k_4, BV	$k_5 = k_6 = 0$

Note. All configurations have an additional blood volume (BV) parameter.

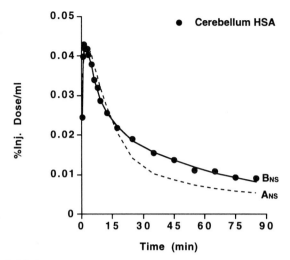

FIGURE 1 Two- and three-compartment model curve fits to cerebellar data: Model fits to the high specific activity cerebellar data displaying the lack of fit by the two-compartment model (A_{NS}). The cerebellar and blocking data were best described by a three-compartment model (B_{NS}).

A variety of configurations were applied to the nonspecific (NS) and specific (SP) data that correspond to the cerebellar or blocking data and to regions with known specific receptor binding, respectively. The different configurations for the NS (Methods A_{NS}, B_{NS}) and SP (Methods A_{SP}, B_{SP}, C_{SP}) data are described in Table 1. Nested models were compared using an F-test with significance assigned to $p < 0.05$. All models were compared using the Akaike information criteria (AIC) (Akaike, 1974) although statistical significance was not evaluated. Regional distribution volumes (DV) were determined and normalized to the cerebellar values (DV_{Ratio}).

III. RESULTS AND DISCUSSION

The metabolism of [^{11}C]WAY 100635 was rapid with unchanged percentages of about 80 and 20% at 2 and 90 min post injection, respectively.

The cerebellar data were not well described by a two-compartment (2C) model (Method A_{NS}) and fit significantly better for all monkeys (F-test) by a three-compartment (3C) model (Method B_{NS}) as shown in Figure 1. The average ($n = 8$) cerebellar 3C DV value, $K_1/k_2 (1 + k_3/k_4)$, was 5.0 ± 2.1 with slow nonspecific binding parameters of 0.02 ± 0.01 for k_3 and 0.02 ± 0.01 for k_4.

Similarly, all blocking data (cerebellum included) were significantly better described (F-test) by a 3C

model than a 2C model. The 3C DV values ($n = 5$ ROIs) were 3.9 ± 0.7 and 5.5 ± 0.8 for 8-OH-DPAT and MPPI, respectively. On average, k_3 and k_4 were similar to the HSA cerebellar values although more variable for the MPPI data: 8-OH-DPAT, 0.03 ± 0.01 and 0.04 ± 0.02; MPPI, 0.03 ± 0.04 and 0.06 ± 0.08. The blocking data yielded frontal DV values that were about 70% lower than the HSA values, a reduction consistent with that reported by Hume *et al.* (1994) for 8-OH-DPAT in rats.

Three curve fitting strategies were applied to the SP data (Table 1). The NS results suggested the use of a 4C model configuration for the SP data. The SP data were fairly well fit by a 4C model when the nonspecific parameters were constrained to the cerebellar values (Method A_{SP}) but not as well when K_1/k_2 was additionally constrained (Method B_{SP}). Therefore, an unconstrained 3C model was applied to the SP data (Method C_{SP}), Figure 2. In general, the 4C models did not perform as well as the 3C model with occasional convergence problems and large individual parameter errors ($>50\%$). The unconstrained 3C model was best across regions and monkeys as compared to the 4C models (F-test). The average 3C results are listed in Table 2. The DV values range from about 19.0 to 7.3 ml/ml (Frt

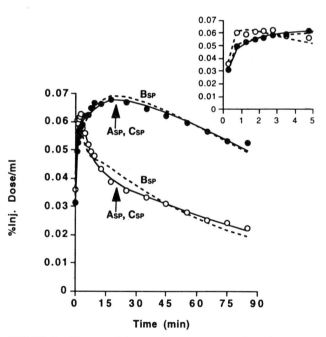

FIGURE 2 Three- and four-compartment model fit to frontal and striatal data: The SP data (Frt, solid circles; Str, open circles) were fairly well fit by a 4C model when the nonspecific parameters were constrained to the cerebellar values (A_{SP}, solid line) but not as well fit with the K_1/k_2 ratio additionally constrained (B_{SP}, dashed line). Therefore, an unconstrained 3C model (C_{SP}, solid line) was applied. The inset graph corresponds to the initial 5 min.

TABLE 2 Three-Compartment Model Results,
[^{11}C]WAY 100635 Monkey Data

Region	K_1/k_2	k_3/k_4	DV (ml/ml)	DV$_{Ratio}$
Frt	3.9 ± 1.5	4.6 ± 2.4	19.0 ± 4.7	4.3 ± 1.0
Temp	4.4 ± 2.1	3.9 ± 2.6	17.6 ± 5.4	3.7 ± 0.7
Str	3.1 ± 1.0	2.0 ± 0.5	8.5 ± 2.7	1.9 ± 0.6
Thal	3.2 ± 1.1	1.3 ± 0.4	7.3 ± 2.7	1.7 ± 0.4
Cer	2.3 ± 0.8	1.2 ± 0.4	5.0 ± 2.1	—

Note. Averages of individual values across monkeys, where
DV $= K_1/k_2(1 + k_3/k_4)$; DV$_{Ratio}$ is DV normalized to the cerebellar
DV value.

to Thal) and follow the rank order of 5-HT$_{1A}$ receptor density. However, for one monkey, the thalamus k_4 value was nearly 0 and $n = 7$ for this region. The BV value was variable across regions and monkeys with an average of about $0.02 \pm 0.02\%$ across all regions.

Alternatives were preliminarily investigated to address the apparent inconsistency of using 3C models for both the NS and SP data. Specifically, speculative models were considered that allowed for (1) irreversible nonspecific binding (Method A_1) and (2) transport of metabolites across the blood–brain barrier (Method A_2). For SP data, Method A_1 is a 4C configuration with the K_1/k_2 ratio constrained to the cerebellar value and $k_6 = 0$ (operationally k_6 was fixed to 1E-6). Method A_2 represents parallel 2C models with transport parameters of K_1 and k_2 for unmetabolized [^{11}C]WAY 100635 and K_1' and k_2' for the radiolabeled metabolites of [^{11}C]WAY 100635.

The F-test results showed that, for the NS data, an irreversible nonspecific binding model (3C model with $k_4 = 0$) was not significantly better than the full 3C model for the cerebellar (7 of 8 monkeys) or 8-OH-DPAT blocking data, although for the MPPI study the model was adequate (4 of 5 ROIs). This speculative model provided adequate curve fits to the SP data (Fig. 3). The AIC values (lower AIC value indicative of a better fit) indicated that Method A_1 was better for the frontal cortex (7 of 8 monkeys) and temporal cortex (5 of 8 monkeys) but equivalent for the striatum and thalamus as compared to the 3C model. The DV values were determined for C_2 and C_3, as $K_1/(k_2+k_5) + K_1/k_2(k_3/k_4)$. The regional DV values were considerably lower than the 3C DV values. However, normalization of the DV values by the four-parameter cerebellar DV value of $K_1/(k_2 + k_3)$ resulted in DV$_{Ratio}$ values of 3.6 ± 1.1, 2.9 ± 0.8, 1.8 ± 0.4, and 1.8 ± 0.4 for the Frt, Temp, Str, and Thal, respectively. These normalized values are in reasonable agreement with the 3C DV$_{Ratio}$ values. These results further support inconsistencies

between the cerebellar and specific-binding kinetics and support the possibility of an irreversible nonspecific binding component.

The evaluation of the metabolite model (Method A_2) was restricted to the cerebellar and blocking data. An input function for the metabolites was not known and was simulated simply using the total concentration of metabolites in plasma. The data were adequately fit for most cases using Method A_2, but occasionally large parameter errors resulted, as did problems with convergence, as reflected by AIC values that were sometimes twice as large as those for the 3C method.

These overall kinetic modeling results indicate an apparent inconsistency between the cerebellar kinetics and the kinetics in specific-binding regions. The cerebellar and blocking data indicated a second kinetically distinguishable brain compartment. Although complete receptor occupancy may not have been achieved during the blocking studies, the cerebellum (a region thought to be devoid of 5-HT$_{1A}$ receptors) still required five parameters. The suitability of a 3C model for the cerebellar, blocking, and specific-binding data casts doubt on what the individual kinetic parameters represent. Nonetheless, the regional DV values follow the rank order of 5-HT$_{1A}$ receptor density (Pazos *et al.*, 1987).

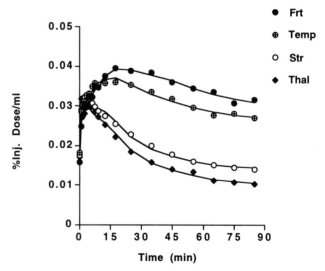

FIGURE 3 Alternative model fit to the regional PET data: Alternative model fit, using Method A_1 (K_1/k_2 constrained, $k_6 = 0$). The F-test results showed that Method A_1 was not significantly better than the 3C model for the cerebellar and 8-OH-DPAT blocking data, although it was adequate for some regions of the MPPI study. The AIC values indicated that Method A_1 was better than the 3C model for the Frt and Temp but equivalent for the Str and Thal.

It is possible that a radiolabeled metabolite, such as [^{11}C]WAY 100634, crosses the blood–brain barrier, contributing to the observed PET signal. Biodistribution studies in rats of [^{11}C]WAY 100634 (the putative metabolite of WAY 100635) resulted in a frontopolar : cerebellar ratio of 1.4 that was not significantly affected by predosing with WAY 100635 (Pike *et al.*, 1995). The poorer fits obtained with the metabolite model (Method A_2) did not support the passage of radiolabeled metabolites across the blood–brain barrier, but these results were complicated because the concentration of all metabolites was used to simulate the metabolite input function.

The model configuration that allowed for irreversible nonspecific binding proved to be more appropriate for the frontal and temporal regions than for the thalamus and striatum. Pike *et al.* (1995) reported a 37% lower tissue ratio in rat caudate as compared to the pontofrontal region after injection of the putative metabolite [^{11}C]-WAY 100634. However, predosing with WAY 100635 (or an α_1 antagonist) did not change these values. It is possible that metabolites bind to receptors in primates.

An appropriate model that bridges the inconsistency between the nonspecific binding kinetics and the kinetics in specific-binding regions was not identified in this chapter, although tracer kinetic modeling did provide adequate fits to the regional [^{11}C]WAY 100635 monkey data. Further *in vivo* evaluation of [^{11}C]WAY 100635 and its putative metabolite [^{11}C]WAY 100634 in primates is needed to fully characterize the kinetics of [^{11}C]WAY 100635, labeled in the 2-methoxy position with ^{11}C.

Acknowledgments

The helpful comments of Drs. Gwenn Smith and David Townsend and technical assistance of Brian Lopresti were genuinely appreciated.

References

Akaike, H. (1974). A new look at the statistical model identification. *IEEE Trans. Automat. Contr.* AC-**19**: 716–723.

Hume, S. P., Ashworth, S., Opaka-Juffry, J., Ahier, R. G., Lammertsma, A. A., Pike V. W., Cliffe I. A., Fletcher, A., and White, A. C. (1994). Evaluation of [O-methyl-^{3}H]WAY-100635 as an in vivo radioligand for 5-HT$_{1A}$ receptors in rat brain. *Eur. J. Pharmacol.* **271**: 515–523.

Kung, M. P., Frederick, D., Mu, M., Zhuang, Z.P., and Kung, H. F. (1995). 4-(2'-Methoxy-phenyl)-1-[2'-(n-2''-pyridinyl)-p-iodobenzamido]-ethyl-piperazine ([125I]p-MPPI) as a new selective radioligand of serotonin-1A sites in rat brain: In vitro binding and autoradiographic studies. (1995). *J. Pharmacol. Exp. Ther.* **272**(1): 429–37.

Mathis, C. A., Simpson, N. R., Mahmood, K., Kinahan, P., and Mintun, M. (1994). [^{11}C]WAY-100635: A radioligand for imaging 5-HT$_{1A}$ receptors with positron emission tomography. *Life Sci.* **55**(20): 403–407.

Pazos, A., Probst, A., and Palacios, J. M. (1987). Serotonin receptors in the human brain—III. Autoradiographic mapping of serotonin-1 receptors. *Neuroscience* **21**: 97–122.

Pike, V. W., McCarron, J. A., Hume, S. P., Ashworth, S., Opacka-Juffry, J., Osman, S., Lammertsma, A. A., Poole, K. G., Fletcher, A., White, A. C., and Cliffe, I. A. (1995). Pre-clinical development of a radioligand for studies of central 5-HT$_{1A}$ receptors in vivo -[^{11}C]WAY-100635. *Med. Chem. Res.* **5**: 208–227.

Stahl, S. M., Gastpar, M., Hesselink, J. M., and Traber, J. (eds.). (1992). Serotonin 1A Receptors in Depression and Anxiety. Raven Press, New York.

Zhuang, Z.-P., Kung, M.-P., Chumpradit, S., Mu, M., Kung, H. F. (1994). Derivatives of 4-(2'-methoxyphenyl)-1-[2'-(N-2''-pyridinyl-p-iodobenzamido)ethyl]piperazine (p-MPPI) as 5-HT$_{1A}$ ligands. *J. Med. Chem.* **37**: 4572–4575.

Measurement of [11C]Raclopride Binding Using a Bolus plus Infusion Protocol

S. HOULE, S. KAPUR, D. HUSSEY, C. JONES, J. DASILVA, and A. A. WILSON

PET Centre, Clarke Institute of Psychiatry
University of Toronto
Toronto, Canada M5T 1R8

The ratio of basal ganglia to cerebellar uptake of [11C]-raclopride is often used as an index of dopamine D_2 receptor density. We describe a bolus plus constant infusion technique and a data analysis approach that provides reliable estimates of the bound-to-free radioligand ratio. The technique does not require arterial blood sampling or correction for metabolites and protein binding. We first develop our method by computer simulation then apply it to PET studies of 12 control subjects and to 15 receptor occupancy studies. We use nonlinear curve-fitting methods to obtain the free and bound time–activity curves. We then solve the differential equation describing the transport of radioligand between the free and bound compartments, but without assuming equilibrium conditions. Because of this, our data analysis technique applies equally well to bolus injection studies. Computer simulations indicate that the free receptor index obtained with our method is not sensitive to changes in cerebral blood flow when applied to both the bolus and the bolus plus infusion methods. Our bolus plus infusion is a simple and reliable technique for clinical research.

I. INTRODUCTION

The basal ganglia (BG)-to-cerebellar ratio of [11C]-raclopride uptake is often used as an index of D_2 receptor density. Many variants of the original "equilibrium" technique introduced by Farde *et al.* (1989) have been used for clinical research. These techniques are advantageous for clinical investigations because neither arterial sampling nor correction for plasma binding

and plasma metabolites is required. Despite their demonstrated usefulness as a clinical research tool, these methods have often been criticized because true equilibrium is never achieved following a bolus injection of [11C]raclopride. True equilibrium can be achieved with a constant infusion. However, it is more practical to combine a bolus injection, as a loading dose, with a constant infusion because equilibrium can be achieved faster in this manner. Such a bolus plus constant infusion (B/I) technique was proposed by Carson *et al.* for cyclofoxy (Carson *et al.*, 1993). We were encouraged by the preliminary results of Minoshima and colleagues (1994) to apply the B/I method to [11C]raclopride. We first tested the B/I method by kinetic model simulations. We then applied the B/I technique to 12 [11C] raclopride PET studies of control subjects and 15 receptor occupancy studies in patients with schizophrenia. We also compared, by model simulation, the bolus only to the B/I method.

II. MATERIAL AND METHODS

A. Kinetic Model

We use the conventional three-compartment model for raclopride with the cerebellum as a reference region devoid of dopamine receptors (Farde *et al.*, 1989). For high specific activity, the rate equations for this model are

$$\frac{dC_f}{dt} = K_1 C_p - (k_2 + k_3)C_f + k_4 C_b \qquad (1)$$

$$\frac{dC_b}{dt} = k_3 C_f - k_4 C_b \qquad (2)$$

where $C_p(t)$ is the arterial plasma concentration of the radiotracer, $C_f(t)$ the concentration of free ligand in the brain, and $C_b(t)$ the concentration specifically bound to dopamine receptors. The rate constant k_3 is proportional to the free receptor density ($B_{max} - B$), where B is the concentration of receptors occupied either by endogenous dopamine or a drug. The ratio k_3/k_4, which is equal to ($B_{max} - B$)/K_d, is a convenient index of the free receptor density. When $dC_b(t)/dt$ equals 0, the ratio k_3/k_4 is equal to the ratio $C_b(t)/C_f(t)$. This equality occurs either at the peak of the $C_b(t)$ curve (Farde *et al.*, 1989) or if true equilibrium exists between the compartments.

B. Computer Simulations

We solved equations (1) and (2) by numerical integration, using published rate constants (Farde *et al.*, 1989). For the bolus plus constant infusion, the arterial plasma input function $C_p(t)$ is the convolution of the arterial plasma curve $C_a(t)$, obtained after bolus injection of a quantity Q of radioligand, with a function representing the bolus plus constant infusion schedule:

$$C_p(t) = C_a(t) \otimes \{Q\delta(t) + Ru(t)\}/A \qquad (3)$$

where $\delta(t)$ is the Kronecker delta and $u(t)$ the unit step function; R is the decay-corrected constant infusion rate (min^{-1}). The total amount of radioligand injected is $A = Q + (R/\lambda)[1 - \exp(-\lambda T)]$, where T is the time at the end of the infusion (normally the end of study) and λ the decay constant of carbon-11.

The time–activity curve in the basal ganglia is $C_{BG}(t) = C_f(t) + C_b(t)$. The data points for the simulated PET scans are obtained by integrating the time–activity curves for each of the scan intervals.

We used these computer simulations to determine the optimal infusion rate for control subjects (Patlak and Pettigrew, 1976; Carson *et al.*, 1993). We also used simulation to assess the effects of (1) receptor occupancy, (2) rate of clearance of the free ligand in the plasma, and (3) varying the parameters K_1 and k_2, which are both dependent on blood flow.

C. Data Analysis

We proceed as follows to calculate the ratio k_3/k_4 from equation (2). We first fit a biexponential function to the cerebellar time activity curve using Marquardt nonlinear least squares method. In all our fitting procedures, we do not include the data points from the first 10 minutes of the study, when there are rapid variations in all time–activity curves as well as significant contribution from the blood in the first minute or two after the bolus injection. By not including these rapidly varying

segments of the curves, we can use simpler fitting functions and achieve more reliable estimates of the fit parameters. We then subtract the fitted cerebellar curve from the basal ganglia curves to obtain the bound ligand time–activity curve. This curve is then fitted with the following function:

$$b(t) = b_0[1 - \exp(-b_1 t)](1 + b_2 t) \qquad (4)$$

where $b_2 \ll b_1$ for a bolus plus constant infusion. This function is the same as that proposed by Lundqvist, Anderson, and Tedroff (1989), except that we use the truncated Taylor expansion ($1 + b_2 t$) instead of $\exp(b_2 t)$. The fitted curve for the bound ligand is differentiated analytically to obtain $dC_b(t)/dt$. We then have a set of linear equations for the time points t_i:

$$\frac{dC_b(t_i)}{dt} = k_3 C_f(t_i) - k_4 C_b(t_i) \qquad (5)$$

We solve this set for k_3 and k_4 and obtain the free receptor index without assuming that $dC_b(t)/dt$ is 0.

D. PET Studies

We use a bolus injection of 300 MBq of [^{11}C]raclopride followed by a constant infusion at a rate of 2.7 MBq/min. We scanned our subjects with a GEMS PC2048-15B camera. We acquired the PET data for 75 min with a time per frame of 1 min for the first 15 min and then 5 min to the end of the study. We corrected the PET data for decay and attenuation. Using ROIs drawn on coregistered MRI studies, we created time–activity curves for the basal ganglia (bound and free) and cerebellum (free). We analyzed the PET data as described previously.

III. RESULTS AND DISCUSSION

We found that near equilibrium conditions could be achieved with $Q = 450$ and $R = 4$ min^{-1}. Figure 1 shows the simulated curves for receptor occupancy ranging from 0 to 90%. The free ligand curves (not shown) also reach a plateau within about 30 min. The values that we found optimal for Q and R are very similar to those of Minoshima *et al.* (1994). These values are not optimal for all subjects because the infusion rate needed to achieve equilibrium is dependent on the peripheral clearance and metabolism of raclopride. Because of individual variations, it is not possible to preselect a single fixed B/I infusion schedule to achieve perfect equilibrium in all subjects within the time span of a [^{11}C]raclopride study (i.e., 45–90 min). Our human PET studies did in fact show that, in practice, complete

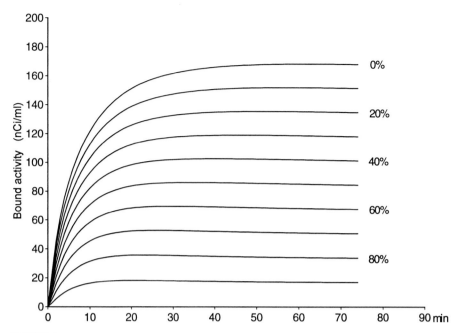

FIGURE 1   Simulated curves for the bound activity $C_b(t)$ for receptor occupancy ranging from 0 to 90%.

equilibrium is not always achieved. Therefore, we include the term $(1 + b_2 t)$ in our fitting function to account for such deviations from ideal equilibrium.

In fact, due to its ability to deal with nonequilibrium situations, our analysis method applies equally well to the bolus technique. Instead of assuming equilibrium at the peak of the bound curve or during the plateau phase, we fit the model to the nonequilibrium situation. We also simulated varying degrees of receptor occupancy for the bolus and the B/I injection techniques. Using our data analysis technique, we found no significant differences between the two methods.

Our simulations also showed that both the B/I and the bolus methods are also insensitive to changes in the values of K_1 alone (from 0.08 to 0.35), to changes in k_2 alone (from 0.33 to 0.38), or to changes in both K_1 and k_2 when the ratio K_1/k_2 was maintained relatively constant. These results indicate that our technique is not sensitive to physiological changes in blood flow.

In studies with high receptor occupancy, the bound time–activity curves tend to be noisy (low signal-to-noise ratio), and in Farde *et al.*'s original technique, it becomes impossible to determine with certainty the point in time for which $dC_b(t)/dt$ is 0. To deal with this situation, previous investigators have used an "area under the curve" approach, which essentially consists of integrating equation (2) to estimate the free receptor density. The integral version of equation (2) is

$$C_b(T_2) - C_b(T_1) = k_3 \int_{T_1}^{T_2} C_f(\tau)d\tau - k_4 \int_{T_1}^{T_2} C_b(\tau)d\tau \qquad (6)$$

If $C_b(t)$ and $C_f(t)$ are both in equilibrium between T_1 and T_2, then the free receptor index is the ratio of the average values of $C_b(t)$ over $C_f(t)$ in that interval, because the left side of equation (3) will be 0. However, because true equilibrium is not achieved after bolus injection of [^{11}C]raclopride, the latter approach is, at best, an approximation of the ideal equilibrium state. The accuracy of that method depends on both the chosen time interval and how much the free and bound time–activity curves deviate from an assumed plateau during that time interval. Our simulations showed that the ratio k_3/k_4 was overestimated by about 10% when T_1 was chosen as 21 min and T_2 as 33 min, as used by Nordström *et al.* (1993). Our data analysis circumvents this problem by making no assumption about the left-hand side of equations (2) and (3).

Figure 2 shows an example of the curves typically obtained in a control subject. The mean value of k_3/k_4 was 2.95 (± 0.3) for both the left and right caudate and putamen in our control subjects. In the receptor occupancy study, as the level of occupancy increases, the fitting function for the bound curve in equation (4) can be replaced by a straight line, $b_0(1 + b_2 t)$, as predicted from our simulations (because we ignore the first 10–15 min of the study in our fitting procedure).

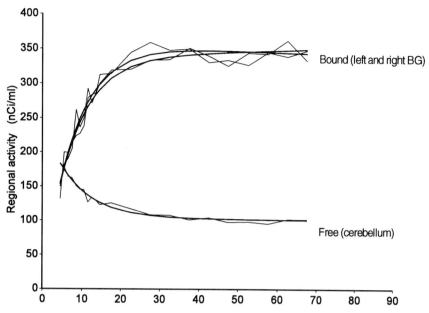

FIGURE 2 Actual and fitted curves for a typical bolus plus infusion study in a control subject.

We have now applied this method in 15 patients with reliable results at receptor occupancy levels ranging from 50 to 90%.

Our approach to modeling is easily extended to other radioligands with kinetics similar to that of raclopride. We have applied our approach to the determination of k_3/k_4 for [^{11}C]SCH 23390 and for [^{18}F]setoperone with equally satisfactory results.

In summary, clinical research requires simple and reliable methods that avoid arterial sampling. The bolus plus infusion method and the data analysis described have met these criteria. It provides reliable estimates of k_3/k_4 and does so without any assumption regarding equilibrium. The technique can be used over the entire range of receptor occupancy and is robust in the face of physiological changes in cerebral blood flow.

Acknowledgment

We thank Astra Arcus AB for their generous supply of the precursor to raclopride.

References

Carson, R. E., Channing, M. A., Blasberg, R. G., Dunn, B. B., Cohen, R. M., Rice, K. C., and Herscovitch, P. (1993). *J. Cereb. Blood Flow Metab.* **13:** 24–42.

Farde, L., Eriksson, L., Blomquist, G., and Halldin, C. (1989). Kinetic analysis of central [^{11}C]raclopride binding to D$_2$–dopamine receptors studied by PET—A comparison to the equilibrium analysis. *J. Cereb. Blood Flow Metab.* **9:** 696–708.

Lundqvist, H., Anderson, J., and Tedroff, J. (1989). Quantitative analysis of receptor binding studies. *In:* "Positron Emission Tomography in Clinical Research and Clinical Diagnosis: Tracer Modeling and Radioreceptors." (C. Beckers *et al.*, Eds.), pp. 65–80. ECSC, EEC, EAEC, Brussels.

Minoshima, S., Koeppe, R. A., Mukhopadhyay, S., Jewett, D., Kuhl, D. E., Kilbourn, M. R., and Frey, K. A. (1994). Equilibrium measurement of [C-11]raclopride distribution volume in the brain using a continuous infusion technique. *J. Nucl. Med.* **35:** 140P.

Nordström, A.-L., Farde, L., Wiesel, F.-A., Forslund, K., Pauli, S., Halldin, C., and Uppfeldt, G. (1993). Central D$_2$-dopamine receptor occupancy in relation to antipsychotic drug effects: A double-blind PET study of schizophrenic patients. *Biol. Psychiatry* **33:** 227–235.

Patlak, C. S., and Pettigrew, K. D. (1976). A method to obtain infusion schedules for prescribed blood concentration time courses. *J. Appl. Physiol.* **40:** 458–463.

The Analysis of Brain PET Radioligand Displacement Studies

A. L. MALIZIA,[1,3] K. J. FRISTON,[1,2] R. N. GUNN,[1] V. J. CUNNINGHAM,[1] S. WILSON,[3] T. JONES,[1] and D. J. NUTT[3]

[1]MRC Cyclotron Unit, Hammersmith Hospital
London W12 0NN, United Kingdom
[2]Wellcome Cognitive Neurology Department
London WCIN 3BG, United Kingdom
[3]Psychopharmacology Unit, University of Bristol
Bristol BS8 1TD, United Kingdom

The voxel based statistical analysis of radioligand displacement studies is a prerequisite for the PET investigation of endogenous ligand release with cognitive activation or other challenges. We describe the application of a method developed for such an analysis that combines a two compartmental kinetic model with the general linear theory as applied in statistical parametric mapping. The data from five normal volunteers who had three [11C] PET scans, one with the tracer alone, one with mid-scan intravenous midazolam displacement, and one with cold flumazenil preloading, indicate that this method is viable for the analysis of such a displacement at cerebral benzodiazepine sites, although its sensitivity still needs to be evaluated.

I. INTRODUCTION

The success of physiological activation work using either H_2O or CO_2 PET in the last five or so years has depended on the ability to generate statistical maps that convey information about increased or decreased hemodynamic demands made by brain areas as they engage in a task. Radioligand work has, however, thus far, concentrated mainly on the description of baseline receptor pharmacokinetic measures and on how these change with disease or therapeutic intervention, much in the same way as FDG PET was originally used in the physiological arena.

Radioligands are now produced that have the potential to be displaced not only by exogenous administration of competing agonists but also by the release of endogenous ligands; for example, [11C]diprenorphine and endogenous opiates or [11C]flumazenil and endozapines (endogenous benzodiazepine ligands). The release of an endogenous ligand can be induced psychologically as in a change in mood, physiologically as in the induction of pain, pathologically as in the induction of a seizure, or pharmacologically, for example, by action on heteroreceptors or upstream neurochemical systems. Although the methodology of measuring pharmacokinetic changes at expected sites of action has been developed for some time, no technique, to date, allows a voxel based "a priori" statistical analysis of ligand displacement. Such a technique would permit the assessment of significant effects, thus opening up functional neurochemistry to PET imaging.

We describe the application of a method that performs such an analysis based on the amalgamation of compartmental kinetic modeling and general linear theory as applied in statistical parametric mapping (Friston *et al.*, 1995b).

II. THEORY

The theory of this method is described separately (Friston *et al.*, 1995c) and at present is restricted to the analysis of effects for ligands like [^{11}C]flumazenil, which can be modeled using a two compartmental model (Koeppe *et al.*, 1991). The essence of the method is that the time-dependent change in tissue ligand concentration, at each voxel, can be modeled by

$$dC_i(t)/dt = \kappa_{1i}C_p(t - \delta_i) - (\kappa_2(t)_i + \lambda) \cdot C_i(t)$$

where C_i is the concentration of ligand in tissue at voxel i, C_p is the free concentration of ligand in the plasma as measured by the arterial sampling, κ_{1i} is the constant characterizing the rate of entry into the tissue at voxel i, $\kappa_2(t)_i$ is the time dependent parameter characterizing the exit of the ligand from the tissue, δ_i is the delay between the peripheral sampling point and the brain voxel i, and λ is the radioactivity decay constant.

Each of κ_{1i}, $\kappa_2(t)_i$, and δ_i can be expanded as a composite of a regionally invariant or canonical value (e.g., κ_1^*), a voxel specific value (e.g., $\Delta\kappa_{2i}$), and a voxel-specific, time-dependent expanded component due to the "activation" (e.g., $\gamma_i \cdot h(t)$, where $h(t)$ is the time course of displacement about which one wants to make an inference and $\gamma_i = 0$ under the null hypothesis). Thus, for a displacement occurring late in the study where effects due to κ_1 would be small because of a very low C_p, the expansions can be written as

$$\kappa_2(t)_i = \kappa_2^* + \Delta\kappa_{2i} + \gamma_i \cdot h(t)$$
$$\kappa_{1i} = \kappa_1^* + \Delta\kappa_{1i}$$
$$\delta_i = \delta^* + \Delta\delta_i$$

The observed counts per frame are approximated to the sum of the canonical values over the time of acquisition, the voxel-specific values, and the time-dependent, voxel-specific component due to the activation. This technique tests whether the voxel-based data are best fitted, in a sum of squares sense, by the inclusion of

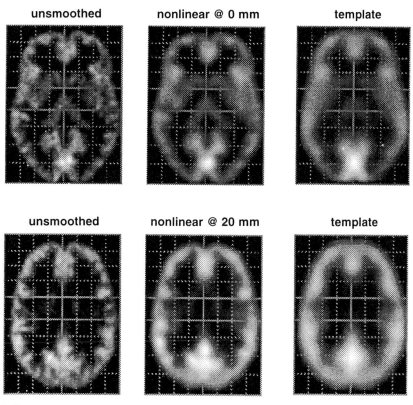

FIGURE 1 Example of 12-parameter affine (linear) normalization of the scans prior to processing. The template is shown on the extreme right, and the normalized images on the left and in the center. See the text for details.

the time-dependent term, the null hypothesis being that its coefficient is 0. This test uses the general linear model and standard statistical inference to generate a *t*-statistical inference to generate a *t*-statistic for all voxels. These statistics constitute a SPM(t).

In addition the parameters κ_2, $V_d(\kappa_{1i}/\kappa_2(t)_i + \lambda)$ and the average relative change in κ_2 (expressed as the difference in the integral of predicted and observed $\kappa_2\delta t$ over the whole scan period) can also be computed. These have to be regarded as rough indices of the same parameters calculated in a kinetic model because of the (first-order) assumptions implicit in the approximations used in this statistical model and the smoothing applied to the images prior to analysis. They can, however, be used as a guide to the relative size of any effect and as a concurrent validation of this model.

III. METHOD

Five healthy male volunteers had three [^{11}C]flumazenil PET scans as part of an ongoing pharmacokinetic–pharmacodynamic experiment. The [^{11}C]flumazenil was prepared by a modification of the method described by Maziere *et al.* (1984). The data was acquired on a CTI-Siemens 953B with the septa retracted; that is, in 3D mode (Spinks *et al.*, 1992). Each scan was acquired for 105 min after the injection of 200–280 MBq of radiotracer. And, 25 frames were recorded (3 × 60 sec, 19 × 180 sec, 3 × 900 sec). In one study, the tracer alone was injected; in another an infusion of 50 μg/kg midazolam was injected intravenously for 5 min between 30 and 35 min; in the third, a loading injection of 2.5–10 μg/kg cold flumazenil was followed by an infusion of 2.5–10 μg/hr cold flumazenil, starting 60 min prior to the pulse of radioligand, thus performing an ''equilibrium'' experiment. In each experiment, a 22-gauge cannula was inserted in the nondominant radial artery and a similar cannula in the contralateral antecubital vein. The infusions were administered using an IMAC pump.

Radioactive counts in arterial blood were continuously monitored using a BGO detector and discrete arterial sampling was used to calibrate the system using a well counter and to determine the free fraction of unmetabolized [^{11}C]flumazenil in plasma. A metabolite corrected input function was thus obtained. The attenuation was measured prior to the scan using germanium rods. Scatter correction was applied using a dual-window method developed in-house (Grootoonk *et al.*, 1993).

The frames were realigned and then the data were spatially normalized (Fig. 1) using a 12-parameter affine transformation that best matched a template [^{11}C]flumazenil image, conforming to standard anatomical space (Talairach and Tournoux, 1988). This technique uses a linear least squares approach (Friston *et al.*, 1995a). Data were then smoothed with a Gaussian kernel (FWHM of 8 mm) and only voxels exceeding 80% of global activity were subject to further analysis. The algorithm requires the time of onset of displacement and the duration of the perturbation. The delay between the start of the infusion and the beginning of the change in slope of the time–activity curve is of the order of one frame. The form of $h(t)$ (the induced time dependent change in k_2) was assumed to be exponential, starting with the infusion.

All scans were, therefore, analyzed (whether in a displacement experiment or not) as if they had a displacement, to assess the robustness of the technique. The prediction was that only scans in which a displacement had actually occurred would show significant differences accounted for by the time-dependent component, and for scans where no displacement had taken place, there would be no significant differences accounted for by this term. The calculated V_d, the $t_{1/2}$ of [^{11}C]flumazenil for the whole scan and the proportional change in mean κ_2 were also calculated.

IV. RESULTS

For all the displacement studies, statistical maps indicated a very significant time-dependent effect in the majority of cortical voxels (e.g., Fig. 2 for one subject). None of the tracer-alone experiments showed such an effect. One preloading experiment showed a spatially limited effect bilaterally on the temporo-occipital border, whose significance is at present unknown. In this experiment, the number of significant voxels was 900 out of 40,000 compared with 20–35,000 in the displacement experiments. The calculated parameters showed an average 15% decrease in V_d in the displacement experiments. While in the preloading experiments V_d changes were proportional to the dose infused. κ_2 changed accordingly in the expected direction. The distribution of increases in k_2 are shown in Figure 3 for one of the subjects.

V. DISCUSSION

This technique was successful in identifying all the studies where a displacement was produced by the exogenous administration of midazolam. It produced no false positives in 9 of the other 10 scans even though

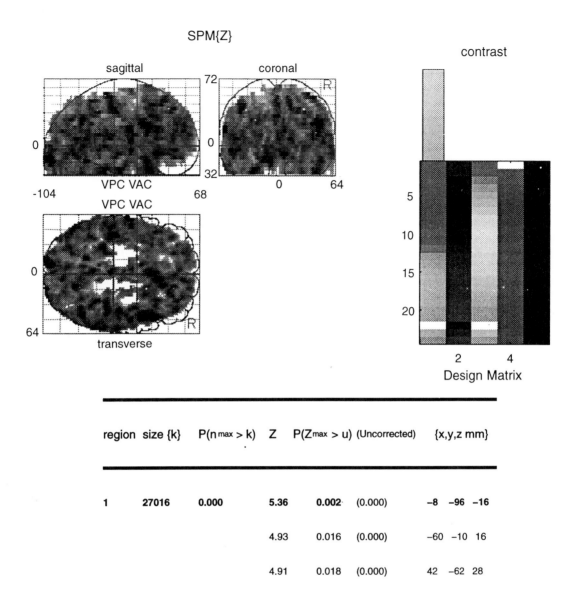

region	size {k}	P(n max > k)	Z	P(Zmax > u)	(Uncorrected)	{x,y,z mm}
1	27016	0.000	5.36	0.002	(0.000)	−8 −96 −16
			4.93	0.016	(0.000)	−60 −10 16
			4.91	0.018	(0.000)	42 −62 28

Threshold = 1.64; Volume [S] = 53333 voxels; df = 19

FWHM = [8.2 9.7 9.8] mm (i.e. 1091 RESELS)

FIGURE 2 Example of SPM{Z} map. The three projections provide a map of all the voxels in which a significant displacement has been detected prior to correction for multiple comparisons. The blocks on the right show the experimental matrix. The table shows that a volume of 27,016 contiguous voxels out of 53,333 had a significant displacement in this study.

the two compartmental fit produced an overestimate of k_2. This overestimate was higher in the preloading studies, confirming the limited validity of a one extravascular compartmental model in the partially blocked state. The volumes of distribution for the whole scan and the $t_{1/2}$ in tissue were decreased and the k_2 was increased in both experimental conditions, compared with the control situation.

The V_d values obtained were smaller than in the corresponding spectral analysis, probably because of the smoothing. Pilot work demonstrated that the choice of displacement time and duration affected the results.

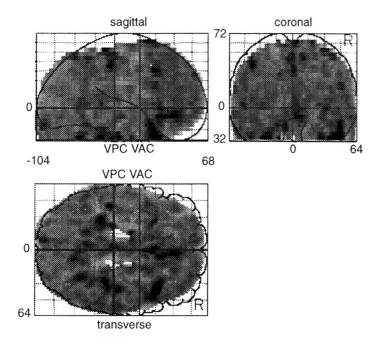

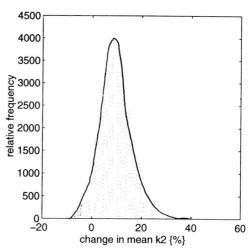

FIGURE 3   The distribution of change in k_2 after displacement is shown in the lower panel. The three projections indicate the areas where this has been most pronounced by an increase in density of blackness.

In this study all the displacements were assumed to start in the second frame of the infusion and last until the end of the scan because negligible amounts of [^{11}C]-flumazenil rebind after displacement, being washed into the blood stream and then dispersed. This technique, however, allows one to look for both tonic and phasic effects in either direction and for any duration of time during the scan, being limited by the temporal resolution of the frames and by the detection noise.

The technique needs to be refined; in particular more studies need to be processed to confirm its robustness, and the model should be expanded to include more than one extravascular compartment. It may, however, signal the dawn for *in vivo* PET neurochemistry activation.

Acknowledgments

ALM is a Wellcome training fellow. KJF is supported by the Wellcome Trust.

References

Friston, K. J., Ashburner, J., Frith, C. D., Poline, J.-B., Heather, J. D., and Frackowiak, R. S. J. (1995a). Spatial registration and normalisation of images. *Hum. Brain Mapping,* in press.

Friston, K. J., Holmes, A. P., Worsley, K. J., Poline, J.-P., Frith, C. D., and Frackowiak, R. S. J. (1995b). Statistical parametric maps in functional imaging: A general linear approach. *Hum. Brain Mapping,* **2:** 189–210.

Friston, K. J., Malizia, A. L., Wilson, S., Cunningham, V. J., Jones, T., and Nutt, D. J. (1995c). The analysis of dynamic radioligand displacement or 'activation' studies. Submitted for publication.

Grootoonk, S., Spinks, T. J., Bloomfield, P. M., Sashin, D., and Jones, T. (1993). The practical implementation and accuracy of dual window scatter correction in a neuroPET scanner with the septa retracted. *In:* IEEE Med Imaging Conference Records, vol. 5, pp. 942–944.

Koeppe, R. A., Holthoff, V. A., Frey, K. A., Kilbourn, M. R., and Kuhl, D. E. (1991). Compartmental analysis of [C-11] flumazenil kinetics for the estimation of ligand transport rate and receptor distribution using positron emission tomography. *J. Cereb. Blood Flow Metab.* **11,** 735–744.

Maziere, M., Hantraye, P., Prenant, C., Sastre, J., and Comar, D. (1984). Synthesis of an ethyl 8-fluoro-5,6-dihydro-5-[C-11]methyl-6-oxo-4H-imidazo[1,5-a][1,4]benzodiazepine-3-carboxylate (RO 15.1788-11C): A specific radioligand for the in vivo study of central benzodiazepine receptors by positron emission tomography. *Int. J. Appl. Radiat. Isot.* **35,** 973–976.

Spinks, T. J., Jones, T., Bailey, D. L., Townsend, D. W., Grootoonk, S., Bloomfield, P. M., Gilardi, M. C., Casey, M. E., Sipe, B., and Reed, J. (1992). Physical performance of a positron emission tomograph for brain imaging with retractable septa. *Phys. Med. Biol.* **8,** 1637–1655.

Talairach, J., and Tournoux, P. (1988). "Co-planar Stereotaxic Atlas of the Human Brain." Thieme, Stuttgart.

53

An Artificial Neural Network Approach to Estimation of the Regional Glucose Metabolism Using PET

CLAUS SVARER,[1] **IAN LAW,**[1] **SØREN HOLM,**[1] **NIELS MØRCH,**[1,2] **STEEN HASSELBALCH,**[1] **LARS K. HANSEN,**[2] **and OLAF B. PAULSON**[1]

[1]*Department of Neurology*
National University Hospital
Rigshospitalet
DK-2100 Copenhagen Ø, Denmark
[2]*CONNECT, Electronics Institute*
Technical University of Denmark
DK-2800 Lyngby, Denmark

In this chapter, a method for fast pixel-by-pixel estimation of parameters in kinetic brain models is introduced. The method is based on artificial neural network (ANN) models. Especially, it is shown how the ANN model can be used to estimate the glucose utilization on a pixel-by-pixel basis in the brain. The data used is derived from dynamic PET scans using the tracer [^{18}F]-fluorodeoxyglucose. Training data for the ANN model is generated by fitting the parameters (rate constants) in Sokoloff's model directly and, from these, calculating the glucose utilization. It is assumed that this method can be used to identify abnormal glucose metabolism in different brain regions for subjects with serious brain disorders. By using the neural estimation procedure, the processing time for a brain scan volume is reduced from 48 hr to 4 min! The neural network method is proposed as a general tool for fast estimation of parameters in kinetic models.

I. INTRODUCTION

The FDG-method for determination of the regional cerebral metabolic rate of glucose (rCMR$_{glu}$) is one of the most widespread applications of positron emission tomography (PET). By investigating the *transient response* to a tracer injection, it is possible to identify fundamental kinetic rate constants on a set of dynamic PET images. The quantification requires known rate constants, k_1–k_3 (k_4) in the correction terms of the Sokoloff *et al.* (1977) and Phelps (1992) autoradiographic method. Although these assumptions may hold to some extent for normal subjects, this cannot be expected to apply in diseased states. Alternatively, the rate constants and the plasma volume, V_p, can be fitted in regions of interest or on a pixel-by-pixel basis for the whole image volume (Sasaki *et al.*, 1986) at a considerable processing expense, and the rCMR$_{glu}$ can thus be calculated.

An effective strategy for reducing the processing time is to use an artificial neural network (ANN) model, trained to invert Sokoloff's model. In this chapter, it is demonstrated how the ANN model can substitute for the tedious parameter-fitting procedures. The ANN model is trained to produce a smooth map, relating a given transient pixel activity to a key parameter of metabolism; namely, the glucose utilization rate R.

The work described in this chapter is a continuation of that presented in the proceedings of NNSP'94 (Fog *et al.*, 1994). Especially, it is shown that the neural network model can *generalize*; that is, the inverse model learned from data on one set of subjects can be used for interpretation of data from other test subjects.

II. SOKOLOFF'S KINETIC MODEL

In the present work we are considering the kinetics of the compound [^{18}F]fluorodeoxyglucose (FDG). The

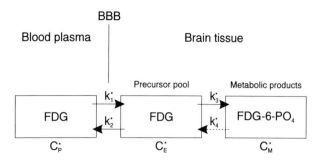

FIGURE 1 Sokoloff's three-compartment model applied to phosphorylization of [^{18}F]fluorodeoxyglucose (FDG). The star on the concentrations signifies that we consider tracer amounts and constants.

kinetics of this tracer are similar to glucose in the initial phases of metabolism. It passes through the blood–brain barrier (BBB) and is phosphorylized intracellularly in a process analogous to glucose. The phosphorylized [^{18}F]fluorodeoxyglucose compound does not enter into the Krebs cycle of glucose metabolism and therefore is effectively trapped. The kinetics can be modeled by a compartemental model involving one compartment representing the tracer density in the arterial blood outside the BBB, C_P^*; one compartment representing the so-called precursor pool, C_E^*; and finally, a compartment representing the intracellular phosphorylized fraction behind the BBB, C_M^*; see Figure 1. In current experiments the arterial concentrations are sampled simultaneously with the scans.

Following the injection of the tracer, hence, the rise of the arterial blood concentration C_P^*, the flow through the BBB starts. The measured PET tracer activity is the sum of the activities of the two compartments to the right of the BBB in Figure 1 and a certain fraction, V_P^*, of the arterial blood concentration. This can be calculated as

$$C_i^* = C_E^* + C_M^* + V_P^* C_P^* \tag{1}$$

The dynamics of the three compartment model is given by

$$\frac{dC_i^*}{dt} = \frac{dC_E^*}{dt} + \frac{dC_M^*}{dt} + V_P^* \frac{dC_P^*}{dt} \tag{2}$$

with

$$\frac{dC_M^*}{dt} = k_3^* C_E^* \tag{3}$$

$$\frac{dC_E^*}{dt} = k_1^* C_P^* - k_2^* C_E^* - k_3^* C_E^* \tag{4}$$

The reverse reaction rate constant k_4^* corresponding

to k_3^* is neglected; it is not identifiable within the measurement time of the present experimental setup.

These linear differential equations describing the response of the activity of the arterial blood ($C_P^*(t')$) are straightforward to integrate yielding the two time-dependent concentrations:

$$C_E^*(t) = k_1^* e^{-(k_2^* + k_3^*)t} \int_0^t e^{(k_2^* + k_3^*)t'} C_P^*(t') \, dt' \tag{5}$$

$$C_M^*(t) = k_1^* k_3^* \int_0^t \left[e^{-(k_2^* + k_3^*)t'} \int_0^t e^{(k_2^* + k_3^*)t''} C_P^*(t'') \, dt'' \right] dt' \tag{6}$$

Following injection these solutions describe the transient activity in terms of the measured blood curve $C_P^*(t)$, the three rate constants (k_1^*, k_2^*, k_3^*) and the plasma volume fraction V_P^*. Conversely, for a given transient $C_P^*(t)$ and for a given measured sum of concentrations $C_i^*(t)$, we may fit the three rate constants and the plasma volume fraction. We use a simple least squares cost function for the fit, hence implicitly assuming Gaussian residuals. Optimization over the four parameters (k_1^*, k_2^*, k_3^*, and V_P^*) is carried out using a second-order Newton scheme.[1]

From these parameters we compute the important glucose utilization parameter R:

$$R = \frac{c_{gl}}{LC} \frac{k_1^* k_2^*}{k_2^* + k_3^*} \tag{7}$$

where c_{gl} is the glucose concentration measured in the blood for each subject and LC is the so-called lumped constant for the model. For LC we use the value 0.55 (Reivich *et al.*, 1985).

Two different approaches have been used when estimating the kinetic constants. In the articles by Sokoloff *et al.* (1977) and Phelps (1992), it is assumed that the parameters are homogeneous in regions and therefore can be fitted using the averaged region activity. Alternatively, the rate constants can be fitted on a pixel-by-pixel basis as proposed in Sasaki *et al.* (1986). However, this approach has not found widespread use because it is rather tedious to fit the kinetic model in all pixels.

III. EXPERIMENTAL SETUP

Data from 10 normal subjects scanned with a Scanditronix PC-4096 PET system were used for training and

---

[1]Based on the solution to the kinetic model, it is straightforward to compute the second-order derivatives.

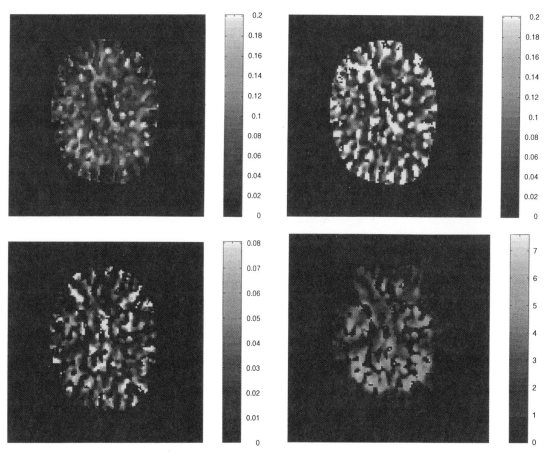

FIGURE 2   Parameters in Sokoloff's model fitted on a pixel-by-pixel basis: Upper left, K_1^*; upper right, K_2^*; lower left, K_3^*; and lower right, R^*. R^* is calculated based on equation (7). Due to noise in the images (each pixel) the fitting procedure is not able to fit the model parameters (rate constants) well in all pixels. In particular, the rate constants K_2^* and K_3^* seem very noisy.

validation of the ANN model. Fifteen brain slices were acquired dynamically after injection of 200 MBq of [^{18}F]-labeled FDG, acquiring 34 frames (10 × 6 sec; 3 × 20 sec; 8 × 60 sec; 5 × 120 sec; 8 × 300 sec) over a period of 1 hr. Arterial samples were drawn simultaneously with the scanning for determination of the tracer input curve.

The images were reconstructed in 128 × 128 matrices (2 mm^2 pixels) by standard filtered back projection (ramp filter with Hann window). Correction for attenuation was based on a separate transmission scan with a rotating Germanium pin source. For further introduction to PET scan techniques, see, for example, Phelps (1992).

The rate constants and the plasma volume were fitted to Sokoloff's model on a pixel-by-pixel basis, using a second-order optimization technique with subsequent calculation of rCMR$_{glu}$. Figure 2 shows a fit of the three rate constants and the calculated glucose utilization R on a pixel-by-pixel basis in a

single slice. We note that these rate constant pictures are rather noisy, reflecting the noise level of the original pixel activity curves, as shown in Figure 3. To provide less noisy data for the neural net training procedure we have averaged and subsampled to yield "superpixels," each averaged over 4 × 4 pixels from the original image. Another reason for subsampling is that it takes approximately 48 hr (on HP9000/735 workstation) to fit the parameters in Sokoloff's model in a full brain volume.

To avoid the tedious fitting procedure, here we investigate the possibility of identifying the *inverse model* of the kinetics: We search for a *map* that provides an estimate of the glucose utilization R in each pixel (Fog *et al.*, 1994). Our basic vehicle will be a simple feed-forward network.

From each of the 10 subjects 500 pixels from the brain volume was randomly sampled. A two-layer fully connected feed-forward ANN model with five hidden units was trained on these data. Each input set con-

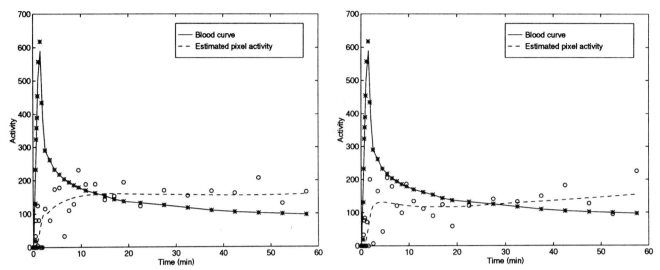

FIGURE 3   The result of simulating the Sokoloff model in two different pixels within the brain. The measured activity data for a single pixel, shown by open circles, is very noisy; noise levels are highest for the first data points where the measuring time is only 5–10 sec. The measured blood curve data is shown by stars. The dashed curve shows the result of a simulation using the estimated model.

sisted of the 34 pixel values in the frames and the corresponding 34 samples of the input blood curve (C_P^*). The network was trained on pixels from 8 of the 10 subjects and a cross-validation technique was applied, using one of the last subjects for choosing the optimized model and the other for evaluation of the generalization ability of the trained network.

Having subsampled the data for the training set does not prevent us from using the network to estimate the glucose utilization on individual pixels.

IV. NEURAL NETWORK OPTIMIZATION

The feed-forward ANN model used comprised five hidden units using *tanh* activation functions and a linear output unit. The network was trained using a pseudo-Gauss Newton method (diagonal Hessian approximation), as described in Svarer *et al.* (1993), and pruned (architecturally optimized) using the optimal brain damage method described in Le Cun *et al.* (1990) to minimize computation and improve generalization. The optimized network architecture was chosen by using a validation set with data from a subject not included in the training or the test sets.

A total of 4,000 examples from eight subjects (500 from each) was used for training the ANN model, and the generalization ability then tested using 8,000 examples from the same group of subjects (1,000 from each). The examples in the training and test set were chosen with the estimated glucose utilization (R) in the interval

(1.0, 12.0). Pixels with R-values outside this interval were typically found outside the brain or were discarded as severe noise outliers. Further, the generalization ability was tested on a data set consisting of 1,500 examples from a subject not included in the training set. The optimized network was chosen using a validation data set consisting of 1,500 examples from yet another subject not used for training nor testing.

From equation (7) it follows that calculation of R involves multiplication by a global factor c_{gl} for each subject: the glucose concentration in the blood. To assist the training problem, the glucose utilization R was divided by this global factor for each subject (it is difficult for a feed-forward net to learn a multiplication). The ANN model was therefore trained to estimate R/c_{gl}.

Further, the data sets used for training and testing the ANN model were normalized to unit variance to help the parameter optimization.

In Figure 4, the results of a pruning session are shown. We see that the network easily generalizes to the (interpolation) test data from the same eight subjects that were used to collect the training set. The minimum validation error occurs for a network with only 75 parameters. This network architecture also generalizes well to the independent test set.

In Figure 5, the left panel shows the direct estimate of the glucose utilization for a subject from the training set (4 × 4 superpixels), and the right panel shows the output from the trained ANN model. The neural network generalizes very well from the 500 examples

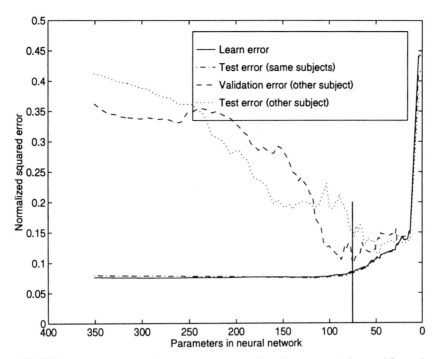

FIGURE 4 Normalized training and test errors (unit variance, mean subtracted for each subject) during a pruning session of the ANN model. The parameters are pruned using the OBD method. For test data from subjects used in the training set, the test error closely follows the training error. The validation error is used for choosing the "optimal" network architecture. This network also generalizes well for the independent test set.

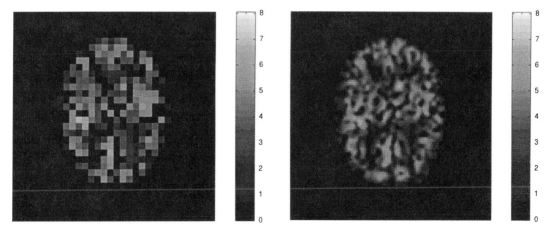

FIGURE 5 Images showing the glucose utilization as determined by fitting the kinetic model (4 × 4 superpixels) using a second Newton scheme (left panel) and as determined by the neural net operating as inverse model for the kinetics (right panel). A total of 500 examples from the 15 slices for a subject is used as a training set, together with 500 examples from each of seven other subjects. The right panel shows the result of evaluating the ANN model on each pixel in the slice. The network generalizes very well for this subject.

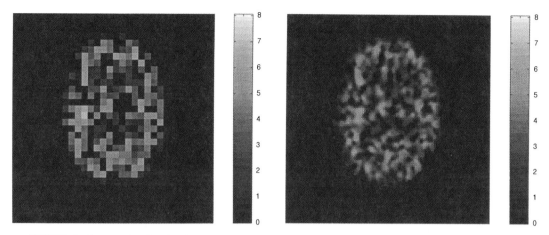

FIGURE 6   Images showing the glucose utilization as determined by fitting the kinetic model (pixel by pixel) using a second Newton scheme (left panel) and as determined by the neural net operating as inverse model for the kinetics (right panel). This subject was not incorporated in the training set.

taken from one subject to the rest of the pixels from the same subject.

Figure 6 shows the estimated glucose utilization for a subject, not used in the training set. At this figure it is seen that the ANN model also generalizes very well to data from subjects not included in the training set.

It is important to note the difference in the computational burden of the two methods. The execution time for the ANN model is orders of magnitude less than the time needed to fit the rate constants in Sokoloff's model by the Newton method. Using the ANN model it is possible to estimate the glucose metabolism in 15 slices of 128×128 pixel images in less than 4 min on the HP9000/735 workstation, compared to about 48 hr required by the fitting procedure.

V. CONCLUSION

We have shown how an artificial neural network model can be trained to learn the inverse model for the three-compartment kinetic model with the estimation of cerebral glucose metabolism as an example. The neural network approach is significantly faster than fitting the kinetic rate constants directly and the generalization ability of the neural network solution seems very good even to subjects not included in the training set. We expect that the ANN model can be extended to estimate the glucose utilization in pixels from patients with neurological disorders, such as Alzheimer's

disease. Furthermore, it can potentially be used as a general tool for kinetic modeling of dynamic PET data.

References

Fog, T., Nielsen, L. H., Hansen, L. K., Holm, S., Law, I., Svarer, C., and Paulson, O. (1994). Neural estimation of kinetic rate constants from dynamic PET-scans. *In:* "Neural Networks for Signal Processing," Vol. IV. IEEE, Piscataway, N.J.

Le Cun, Y., Denker, J. S., and Solla, S. A. (1990). Optimal brain damage. *In:* "Advances in Neural Information Processing Systems," Vol. II. Morgan Kaufmann, San Mateo.

Phelps, M. E. (1992). Positron emission tomography (PET). *In:* "Clinical Brain Imaging, Principles and Applications." (J. C. Maziotta and S. Gilman Eds.), Davis, Philadelphia.

Reivich, M., Alavi, A., Wolf, A., Fowler, J., Russell, J., Arnett, C., MacGregor, R. R., Shiue, C. Y., Atkins, H., Anand, A., Dann, R., and Greenberg, J. H. (1985). Glucose metabolic rate kinetic model parameter determination in humans: The lumped constants and rate constants for [18F]fluorodeoxyglucose and [11C]deoxyglucose. *J. Cereb. Blood Flow Metab.* **5,** 179–192.

Sasaki, H., Kanno, I., Murakami, M., Shishido, F., and Uemuda, K. (1986). Tomographic mapping of kinetic rate constants in the FDG model using dynamic PET. *J. Cereb. Blood Flow Metab.* **6,** 447–454.

Sokoloff, L., Reivich, M., Kennedy, C., Des Rosiers, M. H., Patlak, C. S., Pettigrew, K. D., Sakurada, O., and Shinohara, M. (1977). The C-14-deoxyglucose method for the measurement of local cerebral glucose utilization: Theory, procedures and normal values in the conscious and anesthetized albino rat. *J. Neurochem.* **28,** 897–916.

Svarer, C., Hansen, L. K., and Larsen, J. (1993). On design and evaluation of tapped-delay neural network architectures. *In:* "IEEE International Conference on Neural Networks," Vol. I. IEEE, Piscataway, N.J.

54

Parameter Estimation of the Fluorodeoxyglucose Model with a Neural Network

MICHAEL M. GRAHAM[1] **and FINBARR O'SULLIVAN**[2]

[1]*Department of Radiology (Nuclear Medicine) and*
[2]*Department of Statistics*
University of Washington
Seattle, Washington 98195

An artificial neural network (ANN) is a trainable algorithm that can learn to produce an output appropriate for a given input. Such networks can be applied in a wide variety of pattern recognition tasks, including parameter estimation. The potential advantages of using ANNs for parameter estimation are speed and noise tolerance. The parameter estimation task studied was the five-parameter fluorodeoxyglucose (FDG) model (K_1, k_2, k_3, k_4, and V_p). Training and test data sets were generated from a program that produced both blood time–activity curves (TACs) and tissue TACs using the FDG model. The parameters of both the blood and FDG models were randomized to produce 1,000 data sets for training and six separate 1,000 data sets for testing. One test data set was noise free and the others had 5, 10, 15, 20, and 30% SD normally distributed noise injected into the tissue TAC only. The ANN was a three-layer network trained with back propagation. The input consisted of 20 points from the blood TAC and 20 points from the tissue TAC. Differing numbers of hidden nodes were tested. Training the networks took from a few minutes to several hours using a Macintosh 7100 Power Mac computer. Best results were obtained with three hidden nodes, estimating only glucose metabolic rate. Performance was considerably better than with graphical analysis. This suggests that ANNs may be an effective approach in attempts to generate pixel-by-pixel functional images.

I. INTRODUCTION

Artificial neural networks (ANNs) are a remarkable type of program that can learn to recognize patterns. These programs are beginning to be used successfully for a wide variety of tasks such as character recognition. The reasons ANNs are of interest in the problem of parameter estimation of tracer kinetic modes is that such networks are very fast and are relatively noise tolerant. These characteristics are necessary for the generation of parametric images on a pixel-by-pixel basis. If ANNs can be shown to be effective for generating these images, they are likely to be widely used for this task.

II. METHODS

One of the most common ANNs is the multilayer perceptron network trained with back propagation. This is an appropriate ANN for the task of parameter estimation because the input can be an integral number of values over a wide range and the output is also a number of values over a range. The individual inputs can be the blood activity at different times and the tissue activity at different times. The outputs are the estimated parameters.

The network architecture chosen for this problem is illustrated in Figure 1. The input layer has 40 nodes. Nodes 1–20 are assigned values of the plasma time–activity curve (TAC) with more points from the early part of the curve. The times of the points are not given to the ANN. Similarly, nodes 21–40 are assigned values of the tissue TAC with more early points. Each node in the input layer is connected to each node in the next, hidden layer. A weight is associated with each connection. Thus, the input to each node, j, in the

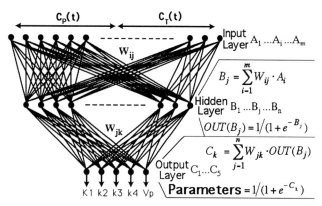

$$B_j = \sum_{i=1}^{m} W_{ij} \cdot A_i$$

$$OUT(B_j) = 1/(1 + e^{-B_j})$$

$$C_k = \sum_{j=1}^{n} W_{jk} \cdot OUT(B_j)$$

$$\textbf{Parameters} = 1/(1 + e^{-C_k})$$

FIGURE 1 Architecture of the artificial neural network used. Plasma and tissue time–activity curves (20 points each) are used as the input vector A. A weight (W_{ij}) is associated with the connection between each node in the input layer and each node in the hidden layer. The input to the next layer, B, is the sum of the product of the weights times the values of the input nodes. The output of the hidden layer is constrained by the function $1/(1 + e^{-B_j})$ to keep the output in a reasonable range. Similarly the input to the last layer is the product of W_{jk} times the output from the hidden layer nodes. The output layer values are calculated in the same way as the output of the hidden layer.

hidden layer is $\sum_{i=1}^{40} W_{ij} \cdot A_i$, where W_{ij} is the weight associated with the connection from node i in the input layer to node j in the hidden layer and A_i is the value of node i in the input layer. In a similar fashion, a set of weights, W_{jk}, connect the hidden layer with the output layer.

Because the weighted sum of all the inputs to a node may be a large number, it is scaled down before producing the output of the node. There are several different possible scaling functions. In this network, the function used is $1/(1 - e^{-NET})$, where NET is the sum of all the weights times the values of the nodes in

the next higher layer. This function produces an output value for each node in the hidden layer and output layer. Forward operation of the ANN is relatively simple. The input vector (plasma and tissue TACs) is applied to the input layer. Using the weights, the values of the hidden and then the output layer are calculated.

The network is trained by adjusting the weights until it produces the desired output. There are several different ways to adjust these weights. The method used for this effort is called the *back propagation method*. Detailed descriptions of this method can be found in almost any text on neural networks such as Wasserman (1989) or Freeman and Skapura (1991). Briefly, the training approach is to present a large number of examples to the ANN including input vectors and target vectors. After each input vector is propagated through the network, the output is compared to the target vector. Based on this comparison, an error signal is generated that is used to adjust the weights. This process is done iteratively with many different examples. Gradually, the network performance improves and reaches a state where it is as accurate as it can get, at which point training is stopped. This process may take many hours of computer time.

A. Generation of Training Examples

It is important to present the network with a wide range of examples, because it is likely to perform best if it has seen an example similar to a given data set. Both the plasma TAC and FDG model parameters (and thus the tissue TAC) were varied. The plasma TAC was generated via a model used for smoothing blood TACs (Graham, 1992). The eight parameters of the model were randomized using a normally distributed random number with a standard deviation of 20%. The plasma TAC was generated for a simulated time of 90 min and was then normalized to have an area under

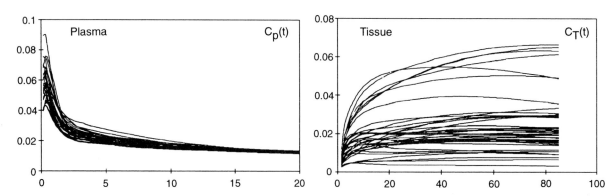

FIGURE 2 Typical plasma and tissue time–activity curves generated to train and test the artificial neural networks.

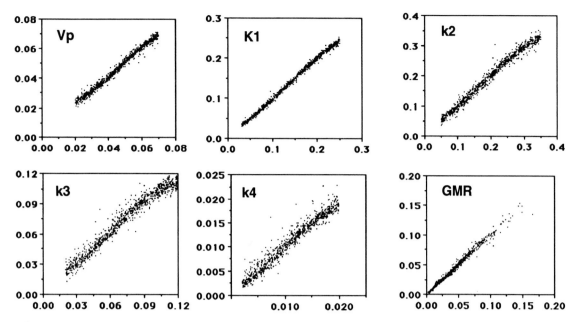

FIGURE 3 Typical performance of a trained artificial neural network. The network contained 20 hidden nodes. It was trained with 1,000 noise-free data sets. The results of testing the ANN with 1,000 independent data sets is shown. Five parameters were estimated and glucose metabolic rate (GMR) was calculated from $K_1 \cdot k_3/(k_2 + k_3)$. In each graph the correct value is plotted on the X-axis and the estimated value on the Y-axis.

the curve of 1.0. The five parameters of the FDG model (plasma volume, K_1, k_2, k_3, k_4) were randomized with uniformly distributed random numbers over the following ranges: V_p, 0.02–0.07; K_1, 0.03–0.25; k_2, 0.05–0.35; k_3, 0.02–0.12; k_4, 0.002–0.02. One thousand example data sets were created for training and several other sets of 1,000 with differing levels of noise were created for testing. Examples of a few training sets are shown in Figure 2.

B. ANN Options

The scaling function used with the ANN has an output range of 0 to 1.0. To take advantage of the full range, it is necessary to scale the values in both the input and target vectors to approximate this range. It was found if the values were not scaled, the ANN could not be adequately trained. If the values were scaled over too large a range, then the ANN output would saturate and consistently underestimate the values of the highest examples.

The most obvious option in constructing the ANN is the number of nodes in the hidden layer. No definite rules exist for determining the optimum number. ANN performance with different numbers of nodes in the hidden layer was one of the main points investigated.

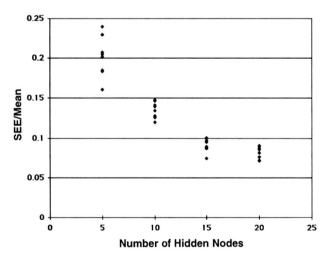

FIGURE 4 Performance of ANNs for estimating glucose metabolic rate, that is, $K_1 \cdot k_3/(k_2 + k_3)$, with different numbers of hidden nodes. Noise-free data were used for training. The standard error of the estimate divided by the mean is depicted as a function of the numbers of hidden nodes. Note that increasing the number of hidden nodes seems to improve the accuracy of the parameter estimates. For each number of hidden nodes, the network was trained eight times, starting with a different set of randomized weights each time. The range of results shows that the final accuracy varies, depending on the starting guess. In general, training should be repeated several times and the best set of weights should be selected for subsequent data analysis.

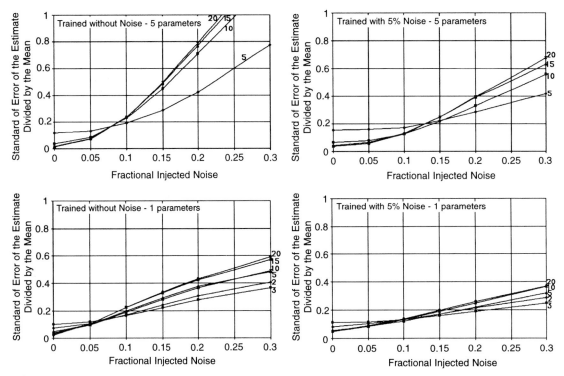

FIGURE 5   These graphs show the performance of artificial neural networks in estimating the glucose metabolic rate. The numbers on the right of each chart are the number of hidden nodes associated with each plotted line. Each point represents the mean result of four to eight repetitions of training with or without noise, estimating either five parameters (K_1, k_2, k_3, k_4, V_p) or one parameter (GMR). The best overall network seems to be the network in the lower right with three hidden nodes, trained with 5% noise, estimating a single parameter.

C. Training the ANN

Two approaches for training were used, with and without noise. The rationale for training with noisy data is that the ANN will ultimately be used to analyze noisy data and it therefore may do better if trained on noisy data. Noise was introduced only into the tissue data. The level of noise indicated is the standard deviation of normally distributed noise applied to 1 min of simulated data. Accordingly, the noise was less for longer, later data points.

ANNs were set up with 5, 10, 15, 20, and 30 hidden nodes with five parameter output nodes. A separate group of ANNs were set up with 2, 3, 5, 10, 15, and 20 hidden nodes with a single output value of FDG metabolic rate (GMR) equal to $K_1 \cdot k_3/(k_2 + k_3)$. The starting weights were randomized between 0 and 1.0. Each ANN was trained eight separate times with different starting weights. The training data sets consisted of 1,000 noise-free plasma and tissue TACs along with the correct parameters and a separate 1,000 TACs and correct parameters with 5% noise applied to the tissue TACs. All ANNs were implemented in Pascal and the programs were run on a Macintosh Power Mac 7100.

Training times varied from a few minutes to several hours.

III. RESULTS

The typical performance of a trained ANN is shown in Figure 3. This network, containing 20 nodes in the hidden layer and 5 output nodes, was trained with 1,000 sets of noise-free data and tested with an independent 1,000 sets of noise-free data. Note that the accuracy of parameter estimation is best for K_1 and worst for k_4. Overall accuracy was expressed as the standard error of the estimate (SEE) divided by the mean (SEE/mean). For this network the SEE/mean for estimating GMR is 7%.

Figure 4 shows the variability in the performance of the ANNs depending on the starting guess for the weights. In addition, it shows that the performance of ANNs improves with larger numbers of hidden nodes. In practice, it would be appropriate to train a selected ANN several times with different starting guesses and select the one with the best performance.

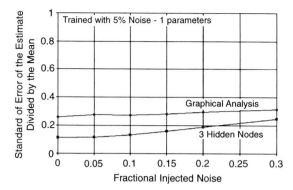

FIGURE 6   The best performance artificial neural network (three hidden nodes, trained with 5% noise, estimating only glucose metabolic rate) performs considerably better than Gjedde–Patlak graphical analysis. This is probably because the ANN looks at the entire curve and takes the k_4 effect into account.

Figure 5 shows the performance of different ANNs in the presence of noise. ANNs trained with noise do better than when trained without noise. The ANNs with a single output parameter (GMR) do better than the networks estimating five parameters. Note that the best ANN seems to be the one with three hidden nodes and a single output. When compared with an alternative method for pixel-by-pixel generation of images of GMR, that is, graphical analysis, (Fig. 6) the best ANN does considerably better.

IV. DISCUSSION

A trainable artificial neural network performs remarkably well in the task of estimating FDG parameters from limited blood and tissue TACs. Although training the network can take several hours, once it is trained it can generate parameter estimates in a fraction of a second. The accuracy of the parameter estimates seems to be better than that achieved with graphical analysis (Gjedde, 1982; Patlak, 1983) and is apparently better than the more conventional methods of parameter optimization. This latter statement is based on a number of attempts to analyze the test data sets with a Marquardt–Levenberg based program for parameter optimization of the FDG model. These attempts met with limited success because the optimizer kept getting caught in local minimae. Even when done with careful manual supervision, the ANN did better than the optimizer program for noisy data sets.

A major reason for the success of this approach is the ability to create many test data sets with a broad range of parameter values. When the trained ANN is used to analyze real data, it is assumed that the model used for generating the test data is an adequate representation of reality. Just as considerable care must be taken in evaluating and validating a model when it is to be used for data analysis, it is essential that similar care be given to evaluating a model used to create test data sets for an ANN. Although this chapter explored the behavior of only the FDG model, it is likely it will do as well with other models as long as they have similar levels of identifiability for their parameters.

Clearly, training with noisy data results in better performance when analyzing noisy data. It is likely that it would be optimum to match the degree of noise in the training data to that expected in analyzing real data. Thus the performance found by training with 5% noise may be improved somewhat by carefully matching the training noise to the expected noise.

Overall, this work suggests that neural networks may be an effective approach in attempts to generate pixel-by-pixel functional images of metabolic rates or of other parameters.

Acknowledgment

This research was supported by N.I.H. Grant CA42045.

References

Freeman, J. A., and Skapura, D. M. (1991). "Neural Networks Algorithms, Applications, and Programming Techniques." Addison-Wesley, New York.

Gjedde, A. (1982). Calculation of cerebral glucose phosphorylation from brain uptake of glucose analogs in vivo: A re-examination. *Brain Res. Rev.* **4:** 237–274.

Graham, M. M. (1992). Parameter optimization programs for positron emission tomography data analysis. *J. Nucl. Med.* **33:** 1069.

Patlak, C. S., Blasberg, R. G., and Fenstermacher, J. D. (1983). Graphical evaluation of blood-to-brain transfer constants from multiple-time uptake data. *J. Cereb. Blood Flow Metab.* **3:** 1–7.

Wasserman, P. D. (1989). "Neural Computing Theory and Practice." Van Nostrand–Reinhold, New York.

55

Redundant-Weighted Integration Method for FDG Parametric Image Creation Using Linear Least Square Estimation

YUICHI KIMURA,[1] HINAKO TOYAMA,[2] TADASHI NARIAI,[1] and MICHIO SENDA[2]

[1]*Tokyo Medical and Dental University, Tokyo, Japan 101*
[2]*PET Center, Tokyo Metropolitan Institute of Gerontology*
Tokyo, Japan

Weighted integration is a practical method that may be used to create parametric images, because its calculation time is much faster than an ordinary nonlinear parameter estimation procedure. Usually, in weighted integration methods, the number of weight functions equals the number of parameters to be estimated. In this study, more weight functions are applied, which means redundant weight functions are used, and parameters are estimated using a linear least squares procedure. A set of simulations was done for the FDG 3K model with various types of weight function (sine, Chebyschev, and Gaussian functions), various numbers of weight functions (from 3 to 20), and various noise levels in the tissue time–activity curve (from 2 to 10% to the maximum value of the true tissue time–activity curve). In the case of Chebyschev or Gaussian functions, the SD of estimated rate constants were decreased with an increase in the number of weight functions. We can conclude that redundant weight functions are effective to reduce noise interference in tissue time–activity curve. The optimal number of weight functions is between 5 and 10, and the Gaussian function is the best of these three types of weight functions.

I. INTRODUCTION

The weighted integration method (WI) is a practical method for creating a parametric image because its calculation time is much faster than that for an ordinary nonlinear parameter estimation method. This research proposes an improved WI on the FDG 3K model for noise reduction in an input signal. In this method, more weight functions are used than the number of estimated parameters, which means redundant weight functions, and an linear least estimation procedure is applied to obtain the estimated rate constants.

II. THEORY

Equations (1)–(3) describe the behavior of FDG transportation (Huang *et al.*, 1980). Here, C_p, C_E, C_M, and C_I denote the tracer activity of FDG in plasma and tissue of FDG–6–P in tissue and in an image from PET, respectively; $\dot{C}_E$ and $\dot{C}_M$ are time derivative:

$$\dot{C}_E = k_1 C_P - (k_2 + k_3) C_E \tag{1}$$
$$\dot{C}_M = k_3 C_E \tag{2}$$
$$C_I = C_E + C_M \tag{3}$$

Both sides of these equations are integrated for linearization and multiplied by an arbitrary differentiable function of W_m. Then we can have the following equation set, in which T denotes the time of the last frame:

$$x \int_0^T W_m(t) C_P(t)\, dt - y \int_0^T W_m(t) C_I(t)\, dt +$$
$$z \int_0^T W_m(t) \int_0^t C_P(\tau) d\tau\, dt \tag{4}$$
$$= W_m(T) C_I(T) - \int_0^T \dot{W}_m(t) C_I(t)\, dt$$

$$x \triangleq k_1 \tag{5}$$
$$y \triangleq k_2 + k_3 \tag{6}$$
$$z \triangleq k_1 k_3 \tag{7}$$

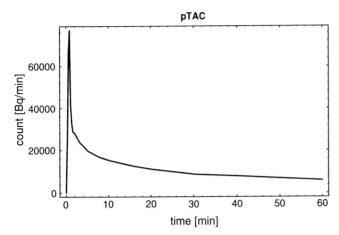

FIGURE 1   Waveform of plasma time–activity curve.

TABLE 1   Results of No Noise Simulation

Number of weights	k_1 (true = 0.102)	k_2 (true = 0.130)	k_3 (true = 0.062)
Weight is Chebyschev function:			
3	0.101	0.127	0.0613
10	0.102	0.132	0.0630
20	0.102	0.130	0.0625
Weight is Gaussian function:			
3	0.101	0.128	0.0618
10	0.102	0.130	0.0622
20	0.101	0.130	0.0623
Weight is sine function:			
3	0.0720	0.146	0.0923
10	0.0541	0.148	0.133
20	0.0146	−0.224	−0.634

Here, more weight functions than the three rate constants are applied to equation (4). Then this linear equation system is obtained:

$$X\theta = Y$$

$$X \triangleq \begin{bmatrix} \int_0^T W_1 C_P dt - \int_0^T W_1 C_I dt & \int_0^T W_1 \int_0^t C_P(\tau)d\tau dt \\ \int_0^T W_2 C_P dt - \int_0^T W_2 C_I dt & \int_0^T W_2 \int_0^t C_P(\tau)d\tau dt \\ \int_0^T W_3 C_P dt - \int_0^T W_3 C_I dt & \int_0^T W_3 \int_0^t C_P(\tau)d\tau dt \\ \int_0^T W_4 C_P dt - \int_0^T W_4 C_I dt & \int_0^T W_4 \int_0^t C_P(\tau)d\tau dt \\ \vdots & \vdots & \vdots \end{bmatrix}$$

$$\theta \triangleq \begin{bmatrix} x \\ y \\ z \end{bmatrix} \qquad (8)$$

$$Y \triangleq \begin{bmatrix} W_1(T)C_I(T) - \int_0^T \dot{W}_1(t)C_I(t)dt \\ W_2(T)C_I(T) - \int_0^T \dot{W}_2(t)C_I(t)dt \\ W_3(T)C_I(T) - \int_0^T \dot{W}_3(t)C_I(t)dt \\ W_4(T)C_I(T) - \int_0^T \dot{W}_4(t)C_I(t)dt \\ \vdots \end{bmatrix}$$

The estimated rate constants can be calculated by using a linear least estimation procedure:

$$\bar{\theta} = (X^T X)^{-1} X^T Y \qquad (9)$$

In this study, three kinds of weight functions were applied:

$$W_m(t) \triangleq \begin{cases} \sin\left(\dfrac{2m\pi t}{T}\right) & \text{sine} \\[2mm] T_m\left(\dfrac{t}{T}\right) & \text{Chebyschev} \\[2mm] \exp\left[-\dfrac{\left\{t - (m-1)\dfrac{T}{n-1}\right\}^2}{2\dfrac{T^2}{n}}\right] & \text{Gaussian} \end{cases}$$

n: total number of weight functions

T: the time of the last frame

III. METHOD

The impulse output from FDG compartment model was calculated using the actual plasma time–activity curve (pTAC) (Fig. 1) and the set of rate constants of $k_1 = 0.102$, $k_2 = 0.130$, and $k_3 = 0.062$. Then interpolated pTAC was resampled with a time interval of 0.6 sec, which was sufficient to pick up the peak in pTAC. By convoluting these two sets of data sequence, the true tissue time–activity curve (tTAC) was calculated, in which the arrangement of the frame times was 0, 1, 2, 3, 4, 6, 8, 10, 12, 14, 16, 21, 26, 31, 36, 41, 46, and 51 min. A simulated tTAC was generated by adding normal distributed random numbers to the true tTAC except $t = 0$ min, because the first data in tTAC can be decided explicitly. The variance was varied from 2 to 10% of the maximum value in the true tTAC.

The computer simulations were done using the true

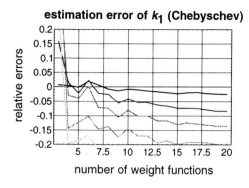

estimation error of k_1 (Chebyschev)

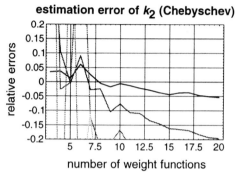

estimation error of k_2 (Chebyschev)

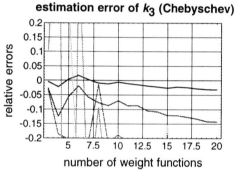

estimation error of k_3 (Chebyschev)

FIGURE 2 Estimation of error using the Chebyschev function as a weight function. The noise level increases from 2 to 10% to the maximum value of tTAC, according to the gray level of the graph. The heavy line denotes a noise level of 2%, and the thin line denotes a noise level of 10%. The vertical axis shows the relative estimation error, which is a mean of 1000 trials of the simulation. Zero means that the true value can be estimated. The horizontal axis shows the number of weight functions.

tTAC and the noise-added tTAC with various types of weight functions: sine, Chebyschev, and Gaussian, and with various numbers of weight functions, from 3 to 20. In the noise-added tTAC, each simulation was repeated 1,000 times to obtain the estimation error.

IV. RESULTS AND DISCUSSION

A. No Noise in tTAC

Table 1 is the result of the simulation for the true tTAC. Except for the sine function, the true value is

estimated. However, in case of the sine function, the estimate includes a large error. This error comes from numerical integration that is a Romberg integral (Press *et al.*, 1988). If the weight function is sine, most of WI calculations cannot converge in this simulation.

B. Noise Simulation

Figures 2 and 4 show the relative estimation error and Figures 3 and 5 show the relative standard deviation on estimated rate constants. The weight function of Figures 2 and 3 is Chebyschev function and of Figures

estimation deviation of k_1 (Chebyschev)

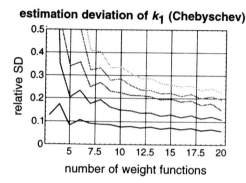

estimation deviation of k_2 (Chebyschev)

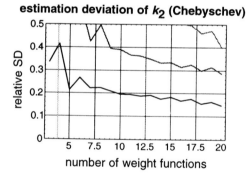

estimation deviation of k_3 (Chebyschev)

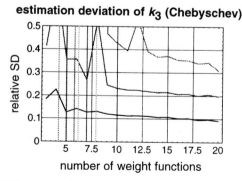

FIGURE 3 Estimation of deviation using the Chebyschev function as a weight function. The noise level is increased from 2 to 10% to the maximum value of tTAC according to the gray level of the graph. The heavy line denotes a noise level of 2%, and the thin line denotes a noise level of 10%. The vertical axis shows the relative standard deviation obtained from 1000 trials of the simulation. The horizontal axis shows the number of weight functions.

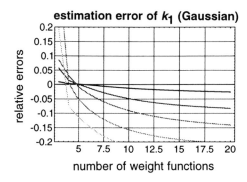

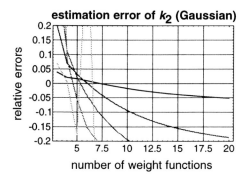

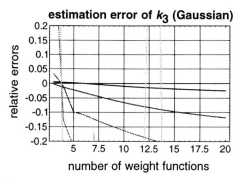

FIGURE 4 Estimation of error using the Gaussian function as a weight function.

ber of weight function, which lies between 5 and 10, from these results.

Little difference is found between Chebyschev and Gaussian weight functions.

C. Calculation Time

Figure 6 shows the calculation time. The program in this study was written in C language and executed on a JS-20/M614 under Solaris 2.4, with a 60-MHz SuperSPARC CPU and a memory of 32 MB/CPU. Using the Gaussian function for weighting, the calculation time was 1.5 times as fast as when using the Chebyschev function for weights equal to 10. And the time

4 and 5, Gaussian function. Horizontal axes denotes the number of weight function to be used. In these figures, heavy lines indicate a noise level of 2% and thin lines, a noise level of 10%.

Figures 3 and 5 show that the standard deviations become smaller as the number of weight functions is increased. And, if the number is only three, which is the minimum number for parameter estimation in FDG 3K model, estimated values have a large deviation. This means that more weight functions are required in WI.

Figures 2 and 4 show a large bias in the estimated parameter; if the number of weight functions is minimum, then increasing the number decreases the bias. As more weight functions are applied, the bias is increased again. This means that there is an optimal num-

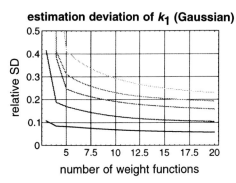

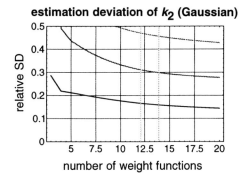

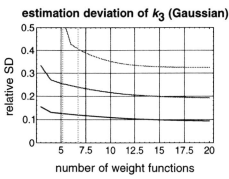

FIGURE 5 Estimation of deviation using the Gaussian function as a weight function.

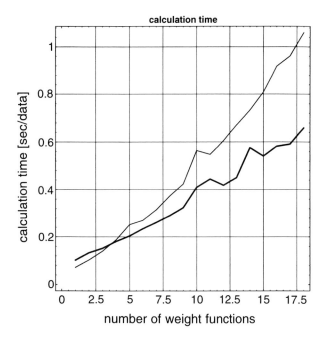

FIGURE 6 Calculation of time per data in sec. The thin and heavy lines denote the Chebyschev function and Gaussian function as weight functions, respectively.

was about 100 times faster than Marquardt method, an ordinary nonlinear parameter estimation procedure.

V. CONCLUSION

1. Redundant weight functions are effective for rate constant estimation in the FDG 3K model to reduce a noise interference in a tissue time–activity curve.
2. The best result can be obtained in this simulation using 10 weight functions.
3. The set of Gaussian functions is faster than the set of Chebyschev functions.

References

Huang, S. C., Phelps, M. E., Hoffman, E. J., *et al.* (1980). Noninvasive determination of local cerebral metabolic rate of glucose in man. *Am. J. Physiol.* **238**, E69–E82.

Press, W. H., Teukolsky, S. A., *et al.* (1988). ''Numerical Recipes in C.'' Sect. 4.3. Cambridge Univ. Press, London/New York.

56

The Application of Fuzzy Control to Compartment Model Analysis for Shortening Computation Time

A. TAGUCHI,[1] H. TOYAMA,[2] Y. KIMURA,[3] Y. MATSUMURA,[1] M. SENDA,[2] and A. UCHIYAMA[1]

[1]*School of Science and Engineering*
Waseda University, Tokyo 169, Japan
[2]*Positron Medical Center*
Tokyo Metropolitan Institute of Gerontology
Tokyo 173, Japan
[3]*Division of Instrumentation Engineering*
Tokyo Medical and Dental University
Tokyo 113, Japan

When we analyze the compartment model with nonlinear least squares (NLS) by the modified Marquardt method, the calculation time and stability of convergence depend on the value of the damping factor λ. In the modified Marquardt method, the λ value is controled by Fletcher's algorithm. In this study, we suggest two methods to control the λ value. One method uses fuzzy control to determine the λ value. The other one is a hybrid method, combining fuzzy control and Fletcher's algorithm. The result showed that the hybrid method computed faster and with better stability of convergence, especially at higher noise levels.

I. INTRODUCTION

PET kinetic data is often analyzed using a compartment model to estimate rate constants. Many methods have been suggested to estimate the model. Among them, the nonlinear least squares (NLS) method is popular and mathematically strict. But, NLS requires much calculation, even if we use the modified Marquardt method, a fast iteration algorithm. In this study, we propose a new method based on fuzzy control to reduce the calculation time and improve the unstableness of convergence due to statistical noise in the Marquardt method. We evaluated the new method on simulation data generated from the blood and obtained in a PET dynamic study of the brain with [18F]FDG and also for actual patient's data with [18F]FDOPA.

II. METHOD

The modified Marquardt method is the most popular iteration algorithm for NLS. In the modified Marquardt method, the next searching point is determined by Fletcher's algorithm. In this study, we modified Fletcher's algorithm and determined the next searching point by fuzzy control.

We show the process to determine the next searching point by the modified Marquardt method. First, we linearize the target model and calculate the sum of squares $\overline{S}$:

$$\overline{S}(x + \Delta x) = \|y - f(x) - J\Delta x\|^2$$

where x are parameter values, y are tissue data, $f(x)$ is the calculated value, and J is the Jacobian matrix.

We also calculate the sum of squares S by using a real target model. Next, we get the reduction of the residual from the previous iteration for actual data (ΔS) and the linearized model ($\Delta \overline{S}$). So we will get the ratio R from ΔS and $\Delta \overline{S}$:

$$R = \frac{\Delta S}{\Delta \overline{S}}$$

The λ value for iteration is determined by U as

$$\lambda(\text{new}) = \lambda(\text{old}) \cdot U$$

In Fletcher's algorithm, three discrete values are employed as U, depending on the value of R, as shown in the following rule:

287

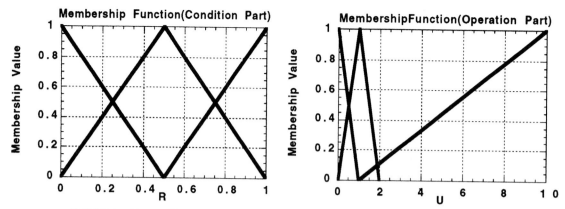

FIGURE 1   The condition part (left) and the operation part (right) of membership function.

$0.0 \leq R \leq 0.25$	Residual decreased minimally.	$U = 2.0$
$0.25 < R < 0.75$	Residual decreased moderately.	$U = 1.0$
$0.75 \leq R$	Residual decreased markedly.	$U = 0.5$

In the present study, we modified the relation between R and U so that U changed continuously from 0.0 to 10.0, corresponding to R according to the membership function of fuzzy control. The membership functions for condition and operation parts are shown in Figure 1. At this time, we use the fuzzy–Singleton method to determine the U value. This method is efficient when we want to get the result in a real number or the operation part is not symmetric. Figure 2 shows the relation between R and U. We got the opportunity to adopt large U value and change the λ value very widely by fuzzy control.

We have developed another method, named the *hybrid method*, that combines Fletcher's algorithm and

fuzzy control. We show the $R-U$ relation in the hybrid method on the right panel of Figure 2.

III. MATERIALS

To evaluate these methods, simulation data for the tissue curve were generated using an actual plasma time–activity curve based on the compartment model of FDG metabolism (Sokoloff, 1986) for the brain with $K_1 = 0.1$, $k_2 = 0.1$, $k_3 = 0.05$, $k_4 = 0.005$. The time–activity curves of plasma and tissue are shown in Figure 3. Adding the Gaussian noise (1, 3, 5, 7, 10%) to the simulation data, we generated 20 curves of the tissue at each noise level during 120 min after administration of $[^{18}F]FDG$. A total of 100 frames of data collected up to 120 min were analyzed by a four-parameter model, and another 100 frames of data up to 45 min were analyzed by a three-parameter model ($k_4 = 0$). The number of iterations was compared among the

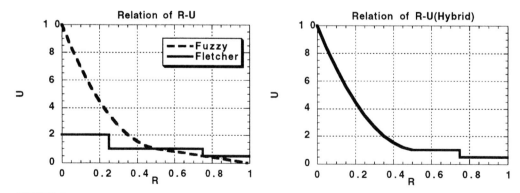

FIGURE 2   Relationships between R and U in Fletcher's algorithm (left, solid line), fuzzy control (left, dotted line), and hybrid method (right, solid line).

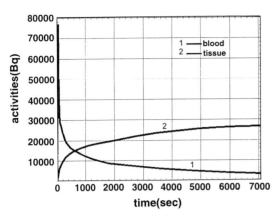

FIGURE 3 Time–activity curves of plasma and brain tissue used in the simulation study. The true values of parameters are $K_1 = 0.1$, $k_2 = 0.1$, $k_3 = 0.05$, and $k_4 = 0.005$.

methods. The initial values are fixed to $K_1 = 0.1$, $k_2 = 0.1$, $k_3 = 0.01$, $k_4 = 0.001$.

The stability of convergence in this parameter estimation was investigated on clinical data for a patient with parkinsonism in an [18F]FDOPA study (Hiroto *et al.*, 1993). Fourteen slices and 20 frames of brain images were collected during 120 min after administration

of [18F]FDOPA. Arterial blood was sampled to get the plasma curve. The regions of interest were in the left and right cerebellar hemispheres, frontal, occipital, caudate, and putamen; and time–activity curves in those regions were generated as shown in Figure 4. A conventional, modified Marquardt method and the hybrid method were applied to these data giving five sets of initial values: 0.01, 0.02, 0.03, 0.04, 0.05 for all parameters. And we looked into how many of the five initial values converged successfully.

IV. RESULT

The number of iterations was scattered at each noise level, as shown for a three-parameter model in Figure 5 and for a four-parameter model in Figure 6. In the fuzzy method, the number of iterations is widely dispersed at every noise level in the three- and four-parameter models. In the Marquardt and hybrid methods, the scatter increased as the noise increased. The mean number of iterations at each noise level is shown in Figures 7 and 8 for three- and four-parameter models, respectively. In the three-parameter model, the fewest iterations was obtained by the modified Marquardt or

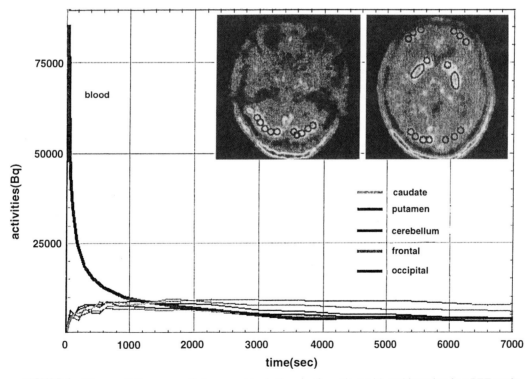

FIGURE 4 Time–activity curves of plasma and brain tissues of a patient with parkinsonism in a PET study with [18F]FDOPA. Regions of interest in the brain are shown in two slices.

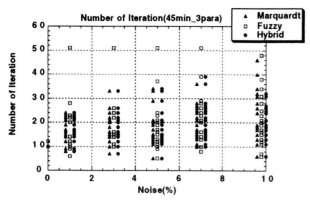

FIGURE 5 A scattergram of the number of iterations at various noise levels of the tissue data by the three methods (▲, Marquardt; □, fuzzy; and ●, hybrid) for a three-compartment, three-parameter model in an [^{18}F]FDG study of the brain.

TABLE 1 Number of Convergences in Parameter Estimation and Estimated Values of the Parameters in the [^{18}F]FDOPA Study of the Brain

	Marquardt	Hybrid	K_1	k_2	k_3	k_4
R. cerb	4	3	0.046	0.061	0.013	0.042
L. cerb	3	4	0.042	0.052	0.0031	0.019
R. front	4	4	0.039	0.095	0.064	0.072
L. front	3	4	0.044	0.12	0.069	0.060
R. occ	4	5	0.057	0.13	0.042	0.050
L. occ	2	5	0.039	0.095	0.045	0.049
R. puta	5	5	0.042	0.056	0.030	0.039
L. puta	4	5	0.049	0.11	0.077	0.043
R. caud	4	4	0.037	0.12	0.21	0.044
L. caud	5	5	0.049	0.34	0.48	0.049
Average	3.8	4.4	—	—	—	—

Note. The same data as shown in Figure 4 were analyzed by conventional modified Marquardt method and proposed hybrid method.

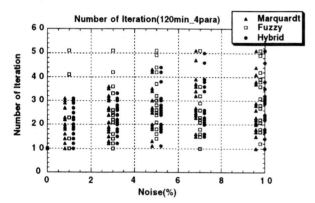

FIGURE 6 A scattergram of the number of iterations at various noise levels of the tissue data by the three methods (▲, Marquardt; □, fuzzy; and ●, hybrid) for a three-compartment, four-parameter model in an [^{18}F]FDG study of the brain.

hybrid method, up to 8% noise. Over 8% noise, fewer iterations were obtained by the fuzzy or hybrid method. The hybrid method always gave the best result for every noise level.

The stability of convergence was investigated by Marquardt and hybrid methods on clinical data for a patient with parkinsonism in an [^{18}F]FDOPA study. The number of convergences in parameter estimation and the estimated values of the parameters are shown in Table 1. The same values for the parameter set was always estimated from five initial values by both methods. The number of successful convergences by the hybrid method was more than that by the Marquardt method.

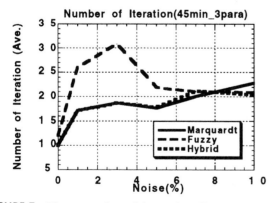

FIGURE 7 The mean values of the number of iterations at various noise levels of the tissue data by the three methods (solid line, Marquardt; broken line, fuzzy; and dotted line, hybrid) for a three-compartment, three-parameter model in an [^{18}F]FDG study of the brain.

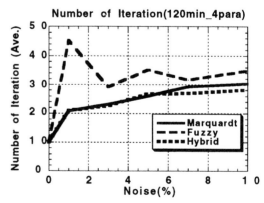

FIGURE 8 The mean values of the number of iterations at various noise levels of the tissue data by the three methods (solid line, Marquardt; broken line, fuzzy; and dotted line, hybrid) for a three-compartment, four-parameter model in an [^{18}F]FDG study of the brain.

V. DISCUSSION

In the fuzzy method, the number of iterations and the scatter increased at low noise levels (<8%). The hybrid method, combining the Fletcher and fuzzy methods in the R-U relation, gave a good result at every noise level. The results show that the value of R oscillates at large R values, and the number of iterations increases, owing to a small λ value independent of the noise level in the fuzzy method. For all simulation and clinical data applied in this study, the estimated values of parameters were independent of the initial values in employing three methods. The hybrid method gave better stability of convergence in parameter estimation on the clinical data with high noise levels, which we suspect is due to low counts.

VI. CONCLUSION

To reduce computation time on parameter estimation, the fuzzy and hybrid methods were proposed to modify Fletcher's algorithm in the Marquardt method. These methods were evaluated using simulation and clinical data. The result of digital simulation showed that the hybrid method was the most useful among three methods applied in this study to reduce the number of iterations at every noise level. From clinical application, it was found that the hybrid method gave more stable convergency than the modified Marquardt method. In conclusion, the hybrid method, combining the fuzzy method and modified Marquardt methods, computed faster and gave good stability of convergence compared to the modified Marquardt method.

References

Hiroto, K., Paul, C., Jacob, R., Gabriel, L., Mirko, D., Alan, C. E., and Albert, G. (1993). Human striatal L-DOPA decarboxylase activity estimated in vivo using 6-[^{18}F]fluoro-DOPA and positron emission tomography: Error analysis and application to normal subjects. *J. Cereb. Blood Flow Metab.* **13:** 43–56.

Sokoloff, L. (1986). Cerebral circulation, energy metabolism and protein synthesis: General characteristics and principles of measurement. *In:* "Positron Emission Tomography and Autoradiography." Raven Press, New York.

57

Generation of Parametric Images Using Factor Analysis of Dynamic PET

JEFFREY T. YAP,[1] MALCOLM COOPER,[1] CHIN-TU CHEN,[1] and VINCENT J. CUNNINGHAM[2]

[1]*Franklin McLean Memorial Research Institute, Department of Radiology*
The University of Chicago, Chicago, Illinois 60637
[2]*Cyclotron Unit, MRC Clinical Sciences Center*
Hammersmith Hospital, London W12 ONN, United Kingdom

The estimation of physiologic parameters from dynamic positron emission tomography (PET) is limited by the validity of the assumed kinetic model. Furthermore, the presence of noise introduces variability that can degrade the precision and accuracy of the parameter estimates. In the case of parametric imaging, the estimation can be especially inadequate because it is performed at the pixel level with much lower counts than averaged regions of interest. These limitations can be reduced or avoided by applying data-driven statistical techniques such as factor analysis to identify the relevant temporal signatures while removing the random variations due to noise. In the first case, principal component analysis (PCA) is used to condition the data prior to applying the conventional parameter estimation, thereby improving the noise limitations. In the second case, the PCA provides the initial solution for the factor analysis, which incorporates prior knowledge to generate factor images, and time factors, which themselves can be considered a form of parametric image, and their associated physiologic time functions. In this regard, data-driven parameter estimation can be performed that avoids the inconsistencies between the actual data and the assumed kinetic model. We have previously applied factor analysis to dynamic neuroreceptor and cerebral glucose metabolism PET studies to generate meaningful factors that differentiate specific from nonspecific binding and normal from diseased tissue function, respectively. In the latter case, a simulated image sequence having a pathophys-
iologic disturbance was generated and analyzed by factor analysis to produce factors consistent with the previous clinical findings. Significant improvements were also achieved in the estimation of the compartmental model rate constants using the PCA processed data as compared to the raw simulated sequence.

I. INTRODUCTION

Estimation of physiologic parameters from dynamic PET data is conventionally performed by compartmental modeling or graphical analysis. Although both methods have certain advantages, they are subject to estimation errors due to noise and may require preconditioning the data. Generation of parametric images is particularly noise limited because the estimation is performed on individual pixel time–activity curves. Furthermore, both methods require model assumptions that may not be valid in some cases, leading to erroneous physiologic parameters. These limitations may be overcome by extracting the relevant temporal dynamics prior to the parameter estimation, using data-driven statistical methods such as factor analysis. We have previously applied factor analysis to dynamic PET studies, using [^{18}F]fallypride (Mukherjee *et al.*, 1993), [^{11}C]diprenorphine, and [^{18}F]FDG to generate novel parametric images and kinetic functions (factor images and time factors) that differentiate specific and

Gray matter   **White matter**   **Gray+White**   **Gray+White+ROI**

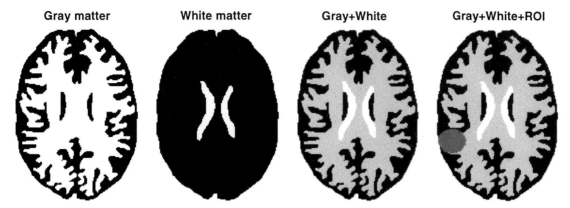

FIGURE 1   Spatial maps based on the Hoffman brain phantom.

nonspecific binding in dopamine D2 receptors and opiate receptors as well as characterize normal and abnormal tissue function in brain tumors (Yap *et al.*, 1994). In this work, the factor analysis results will be compared to conventional methods, using a simulated image sequence with known spatial distribution and kinetic parameters.

II. MATERIALS AND METHODS

A simulation study was designed to generate a pathophysiologic image sequence comparable to the [^{18}F]-FDG brain tumor case acquired on a PETT VI tomogram (Ter-Pogossion *et al.*, 1982). The digital Hoffman brain phantom was used to define the spatial distribution of a normal brain (Hoffman *et al.*, 1990). Since the Hoffman data are already separated into gray matter and white matter images, each of these was used as a spatial map for the two tissue types (Fig. 1). An abnormal structure was introduced by manually defining a region of interest (ROI) and using this as a third spatial map, representing a pathophysiologic condition. In this example, a circular region was used to simplify the visualization of the ROI. However, because the factor analysis extracts the information based on the temporal kinetics rather than the spatial distribution, the analysis would work equally well with an irregular or dispersed ROI, excluding partial volume effects.

The temporal functions for each tissue type are generated from the three-compartment model for [^{18}F]-FDG developed by Sokoloff *et al.* (1977) and modified by others (Phelps *et al.*, 1979). Given a plasma input function $C_p(t)$, the time course of each tissue pixel, $C_i(t)$, is described by

$$C_i(T) = \frac{K_1}{(\alpha_2 - \alpha_1)} \int_0^T [(k_3 + k_4 - \alpha_1)e^{-\alpha_1(T-t)}$$
$$- (k_3 + k_4 - \alpha_2)e^{-\alpha_2(T-t)}] \cdot C_p(t)\, dt \quad (1)$$

where

$$\alpha_{2,1} = \frac{1}{2}\left[(k_2 + k_3 + k_4) \pm \sqrt{(k_2 + k_3 + k_4)^2 - 4k_2k_4}\right] \quad (2)$$

Previously reported values (Phelps *et al.*, 1979) of the rate constants K_1, k_2, k_3, and k_4 were used to generate pixel time–activity curves representing the gray matter (102, .13, .062, .0068) and white matter (.054, .109, .045, .0058). Because it was believed that the second factor in the brain tumor case (Fig. 2) involved normal transport across the blood–brain barrier with diminished phosphorylation, the time–activity curves within the ROI were defined with the same K_1, k_2, and k_4 values as gray matter but with half the k_3 value (.031). Noise was added independently to each pixel time–activity curve according to the Poisson distribution to simulate typical count statistics.

Principal component analysis (PCA) was applied to the raw pixel time–activity curves to identify the statistically significant temporal variations and remove the random variations due to noise. This resulted in a new, reduced set of variables, known as principal components (PCs), which consist of a small number of temporal basis functions and coefficient images. These PCs can be used to provide an initial solution for the factor analysis and can also be recombined to generate a new preprocessed image sequence with reduced noise (Barber, 1980). In the latter case, the rate constants were then estimated for all of the raw and PCA processed pixel time–activity curves by performing nonlinear least squares curve fitting of the model defined by equa-

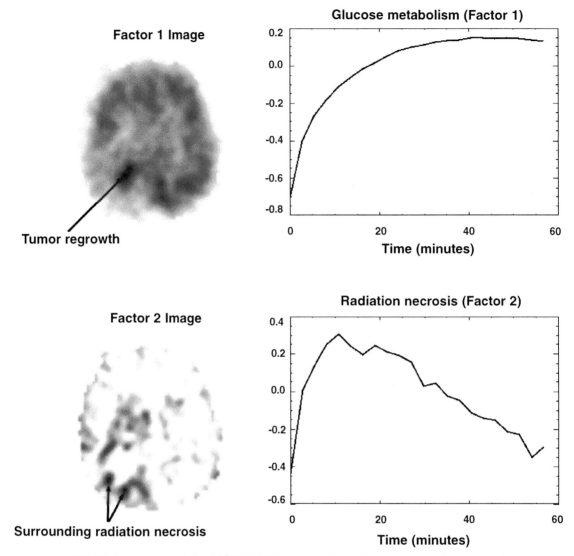

FIGURE 2 Factor analysis of [¹⁸F]FDG PET study with a brain tumor and radiation necrosis.

tion (1). In this manner, the information content of the PCA data could be assessed in terms of its accuracy and precision.

The goal of the factor analysis (as opposed to the PCA) is to transform the original PCs into the ideal set of factor images and time functions that maximally represent the underlying biochemistry or physiology. Our preliminary studies suggest that this may be attainable and has promising implications for characterizing tissue function and radioligand binding. To obtain these optimal solutions, various forms of *a priori* knowledge are incorporated to constrain the analysis. General imaging properties such as positivity and simple structure are imposed as constraints in the factor rotation to obtain a domain-independent solution (Samal *et al.*,

1987). Specific *a priori* knowledge, such as the input function and kinetic models can also be incorporated to obtain a case-specific solution (Nijran and Barber, 1986 and Yap *et al.*, 1994).

III. RESULTS AND DISCUSSION

Factor analysis was applied to the dynamic [¹⁸F]-FDG brain PET study of a clinical patient with previous cerebral glioma and consequent radiation therapy to assess the presence of tumor regrowth or radiation necrosis or both. For this case, an active hypermetabolic tumor was identified as having the same dynamics

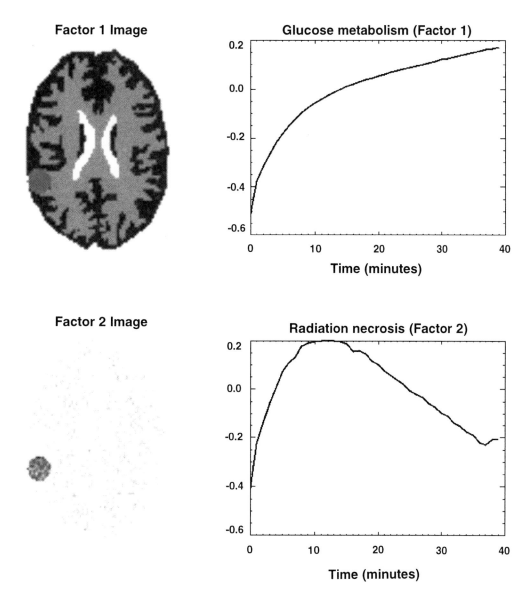

FIGURE 3 Factor analysis of simulated data with necrotic region of interest.

as glucose metabolism in normal gray and white matter but with increased magnitude, as is indicated by the first factor (Fig. 2). Furthermore, a second significant factor revealed a unique time factor believed to be associated with radiation necrosis, as can be seen in the second factor image, where the areas surrounding

TABLE 1 Estimated Rate Constants for the Sample Pixel Time–Activity Curve Shown in Figure 4 and Average Values for All Pixels Within the Defined Circular Region of Interest

	K_1	k_2	k_3	k_4	χ^2
True values	.102	.130	.031	.0068	—
Raw pixel	.097 ± .00030	.11 ± .0012	.026 ± .0011	.0059 ± .0019	404
PCA pixel	.093 ± .00022	.11 ± .0010	.033 ± .00091	.0010 ± .0012	48
Avg. raw values	.103 ± .0072	.14 ± .041	.039 ± .032	.0022 ± .035	352
Avg. PCA values	.094 ± .0045	.12 ± .023	.031 ± .017	.0051 ± .020	72

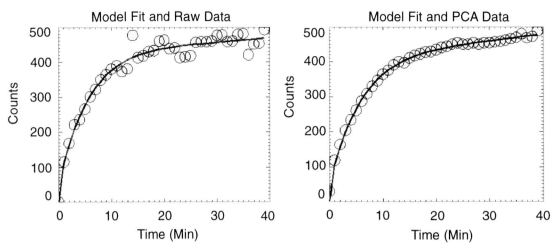

FIGURE 4   Comparison of compartmental model fit to raw and PCA processed data.

the tumor regrowth are highlighted. The factor analysis of the simulated image sequence with known disease involving diminished phosphorylation identified the same factors. In particular, the second factor image of the simulated sequence clearly identifies the appropriate ROI and its time factor has a similar shape as the clinical case (Fig. 3). This demonstrates the ability of the factor analysis to generate meaningful results that are consistent with the predictions based on the compartmental model. However, because these methods provide a unique representation of the data that is not simply described by existing kinetic models, the next step will be to develop quantitative measures that best characterize the isolated functional information provided by each of the factors.

The image sequence generated from the PCA of the simulated data had significantly less noise, thereby improving the fit of the compartmental model at the pixel level (Fig. 4). This is also indicated by a reduction of the χ^2 goodness-of-fit measure by a factor of 8.4 for the pixel time–activity curve shown and by an average of 4.9 for all the pixels within the necrotic ROI (Table 1). As a direct result, the precision of the estimated rate constants is improved, as is indicated in reduction of the standard deviation by a factor of up to 1.9. Furthermore, in some cases the accuracy may also be improved, especially the defining parameter for this study, k_3. Similar gains can be achieved in other types of studies, such as neuroreceptor binding, as well as by using other methods, such as graphical analysis (Yap *et al.*, 1995). Although reduction of data variance can be accompanied by the introduction of bias, in this study significant gains were achieved in both the accuracy and the precision of the rate constant of interest. However, in future studies, a series of simulations need to be performed over the range of all parameters

to rigorously characterize the gains and losses of the methods.

References

Barber, D. C. (1980). The use of principal components in the quantitative analysis of gamma camera dynamic studies. *Phys. Med. Biol.* **24**(2): 385–395.

Hoffman, E., Cutler, P., Digby, W., and Mazziotta, J. (1990). 3-d phantom to simulate cerebral blood flow and metabolic images for PET. *IEEE Trans. Nuc. Sci.* NS-**37**: 616–620.

Mukherjee, J., Yang, Z.-Y., Das, M. K., Kronmal, S., Brown, T., and Cooper, M. (1993). [^{18}F]fallypride as an improved pet radiotracer for dopamine D2 receptors. *J. Nuc. Med.* **34**(5): 243.

Nijran, K. S., and Barber D. C. (1986). Factor analysis of dynamic function studies using a priori physiological information. *Phys. Med. Biol.* **31**(10): 1107–1117.

Phelps, M. E., Huang, S. C., Hoffman, E. J., Selin, C. J., Sokoloff L., and Kuhl, D. E. (1979). Tomographic measurement of local cerebral glucose metabolic rate in humans with [F-18]1-fluoro-2-deoxy-d-glucose: Validation of method. *Ann. Neurol.* **6**: 371–388.

Samal, M., Karny, M., Surova, H., Penicka, P., Marikova, E., and Diensbier, Z. (1987). Rotation to simple structure in factor analysis of dynamic radionuclide studies. *Phys. Med. Biol.* **32**(3): 371–382.

Sokoloff, L., Reivich, M., Kennedy, C., DesRosiers, M. H., Patlak, C. S., Pettigrew, K. D., Sakurada, D., and Shinohara, M. (1977). The (14C) deoxyglucose method for the measurement of local cerebral glucose utilization: theory, procedure, and normal values in the conscious and anesthetized albino rat. *J. Neurochem.* **28**: 897–916.

Ter-Pogossian, M. M., Ficke, D. C., Hood, J. T., Yamamoto, M., and Mullani, N. A. (1982). PETT VI: A positron emission tomograph utilizing cesium fluoride scintillation detectors. *J. Comput. Assist. Tomogr.* **6**: 125–133.

Yap, J. T., Chen, C.-T., Cooper, M., and Treffert, J. D. (1994). Knowledge-based factor analysis of multidimensional nuclear medicine image sequences. *Proc. SPIE,* **Vol. 2168**: 289–297.

Yap, J. T., Chen, C.-T., and Cooper, M. (1995). Estimation of physiological parameters using knowledge-based factor analysis of dynamic nuclear medicine image sequences. *Proc. SPIE,* **Vol. 2433**: 209–231.

58

Parametric Imaging by Mixture Analysis in 3D Validation for Dual-Tracer Glucose Studies

FINBARR O'SULLIVAN, MARK MUZI, MICHAEL M. GRAHAM, and ALEXANDER SPENCE

University of Washington Medical Center
Seattle, Washington 98195

A technique for constructing parametric images from three-dimensional dynamic positron emission tomography (PET) studies is presented. The approach is based on a mixture analysis model in which the time–activity curve (TAC) at a given volume element (voxel) is expressed as a weighted sum of sub-TACs corresponding to homogeneous tissues represented there. Estimates of metabolic parameters at a voxel are defined as a weighted sum of the parameters associated with the individual sub-TACs. Segmentation plays a key role in the methodology. We present an overview of the implementation of the approach illustrated by application to a dual-tracer study designed to measure the local cerebral glucose lumped constant.

I. INTRODUCTION

The quantitative analysis of dynamic PET data to obtain estimates of tissue characteristics, such as blood flow, energy consumption, or receptor density, usually relies on fitting an appropriate kinetic model to the radiotracer time course data. If this analysis is carried out on a voxel-by-voxel basis, maps of tissue function can be obtained. A number of approaches to constructing such maps or *parametric images* have been proposed in the literature. The most well known techniques are for blood flow quantitation with ^{15}O water (Bol *et al.*, 1990; Herscovitch *et al.*, 1983; Huang *et al.*, 1983) and glucose metabolic rate estimation with FDG (Blomqvist, 1984; Gjedde, 1981; Patlak *et al.*, 1983). These methods rely on simplifications of an appropriate kinetic model that allow key parameters to be approximately determined by direct formulas.

A general approach to the construction of parametric images was proposed by Herholtz (1988). His method is based on directly fitting the kinetic radiotracer model to regionally averaged time course data. A spatially adaptive averaging technique is applied to obtain the time–activity curve (TAC) data corresponding to each voxel. The kinetic analysis of the TAC data yields a set of parameters for the voxel. Some limitations of the approach are (1) the assumption that the time course data at the voxel are sufficiently homogeneous to allow the application of the radiotracer model (Lucignani *et al.*, 1993; Schmidt *et al.*, 1991) and (2) the computational requirement of having to separately fit the radiotracer model to TAC data for each voxel in the volume under consideration. An alternative approach, based on a mixture analysis, was proposed by O'Sullivan (1993, 1994). This approach directly addresses the inhomogeneity of PET data. In addition, the computational burden of fitting a complex radiotracer model is not a practical limitation for the method. Here we present a summary of the current implementation of the mixture analysis technique. The methodology is illustrated by application to data from a dual-tracer glucose utilization study.

II. MATERIALS AND METHODS

A. Algorithm Description

A dynamic PET study provides estimates of the total radiotracer activity in a tissue volume over a specific time frame. The data are represented as an array

$$z_i(t), \quad \text{for } i = 1, 2, \ldots, I \quad \text{and} \quad t = 1, 2, \ldots, T$$

where $z_i(t)$ is the radiotracer activity estimated over the ith volume element in the tissue and the tth time bin of data acquisition. The voxels are 3D rectangles arranged in a regular lattice on cross-sectional slices throughout the tissue being imaged. The coordinates of the centers of these rectangles are denoted $\{x_i, i = 1, 2, \ldots, I\}$. The total number of voxel (I) and time (T) bins depends on the imaging protocol and on the tomograph.

The basis of the parametric imaging method is a mixture model that represents voxel-level time course data as a convex linear combination of a number of underlying component time courses. In a K-component mixture model the approximation of data is expressed by the equation

$$z_i(t) \approx \sum_{k=1}^{K} \pi_k(x_i)\mu_k(t) \qquad (1)$$

where $\mu_k(t)$ represents the kth *sub-TAC* in the model and $\pi_k(x_i)$ is the mixing fraction defining fractional contribution of the kth sub-TAC at the ith voxel. Parametric images are constructed by first fitting the radiotracer model to each sub-TAC (this yields a set of kinetic parameters, $\theta^{(k)}$, corresponding to each) and then mapping kinetic parameters at individual voxels in accordance with the relative contribution of the various sub-TACs at the voxel; that is, the parameter mapped at the ith voxel is $\theta(x_i) = \sum_{k=1}^{K} \pi_k(x_i)\theta^{(k)}$.

The mixture model representation in equation (1) shows a lack of uniqueness, and this complicates the implementation of the approach (O'Sullivan, 1993). After experimentation with a number of alternative schemes (O'Sullivan, 1993), we have fixed on an approach that requires the mixing fractions to be constrained by a segmentation model. The tissue volume under study is segmented into a set of K disjoint connected regions, $R_1, R_2, \ldots, R_K$. Let I_{R_k} be the indicator function associated with the kth region in the segmentation ($I_{R_k}(x)$ is 0 except if x is in R_k, in which case it is 1). In the present implementation the mixing fractions are obtained by blurring and renormalizing region indicators of the segmentation; that is,

$$\pi_k(x_i) = \frac{s_h * I_{R_k}[x_i]}{\sum_{k'} s_h * I_{R_{k'}}[x_i]}$$

for $k = 1, 2, \ldots, K$. Here the $*$ indicates convolution between a blurring function, s_h, and the region indicator. The blurring function is taken to be of the form $s_h(x) = s(x/h)$, where s is the point spread or resolution function measured at a representative point in the field of view. The one-dimensional parameter h controls the smoothness of the mixing fractions in the model. Reso-

lution constraints of the tomograph as well as tissue heterogeneity both contribute to mixing.

The parameters (h and μ_k) are simultaneously adjusted to minimize the total weighted residual sum of squares (WRSS) misfit of the model:

$$\text{WRSS}[\mu, h] = \sum_t \sum_i w_t[z_i(t) - \sum_{k=1}^{K} \pi_k(x_i)\mu_k(t)]^2$$

The weights are inversely proportional to the total count in the tth time bin. The optimization of the sub-TACs conditional on h is achieved using a quadratic programming code. This code constrains the sub-TACs to be nonnegative.

The segmentation of the tissue volume is achieved by a variation on the split-and-merge scheme of Chen *et al.* (1991). First recursive *splitting* is used to reduce the tissue volume to a large number of rectangular subregions with the property that the data within each region has a high degree of homogeneity (low sum of squares deviation from the mean). This is followed by a *merging* process that recursively combines regions that are spatially contiguous and whose combination leads to the smallest increase in regional inhomogeneity.

B. Dual-Tracer Glucose Imaging

A dual-tracer glucose imaging protocol is being used to study glucose utilization in brain tumors at our institution. The protocol involves injection of ^{11}C glucose (GLC) followed by [^{18}F]fluorodeoxyglucose (FDG), see Figure 1. The primary focus is on evaluation of the local cerebral lumped constant (LC). Previous work has shown that the increased uptake of FDG in metabolically active brain tumors may well be explained in terms of an elevated lumped constant in the tumor rather than a substantially elevated glucose metabolic rate (Spence *et al.*, 1990).

Blomqvist *et al.* (1990) and Phelps *et al.* (1979) have defined two-compartment models appropriate for application to the GLC and FDG tracers. Let $q_{pC}(t)$ be the concentration (activity/ml) of the ^{11}C label in plasma at time t and let $q_{1C}(t)$ and $q_{2C}(t)$ be the concentrations (activity/ml) of the ^{11}C label in the cellular components in the original and phosphorylated forms, respectively. The corresponding quantities for the ^{18}F label are denoted $q_{pF}(t)$, $q_{1F}(t)$, and $q_{2F}(t)$. The state equations for the GLC tracer are

$$\frac{dq_{1C}}{dt}(t) = K_{1C}q_{pC}(t - \tau_C) - (k_{2C} + k_{3C} + \lambda_C)q_{1C}(t)$$

$$\frac{dq_{2C}}{dt}(t) = k_{3C}q_{1C}(t) - (k_{4C} + \lambda_C)q_{2C}(t) \qquad (2)$$

For the FDG tracer, we have

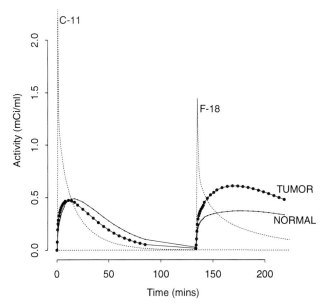

FIGURE 1 Dual-tracer glucose imaging protocol. The plasma activity corresponding to GLC and FDG are shown by the dashed lines. Hypothetical time courses associated with (metabolically active) tumor and normal tissue are shown. The asterisks indicate the midpoints in the time bins used for dynamic PET data acquisition.

$$\frac{dq_{1F}}{dt}(t) = K_{1F}q_{pF}(t - \tau_F) - (k_{2F} + k_{3F} + \lambda_F)q_{1F}(t)$$

$$+ k_{4F}q_{2F}(t) \qquad (3)$$

$$\frac{dq_{2F}}{dt}(t) = k_{3F}q_{1F}(t) - (k_{4F} + \lambda_F)q_{2F}(t)$$

Note that these model equations are a little nonstandard because they include, via the parameters λ_C and λ_F, decay of the C and ^{18}F isotopes over the duration of the study (both of these are known, of course). The flux ratios

$$MR_C = \frac{K_{1C}k_{3C}}{k_{2C} + k_{3C}}$$

$$MR_F = \frac{K_{1F}k_{3F}}{k_{2F} + k_{3F}}$$

are used to define estimates of metabolic rates using GLC and FDG. The lumped constant (LC) and phosphorylation ratio (PR) are of primary interest

$$LC = \frac{MR_F}{MR_G}$$

$$PR = \frac{k_{3F}}{k_{3C}}$$

C. Application and Validation Studies

A dual-tracer glucose study was conducted on a patient with a brain tumor. The parametric images obtained from the study will be presented. A number of studies have been conducted to validate the approach. Numerical simulations for homogeneous tissues have been used to explore the mean square error in the measurement of the lumped constant and other parameters as a function of the time lag between the injections of GLC and FDG. Simulations of dynamic PET data, incorporating mixing due to tomograph resolution and tissue heterogeneity, have been carried out to compare the accuracy of regionally averaged mixture analysis parametric images relative to standard ROI analysis; that is, estimates obtained from kinetic analysis applied to regionally averaged but heterogeneous time course data. A corresponding set of studies have been conducted using actual patient data. In this latter case the ground truth is not known; however, the correlation between the estimates obtained by both methods is still of interest.

III. RESULTS AND DISCUSSION

Figure 2 (Colorplate) shows transverse, sagittal, and coronal (mid-volume planes) images of four main parameters (MR_{GLC}, MR_{FDG}, LC, and PR). The analysis of entire volume of data (35 planes with 128×128 voxels per plane) took 90 min on a DEC-Alpha computer. The tumor region is outlined by elliptical contours on the transverse and coronal lumped constant scans. This particular tumor has been treated and shows suppressed metabolic activity, see the flux images (MR_{GLC} and MR_{FDG}). The lumped constant is substantially elevated in the tumor region, roughly 1.7 times greater than normal tissue. The phosphorylation ration is also seen to be elevated in the tumor region. This is consistent with previous work reported by Spence *et al.* (1990).

For realistic noise levels, the regionally averaged LC parameter was estimated with a percent of standard deviation on the order of 10 to 20%. Typical percent differences between the regionally averaged LC parametric image and the LC obtained by application of standard ROI analysis to those same regions were on the order of 20 to 30% for both normal brain and tumor regions. The differences between the methods appeared to be well correlated to the degree of apparent heterogeneity in the regional data. Similar error characteristics were obtained for the metabolic rates of FDG and GLC.

Our results indicate that the mixture analysis scheme

is a computationally efficient and reliable approach to constructing 3D parametric images of the lumped constant and phosphorylation ratio parameters in the context of the dual-tracer glucose studies. The approach relies on no particular simplifications of the radiotracer model; hence, there is good potential for adapting the approach to other contexts in which quantitative parametric images are of interest.

We have prepared a separate manuscript describing the details of the implementation and validation of the approach. This manuscript is available from the authors on request.

Acknowledgments

This work was supported by the National Institutes of Health under Grants CA-57903, CA-42593 and CA-42045.

References

Blomqvist, G. (1984). On the construction of functional maps in positron emission tomography. *J. Cereb. Blood Flow Metab.* **4:** 629–632.

Blomqvist, G., Stone-Elander, S., Halldin, G., Roland, P. E., Widen, L., Linqvist, M., Sivahm, C. G., Langstrom, B., and Wissel, L. A. (1990). Positron emission tomographic measurement of cerebral glucose utilization using [1−^{11}C]D-glucose. *J. Cereb. Blood Flow Metab.* **10:** 467–483.

Bol, A., Vanmeickenbeke, P., Michel, C., Cogneau, M., and Goffinet, A. M. (1990). Measurement of cerebral blood flow with a bolus of oxygen-15-labeled water: Comparison of dynamic and integral methods. *Eur. J. Nucl. Med.* **17:** 234–241.

Chen, S.-Y., Lin, W.-C., and Chen, C.-T. (1991). Split-and-merge image segmentation based on localized feature analysis and statistical tests. *Graphical Models Image Processing* **53:** 457–475.

Gjedde, A. (1981). High- and low-affinity transport of D-glucose from blood to brain. *J. Neurochem.* **36:** 1463–1471.

Herholtz, K. (1988). Nonstationary spatial filtering and accelerated curve fitting for parametric imaging with dynamic PET. *Eur. J. Nucl. Med.* **14:** 477–484.

Herscovitch, P., Markham, J., and Raichle, M. A. (1983). Brain blood flow measured with intravenous H$_2^{15}$O. I. Theory and error analysis. *J. Nucl. Med.* **24:** 782–789.

Huang, S. C., Carson, R. E., Hoffman, E. J., Carson, J., MacDonald, N., Barrio, J. R., and Phelps, M. E. (1983). Quantitative measurement of local cerebral blood flow in humans by positron computed tomography and [O-15]-water. *J. Cereb. Blood Flow Metab.* **3:** 141–153.

Lucignani, G., Schmidt, K. C., Moresco, R. M., Striano, G., Colombo, F., Sokoloff, L., and Fazio, F. (1993). Measurement of regional cerebral glucose utilization with fluorine-18-FDG and PET in heterogeneous tissues: Theoretical considerations and practical procedure. *J. Nucl. Med.* **34:** 360–369.

O'Sullivan, F. (1993). Imaging radiotracer model parameters in PET: A mixture analysis approach. *IEEE Trans. Med. Imaging* **12:** 399–412.

O'Sullivan, F. (1994). Metabolic images from dynamic positron emission tomography studies. *Statistical Methods Med. Res.* **3:** 87–101.

Patlak, C. S., Blasberg, R. G., and Fenstermacher, J. D. (1983). Graphical evaluation of blood-to-brain transfer constants from multiple-time uptake data. *J. Cereb. Blood Flow Metab.* **3:** 1–7.

Phelps, M. E., Huang, S. C., Hoffman, E. J., Selin, C., Sokoloff, L., and Kuhl, D. E. (1979). Tomographic measurement of local cerebral glucose metabolic rate in humans with [F-18]2-fluoro-2-deoxy-D-glucose: Validation of method. *Ann. Neurol.* **6:** 371–388.

Schmidt, K., Mies, G., and Sokoloff, L. (1991). Model of kinetic behavior of deoxyglucose in heterogeneous tissues in brain: A reinterpretation of the significance of parameters fitted to homogeneous tissue models. *J. Cereb. Blood Flow Metab.* **11:** 10–24.

Spence, A. M., Graham, M. M., Muzi, M., Abbott, G. L., Krohn, K. A., Kapoor, R., and Woods, S. D. (1990). Deoxyglucose lumped constant estimated in a transplanted rat astrocytic glioma by the hexose utilization index. *J. Cereb. Blood Flow Metab.* **10:** 190–198.

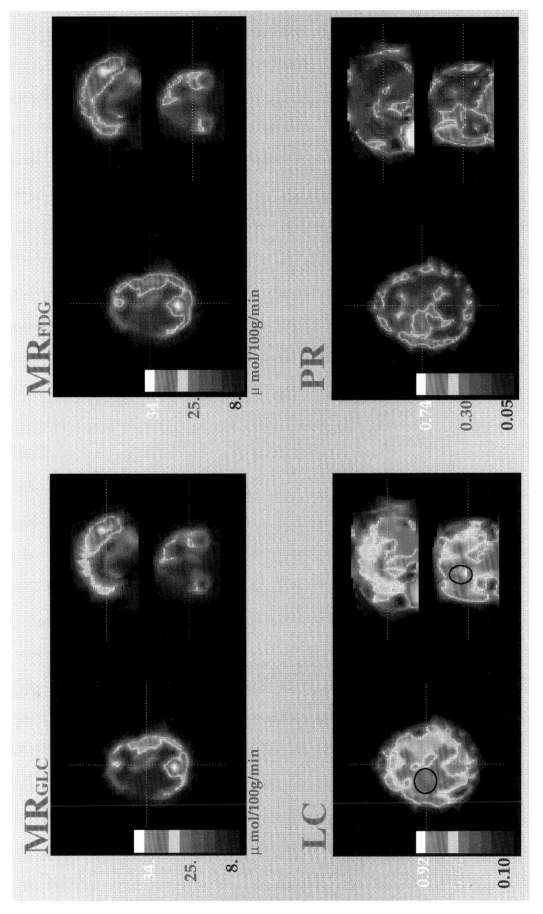

FIGURE 2 Parametric images of glucose utilization constants defined in Section II.B in the text. Each panel shows transverse, sagittal, and coronal (mid-volume) planes. For GLC, the flux constant is multiplied by the plasma glucose concentration to obtain a metabolic rate estimate. For FDG, the flux is also divided by the mean lumped constant for normal brain (0.58) so the result reflects an estimated regional glucose metabolic rate computed with FDG.

59

A Cluster Analysis Approach for the Characterization of Dynamic PET Data

JOHN ASHBURNER,[1] **JANE HASLAM,**[2] **CHRIS TAYLOR,**[2] **VINCENT J. CUNNINGHAM,**[1] **and TERRY JONES**[1]

[1]*Cyclotron Unit, Hammersmith Hospital, London W12 0NN, United Kingdom*
[2]*Medical Biophysics, Medical School, Manchester, United Kingdom*

Cluster analysis is one of several data-led techniques that are of potential value in the analysis of PET data. This technique can be used to partition the large number of pixel time–activity curves (TACs, each of which is considered as a vector), obtained from a dynamic scan into a smaller number of clusters (each described by a multinormal distribution about a mean). Effectively each cluster represents a characteristic "shape" of a time–activity curve. The likelihood of any pixel vector belonging to a given cluster can be computed. This then enables a corresponding partition or segmentation of the dynamic image set into images of the spatial distribution of each of the clusters. Since the cluster means are derived from many pixels, they exhibit a much improved signal-to-noise ratio. This partitioning requires no knowledge of the plasma input function. However, because the cluster means are in the same space as the original data, further model analysis and characterization of the cluster means relative to an input function is possible.

We have applied the technique to a number of areas of PET and will give examples of its application to [^{11}C]flumazenil in brain. However, problems are associated with its general application, and the technique does not always give a convincing partition of the images. The cluster model may not always be appropriate, in that the real data may form a continuum and not distinct clusters. The technique is nonetheless of great value as an exploratory tool in the characterization of dynamic data sets.

I. INTRODUCTION

The purpose of the work described here was to investigate the application of cluster analysis to the characterization of dynamic PET images. In this context, it may be seen as a segmentation technique aimed at identifying a limited number of underlying TACs present in the raw data and the likelihood of individual pixel TACs belonging to them. It was anticipated that parametric images of these distributions could then be produced that would lead to a spatial segmentation of the images and aid the definition of regions of interest for further analysis. We first describe a clustering algorithm, based on a mixture model (Hartigan, 1975) and modified to accommodate dynamic PET data. Examples of its application to [^{11}C]flumazenil studies will be shown that illustrate its potential as a segmentation tool, together with a discussion of the assumptions implicit in the modified algorithm and some inherent limitations.

II. METHODS

Let the dynamic PET data be represented by a matrix A that has m rows and n columns. Each column of A represents a time frame of data, and each row represents a pixel vector (pixel TAC). The elements of A contain counts per frame per voxel, rather than counts per second per voxel.

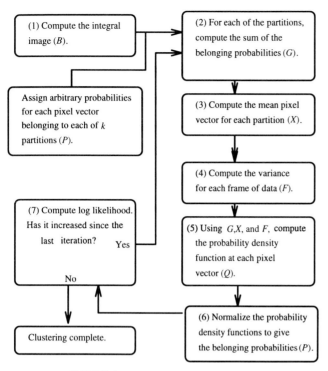

FIGURE 1   Flow diagram for clustering.

It is assumed that the dynamic data has a known number (k) of characteristic underlying TAC shapes and that each pixel vector constitutes one of these shapes scaled by a constant, with superimposed Gaussian noise. The noise is assumed to be stationary within each column of A but can vary from column to column. These assumptions will be discussed later.

The objective is to partition the data according to its probability of belonging to each of k clusters (P), based purely on the shape of the pixel vectors. The clusters are each described by a multinormal distribution, the parameters of which are

- A mean pixel vector (X),
- A diagonal covariance matrix that is common to all clusters (F),
- The number of pixel vectors that constitute the distribution (G).

The algorithm is illustrated in Figure 1, and the individual stages are expanded in the following equations. It is based on estimating the likelihood of each pixel vector being drawn from each of the distributions and updating the distributions according to the properties of the pixels of which they are composed.

Compute the integral image B of the dynamic image A:

$$b_i = \sum_{j=1}^{n} a_{i,j}, \qquad i = 1, \dots, m \qquad (1)$$

Compute the number of pixel vectors associated with each partition (G):

$$g_l = \sum_{i=1}^{m} p_{i,l}, \quad l = 1, \dots, k \qquad (2)$$

Compute the mean pixel vector for each of the partitions (X):

$$x_{j,l} = \frac{\sum_{i=1}^{m} a_{i,j} p_{il} b_i}{\sum_{i=1}^{m} p_{i,l} b_i b_i},$$
$$j = 1, \dots, n, \qquad l = 1, \dots, k \qquad (3)$$

Compute a variance for each frame (F):

$$f_j = \frac{\sum_{l=1}^{k} \sum_{i=1}^{m} (a_{i,j} - x_{j,l} b_i)^2 p_{i,l}}{m}, \qquad j = 1, \dots, n \quad (4)$$

Compute the probability densities (Q) at each pixel vector for each cluster:

$$q_{i,l} = \frac{g_l}{\sqrt{\prod_{j=1}^{n} 2\pi f_{j,l}}} e^{-0.5 \sum_{j=1}^{n} (a_{i,j} - x_{j,l} b_i)^2 / f_{j,l}},$$
$$i = 1, \dots, m, \quad l = 1, \dots, k \qquad (5)$$

Compute the belonging probabilities (P):

$$p_{i,l} = \frac{q_{i,l}}{\sum_{l_1=1}^{k} q_{i,l_1}}, \qquad i = 1, \dots, m, \quad l = 1, \dots, k \quad (6)$$

The likelihood is given by $\prod_{i=1}^{m} \sum_{l=1}^{k} q_{i,l}$. In practice, we compute the log likelihood:

$$\text{log likelihood} = \sum_{i=1}^{m} \log\left(\sum_{l=1}^{k} q_{i,l}\right) \qquad (7)$$

If the log likelihood has increased significantly since the previous iteration, then repeat the process from equation (2).

III. RESULTS AND DISCUSSION

A. Comments on the Algorithm

The principal difference between the algorithm used in the present application of cluster analysis and the mixture model algorithm described by Hartigan (1975) is that here we are concerned with the shapes of the pixel TACs (vectors) and not their absolute scaling. In dynamic PET data, the observed absolute scaling is determined by the delivery of the tracer, and other factors (such as binding) that may be more readily visualized by simple integral images of the data. The distribution of particular dynamics is, however, more difficult to visualize. If we were to use the original

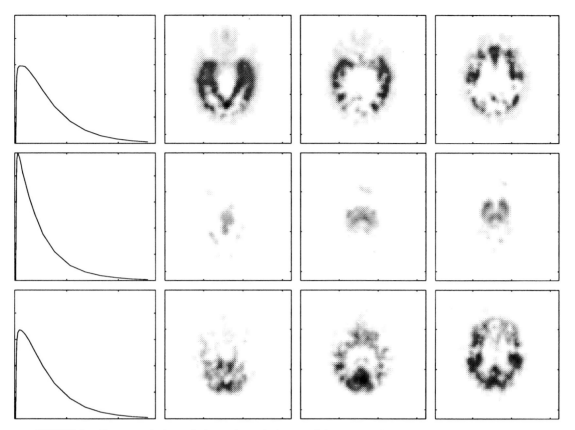

FIGURE 2   Cluster analysis applied to a dynamic flumazenil image. The three rows represent the clusters, and the columns are selected planes from the volume. The images are the likelihoods of belonging to each of the clusters, multiplied by the integral image. They have been smoothed slightly to improve visualization. The plot on the left is the cluster mean.

algorithm, the partitioning of the images would be dominated by effects of magnitude, and the more subtle variation in curve shapes would be largely ignored. The approach here attempts to overcome this problem. The modification to the algorithm is effected by the computation of the integral image in equation (1), and its inclusion in equations (3) and (4) of the algorithm.

Note however, that, as a consequence of these modifications, the dimensionality of the problem is reduced, because all the data are effectively mapped to the same hyperplane (see the expression $a_{i,j} - x_{j,l}b_i$ in equations (4) and (5)). Strictly, it is necessary to consider clustering on this hyperplane, rather than the original n-dimensional space. The present algorithm assumes that the statistical noise is independent between frames. However, because of the loss of dimensionality, a small negative covariance is introduced that is not accounted for. In early implementations of the algorithm, these covariances were accounted for by computing the whole covariance matrix for each cluster at each iteration. However, the current implementation assumes that off-diagonal elements in the covariance matrixes are 0, thus increasing stability by reducing the number of unknowns in the model and also, incidentally, greatly reducing computing time. The effects of these approximations relating to the dimensionality may however be small, particularly when there is a relatively large number of frames.

A further assumption within the present model is that the noise is stationary (i.e., it does not vary across the image). Although this is not the case with filtered back projected PET data, it was felt to be a necessary constraint because, without it, the partitioning of the images would be based partially on the amount of statistical noise in different regions.

An area to be cautious about when applying the technique to filtered back projected PET data is frames with only a few counts (background frames, for example). Most of the voxel values are very close to 0, with a few exceptions where there are streaks in the image. The high number of near 0 values results in an apparently low variance for these frames. Because of this

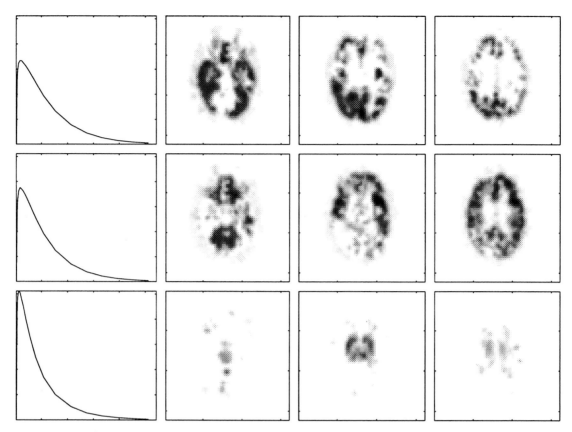

FIGURE 3   Cluster analysis applied to a flumazenil image containing an epileptic focus.

low variance, the streaks appear to the algorithm as separate clusters. For better results, it was found necessary to exclude low count frames from the computations or combine adjacent frames.

B. Examples

As an illustration, we applied the algorithm to the whole volume of a dynamic [^{11}C]flumazenil image. Because of the memory requirements of our implementation, the original 128 × 128 images were reduced to 64 × 64 images, by combining adjacent pixels. The results from searching for three clusters are shown in Figure 2.

Although the top and bottom cluster means appear visually similar, the top curve exhibits a slightly slower washout of the tracer. The middle cluster appears to reflect nonspecific binding.

A second, similar example illustrates the use of flumazenil in an epilepsy patient. In Figure 3, there is an obvious asymmetry in the pattern of clustering. The epileptic focus can be seen as a decreased rate of washout on the lower left side of the images in the center column.

C. Computation Time

A major consideration is the amount of computation required for this iterative algorithm. For best results, it is necessary to include as much of the image volume as possible in the computations. Our implementation requires $5mn + 6m + 3km + 8kmn + 2kn$ floating point operations per iteration (m pixel vectors of length n and k clusters), so a typical data set (e.g., 25 frames, 31 planes of 64 × 64 images, searching for 8 clusters with 64 iterations) will take on the order of 1.5e + 10 floating point operations.

D. Problems with the Model

For most PET images, we cannot assume that only a few underlying TAC shapes exist. Even if we were to approximate the TACs to a simple compartmental model, because the parameters of the model over the whole image volume do not take a number of discrete values but rather a whole continuum of values, we would expect a continuous range in the shape of the pixel vectors. In this case, the cluster means would be placed in the data space in such a way that they would

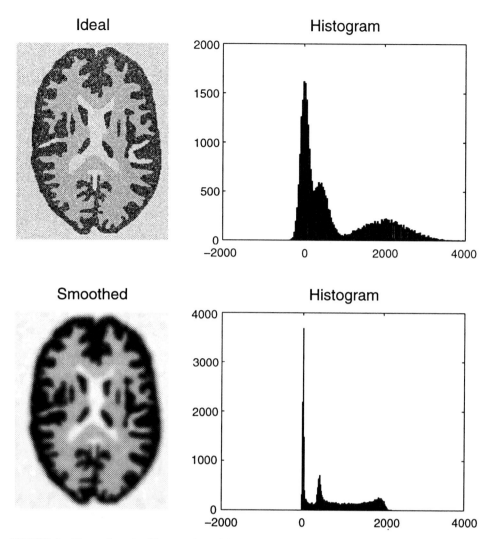

FIGURE 4   Illustration of spillover and partial volume effects on the histogram distribution. Images and histograms were created using ANALYZE software (Robb and Hanson, 1991).

best represent the variation in the data. Where there are discrete organs within the image volume, the resulting pattern of clusters is more likely to have true physiological meaning. In this case, it is interesting to draw an analogy with techniques such as PCA and factor analysis where similar considerations apply.

Another factor leading to a continuum of data is the effect of partial volume and spillover due to the point-spread function in the images. This is illustrated by a simple one-dimensional example in Figure 4. The histogram of the unsmoothed image follows the sum of three normal distributions. However, when this image is convolved with a Gaussian kernel, the histogram becomes severely distorted away from a sum of normal distributions. Any classification by an algorithm searching for three normal distributions would produce a rather poor fit to the data.

In our experience movement artifacts can account for much of the variation in TAC shape. For any meaningful results to be obtained, it is essential that these effects be eliminated.

The number of clusters to search for is specified by the user. The optimum number is usually found by trial and error and is determined by what the user requires from the data. The preceding factors need to be taken into consideration when attempting to interpret the results of the analysis.

IV. SUMMARY

This form of cluster analysis has yet to be widely evaluated in PET. Initial tests suggest that it may prove itself to be a useful tool in the characterization of certain dynamic PET data sets.

A final caution: "It is worth keeping in mind, when contemplating the use of one of these techniques, that its descriptive use carries no penalty but an inferential extension may be founded on an inappropriate model and may therefore lead to incorrect conclusions" (Krzanowski, 1988).

Acknowledgments

We would like to thank Matthias Koepp, Mark Richardson, Andrea Malizia, Susan O'Reilly, and others for providing data for testing the algorithms and also for their useful feedback. We would also like to thank Julian Matthews and Karl Friston for their helpful input in the early stages of the work.

References

Hartigan, J. A. (1975). "Clustering Algorithms," pp. 113–129. Wiley, New York.

Krzanowski, W. J. (1988). "Principles of Multivariate Analysis: A Users Perspective," pp. 261–264. Clarendon Press, Oxford.

Robb, R. A. and Hanson, D. P. (1991). A software system for interactive and quantitative visualization of multidimensional biomedical images. *Australasian Phys. Eng. Sci. Med.* **14**(1): 9–30.

60

Patlak Analysis Applied to Sinogram Data

R. P. MAGUIRE, C. CALONDER, and K. L. LEENDERS

Paul Scherrer Institute, CH 5232 Villigen PSI, Switzerland

The determination of tissue time–activity course in PET is normally performed by region of interest (ROI) analysis of reconstructed images. However, in some cases, the same analysis may be performed equally well on the data in sinograms before reconstruction, avoiding the reconstruction of large time sequence data sets, especially important in the 3D mode. Linearization, by remapping the time–activity data, as performed in Patlak analysis (Gjedde, 1982; Patlak et al., 1983), creates the conditions that enable parameters, estimated pixel by pixel in the sinogram data set, to be reconstructed to form parametric images of the influx rate constant K_{mr} and volume of distribution V_d for tracer substances. A further advantage of sinogram analysis is that the elements of the sinogram contain integrated detector counts over the acquisition period and can be considered random variables with a known (Poisson) population density function. A general theory and a validation of this technique for the tracer [^{18}F]fluorodeoxyglucose is presented.

I. INTRODUCTION

After application of a tracer substance, PET measures the tracer time course by registering coincident counts along lines of response (LOR) between detector crystals. The counts can be reorganized into a set of plane projections of the object's activity concentration, stored as a sinogram, which can be reconstructed using standard filtered back projection algorithms to form a set of two-dimensional images of the distribution of the tracer at different time points, in the organs of interest. Time–activity data drawn from the reconstructed images are normally analyzed in the light of a mathematical model that explains the uptake of the tracer in terms of the input arterial activity concentration and exchange between different tissue compartments. However, the process of reconstruction is costly in terms of CPU time. It is also difficult to construct a probability distribution for the individual pixel values in the reconstructed image because the probability density function is not well known. It is, therefore, enticing to attempt to analyze the raw data before reconstruction to determine the physiological parameters of interest before creating images. Sinograms of the physiological parameters, rather than the counts, can subsequently be reconstructed to form images of the parameters directly.

II. MATERIALS AND METHODS

A. Theory

A full set of plane parallel projections of the activity distribution measured along a LOR during the acquisition period forms the basis data set for the measurement, and the object of the reconstruction process is to invert the projections to regain an estimation of the activity concentration at a point in space. Equation (1) shows the relationship between the radon transform $\lambda_\Phi(x_r)$ at angle Φ of the 2D activity distribution $\mu(\mathbf{r})$. It is equivalent to a plane projection along the direction y_r through the object (Barrett *et al.*, 1981):

$$\lambda_\Phi(x_r) = \int_l \mu(\mathbf{r})\, dy_r \qquad (1)$$

From the Patlak derivation, we expect the following relationship to be true for time points after equilibrium between the irreversible compartments in tissue, K_{mr} is the influx rate constant and P is the partition coefficient or apparent volume of distribution, V_d, of the reversible compartments:

$$\frac{\mu(\mathbf{r}, t)}{C_p(t)} = K(\mathbf{r})\, \theta + P(\mathbf{r}) \quad (2)$$

where

$$\theta = \frac{\int_0^t C_p(\tau)\, d\tau}{C_p(t)} \quad (3)$$

Equation (4) extends (1) by introducing variation in time into the radon transform:

$$\lambda_\Phi(x_r, t) = \int_l \mu(\mathbf{r}, t)\, dy_r \quad (4)$$

Rearranging and substituting (2) in (4),

$$= \int_l (K(\mathbf{r})\, \theta + P(\mathbf{r}))\, C_p(t)\, dy_r \quad (5)$$

Since $\dot{C}_p(t)$ and θ are independant of $\mathbf{r}$,

$$\frac{\lambda_\Phi(x_r, t)}{C_p(t)} = \theta \int_l K(\mathbf{r})\, dy_r + \int_l P(\mathbf{r})\, dy_r \quad (6)$$

which can be fitted to the linear model in exactly the same way as proposed by Patlak for the activity concentration values to determine

$$\kappa_\Phi(x_r) = \int_l K(\mathbf{r})\, dy_r \quad (7)$$

$$\pi_\Phi(x_r) = \int_l P(\mathbf{r})\, dy_r \quad (8)$$

In comparison with (1), $\kappa(x_r)$ and $\pi(x_r)$ can be seen to be the 2D projections of the uptake rate constant and partition coefficient, respectively. These 2D projections can be back projected using standard back projection algorithms to create 2D images of these two parameters.

The variance of $\kappa(x_r)$ and $\pi(x_r)$ can be estimated during linear regression. In a summation image $b(\mathbf{r})$, which is a first-order approximation to back projection, where the projections are smeared in space and added together, the following holds:

$$b(\mathbf{r}) = \sum \lambda_\Phi(x_r) \quad (9)$$

so that variances could be combined in the following way (Fischer et al., 1993).

$$\sigma_{b(r)}^2(\mathbf{r}) = \sum \sigma_{\lambda_\Phi(x_r)}^2(x_r) \quad (10)$$

However, this equation is not exact for filtered back projection, where the weightings employed during fil-

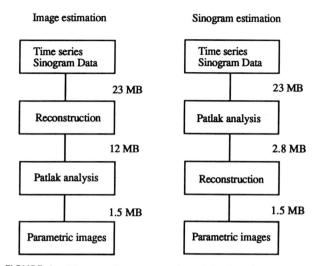

FIGURE 1 Diagramatic representation of the data flow. The data amounts have been estimated for 16 time frames, 47 2D planes each of 192 views with 160 radial elements and for estimation of rCMR$_{glu}$, the regional cerebral glucose consumption, and V_d, the volume of distribution of the equilibrating compartments.

tering would have to be taken into consideration when combining variances.

In practice, corrections are normally made during reconstruction for attenuation of the source object, variations in the efficiency of detectors, and dead time of the instrument. Since all these corrections are applied independent of pixel value and are, in effect, constant scaling factors, it is immediately apparent that they can be applied before or after fitting the projection data, depending on convenience. The decay correction must be applied before fitting because it is a nonlinear function of time. Note that we have not addressed the issue of scatter correction, which may be a function time and may depend both on the value of individual pixels and not be independent for each pixel.

B. Method

We chose to validate the preceding ideas using the tracer FDG, which, according to the published model data (Sokoloff, 1978), approaches closely an ideal tracer in the sense of the Patlak analysis. Indeed, the tracer model that we will assume is exclusively for estimation of time series data up to 48 min and so does not include a rate constant to account for backflow of phosphorylized FDG.

Five normal subjects were scanned for 48 min after injection of approximately 200 MBq [^{18}F]fluorodeoxyglucose using a protocol of frames of 3×1 min, 10×3 min, and 3×5 min. During the study 20 5 ml blood samples were collected and analyzed for plasma activity concentration. PET measurement was performed on a Siemens ECAT 933/04-16 (Siemens-CTI, Knoxville, Tennessee) with seven concurrent acquisition planes resulting in a set of 16 sinograms for each of the planes. Plasma activity was measured using a NaI well counter (Berthold LB 951 G).

The acquired data was back projected—standard filtered Fourier back projection, using a standard ramp and a Hanning apodizing function with a cutoff at 0.5 cycles per pixel to create cross-sectional slices of the activity concentration distribution for each time frame. This reconstructed data was then fitted (Press *et al.*, 1987) on a pixel-by-pixel basis to the linear model of uptake as specified by the Patlak technique and images of $rCMR_{glu}$ and V_d, and their variances were calculated. This calculation is referred to here as *image estimation*.

The sinogram data were also fitted on a pixel-by-pixel basis for K_{mr} and partition coefficients in the same way as for the images and were subsequently back projected—referred to here as *sinogram estimation*. The same filter and back projection algorithm was used in the reconstruction of the parametric images as in the reconstruction of the time series images of the count rate.

For both the sinogram and the image based analyses, the initial time for the fitting range was varied between 4.5 and 31.5 min, representing inclusion of between 13 and 3 frames of time series data, respectively. The data amounts shown in Figure 1 represent the normal protocol of 16 frames. Naturally, the data reduction

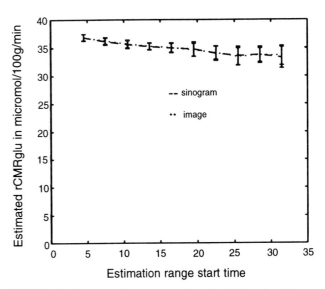

FIGURE 3   The variation in the estimated $rCMR_{glu}$ for different time ranges of regression. The error bars are the standard deviations of the mean between ROIs for all subjects.

gained is related to the number of frames chosen, and this technique lends itself to protocols with higher time resolution and, hence, greater data reduction.

The reconstructed K_{mr} values were converted to $rCMR_{glc}$ units using the measured concentration of glucose in blood and the lumped constant for the uptake of FDG of 0.52. Both reconstructed data sets were analyzed with a set of four regions of interest (ROIs), which comprised the caudate nucleus (a small region surrounded by low-uptake white matter) and a region of the insular cortex (a larger region that is homogeneous).

The variances of K_{mr} and V_d estimated from the fits were also back projected; however, the filter weightings were not taken into account (see equation (10)).

III. RESULTS AND DISCUSSION

The very good correlation between the two methods is shown in Figure 2. The difference between the two methods is <5% for both parameters for ranges, which include times <20 min after injection.

There is, however, a dependence of the estimated parameters on the time range over which linear regression is performed. Figure 3 shows the variation in the mean of the estimation of $rCMR_{glu}$ across all subjects and regions. The estimation consistently decreases with estimation range starting time.

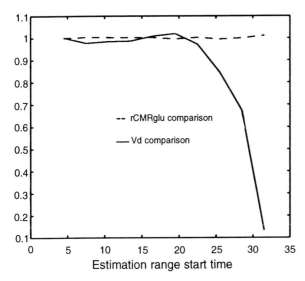

FIGURE 2   The mean of the ratio of $rCMR_{glu}$ and V_d values between the two methods shown for estimations using different starting times for the linear portion of the curve. The mean is taken for all regions and studies.

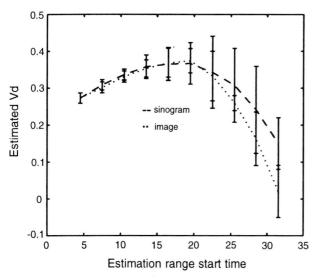

FIGURE 4   The variation in the estimated V_d for different time ranges of regression.

TABLE 2   A Comparison of the Standard Deviations of V_d as Estimated by the Variation Between V_d Values in Different Studies (between studies) and by Back Projecting the Variance (single study), Both Standard Deviations are Calculated for a Mid-scan Time Point of 10.5 min

	Image σ		Sinogram σ	
	Between studies	Single study	Between studies	Single study
Insular left	0.11	0.09	0.11	0.40
Insular right	0.13	0.13	0.13	0.42
Caudate left	0.05	0.12	0.06	0.31
Caudate right	0.13	0.12	0.13	0.41

In the V_d estimation, shown in Figure 4, both methods remain consistent in their estimation up to a starting time of 20 min. After this point, the estimations diverge rapidly. There is also strong variation in the estimation of V_d by both methods over time. This is a characteristic of the Patlak methodology rather than the fitting method.

Tables 1 and 2 show a comparison of the standard deviation of the estimates for an estimation range starting at 10.5 min. Errors calculated by back projecting the variances are larger than those estimated by comparing the variance across subjects, indicating that the back projected variance is not a good estimator of the

accuracy of the calculated rCMR$_{glu}$ and V_d values. The results of the validation study clearly show that the method is applicable to 2D data data sets.

Since the calculation of the parameters is independent for each pixel in a data set, it is possible to perform the analysis on each pixel independently. This means that the technique is ideally suited to a parallelization on a pixel-by-pixel basis.

Variations in the estimated parameters with range of regression is to be expected in the light of the statistical variation present in the raw data. We found that starting times for the range should be <20 min, which is consistent with the time required for the equilibration of the reversible compartments of the model.

The estimation of the variance by back projection of the estimated sinogram variances was not shown to correlate well with intersubject variability, presumably because of the noise associated with the sinogram estimate and the weightings applied, which render equation (10) invalid. A more thorough investigation of the error estimates needs to be carried out.

The main advantage of the method is that it allows the calculation of physiological parameters before reconstruction, reducing the number of images to be reconstructed by a factor equal to the number of frames acquired. Since the accuracy of the parameters calculated will depend on both the accuracy of the determination of the activity concentration at each time point and the amount of information about time in the data, it well may be advantageous to increase the number of time points acquired. This algorithm allows the implementation of a protocol involving more time points without compromising on reconstruction times for the whole data set.

The assumptions of the method are exactly the same as those applied to any Patlak analysis, and so it can be applied to the modeling of any tracer that fulfills the original criteria.

TABLE 1   A Comparison of the Standard Deviations of rCMR$_{glu}$ as Estimated by the Variation Between rCMR$_{glu}$ Values in Different Studies (between studies) and by Back Projecting the Variance (single study), Both Standard Deviations are Calculated for a Mid-scan Time Point of 10.5 min

	Image σ		Sinogram σ	
	Between studies	Single study	Between studies	Single study
Insular left	7.84	2.19	7.28	9.02
Insular right	5.98	2.68	5.94	9.65
Caudate left	5.72	2.62	5.73	7.09
Caudate right	7.98	2.93	7.59	9.31

The method also can be extended to other estimation methods where the condition of linear dependence of the parameters of interest on the projection integrals is held (e.g., Blomquist, 1984; Van den Hoff *et al.*, 1993).

References

Barrett, H. H., and Swindell, W. (1981). "Radiological Imaging," Vol. 2, p. 379. Academic Press, New York.

Blomquist, G. (1984). On the construction of functional maps in positron emission tomography. *J. Cereb. Blood Flow* **4:** 629–632.

Fischer, L. D., and van Belle, G. (1993). "Biostatistics, A Methodology for the Health Sciences." Wiley, New York.

Gjedde, A. (1982). Calculation of cerebral glucose phosphorylation from brain uptake of glucose analogs in vivo: A re-examination. *Brain Res. Rev.* **4:** 237–274.

Patlak, C. S., Blasberg, R. G., and Fenstermacher, J. D. (1983). Graphical evaluation of blood-to-brain transfer constants from multiple-time uptake data. *J. Cereb. Blood Flow Metab.* **3:** 1–7.

Press, W. H., Flannery, B. P., Tevkolsky, S. A., and Vetterling, W. T. (1987). "Numerical Recipes in C (The Art of Scientific Computing)," 2 ed., Cambridge Univ. Press, Cambridge.

Sokoloff, L. (1978). Mapping cerebral functional activity with radioactive deoxyglucose. *Trends Neurosci.* **1:** 75–79.

Van den Hoff, J., Burchert, W., Müller-Schavenberg, W., Meyer, G.-J., and Hundeshagen, H. (1993). Accurate local blood flow measurements with dynamic PET: Fast determination of input function delay and dispersion by multilinear minimization. *J. Nucl. Med.* **34:** 1770–1777.

61

A Graphical Method of Determining Tracer Influx Constants in the Presence of Labeled Metabolites

DAVID A. MANKOFF,[1] MICHAEL M. GRAHAM,[1] and ANTHONY F. SHIELDS[2]

[1]*Division of Nuclear Medicine, University of Washington, Seattle, Washington 98195*
[2]*Department of Medicine and Veterans Affairs Medical Center and University of Washington, Seattle, Washington*

The graphical analysis technique of Patlak, Blasburg, and Fenstermacher (1983) and Gjedde (1982) is a popular tool for estimating blood-to-tissue influx constants from multiple-time uptake data. We present a convenient extension of this technique that can be applied to tracers with significant quantities of labeled metabolites in the blood, which cause errors in the standard graphical analysis. The extended graphical method applies when the intact tracer is irreversibly trapped in tissue and the labeled metabolites are not. Under these conditions, the following relationship holds:

$$A/C_{tot} = K_x \int C_x d\tau/C_{tot} + V_{0x}C_x/C_{tot}$$
$$+ \Sigma(V_{0mi})C_{mi}/C_{tot} + V_b$$

where A is the measured tissue activity; C_{tot}, C_x, and C_{mi} are the measured total, tracer, and ith metabolite plasma concentrations; V_{0x} and V_{0mi} are virtual volumes of distribution for the tracer and ith metabolite; V_b is the partial volume contribution of blood activity; and K_x is the tracer influx constant (desired value). To determine K_x, the parameters K_x, V_{0x}, V_b, and the V_{0mi} must be estimated, which can be accomplished using linear estimation methods. The problem can usually be simplified to the estimation of three or four parameters, including the tracer influx constant. We conclude that the extended graphical analysis approach provides a simple and efficient method for estimating tissue transfer constants for tracers with labeled metabolites.

I. INTRODUCTION

Radiopharmaceutical imaging is frequently complicated by the presence of labeled metabolites. The me-
tabolites will usually have a different distribution pattern than the intact tracer and therefore can cause errors in the quantitative kinetic analysis. When the blood concentrations of the tracer and its metabolites are known through blood sampling and metabolite analysis, tracer kinetic modeling can be used to separate the contributions of tracer and metabolites to the image and to estimate physiologic parameters based on the dynamic distribution of the tracer of interest. Models accounting for the behavior of the intact tracer and its metabolites are, by necessity, more complex and generally ill-suited for the routine estimation of physiologic parameters. Therefore, a method capable of simplifying the quantitative analysis of such tracers without ignoring the contribution of labeled metabolites would be highly desirable.

The graphical analysis method of Patlak (Patlak and Blasberg, 1985; Patlak *et al.*, 1983) and Gjedde (1982) has been applied to tracers that can be characterized by models with a single compartment of irreversible or nearly irreversible trapping. In this analysis, a transformation of the data leads to a simple graphical relationship that can be used to estimate the steady-state flux of the traced substance into the compartment with irreversible trapping. Previous investigators have suggested methods for adapting graphical analysis to handle labeled metabolites (Martin *et al.*, 1989; Patlak and Blasberg, 1985; Willemsem *et al.*, 1995). We present a general extension of the graphical anlaysis method that requires no tissue subtraction to correct for labeled metabolites and is applicable under the condition that none of the labeled metabolites is irreversibly trapped in the tissue of interest. Examples of tracers (metabolites) to which this method is potentially applicable

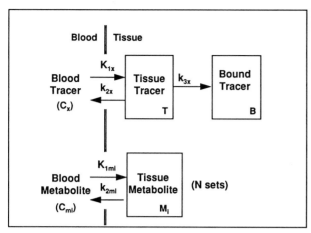

Total Plasma Activity = C_{tot} = C_x + ΣC_{mi}

Total Image Activity = A = T + B + ΣM_i + $V_b(C_{tot})$

FIGURE 1   Compartmental model for graphical estimation of influx constants for systems with labeled metabolites, irreversible trapping of intact tracer, and no irreversible trapping of the metabolites.

include 2-[^{11}C]thymidine (thymine, CO_2) (Mankoff *et al.*, 1994; Shields *et al.*, 1990; Vander Borght *et al.*, 1991), [^{18}F]fluorodopa (3-O-MFD) (Huang *et al.*, 1991; Martin *et al.*, 1989), and 1-[^{11}C]tyrosine (L-dopa, CO_2) (Willemsem *et al.*, 1995).

We present the theory and background for this method as well as suggestions for implementation.

II. BACKGROUND AND THEORY

A. Assumptions

We confine our discussion to the tracers that can be described by the model shown in Figure 1. The following assumptions are made for the subsequent mathematical development of the extended graphical method:

Standard graphical analysis assumptions for intact tracer:

1. Both the blood and tissue tracer activities over time are known. The blood is the only source of the tracer.

2. Tracer kinetics can be described by an exchangeable tissue compartment plus a single compartment into which flow is unidirectional (i.e., trapping). Unlike standard graphical analysis, labeled metabolites in the blood are allowed under the conditions described in the second set of assumptions.

3. The system obeys first order kinetics for transfer between compartments.

4. There exists a time, t^*, after injection when the intact tracer compartments reach a quasi-steady state and the exchangeable compartment is in near equilibrium with the blood. At this time, the relative rate of change of the plasma tracer concentration is much less than the rate constant for efflux from the exchangeable compartment. Using the parameter names illustrated in Figure 1, this is equivalent to the following statement for $t > t^*$:

$$\frac{dC_x/dt}{C_x} \ll k_{2x} + k_{3x} \qquad (1)$$

Additional assumptions for labeled metabolites:

5. The blood concentrations of the tracer and its metabolites (denoted m_i) are known over time. Only the sum of the tissue concentrations of the tracer and its metabolites is known, as would be the case in radionuclide imaging.

6. The blood is the most significant source of metabolites for the tissue of interest. In other words, the flux of metabolites from the blood to the tissue of interest is much greater than the local rate of metabolite generation. It is, therefore, assumed that a tissue other than the tissue of interest is principally responsible for the generation of metabolites. This assumption allows us to model the tracer and metabolites as having independent compartment sets, as illustrated in Figure 1.

7. The metabolites undergo only reversible exchange between blood and tissue; that is, none of the metabolites is irreversibly trapped in the tissue.

8. There exists a time, t^*, after injection when each compartment set reaches quasi-steady state. In addition to equation (1), we also require that, for $t > t^*$ (refer to Figure 1),

$$\frac{dC_{mi}/dt}{C_{mi}} \ll k_{2mi} \qquad \text{for all } i \qquad (2)$$

B. Mathematical Development

Under the preceding assumptions, the standard graphical relationship holds for each independent compartment set. For the intact tracer, the following holds:

$$\frac{A_x}{C_x} = K_x \frac{\int C_x d\tau}{C_x} + (V_{0x} + V_b) \qquad (3)$$

where K_x is the tracer influx constant, V_{0x} is the volume of distribution for the intact tracer, and A_x is the time-varying portion of tissue activity attributable to the intact tracer. The steady state flux of the tracer into the trapped compartment is given by K_x times the concentration of the native (i.e., nonlabeled) substance being traced.

For the ith metabolite, because there is no irreversible trapping, k_{3mi} is 0, and thus K_{mi} is 0. Therefore, the following simple relationship holds:

$$\frac{A_{mi}}{C_{mi}} = V_{0mi} + V_b \quad (4)$$

where C_{mi} is the blood concentration of the ith metabolite, A_{mi} is the portion of the tissue activity arising from the ith metabolite, and V_{0mi} is the distribution volume for the ith metabolite. Adding together equations (3) and (4) for all metabolites and rearranging the terms, we obtain the following relationship:

$$\frac{A}{C_{tot}} = K_x \frac{\int C_x d\tau}{C_{tot}} + V_{0x} \frac{C_x}{C_{tot}} + \sum V_{0mi} \frac{C_{mi}}{C_{tot}} + V_b \quad (5)$$

where A is the total tissue activity $= A_x + \sum A_{mi}$ and C_{tot} is the total blood activity $= C_x + \sum C_{mi}$.

Equation (5) describes a relationship between the normalized tissue activity and a linear combination of basis functions: $\int C_x d\tau / C_{tot}$, C_x / C_{tot}, several C_{mi}/C_{tot}, and 1, with a set of parameters K_x (tracer influx constant and parameter of interest), V_{0x}, several V_{0mi}, and V_b. It contains a new definition for normalized time: $\int C_x d\tau / C_{tot}$. The extended graphical method requires a decreased number of parameters to be estimated, and furthermore, it reduces parameter estimation to a linear estimation process rather than a nonlinear optimization process, as would be required by compartmental analysis.

C. Special Cases

In general, one is interested in the influx constant and not the volume terms in equation (5); therefore, simplifications are usually possible.

1. Special Case: Dominant Metabolite

Under the condition that there is a single dominant metabolite, equation (5) can be rewritten as follows:

$$\frac{A}{C_{tot}} = K_x \frac{\int C_x d\tau}{C_{tot}} + V_1 \frac{C_m}{C_{tot}} + V_2 \quad (6)$$

where the subscript m refers to the dominant metabolite and

$$V_1 = V_{0m} - V_{0x} \quad (7)$$
$$V_2 = V_b + V_{0x} \quad (8)$$

In this case, only three parameters need to be estimated, K_x, V_1, and V_2.

2. Special Case: Constant Ratio of Tracer and Metabolites in Blood

Under the condition that the tracer and its metabolites reach constant relative activities in the blood after time, t^*, even further simplifications are possible. Under these conditions,

$$\frac{A}{C_{tot}} = K_x \frac{\int C_x d\tau}{C_{tot}} + V \quad (9)$$

where

$$V = V_{0x} \frac{C_x}{C_{tot}} + \sum V_{0mi} \frac{C_{mi}}{C_{tot}} + V_b \quad (10)$$

which is a constant by virtue of the fact that C_x / C_{tot} and all the C_{mi}/C_{tot} are constant for $t > t^*$. The estimation of K_x is reduced to a simple line fit, as in conventional graphical analysis. This relationship looks very similar to the original graphical relationship, except for the new definition of normalized time, $\int C_x d\tau / C_{tot}$, which takes into account the presence of labeled metabolites.

3. Special Case: Small Amount of Metabolite Trapping

We also consider the case where one of the metabolites, denoted by subscript m^*, undergoes irreversible trapping in the tissue. In this situation, the following equation applies:

$$\frac{A}{C_{tot}} = K_x \frac{\int C_x d\tau}{C_{tot}} + V_{0x} \frac{C_x}{C_{tot}}$$
$$+ \sum V_{0mi} \frac{C_{mi}}{C_{tot}} + V_b + K_{m^*} \frac{\int C_{m^*} d\tau}{C_{tot}} \quad (11)$$

where K_{m^*} is the blood–tissue transfer constant for the trapped metabolite. In general, it will be difficult to mathematically separate the contribution of the trapped metabolite from the tracer of interest. The shape of the trapped metabolite normalized time, $\int C_{m^*} d\tau / C_{tot}$, is likely to be similar to the tracer of interest normalized time, $\int C_x d\tau / C_{tot}$, late after the injection, when the graphical approach applies. In this situation, K_x cannot be estimated independently of K_{m^*}; however, if only a small amount of metabolite trapping occurs, then approximate methods of estimating K_x can be used. We have used the following approach:

1. Identify the expected range of K_{m^*} and assume a fixed value for K_{m^*} in the center of the range of expected values.

2. Estimate K_x using the relationship

$$\left(\frac{A}{C_{\text{tot}}} - K'_{m*}\frac{\int C_{m*}d\tau}{C_{\text{tot}}}\right) = K_x\frac{\int C_x d\tau}{C_{\text{tot}}}$$
$$+ V_{0x}\frac{C_x}{C_{\text{tot}}} + \sum V_{0mi}\frac{C_{mi}}{C_{\text{tot}}} + V_b \tag{12}$$

where K'_{m*} is the assumed flux constant for the trapped metabolites. This relationship can be simplified if either of the first two special cases applies.

3. The range of possible errors in K_x resulting from this approach can be estimated by substituting the endpoints of the estimated range of possible values for K'_{m*} in equation (12).

III. IMPLEMENTATION CONSIDERATIONS

In general, the parameters in the extended graphical analysis relationship (equation (5)) can be obtained using linear estimation methods. The basis functions $\int C_x d\tau/C_{\text{tot}}$, C_x/C_{tot}, C_{mi}/C_{tot}, and 1, sampled at a number of discrete time points, form the design matrix for a set of linear equations. For N metabolites, $N + 3$ parameters will have to be estimated, and if there are M time points (for $t > t_0$) where plasma and tissue measurements are made, the design matrix will be an $M \times (N + 3)$ rectangular matrix as follows:

$$\begin{bmatrix} \dfrac{\int_{t_0}^{t_1} C_x d\tau}{C_{\text{tot}}(t_1)} & \dfrac{C_x(t_1)}{C_{\text{tot}}(t_1)} & \dfrac{C_{m1}(t_1)}{C_{\text{tot}}(t_1)} & \cdots & \dfrac{C_{mN}(t_1)}{C_{\text{tot}}(t_1)} & 1 \\ \vdots & \vdots & \vdots & \vdots & \vdots & \vdots \\ \dfrac{\int_{t_0}^{t_M} C_x d\tau}{C_{\text{tot}}(t_M)} & \dfrac{C_x(t_M)}{C_{\text{tot}}(t_M)} & \dfrac{C_{m1}(t_M)}{C_{\text{tot}}(t_M)} & \cdots & \dfrac{C_{mN}(t_M)}{C_{\text{tot}}(t_M)} & 1 \end{bmatrix}$$
$$M \times (N + 3)$$

$$\begin{bmatrix} K_x \\ V_{0x} \\ V_{0m1} \\ \vdots \\ V_{0mN} \\ V_b \end{bmatrix} = \begin{bmatrix} \dfrac{A(t_1)}{C_{\text{tot}}(t_1)} \\ \vdots \\ \dfrac{A(t_M)}{C_{\text{tot}}(t_M)} \end{bmatrix} \tag{13}$$
$$(N + 3) \times 1 \qquad M \times 1$$

where the $(N + 3) \times 1$ column vector on the left represents the vector of parameters to be estimated, and the $M \times 1$ vector on the right side of the equation is the normalized tissue activity sampled at M time points.

This equation can be solved, for example, by singular-value decomposition of the design matrix (Press *et al.*, 1988).

When the second special case applies (constant ratio of tracer and metabolites in the blood after time t^*), then the slope of a line fit of A/C_{tot} vs. $\int C_x d\tau/C_{\text{tot}}$ will provide an estimate of K_x.

When metabolite trapping is present to a small extent, the approximate method as given by equation (12) must be used. In this case, the normalized tissue activity vector in equation (13) is replaced according to the left side of equation (12), where a term accounting for metabolite trapping is subtracted from the normalized tissue activity at each time point. If either of the first two special cases applies, the resulting equation may be simplified accordingly.

IV. DISCUSSION

In the original papers on the graphical technique of Patlak and Gjedde (Gjedde, 1982; Patlak and Blasberg, 1985; Patlak *et al.*, 1983), the authors presented a convenient method for estimating blood–tissue transfer constants for tracers that are irreversibly trapped in tissue. The original formulations required that no labeled metabolites be present outside of the compartment where the tracer is trapped. We have presented a specific extension of the graphical analysis method that applies when the blood concentrations of the metabolites are known and the metabolites are not irreversibly trapped in the tissue. The result is a simple graphical estimation problem requiring only linear estimation of a small number of parameters, where the estimation can be handled using linear estimation methods; and under certain conditions, a simple two-dimensional linear regression can be used. We have also presented an approximate estimation method that can be used when one of the metabolites is trapped in tissue to a small extent.

Preliminary simulations of a particular tracer, 2-[^{11}C]thymidine (data not presented), have shown that the extended graphical method estimates of the tracer influx constant are comparable to those obtained with compartmental analysis. A moderate amount of local tracer degradation can be tolerated without significantly limiting the accuracy of the influx constant estimates; however, trapping of any of the metabolites can cause significant errors in the estimates, which can be partially, but not completely, corrected by assuming a fixed value for the influx constant for metabolite trapping. More work is needed to test the performance of the extended graphical method under more realistic simulations, including different tracers and models, a range of physiologic states (i.e., a range of parameter values), and statistical noise, as would be encountered in patient studies. In addition, the more difficult task of verifying the accuracy of the method applied to patient images must be undertaken.

V. CONCLUSIONS

We have presented an extension of the standard graphical analysis method that applies to systems with labeled metabolites. This method provides a computationally efficient tool for estimating tracer blood–tissue transfer constants for appropriate tracers and therefore may be useful in pixelwise image analysis.

Acknowledgments

The authors wish to thank Drs. Kenneth A. Krohn and Finbarr O'Sullivan, and Jeanne M. Link and Mark Muzi for helpful discussions. This work was supported in part by NIH Grants CA39566 and CA42045, the Medical Research Service of the Department of Veterans Affairs, and the Mallinckrodt Fellowship of the Society of Nuclear Medicine.

References

Gjedde A. (1982). Calculation of cerebral glucose phosphorylation from brain uptake of glucose analogs *in vivo*: A re-examination. *Brain Res. Rev.* **4:** 237–274.

Huang, S.-C., Yu, D.-C., Barrio, J. R., Grafton, S., Melega, W. P., Hoffman, J. M., Satyamurthy, N., Mazziotta, J. C., and Phelps, M. E. (1991). Kinetics and modeling of L-6-[F-18]Fluoro-DOPA in human Positron Emission Tomographic studies. *J. Cereb. Blood Flow Metab.* **11:** 898–913.

Mankoff, D. A., Shields, A. F., Lee, T. T., and Graham, M. M. (1994). Tracer kinetic model for quantitative imaging of thymidine utilization using [C-11]thymidine and PET [Abstract]. *J. Nucl. Med.* **35:** 138P.

Martin, W. R. W., Palmer, M. R., Patlak, C. S., and Calne, D. B. (1989). Nigrostriatal function in humans studies with Positron Emission Tomography. *Annal. Neurol.* **26:** 535–542.

Patlak, C. S., and Blasberg, R. G. (1985). Graphical evaluation of blood-to-brain transfer constants from multiple-time uptake data. Generalizations. *J. Cereb. Blood Flow Metab.* **5:** 584–590.

Patlak, C. S., Blasberg, R. G., and Fenstermacher, J. D. (1983). Graphical evaluation of blood-to-brain transfer constants from multiple-time uptake data. *J. Cereb. Blood Flow Metab.* **3:** 1–7.

Press, W., Flannery, B., Teukolsky, S., and WT., V. (1988). Numerical Recipes in C. Cambridge University Press, New York.

Shields, A. F., Lim, K., Grierson, J., Link, J., and Krohn, K. A. (1990). Utilization of labeled thymidine in DNA synthesis: studies for PET. *J. Nucl. Med.* **31:** 337–342.

Vander Borght, T., Labar, D., Pauwels, S., and Lambotte, L. (1991). Production of [2-^{11}C]thymidine for quantification of cellular proliferation with PET. *Appl. Radiat. Isotopes.* **42:** 103–104.

Willemsem, A. T. M., van Waarde, A., Paans, A. M. J., Pruim, J., Luurtsema, G., Go, K. G., and Vaalburg, W. (1995). *In vivo* protein synthesis rate determination in primary or recurrent brain tumors using L-[1-C-11]-tyrosine and PET. *J. Nucl. Med.* **36:** 411–419.

62

Quantitative Imaging of [11C]Benztropine in the Human Brain with Graphic Analysis and Spectral Analysis

T. FUJIWARA,[1] M. MEJIA,[1] M. ITOH,[1] K. YANAI,[2] K. MEGURO,[3] H. SASAKI,[3] S. ONO,[4]
H. ITOH,[4] H. FUKUDA,[4] R. IWATA,[5] T. IDO,[5] H. WATABE,[6] V. J. CUNNINGHAM,[7]
J. ASHBURNER,[7] and T. JONES[7]

Divisions of [1]Cyclotron Nuclear Medicine and [5]Radiopharmaceutical Chemistry
Cyclotron and Radioisotope Center
Tohoku University, Sendai 980–77, Japan
Departments of [2]Pharmacology I and [3]Geriatric Medicine
Tohoku University School of Medicine
Sendai 980–77, Japan
[4]Department of Radiology and Nuclear Medicine
Institute of Development, Aging and Cancer
Tohoku University, Sendai 980–77, Japan
[6]Department of Investigative Radiology
National Cardiovascular Center Research Institute
Suita 565, Japan
[7]MRC Clinical Sciences Centre
Hammersmith Hospital, London, W12 ONN, United Kingdom

Patlak graphical analyses are frequently used for the quantitative study of receptor distribution in the human brain, when the specific binding of the tracer is apparently irreversible over the time course of the study. An alternative approach is provided by spectral analysis, which allows the unit impulse response function, and hence an estimate of the irreversible disposal rate constant, to be derived. The latter technique also can be used to obtain estimates of the total volume of distribution when the binding is reversible. We have compared these two techniques and applied them to the quantitative estimation of muscarinic cholinergic receptor distribution in human brain with [11C]benztropine PET. After transmission scanning, [11C]benztropine was injected into three healthy male volunteers and serial tomographic scans were performed using a Siemens-CTI 931 PET scanner. Arterial blood samples were drawn rapidly and plasma was separated and counted. Selected plasma samples were also analyzed for percentage of unchanged tracer. [11C]benztropine binding was analyzed at the pixel level by both the Patlak method and spectral analysis to give quantitative parametric images of [11C]benztropine uptake. Estimates of the irreversible disposal rate constant were obtained from the terminal slope of the equivalent Patlak plot and from the value of the unit impulse response function at a late time (60 min). Very close correlation was found at the pixel level between the two estimates. Overall, estimates obtained by spectral analysis were about 90% of those obtained by the Patlak analysis, reflecting some reversibility in the binding measured over the scan period.

I. INTRODUCTION

Positron emission tomography has been widely used for investigating the neuroanatomical distribution of radiolabeled neurotransmitter-specific receptor ligands. The generation of quantitative functional or parametric images of binding requires analytical techniques that are robust and also sufficiently rapid to allow routine implementation at the pixel level. For processes that are apparently irreversible over the time course of the study, Patlak analysis (Patlak *et al.*, 1983)

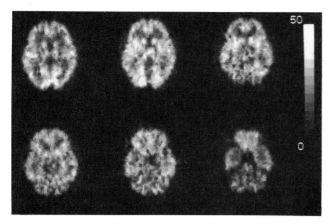

FIGURE 1 Parametric images of spectral analysis of [¹¹C]benztropine. Total volume of distribution.

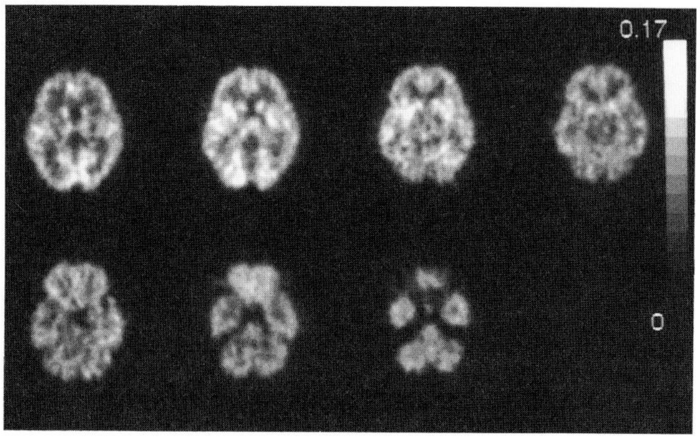

FIGURE 3 Parametric images of spectral analysis of [¹¹C]benztropine. Unit impulse response function at 60 min (min^{-1}).

provides such a technique. An alternative, however, is to use spectral analysis (Cunningham *et al.*, 1993a, 1993b), which is a linear technique and hence computationally rapid and has the further advantage that it makes no a priori assumption of the nature or number of kinetic components in the data. It allows the unit impulse tissue response function to be obtained for each pixel time–activity curve. For irreversible processes, this function should plateau in the limit at late times (equivalent to the derivative of the terminal slope of a Patlak plot), and an estimate of the irreversible disposal rate constant can be obtained from this plateau value. For reversible processes, the function approaches 0 at late times. In this case, an image of the total volume of distribution can be used as a quantitative index of binding. This is given by the integral of the unit impulse response function. We have applied both these techniques to PET studies using [¹¹C]benz-

tropine to compare their application to the quantitative estimation and imaging of muscarinic cholinergic receptor distribution in human brain.

II. MATERIALS AND METHODS

Three normal adult male volunteers were studied. [¹¹C]benztropine was synthesized as described by Dewey *et al.* (1990). After transmission scanning, 740 MBq of [¹¹C]benztropine was injected intravenously. Following the injection, serial tomographic scans were performed using a Siemens-CTI 931/04-12 PET scanner. A sequence of 22 scans covered 90 min (1 min × 2; 2 min × 4; 5 min × 16). Arterial blood samples were drawn rapidly and plasma was separated and counted. Selected plasma samples (5, 10, 15, 30, and 60 min post injection) were analyzed for the percentage of unchanged tracer. Spectral analysis of the data was

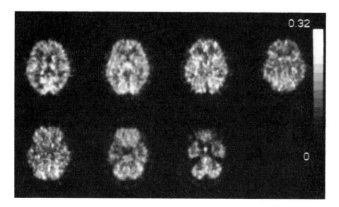

FIGURE 2 Parametric images of spectral analysis of [¹¹C]benztropine. Unit impulse response function at 1 min (min^{-1}).

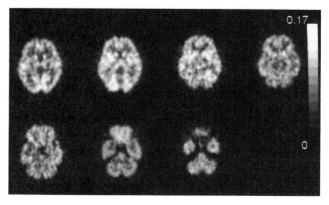

FIGURE 4 Pixel-by-pixel Patlak slope images of [¹¹C]benztropine (ml/g/min).

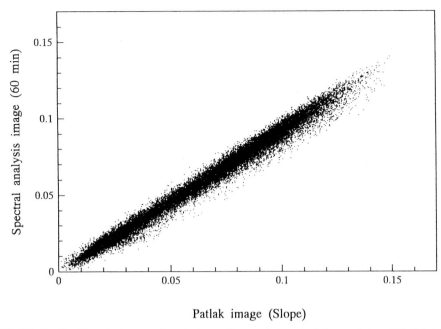

FIGURE 5   Pixel-by-pixel comparison between the spectral analysis image data and Patlak image data.

carried out as described by Cunningham *et al.* (1993a, b) to give estimates of the total volume of distribution and values of the unit impulse response functions at 1 min and 60 min. Under the assumption of (near) irreversibility, the 60 min values of the unit impulse response function were compared with estimates of the irreversible disposal rate constant obtained by Patlak analysis (Patlak *et al.*, 1983). Data collected between 5 and 60 min (real time) were used for the determination of the slope of the Patlak analysis.

III. RESULTS AND DISCUSSION

Parametric images of [^{11}C]benztropine calculated by spectral analysis of data from one subject are shown in Figures 1–3. Figure 1 shows the total volume of distribution. These images were derived by integrating (to infinity) the unit impulse response function derived from data collected over 90 min. The images are relatively noisy because of the extrapolation associated with the large volume of distribution. This, in turn, suggests that it may be reasonable to assume near irreversible behavior during time period of the scan. It was, therefore, of interest to compare parametric images of the unit impulse response function at a late time (60 min) with the corresponding Patlak analysis. In this irreversible case, images of the unit impulse response function at early times (Fig. 2) are dominated by delivery, whereas values of the function at late times approach the irreversible disposal rate constant and are equivalent to the terminal limiting slope of a Patlak plot (Fig. 4). The 60 min response images and the Patlak slope images were used for pixel-by-pixel comparison. Figure 5 shows the correlation between 60 min response images and the slope images of all slices. Good correlation of the two different parametric images was observed, and the square of the correlation coefficient (r^2) was 0.982. The squares of other two studies were 0.977 and 0.986. The values of slopes were 0.913, 0.889, and 0.855; and the intercepts were -0.0004, 0.0002, and -0.0011, respectively. This small difference probably reflects the assumption of irreversibility, as opposed to analyses involving relatively large but finite volumes of distribution.

The muscarinic cholinergic system plays an essential role in many memory and cognitive functions. Dewey and his colleagues reported imaging of muscarinic cholinergic receptors in the human brain using [^{11}C]benztropine (Dewey *et al.*, 1990). They analyzed [^{11}C]benztropine distribution by drawing region of interests on the images. The work presented here is concerned with the quantitation of muscarinic cholinergic receptors carried out on a pixel-by-pixel basis. The generation of such parametric images has great advantages both for the visualization and the subsequent analysis of receptor binding. Several methods of analyzing PET data have been developed and compartmental models are often used. Model parameters can be determined by a nonlinear least squares fit to the experimental data. However, parameter estimation often yielded uncertain results. The Patlak method of analysis applicable to ligands that are trapped in tissue for the duration of the experiment therefore was applied. This method is robust and, because of the simplicity of the calculation, greatly facilitates the intercomparison of experimental data. Spectral analysis identifies the components in PET tissue radioactivity data with no prior assumptions of a specific kinetic model and no assumptions about tissue equilibrium or product loss.

The value of [^{11}C]benztropine uptake of spectral analysis were lower than those of graphical analysis. This may be derived from the procedure of graphical analysis of this study. The graphical method assumes that the binding process is essentially irreversible. Although the graphic plots of [^{11}C]benztropine became fairly linear, there was some uncertainty of determination of linear part of plots on a pixel-by-pixel basis. Since the total count of the later part of dynamic scans became low and images became noisy, the earlier part of dynamic scans were included for calculation of the graphic plots in this preliminary study. This difference

may be overcome to chose more adequate dynamic scan sequences. The current work demonstrates the expected close correlation between the Patlak approach and late images of the impulse response function using spectral analysis but suggests that the latter may be advantageous here because it can also be used to generate volumes of distribution if the assumption of irreversibility is considered inappropriate.

References

Cunningham, V. J., and Jones, T. (1993a). Spectral analysis of dynamic PET studies. *J. Cereb. Blood Flow Metab.* **13:** 15–23.

Cunningham, V. J., Ashburner, J., Byrne, H., and Jones, T. (1993b). Use of spectral analysis to obtain parametric images from dynamic PET studies. *In:* "Quantification of Brain Function. Tracer Kinetics and Image Analysis in Brain PET" (K. Uemura, N. A. Lassen, T. Jones, and I. Kanno, Eds.), pp. 101–108. Elsevier Science Publishers, Amsterdam, Netherlands.

Dewey, S. L., Macgregor, R. R., Brodie, J. D., Bendriem, B., King P. T., Volkow N. D., Schlyer, D. J., Fowler J. S., Wolf, A. P., Gatley, S. J., and Hitzemann, R. (1990). Mapping muscarinic receptors in human and baboon Brain Using [N-11C-methyl]-benztropine. *Synapse* **5:** 213–223.

Patlak, C. S., Blasberg, R. C., and Fenstermacher, J. D. (1983). Graphical evaluation of blood-to-brain transfer constants from multiple-time uptake data. *J. Cereb. Blood Flow Metab.* **3:** 1–7.

63

Kinetic Analysis Summary

RICHARD E. CARSON

I. INTRODUCTION

Kinetic analysis is at the heart of the quantification of brain function with PET. A wide variety of methods have been developed to convert the tracer radioactivity concentration values provided by the scanner to measurements of physiological parameters. The issues to be considered in the development and application of tracer methods include choices of tracer administration and data acquisition schemes; measurement of the input function with corrections for metabolites, if necessary, development of the most appropriate kinetic analysis techniques, including compartment modeling and graphical or spectral analysis; and the use of parameter estimation schemes for rapid calculation of the physiological parameter(s) of interest on a pixel-by-pixel basis.

The kinetic analysis session of Brain PET '95 had 30 papers covering a wide range of topics. Many authors showed new methods to measure physiological parameters or refinements in existing methods to measure parameters with more accuracy, less variability, or with simpler acquisition or analysis protocols. These papers dealt with cerebral blood flow, glucose metabolism, F-DOPA uptake and metabolism, and receptor ligand interactions. In addition, new methods for rapid parameter estimation from kinetic data were introduced. Other techniques simultaneously analyzed the entire image volume to improve the quality of kinetic estimates. New graphical analysis methods were also presented. The papers in this session are summarized here.

II. CEREBRAL BLOOD FLOW

New methods and analyses for the measurement of cerebral blood flow were presented in seven papers. The goal of two papers (Carson, Yan, and Shrager,

Chapter 36; Watabe *et al.*, Chapter 37) was to determine absolute cerebral blood flow without measurement of an arterial input function. These methods used the Kety one-compartment model to extract information about the input function from pixel time–activity curves throughout the brain. Measurement of regional dispersion and delay, important parameters in the estimation of CBF, was performed by Murase *et al.*, Chapter 39. Toussaint and Meyer (Chapter 38) performed a sensitivity analysis of dispersion, delay, and the initial volume of distribution for CBF studies. In a second paper (not submitted for publication), these authors evaluated the effect of including the initial volume of distribution as a fitted parameter in analyzing [^{15}O]water dynamic data. Andersson *et al.* (not submitted for publication) proposed a revised autoradiographic flow method that uses a variable value for the distribution volume of water to account for the effects of tissue heterogeneity. Mejia *et al.* (Chapter 40) proposed a new formulation for converting brain tissue data to relative CBF measurement.

III. GLUCOSE METABOLISM

Two papers showed methods for the measurement of the glucose metabolic rate with FDG. Halber *et al.* (Chapter 41) evaluated a linear normalization scheme for FDG measurements to permit intersubject comparison. A new methodology for analysis of double injection FDG studies was presented by Reutens *et al.* (Chapter 42).

IV. FDOPA

A wide variety of approaches have been developed for the analysis and application of the tracer FDOPA.

321

Six papers were presented in the kinetic analysis session. Dhawan *et al.* (Chapter 43) presented the modeling issues associated with combined studies of FDOPA and O-MFD, a metabolite that crosses the blood–brain barrier. Vontobel *et al.* (Chapter 44) evaluated the effects of various assumptions concerning the relative kinetic constants of FDOPA and O-MFD on FDOPA results. Holden *et al.* (Chapter 45) presented findings on the relationship between the O-MFD distribution volume and the ratio of FDOPA uptake slopes from plasma or occipital input functions. The ability of various kinetic constants to discriminate normal controls from patients with Parkinson's disease was evaluated by Ishikawa *et al.* (Chapter 46) and Shiraishi *et al.* (Chapter 47). The effects of the COMT inhibitor entacapone was also presented by Ishikawa *et al.* (Chapter 46).

V. RECEPTOR MODELING

A variety of issues associated with receptor modeling were presented in five papers. Different methods for estimating the total receptor concentration B_{max} were presented by Delforge *et al.* (Chapter 48), ranging from the complex multi-injection technique to simple single-scan methods. Morris, Fischman, and Alpert (Chapter 49) demonstrated the importance of accurate compartment modeling of both hot and cold ligands in studies using multiple injections. The initial characterization of a ligand that binds to the serotonin-1A site was presented by Price *et al.* (Chapter 50). Houle *et al.* (Chapter 51) described the use of bolus plus infusion administration of [^{11}C]raclopride with a new data analysis scheme. The ability to detect the release of endogenous ligand via its displacement of radioligands was presented in Chapter 52 by Malizia *et al.* A simulation study of this approach was also presented by Morris *et al.* (Chapter 82) in the Statistical Analysis session. This issue was the topic of a breakout session in which there was substantial interest in developing techniques to measure stimulus-induced neurotransmitter release. Much work lies ahead to determine the sensitivity for measurement of endogenous ligand release and to choose optimal methodology.

VI. PARAMETER ESTIMATION

The Kinetic Analysis session included four papers describing new methods for rapid estimation of kinetic parameters. Two papers (Svarer *et al.*, Chapter 53; Graham and O'Sullivan, Chapter 54) demonstrated the use of neural nets to perform estimation of the kinetic

parameters of FDG. These authors first trained their neural nets on a wide range of data (input functions and tissue time–activity curves) and could then rapidly produce functional images of the rate constants. The issues associated with the use of neural nets were further discussed in a breakout session. Kimura *et al.* (Chapter 55) presented a new weighted integration method for rapid calculation of kinetic constants using more than the minimum number of weighting functions. Methods for reducing computation time for iterative least squares were shown by Taguchi *et al.* (Chapter 56).

VII. IMAGE AND VOLUME KINETIC ANALYSIS

Three papers presented four-dimensional techniques; that is, approaches that analyzed the complete data set simultaneously, taking advantage of the fact that many pixels share similar kinetic properties. By pooling data across "similar" pixels, significant noise reduction can be realized. Factor analysis of dynamic receptor data was presented by Yap *et al.* (Chapter 57). O'Sullivan *et al.* (Chapter 58) showed the most recent developments in the mixture analysis approach. A third method, cluster analysis, was applied to PET kinetic data in Chapter 59 by Ashburner *et al.*

VIII. GRAPHICAL ANALYSIS

A variety of graphical analysis methods have been widely applied for various PET tracers. Three chapters were presented further developing these techniques. Maguire, Calonder, and Leenders (Chapter 60) demonstrated the ability to estimate the slope of the Patlak plot directly from sinogram data. Mankoff, Graham, and Shields (Chapter 61) extended previous graphical approaches for tracers with labeled metabolites. Patlak slope data was compared to spectral analysis on pixel-by-pixel data by Fujiwara *et al.* (Chapter 62).

IX. SUMMARY

PET methods for kinetic analysis can be very complex due to the many subtleties associated with the use of each tracer. Techniques range from simple ratio methods that provide indices of physiological function to complex multi-injection, multitracer techniques for absolute quantification. The choice of the most appropriate data analysis method depends on the biological question. The Kinetic Analysis session of Brain PET

'95 presented a broad overview of current issues in the development and application of tracer methods. New PET tracers are continuously being developed for the measurement of an increasing number of regional physiological characteristics. The approaches embodied in the chapters in the Kinetic Analysis session will continue to be of prime importance in the successful application of current and new PET tracers.

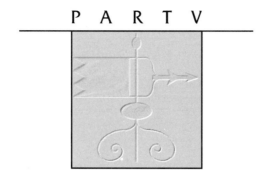

STATISTICAL ANALYSIS

64

A Unified Statistical Approach for Determining Significant Signals in Location and Scale Space Images of Cerebral Activation

K. J. WORSLEY,[1] S. MARRETT,[2] P. NEELIN,[2] and A. C. EVANS[2]

[1]*Department of Mathematics and Statistics, McGill University, Montreal, Quebec, Canada H3A 2K6*
[2]*McConnell Brain Imaging Centre, Montreal Neurological Institute, Montreal, Quebec, Canada H3A 2B4*

We present a unified P-value for assessing the significance of peaks in statistical fields searched over regions of any shape or size. We extend this to 4D scale space searches over smoothing filter width as well as location. The results are usable in a wide range of applications, including PET and fMRI, but are discussed with particular reference to PET images that represent changes in cerebral blood flow (CBF) elicited by a specific cognitive or sensorimotor task.

I. INTRODUCTION

We present a unified statistical theory for assessing the significance of apparent signals observed in noisy difference images. The results are usable in a wide range of applications, including PET and fMRI, but are discussed with particular reference to PET images that represent changes in cerebral blood flow (CBF) elicited by a specific cognitive or sensorimotor task. Our first result, derived by Worsley (1995), is an estimate of the P-value for local maxima of Gaussian, T, χ^2, and F fields over search regions of any shape or size in any number of dimensions. This unifies the P-values for large search areas in 2D (Friston *et al.*, 1991), large search regions in 3D (Worsley *et al.*, 1992), and the usual uncorrected p-value at a single pixel or voxel. This makes it possible to restrict the search to small anatomical regions, such as the cingulate gyrus or caudate nucleus, or two-dimensional regions, such as a slice or the cortical surface, or even single voxels. The results are also generalizable to 4D searches in time as well as space, which may be useful for fMRI.

Our second result is an extension to searches over

smoothing filter width or scale space. PET images of CBF in an activation study are usually smoothed to a resolution much less than that attainable by the PET camera. In many studies the choice of this smoothing is arbitrarily fixed at a 20 mm FWHM, and the resulting statistical field or parametric map is searched for local maxima. Poline and Mazoyer (1994) have proposed a 4D search over smoothing kernel widths as well as location to find local maxima in 1D scale space as well as 3D location space. If the peaks are well separated, this allows us to estimate the size of regions of activation as well as their location. We avoid repeating the smoothing and statistical analysis on all scans in an experiment by smoothing just the highest resolution statistical field and then correcting its standard deviation. Only a small number of "fixels," or filter pixels, are required because the 4D image is very smooth in the scale direction. The result, derived by Siegmund and Worsley (1995), is a unified P-value for the 4D local maxima that makes it possible to assess the significance of the regions of activation. The price paid for searching in scale space is a small increase in the critical threshold, but this is offset by the increased sensitivity to detect peaks of all widths.

II. PREVIOUS RESULTS FOR LARGE SEARCH REGIONS

In many PET activation studies, the researcher wishes to compare the CBF under one condition with that under another, or the response of CBF to a covariate such as stimulus intensity. In either case, the problem can be analyzed as a multiple regression, in which

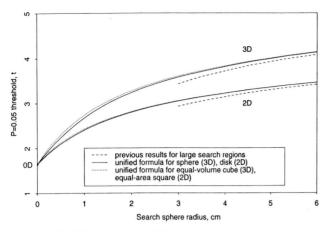

FIGURE 1   Max *Z*, FWHM = 20 mm, *P* = 0.05.

TABLE 1   Examples from a Voxel Atlas, FWHM = 20 mm, *P* = 0.05

Search region	V_0	V_1, cm	V_2, cm^2	V_3, cm^3	*t*
Single voxel	1	0	0	0	1.64
Globus pallidus	0	8	9	2	2.78
Head of caudate	0	12	19	5	3.02
Thalamus	1	10	21	9	3.05
Putamen	1	15	27	9	3.15
Cingulate	0	26	39	12	3.27
Occipital lobe	−1	21	92	57	3.55
Temporal	0	34	147	104	3.71
Parietal	1	30	148	116	3.72
Frontal	1	39	214	189	3.84
4 mm shell	2	1	829	127	4.04
Whole brain	1	41	428	1227	4.23

the test statistic of interest is a *T* or *Z* statistic evaluated at each voxel (Friston *et al.*, 1995). These images, often called *statistical parametric maps* (SPM), are then searched for local maxima that might indicate the presence of significant activation. The main problem is to control false positives; that is, the detection of significant peaks when in fact no activation is present.

If the images are finely sampled, that is, the voxel size is small relative to the FWHM of the PET camera, then the image can be approximated by a continuous image or *random field*, in which the voxel values are the values of the random field sampled on a lattice of equally spaced points. Local maxima of the voxels are then closely approximated by local maxima of the continuous random field. The *P*-value of these (continous) local maxima has a long history in the statistics literature. Early results for two-dimensional random fields, appearing in 1945, were motivated by studies of waves on the ocean surface. More powerful results for arbitrary numbers of dimensions were derived by Russian probabilists in the 1970s, culminating in the papers and book by Robert Adler (Adler, 1981). The result for a stationary Gaussian random field smoothed by a Gaussian point spread function in two dimensions is

$$P(\text{Max } Z \geq t) \approx \frac{\text{Area}}{\text{FWHM}^2} \frac{(4 \log_e 2)}{(2\pi)^{3/2}} t e^{-1/2 t^2} \quad (1)$$

where Area is the area of the search region and FWHM is the full-width at half-maximum of the (Gaussian) point spread function. This result was discovered independently by Friston *et al.* (1991), after correction by a factor of $\pi/4$. The result for three dimensions is

$$P(\text{Max } Z \geq t) \approx \frac{\text{Volume}}{\text{FWHM}^3} \frac{(4 \log_e 2)^{3/2}}{(2\pi)^2} (t^2 - 1) e^{-1/2 t^2} \quad (2)$$

where Volume is the volume of the search region (see Fig. 1). These results (1) and (2) are accurate only for large peak heights and large volumes, and no exact *P*-value exists.

Considerable debate has centered on whether the standard deviation of a CBF subtraction should be estimated by the standard deviation at a voxel or whether the voxel standard deviations can be pooled over all voxels to give a more stable estimator. The former

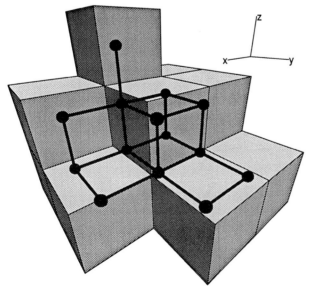

FIGURE 2 $P = 14$, $E = 21$, $F = 9$, $C = 1$; $V_0 = 1$, $V_1 = 6\delta$, $V_2 = 6\delta^2$, $V_3 = 1\delta^3$.

TABLE 2   EC Densities for Different Types of Fields

Gaussian field

$$\rho_0(t) = \int_t^\infty \frac{1}{(2\pi)^{1/2}} e^{-1/2u^2} du$$

$$\rho_1(t) = \frac{(4 \log_e 2)^{1/2}}{2\pi} e^{-1/2t^2}$$

$$\rho_2(t) = \frac{(4 \log_e 2)}{(2\pi)^{3/2}} t e^{-1/2t^2}$$

$$\rho_3(t) = \frac{(4 \log_e 2)^{3/2}}{(2\pi)^2} (t^2 - 1) e^{-1/2t^2}$$

T-field with ν degrees of freedom, $\nu \geq d$

$$\rho_0(t) = \int_t^\infty \frac{\Gamma\left(\frac{\nu+1}{2}\right)}{(\nu\pi)^{1/2} \Gamma\left(\frac{\nu}{2}\right)} \left(1 + \frac{u^2}{\nu}\right)^{-1/2(\nu+1)} du$$

$$\rho_1(t) = \frac{(4 \log_e 2)^{1/2}}{2\pi} \left(1 + \frac{t^2}{\nu}\right)^{-1/2(\nu-1)}$$

$$\rho_2(t) = \frac{(4 \log_e 2)}{(2\pi)^{3/2}} \frac{\Gamma\left(\frac{\nu+1}{2}\right)}{\left(\frac{\nu}{2}\right)^{1/2} \Gamma\left(\frac{\nu}{2}\right)} t \left(1 + \frac{t^2}{\nu}\right)^{-1/2(\nu-1)}$$

$$\rho_3(t) = \frac{(4 \log_e 2)^{3/2}}{(2\pi)^2} \left(\frac{\nu-1}{\nu} t^2 - 1\right) \left(1 + \frac{t^2}{\nu}\right)^{-1/2(\nu-1)}$$

χ^2-field with ν degrees of freedom

$$\rho_0(t) = \int_t^\infty \frac{u^{1/2(\nu-2)} e^{-1/2u}}{2^{\nu/2} \Gamma\left(\frac{\nu}{2}\right)} du$$

$$\rho_1(t) = \frac{(4 \log_e 2)^{1/2}}{(2\pi)^{1/2}} \frac{t^{1/2(\nu-1)} e^{-1/2t}}{2^{1/2(\nu-2)} \Gamma\left(\frac{\nu}{2}\right)}$$

$$\rho_2(t) = \frac{(4 \log_e 2)}{(2\pi)} \frac{t^{1/2(\nu-2)} e^{-1/2t}}{2^{1/2(\nu-2)} \Gamma\left(\frac{\nu}{2}\right)} [t - (\nu - 1)]$$

$$\rho_3(t) = \frac{(4 \log_e 2)^{3/2}}{(2\pi)^{3/2}} \frac{t^{1/2(\nu-3)} e^{-1/2t}}{2^{1/2(\nu-2)} \Gamma\left(\frac{\nu}{2}\right)} [t^2 - (2v - 1)t + (\nu - 1)(\nu - 2)]$$

F-field with k and ν degrees of freedom, $k + \nu > d$

$$\rho_0(t) = \int_t^\infty \frac{\Gamma\left(\frac{\nu+k}{2}\right)}{\Gamma\left(\frac{\nu}{2}\right) \Gamma\left(\frac{k}{2}\right)} \frac{k}{\nu} \left(\frac{ku}{\nu}\right)^{1/2(k-2)} \left(1 + \frac{ku}{\nu}\right)^{-1/2(\nu+k)} du$$

$$\rho_1(t) = \frac{(4 \log_e 2)^{1/2}}{(2\pi)^{1/2}} \frac{\Gamma\left(\frac{\nu+k-1}{2}\right) 2^{1/2}}{\Gamma\left(\frac{\nu}{2}\right) \Gamma\left(\frac{k}{2}\right)} \left(\frac{kt}{\nu}\right)^{1/2(k-1)} \left(1 + \frac{kt}{\nu}\right)^{-1/2(\nu+k-2)}$$

$$\rho_2(t) = \frac{(4 \log_e 2)}{2\pi} \frac{\Gamma\left(\frac{\nu+k-2}{2}\right)}{\Gamma\left(\frac{\nu}{2}\right) \Gamma\left(\frac{k}{2}\right)} \left(\frac{kt}{\nu}\right)^{1/2(k-2)} \left(1 + \frac{kt}{\nu}\right)^{-1/2(\nu+k-2)}$$

$$\times \left[(\nu - 1) \frac{kt}{\nu} - (k - 1)\right]$$

$$\rho_3(t) = \frac{(4 \log_e 2)^{3/2}}{(2\pi)^{3/2}} \frac{\Gamma\left(\frac{\nu+k-3}{2}\right) 2^{-1/2}}{\Gamma\left(\frac{\nu}{2}\right) \Gamma\left(\frac{k}{2}\right)} \left(\frac{kt}{\nu}\right)^{1/2(k-3)} \left(1 + \frac{kt}{\nu}\right)^{-1/2(\nu+k-2)}$$

$$\times \left[(\nu - 1)(\nu - 2)\left(\frac{kt}{\nu}\right)^2 - (2\nu k - \nu - k - 1)\left(\frac{kt}{\nu}\right)\right]$$

$$+ (k - 1)(k - 2)\bigg]$$

leads to a T-statistic image with degrees of freedom depending on the number of scans (Friston *et al.*, 1991), whereas the latter leads to a Z-statistic (Worsley *et al.*, 1992). The choice ultimately hinges on a trade-off between specificity and sensitivity. The T-statistic has good specificity but lower sensitivity, due to the extra variability of the voxel standard deviation; attempts to alleviate this by pooling standard deviations across conditions may bias the specificity. The Z-statistic has

a higher sensitivity due to its stable standard deviation, but its specificity is susceptible to fluctuations in the true voxel standard deviation. For a discussion of this issue, see Worsley *et al.* (1995a).

Early work with the T-statistic image was hampered by the lack of an accurate formula for the P-value of local maxima. Friston *et al.* (1991) suggested converting the T-statistic map to a Z-statistic map by probability integral transforms. Although the resulting map is

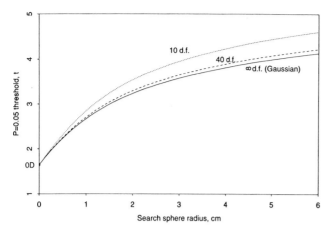

FIGURE 3 3D Max Gaussianized T, FWHM = 20 mm, $P = 0.05$.

only for large search regions (see Fig. 1). This was overcome by results derived in Worsley (1995), which gives a "unified" formula for Gaussian fields that combines the previous two- and three-dimensional results (1) and (2) with analogous zero- and one-dimensional results to give a P-value that is accurate for search regions of (almost) any shape or size:

$$P(\text{Max } Z \geq t) \approx \text{Euler characteristic} \frac{1}{(2\pi)^{1/2}} \int_t^\infty e^{-1/2u^2} \, du$$

$$+ \frac{2 \text{ Caliper diameter}}{\text{FWHM}} \frac{(4 \log_e 2)^{1/2}}{(2\pi)} e^{-1/2t^2}$$

$$+ \frac{(1/2) \text{ Surface area}}{\text{FWHM}^2} \frac{(4 \log_e 2)}{(2\pi)^{3/2}} t e^{-1/2t^2}$$

$$+ \frac{\text{Volume}}{\text{FWHM}^3} \frac{(4 \log_e 2)^{3/2}}{(2\pi)^2} (t^2 - 1) e^{-1/2t^2}$$

$$(4)$$

The formula (4) is most accurate when the boundary of the search region is smooth relative to the smoothness of the image; it is too conservative for highly convoluted search regions such as the cortex. Instead we suggest using (4) with the convex hull of highly convoluted search regions, which produces a less conservative and more accurate P-value.

The coefficient of the first term in (4) is the Euler characteristic (EC) of the search region, which is 1 for connected regions with no holes. For a convex search region, the caliper diameter is the average, over all rotations, of the height, length, and width of a bounding box placed around the search region. Values of these region size measures for a sphere and for a box are

Gaussian at every voxel, its joint distributional behavior is different from a Gaussian field and the P-value (2) is too small, especially for low degrees of freedom. This problem was solved in Worsley (1994), which gives an accurate formula for the P-value of T-field local maxima. For three dimensions, the result is

$$P(\text{Max } T \geq t)$$

$$\approx \frac{\text{Volume}}{\text{FWHM}^3} \frac{(4 \log_e 2)^{3/2}}{(2\pi)^2} \left(\frac{\nu - 1}{\nu} t^2 - 1 \right) \left(1 + \frac{t^2}{\nu} \right)^{-1/2(\nu-1)}$$

$$(3)$$

where ν is the degrees of freedom. This result was reported in the last PET Brain '93 meeting in Akita (Worsley *et al.*, 1993).

III. SEARCH REGIONS OF ANY SHAPE OR SIZE

Progress since the Akita meeting has been made on two fronts. The first is the problem of small search regions. The P-value formulas given so far are accurate

		Sphere, radius r	Box, $a \times b \times c$
Euler characteristic,	$V_0 =$	1	1
2 Caliper diamater,	$V_1 =$	$4r$	$a + b + c$
(1/2) Surface area,	$V_2 =$	$2\pi r^2$	$ab + bc + ac$
Volume,	$V_3 =$	$(4/3)\pi r^3$	abc

Note that, for a box, twice the caliper diameter is the measure of size frequently used by airlines for luggage. $P = 0.05$ thresholds found by equating (4) to 0.05 and solving for t are plotted against search region size in Figure 1. Note that thresholds for the equal-volume cube and equal-area square are slightly higher than for the sphere and disk, respectively.

For voxel data, such as search regions taken from a voxel atlas, the size measures can be calculated as follows. The voxel size δ must be the same in all dimensions. The voxels inside the search region are treated as points on a lattice, and P is the number of such points, E the number of "edges" joining adjacent

TABLE 3 Scale Space Gaussian Field

$$\rho_0(t) = \frac{1}{(2\pi)^{1/2}} \left\{ \sqrt{\frac{3}{4\pi}} (-\log_e r) \, e^{-1/2t^2} + \int_t^\infty e^{-1/2u^2} \, du \right\}$$

$$\rho_1(t) = \frac{(4 \log_e 2)^{1/2}}{(2\pi)} \left\{ \sqrt{\frac{3}{4\pi}} (1 - r) \, t + \frac{1+r}{2} \right\} e^{-1/2t^2}$$

$$\rho_2(t) = \frac{(4 \log_e 2)}{(2\pi)^{3/2}} \left\{ \sqrt{\frac{3}{4\pi}} \frac{1 - r^2}{2} \left(t^2 - \frac{1}{3} \right) + \frac{1 + r^2}{2} t \right\} e^{-1/2t^2}$$

$$\rho_3(t) = \frac{(4 \log_e 2)^{3/2}}{(2\pi)^2} \left\{ \sqrt{\frac{3}{4\pi}} \frac{1 - r^3}{3} (t^3 - t) + \frac{1 + r^3}{2} (t^2 - 1) \right\} e^{-1/2t^2}$$

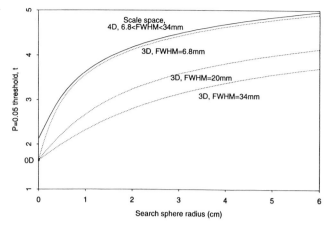

FIGURE 4 Scale space, $P = 0.05$.

points on the lattice, F is the number of "faces" joining a square of four adjacent points, and C is the number of "cubes" joining a cube of eight adjacent points, all of which are inside the search region (see Fig. 2). Then,

Euler characteristic,	$V_0 = (P - E + F - C)$
2 Caliper diamater,	$V_1 = (E - 2F + 3C)\delta$
(1/2) Surface area,	$V_2 = (F - 3C)\delta^2$
Volume,	$V_3 = C\delta^3$

Table 1 gives $P = 0.05$ thresholds for some structures selected from a voxel atlas (Evans *et al.*, 1991). Note that the large surface area of the 4 mm thick shell covering the outer cortex produces a larger threshold than the frontal lobe, even though the frontal lobe has a larger volume. Further details are given in Worsley *et al.* (1995a).

IV. UNIFIED *P*-VALUE FOR *Z*, *T*, χ^2, AND *F* FIELDS

The result (3) can be generalized to other types of random fields, such as a *T*-field. We define the *d*-dimensional *resel count* as

$$R_d = V_d/\text{FWHM}^d, \qquad d = 0, \ldots, 3 \qquad (5)$$

Then the unified formula is

$$P(\text{Max} \geq t) \approx \sum_{d=0}^{3} R_d \rho_d(t) \qquad (6)$$

where $\rho_d(t)$ is the *d*-dimensional *EC density*, which depends on the threshold t and the type of random field. Table 2, based on results in Worsley (1994), gives the EC densities for a Gaussian field (which matches the previous formula (4)), a *T*-field (which generalizes the earlier result (3)), a χ^2-field, and an *F*-field. $P = 0.05$ thresholds for a *T*-field, transformed to a Gaussian scale, are shown in Fig. 3. Note that the Gaussian is a good approximation for 40 or more degrees of freedom.

V. UNIFIED *P*-VALUE FOR SCALE SPACE SEARCHES

The second theoretical development since the Akita meeting is a formula for the *P*-value of 4D scale space local maxima (Seigmund and Worsley, 1995). We assume that the Gaussian images can be modeled as white noise convolved with a Gaussian filter or point response function and let $r = (\text{min FWHM})/(\text{max}$

TABLE 4 Significant Peaks in Coghill *et al.* (1994)

Peaks	Location (mm) in scale space						Fixed scale	
	x	*y*	*z*	FWHM	Max	*P*	Max	*P*
Increases:								
R. SII/anterior insula	35	−2	10	22.7	6.56	0.0000	5.65	0.0006
R. SMA (Inferior)	4	−2	54	22.7	6.22	0.0001	5.00	0.014
R. thalamus	11	−19	−3	17.4	5.73	0.0012	5.36	0.0025
L. anterior insula	−33	13	7	6.8	4.86	0.0824	3.72	1.96
R. SI	24	−28	57	19.9	4.77	0.12	4.02	0.72
L. putamen	−25	5	0	19.9	4.76	0.12	4.57	0.089
R. caudate	−12	−2	15	6.8	4.73	0.14	—	—
Decreases:								
R. posterior cingulate	5	−59	25	15.2	4.86	0.082	5.14	0.0072
M. posterior cingulate	1	−42	30	11.6	4.54	0.31	—	—

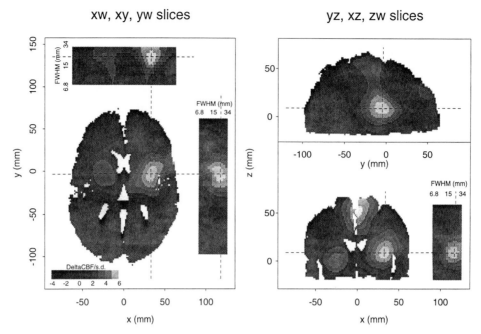

FIGURE 5   Scale space slices.

FWHM) be the ratio of the FWHM limits. Then the unified *P*-value, again accurate for search regions of almost any shape or size, is the same as (6) but with the EC densities given in Table 3. $P = 0.05$ thresholds are given in Figure 4 and compared to the equivalent thresholds for a fixed FWHM search. The price paid for searching in scale space is an increase in threshold of about 0.8 over the threshold for a fixed 20 mm FWHM search.

The practical issues of searching scale space are dealt with in some detail in Worsley *et al.* (1995b), which shows that only a small number of filter widths or "fixels" are needed (≈ 13), equally spaced on a log scale; only the highest resolution Gaussian image needs to be smoothed, not all the data; and the standard deviation can be corrected by using the spatial correlation function. A drawback to the method is that close sharp foci are detected as one large region. In this case, we suggest that peaks should be inspected for "bifurcations" in scale space slices.

An example of an application to an experiment in pain perception (Coghill *et al.*, 1994) is shown in Table 4. The data were smoothed from 6.8 to 34 mm FWHM ($r = 5$) and searched inside the whole brain search region, whose volume measures are given in the last line of Table 1. The formulas (5) and (6) and Table 3 were used to calculate *P*-values for 4D scale space peaks. Note that the scale space peaks are nearly always larger and more significant than the peaks from

a fixed scale search at 20, 20, and 7.4 mm FWHM in the *x*, *y*, and *z* directions. More importantly, two small foci were discovered in the scale space search that were overlooked in the fixed scale search, presumably because they were oversmoothed. Figure 5 shows scale space slices through the largest peak, which indicate a bifurcation that suggests that the largest peak is in fact composed of two smaller foci 2 cm apart in the *y* direction. Further details are given in Worsley *et al.* (1995b).

References

Adler, R. J. (1981). "The Geometry of Random Fields." Wiley, New York.

Coghill, R. C., Talbot, J. D., Evans, A. C., Meyer, E., Gjedde, A., Bushnell, M. C., and Duncan, G. H. (1994). Distributed processing of pain and vibration by the human brain. *J. Neurosci.* **14:** 4095–4108.

Evans, A. C., Marrett, S., Torrescorzo, J., Ku, S., and Collins, L. (1991). MRI-PET correlative analysis using a volume of interest (VOI) atlas. *J. Cereb. Blood Flow Metab.* **11**(2): A69–A78.

Friston, K. J., Frith, C. D., Liddle, P. F., and Frackowiak, R. S. J. (1991). Comparing functional (PET) images: The assessment of significant change. *J. Cereb. Blood Flow Metab.* **11:** 690–699.

Friston, K. J., Holmes, A. P., Worsley, K. J., Poline, J.-B., Frith, C. D., and Frackowiak, R. S. J. (1995). Statistical parametric maps in functional imaging: A general approach. *Hum. Brain Mapping* **2:** 189–210.

Poline, J. B., and Mazoyer, B. M. (1994). Enhanced detection in brain activation maps using a multifiltering approach. *J. Cereb. Blood Flow Metab.* **14:** 639–642.

Siegmund, D. O., and Worsley, K. J. (1995). Testing for a signal with unknown location and scale in a stationary Gaussian random field. *Ann. Statistics* **23:** 608–639.

Worsley, K. J., Evans, A. C., Marrett, S., and Neelin, P. (1992). A three dimensional statistical analysis for CBF activation studies in human brain. *J. Cereb. Blood Flow Metab.* **12:** 900–918.

Worsley K. J., Evans, A. C., Marrett, S., and Neelin, P. (1993). Detecting and estimating the regions of activation in CBF activation studies in human brain. *In:* "Quantification of Brain Function: Tracer Kinetics and Image Analysis in Brain PET" (K. Uemura, N. Lassen, T. Jones, and I. Kanno, Eds.), pp. 535–548. Elsevier Science Publ., BV., Amsterdam.

Worsley, K. J. (1994). Local maxima and the expected Euler characteristic of excursion sets of χ^2, F, and t fields. *Adv. Appl. Probability* **26:** 13–42.

Worsley, K. J. (1995). Estimating the number of peaks in a random field using the Hadwiger characteristic of excursion sets, with applications to medical images. *Ann. Statistics* **23:** 640–669.

Worsley, K. J., Marrett, S., Neelin, P., Vandal, A. C., Friston, K. J., and Evans, A. C. (1995a). A unified statistical approach for determining significant signals in images of cerebral activation. Submitted for publication.

Worsley, K. J., Marrett, S., Neelin, P., and Evans, A. C. (1995b). Searching scale space for activation in PET images. Submitted for publication.

Nonparametric Analysis of Statistic Images from Functional Mapping Experiments

A. P. HOLMES,[1,2] **R. C. BLAIR,**[3] **J. D. G. WATSON,**[4,5] **and I. FORD**[1]

[1]*Department of Statistics, University of Glasgow, Glasgow, United Kingdom*
[2]*Wellcome Department of Cognitive Neurology, Institute of Neurology, London WCIN 3BG, United Kingdom*
[3]*Department of Epidemiology and Biostatistics, College of Public Health*
University of South Florida, Tampa, Florida
[4]*Medical Research Council Cyclotron Unit, Hammersmith Hospital, London W12 ONN, United Kingdom*
[5]*Department of Anatomy, University College, London, United Kingdom*

The analysis of functional mapping experiments in PET and fMRI involves the formation and assessment of images of statistics. Existing methods are predominantly parametric, requiring a multitude of assumptions and relying on various approximations. In contrast to the parametric (and simulation) approaches, we present a nonparametric procedure that is intuitive, flexible, and (almost) exact (valid and not conservative), given minimal assumptions regarding the mechanisms generating the data. These randomization and permutation tests are simple extensions of widely accepted univariate exact nonparametric statistical procedures to the multiple comparisons problem of assessing a statistic image. These methods can consider any voxel statistic, including "pseudo" t-statistic images computed with smoothed variance estimates. For t-statistic images of low degrees of freedom, this appears to give the nonparametric methods greatly improved power over their conservative parametric counterparts. This suggests the use of nonparametric methods with "pseudo" statistics for analyzing low degree-of-freedom statistic images, such as those from single-subject analyses. Further, the guaranteed validity and flexibility of the nonparametric method make it attractive in situations where parametric methods are unavailable or the requisite assumptions or approximations untenable.

I. INTRODUCTION AND MOTIVATION

Pixel-by-pixel analyses of functional mapping experiments in PET involve the formation and assessment of statistic images. Current approaches are predominantly parametric: Distributional forms are assumed for the voxel values of the preprocessed data, and voxel hypotheses are formulated in terms of the parameters of these assumed distributions. Statistics with known null distribution are formed. These statistic images are then regarded as lattice representations of continuous random fields, whose properties are then used to assess the significance of the statistic image (Friston *et al.*, 1991; Worsley *et al.*, 1992; Worsley, 1994; Friston *et al.*, 1995).

These parametric approaches rely on a multitude of assumptions and approximations. "Noisy" statistic images (such as *t*-statistic images with low degrees of freedom, DF) are not well approximated by similar continuous fields. Essentially the continuous fields have features smaller than the voxel spacing, leading to extremely conservative tests (Worsley *et al.*, 1993). In general, it is not known how departures from the assumptions affect the validity of the tests, and it is difficult to assess the validity of the assumptions with the small sample sizes available in PET functional mapping experiments.

In contrast to parametric approaches, a nonparametric approach assesses simple hypotheses regarding the data using minimal assumptions in a computationally intensive manner (Good, 1993). Exact nonparametric statistical techniques are not new. Their origins are alongside classical statistical techniques, but their full potential has been realized only recently, as the necessary computing power has become available.

In this short chapter, an heuristic argument will be

developed for the multiple comparisons problem (MCP) of assessing functional mapping experiments. We will concentrate on illustration and discussion. For a rigorous treatment of the methodology as applied to PET, including algorithms, see Holmes *et al.* (1996).

II. METHOD

A nonparametric test can be constructed wherever a statistic is computed on the basis of some labeling of the data and where a probabilistic justification for relabeling exists. This probabilistic justification for relabeling comes from the null hypothesis, together with either an initial randomization (of labels to data epochs) or from weak distributional assumptions, leading to (re)randomization and permutation tests, respectively.

A. Randomization and Permutation Distributions for Statistic Images

1. Randomization: A Multisubject Activation Study

In the randomization approach, "labels" are randomly allocated to scan epochs before the data are acquired. The possible relabelings then are all those that could have arisen from the initial randomization of conditions to scan epochs.

For example, consider the following multisubject activation experiment with n subjects each scanned m times under both "baseline" (B) and "activation" (A) conditions, with conditions presented alternately. Half the subjects were randomly selected to be scanned ABAB . . . , the remaining half being scanned BABA . . . There are $_nC_{n/2}$ ways of choosing $n/2$ subjects from n, so there are $N = {}_{2m}C_m$ possible labelings of the scan epochs as A or B.

Under the null hypothesis $\mathcal{H}$, *each scan would have been the same whatever the condition*, and regarding the data as fixed, the N statistic images corresponding to these N possible labelings of the scans are all equally likely. This gives us the randomization distribution for the entire statistic image: the null sampling distribution of the statistic image given the data.

2. Permutation: A Single-Subject Correlational Study

Consider a single subject correlational study,[1] where a single variable is associated with each scan, some measure of performance, for example. In the absence of random allocation, a nonparametric model must be assumed. For example, a nonparametric general linear model is

$$Y_{jk} = \mu_k + \zeta_k S_j + \beta_k X_k + \varepsilon_{jk}$$

where Y_{jk} is the measured rCBF, or regional activity (rA), at voxel k of scan $j(= 1, \ldots, m)$; and X_j and S_j the gCBF (gA) and scores for the jth scan, respectively. The errors ε_{jk} will be assumed to be drawn from some *unspecified* distribution centered around 0. Here, the "labels" are the scores themselves. Under $\mathcal{H}$: $\zeta = 0$ (i.e., scans and scores are independent), any permutation of the scores is as likely as that observed and gives an equally likely statistic image. The $N = m!$ statistic images corresponding to the possible permutations of the scores constitute the permutation distribution for the statistic image: the null sampling distribution (given the data).

In the situation where the number of possible relabelings is too large to be computationally feasible, approximate randomization–permutation distributions can be constructed using a random sample of the possible permutations. Despite the name, the resulting tests are still exact. A loss of power is associated with estimating the randomization–permutation distribution, but this loss is minimal for large samples of relabelings, and many authors propose 1,000 as adequate.

B. Nonparametric Tests for Images

From this distribution for the whole statistic image, randomization–permutation distributions for any statistic summarizing a statistic image can be obtained.

1. Single-Threshold Test

The simplest form of test for a statistic image is a single-threshold test, where a threshold is set and the voxel hypotheses rejected for voxels with suprathreshold statistics. To maintain (weak) control over experimentwise Type I errors, the threshold must be set such that under the null hypothesis, the probability that any voxel statistic exceeds the threshold by chance alone, is less than a specified error level α (usually taken to be 0.05). Clearly, this depends on the value of the maximal statistic. The distribution of the maximal statistic is required, and a valid test is achieved with a threshold in the $100(1 - \alpha)$th percentile of this distribution.

In the nonparametric framework, the null sampling distribution, given the data, of the maximal statistic, is easily found by taking the maximal statistic of each of the N members of the randomization–permutation distribution for the statistic image. The critical threshold is then the $([\alpha N] + 1)$ largest member of the randomization–permutation distribution of the maximal statis-

---

[1]Usually called *parametric* designs, a terminology we shall not use, for obvious reasons.

tic.[2] Any voxels in the observed statistic image with statistics exceeding this threshold may have their null hypotheses rejected.

Note that the set of voxels over which the test is performed (the region over which the maximal statistic is searched) is arbitrary, provided it is specified *a priori*. Subsets of the whole image space can be tested, perhaps reflecting prior hypotheses, leading to increased power over the region of interest.

Further, it can be shown that this test maintains control over experimentwise Type I errors in the strong sense (Holmes *et al.*, 1996). Loosely speaking, this means that the test has ''localizing'' power, the results of the test at individual voxels can be reported.

Adjusted *p*-values for each voxel are computed as the proportion of the randomization–permutation distribution exceeding the voxels statistic. Because the voxel statistic is arbitrary and the critical threshold dependent on the actual data, it is preferable to report adjusted *p*-values rather than voxel statistics and a critical threshold.

It should be noted that, because the data are regarded as fixed, inference is restricted to the data; that is, to the subjects studied at the time of the study. In this respect, results should be treated as ''case reports'' rather than definitive results for some hypothetical population.

2. Other Tests

It is not difficult to see that these arguments are not limited to the cases presented here. For example, by summarizing statistic images by the size of the largest cluster of voxels with statistics exceeding a given threshold, a nonparametric suprathreshold cluster size test is obtained (Poline and Mazoyer, 1993; Roland *et al.*, 1993; Friston *et al.*, 1994).[3] Future tests may consider the maximum *suprathreshold cluster exceedence mass* (the integral of the image less the threshold over the cluster) as a summary statistic. Indeed, the preceding arguments guarantee that any maximal summary statistic for the statistic image leads to a test with weak control over Type I error.

C. ''Pseudo'' *t*-Statistics

Note that any voxel statistic can be used. Because the ''noise'' in low DF *t*-statistic images comes from the estimated variance image used in their computation, consider ''pseudo'' *t*-statistic images constructed with such a smoothed variance estimate: This effectively smooths the noise but not the signal! Neighboring voxels are not independent, so the voxel distribution of ''pseudo'' *t*-statistic images is intractable, precluding parametric analysis.

III. RESULTS

A. Multistudy Activation Study

The multisubject activation experiment we shall use for illustration is that reported by Watson *et al.* (1993). The experiment was designed to accurately locate the motion area (area V5) of the visual cortex by comparing

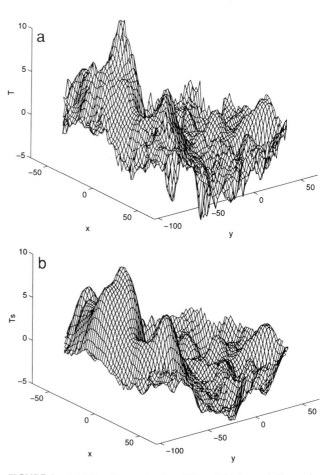

FIGURE 1   (a) ''Raw'' (voxel values T_k), and (b) ''pseudo'' *t*-statistic images (voxel values T_k^s) for the ''V5'' study. These are shown for the AC–PC plane only, using mesh plots to illustrate smoothness. The x–y plane is graduated in Talairach coordinates. Note that the mean difference image is smooth but that the statistic image is relatively noisy.

---

[2] Where [·] denotes the floor function.

[3] It should be noted that suprathreshold cluster tests do not control experimentwise Type I errors in the strong sense at the voxel level: Only entire suprathreshold clusters of significant size can be reported. Strong control may be ''loosely'' claimed at the cluster level.

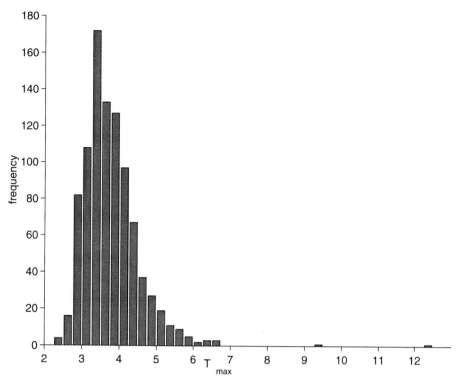

FIGURE 2   Randomization distribution of the maximal "pseudo" t-statistic for the multisubject activation study.

a "baseline" state during which subjects viewed a stationary checkerboard pattern (B), with an "active" state during which the pattern was in motion. In the study, $n = 12$ subjects were scanned $m = 6$ times under each of the two conditions, with conditions being randomly assigned to scan epochs as described in the methods section. After reconstruction, realignment within subjects, stereotactical normalization, and smoothing with a Gaussian kernel of FWHM 10 mm $\times$ 10 mm $\times$ 12 mm the images are ready for statistical analysis.

As a voxel statistic, consider a t-statistic on mean subject difference images, with global changes normalized by proportional scaling. This statistic is simple, robust, and illustrates the problems with t-statistic images of low degrees of freedom.

1. Statistic Images

The normalized data have voxel values $Y'_{ijqk} = Y_{ijqk}/(\overline{Y}_{ijq\bullet}/50)$, where in addition to the previously introduced notation, i subscripts the subjects.[4] The subject mean difference images have voxel values $\Delta_{ik} =$ $\overline{Y}'_{i\bullet Ak} - \overline{Y}'_{i\bullet Bk}$. A one-sample t statistic is computed at each voxel with voxel values $T_k = \overline{\Delta}_{\bullet k}/\sqrt{S_k^2/n}$, where S_k^2 is the estimated variance of the mean subject difference at voxel k (Fig. 1(a)).[5] Under appropriate assumptions and voxel null hypotheses,[6] the voxel t values are distributed as a Student's t-distribution with $n - 1$ degrees of freedom.

"Pseudo" t-statistic images, with voxel values T_k^s, were computed with a smoothed variance estimate obtained by convolving the estimated variance image S_k^2 with a Gaussian kernel of 10 mm $\times$ 10 mm $\times$ 6 mm FWHM (Fig. 1(b)). This filter size was arbitrarily chosen to be just less than the resolution of the reconstructed images, truncated in the Z-direction to avoid excessive edge effects. (Experience suggests that the size of the kernel is not critical.)

2. Randomization Distributions, Single-Threshold Test

Considering the $N = 12$, $\mathscr{C}_6 = 924$ possible rerandomizations of the labelings, the randomization distri-

---

[4]The usual statistical "bar and bullet" notation indicating that the mean has been taken over all values of the parameter replaced by the bullet.

[5]$S_k^2 = \dfrac{\sum_{i=1}^n (\Delta_{ik} - \overline{\Delta}_{\bullet k})^2}{(n-1)}$.

[6]$\Delta_{ik} \sim \mathcal{N}(\mu_k, \sigma_k^2)$ and $\mathscr{H}_k$: $\mu_k = 0$.

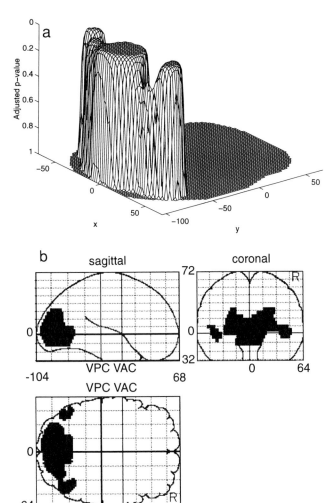

for imaging transient events. During each of 12 scans, the subject was presented with short sentences of random content in varying temporal patterns and was instructed to press a button for the duration of the stimulus. The button-press data was combined with the head curve to compute scores for each scan reflecting the amount of activity occurring during self-reported stimulation. Areas with rCBF positively correlated with the score are assumed to be those activated by the stimulus.

The voxel statistic considered was the t-statistic for $\mathcal{H}_k: \zeta_k = 0$ vs. $\overline{\mathcal{H}}_k: \zeta_k > 0$. Again, "pseudo" t-statistics were constructed by smoothing the estimated residual

FIGURE 3 Multisubject activation study: (a) Adjusted p-value image for the AC–PC plane, and (b) projections of the significantly activated region, $p < 0.05$. The latter corresponds to thresholding the observed "pseudo" t-statistic image at 5.083, the 47th largest member of the randomization distribution for the maximal statistic.

bution of the maximal t-statistic searched over the intracerebral volume was computed (Fig. 2). The maximal statistic of the "observed" statistic image is the largest of these, so a p-value for the omnibus null hypothesis is $p = 1/924$. Adjusted p-values and significant regions at $\alpha = 0.05$ are shown in Figure 3. The result of the corresponding parametric analysis is shown in Figure 4.

B. Single-Subject Activation Study

To illustrate the single subject correlation analysis consider one of the subjects (subject 1) studied by Silbersweig *et al.* (1994) in developing their methodology

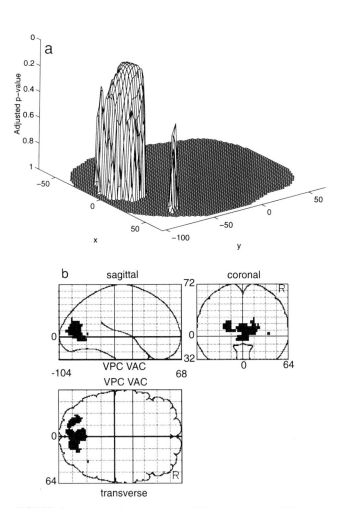

FIGURE 4 Results of a parametric SPM-type analysis (Friston *et al.*, 1995): The "raw" t-statistic image (computed with unsmoothed estimated variance image) was "Gaussianized" by replacing each voxel statistic with an equally extreme Z-score. Adjusted p-values were then computed using the expected Euler characteristic for a similar continuous Gaussian random field, as per Worsley *et al.* (1992). (Smoothness was estimated directly from the statistic image.) Shown are (a) the adjusted p-value image for the AC–PC plane, and (b) projections of the significantly activated region, $p < 0.05$.

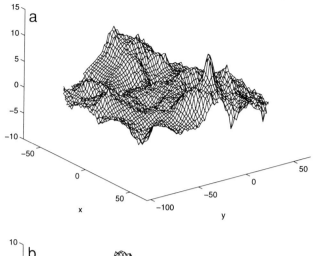

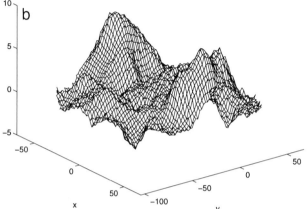

FIGURE 5   Mesh plots for the AC–PC planes of (a) the "raw" and (b) "pseudo" t-statistic images for $\mathcal{H}_k$: $\zeta_k = 0$.

A. Advantages and Disadvantages

The advantages of these methods are numerous:

Minimal assumptions. In contrast to current parametric methods, the randomization approach relies only on an initial random allocation in the design of the experiment. The permutation approach relies on weak distributional assumptions.

Validity. Given the data, the nonparametric tests maintain weak and strong control over experimentwise Type I errors. Further, the tests are (almost) exact.

Applicability. A nonparametric test can be constructed in most situations. All that is required is the concept of a "label" and a probabilistic justification for rerandomizing or permuting them.

Flexibility. Any voxel statistic can be considered. The statistic image may be assessed over any prespecified region, using any statistic summarizing the statistic image over that region.

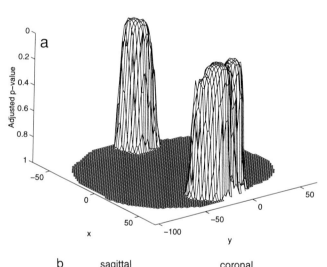

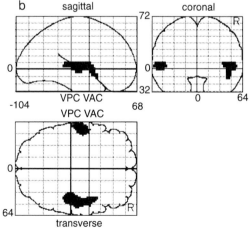

FIGURE 6   Single-subject correlation study: (a) Adjusted p-value image for the AC–PC plane, and (b) projections of the significantly activated region, $p < 0.05$.

variance image (Fig. 5). In addition to the actual allocation of scores to scans, 999 random permutations of the scores were chosen (without replacement) from the 12! possible ones. The maximum "pseudo" t-statistic was computed for each, giving the approximate permutation distribution, from which approximate adjusted p-values were computed (Fig. 6). Again, the result of the corresponding parametric analysis is shown in Figure 7.

V. DISCUSSION

In this short chapter, nonparametric randomization and permutation techniques for assessing functional mapping experiments have been described. The feasibility, flexibility, attractiveness, and power of the methods have been demonstrated, with particular emphasis on "noisy" statistic images.

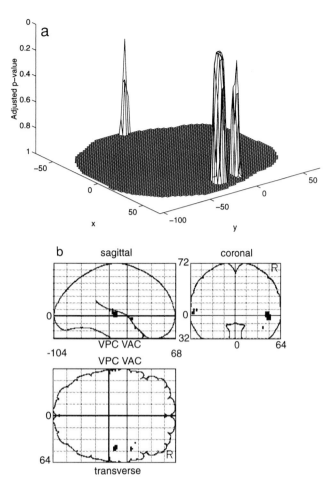

FIGURE 7 Single-subject correlation study. Results of a parametric SPM-type analysis of the "raw" *t*-statistic image. See legend to Figure 4 for details. Shown are (a) the adjusted *p*-value image for the AC–PC plane and (b) projections of the significantly activated region, $p < 0.05$.

Power. For *t*-statistic images with low degrees of freedom, the ability to consider "pseudo" *t*-statistics makes the nonparametric tests more powerful than parametric random field methods on the "raw" *t*-statistic image.

However, there are two notable disadvantages.

Computational burden. A statistic image has to be computed for each possible relabeling.

Number of labelings. The null sampling distributions are discrete, so adjusted *p*-values can be estimated accurately only when a large number of possible relabelings are available. This can be restrictive for some designs. (A single-subject activation experiment with two conditions presented alternatively over 12 scans only has $2^6 = 64$ possible relabelings if one is prepared to permute labels only within successive pairs.)

B. Power

In general, parametric methods outperform nonparametric methods when the assumptions of the former are true, the discrepancy being greater for small sample sizes (corresponding to small numbers of possible relabelings). However, present experience suggests that the approximations inherent in the parametric methods for assessing statistic images leave them comparable with the nonparametric methods. Further, for noisy *t*-statistic images of low degrees of freedom, the ability to consider "pseudo" statistics results in nonparametric tests that outperform their parametric counterparts.

C. Conclusions

The nonparametric methods presented are extremely flexible and always valid, given minimal assumptions. They are particularly powerful for *t*-statistic images of low degrees of freedom due to their ability to consider "pseudo" *t*-statistic images computed with a smoothed estimated variance image.

Therefore, these methods have three main fields for application:

- Analysis of studies with noisy statistic images, such as single subject studies where the *t*-statistic images have low degrees of freedom.
- Analysis in situations where parametric theory breaks down, is unavailable, or where the assumptions are untenable.
- Validation of existing methods.

References

Friston, K. J., Frith, C. D., Liddle, P. E., and Frackowiak, R. S. J. (1991). Comparing functional (PET) images: The assessment of significant change. *J. Cereb. Blood Flow Metab.* **11:** 690–699.

Friston, K. J., Worsley, K. J., Frackowiak, R. S. J., Mazziotta, J. C., and Evans, A. C. (1994). Assessing the significance of focal activations using their spatial extent. *Hum. Brain Mapping* **1:** 214–220.

Friston, K. J., Holmes, A. P., Worsley, K. J., Poline, J. P., Frith, C. D., and Frackowiak, R. S. J. (1995). Statistical parametric maps in functional imaging: A general approach. *Hum. Brain Mapping* **2:** 189–210.

Good, P. (1993). "Permutation Tests: A Practical Guide to Resampling Methods for Testing Hypotheses." Springer-Verlag, New York.

Holmes, A. P., Blair, R. C., Watson, J. D. G., and Ford, I. (1996). Non-Parametric Analysis of Statistic Images from Functional Mapping Experiments. *J. Cereb. Blood Flow Metab.* **16:** 7–22.

Poline, J.-B., and Mazoyer, B. M. (1993). Analysis of Individual Positron Emission Tomography Activation Maps by Detection of High Signal-to-Noise Ratio Pixel Clusters. *J. Cereb. Blood Flow Metab.* **13:** 425–437.

Roland, P. E., Levin, B., Kawashima, R., and Åkerman, S. (1993). Three-dimensional analysis of clustered voxels in ¹⁵O-butanol brain activation images. *Hum. Brain Mapping* **1:** 3–19.

Silbersweig, D. A., Stern, E., Schnorr, L., Frith, C. D., Ashburner, J., Cahill, C., Frackowiak, R. S. J., and Jones, T. (1994). Imaging transient, randomly-occurring neuropsychological events in single subjects with positron emission tomography: An event-related countrate correlational analysis. *J. Cereb. Blood Flow Metab.* **14:** 771–782.

Watson, J. D. G., Myers, R., Frackowiak, R. S. J., Hajnal, J. V., Woods, R. P., Mazziotta, J. C., Shipp, S., and Zeki, S. (1993). Area V5 of the human brain: Evidence from a combined study using positron emission tomography and magnetic resonance imaging. *Cereb. Cortex* **3:** 79–94.

Worsley, K. J., Evans, A. C., Marrett, S., and Neelin, P. (1992). A Three-Dimensional Statistical Analysis for CBF Activation Studies in Human Brain. *J. Cereb. Blood Flow Metab.* **12:** 900–918.

Worsley, K. J., Evans, A. C., Marrett, S., and Neelin, P. (1993). Detecting and estimating the regions of activation in CBF activation studies in human brain. *In* "Quantification of Brain Function: Tracer Kinetics and Image Analysis in Brain PET" (K. Uemura *et al.*, Eds.), pp. 535–544. Elsevier Science Publ., BV.

Worsley, K. J. (1994). Local maxima and the expected Euler characteristic of excursion sets of χ^2, F, and t fields. *Adv. Appl. Probability* **26:** 13–42.

Individual Detection of Activations Using Amplitude and Size Information

Evaluation of a New Algorithm

F. CRIVELLO,[1] J.-B. POLINE,[2] N. TZOURIO,[1] L. PETIT,[1] E. MELLET,[1] M. JOLIOT,[1] L. LAURIER,[1] E. TALARICO,[1] and B. MAZOYER[1]

[1]*Groupe d'Imagerie Neurofonctionnelle*
Service Hospitalier Frédéric Joliot, CEA-DRM, 91401 Orsay
and EA 1555, Université Paris 7, Paris, France
[2]*The Wellcome Department of Cognitive Neurology*
Institute of Neurology, London WCIN 3BG, United Kingdom

We present an experimental evaluation of a new algorithm for the detection of activated areas in brain functional maps. The new algorithm, HMSD, is based on a hierarchical multiscale description of the difference image in terms of connected objects. The size and magnitude of each object are simultaneously tested with respect to a bidimensional frequency distribution derived using Monte-Carlo simulations under the null hypothesis. In the present work, HMSD was applied to the analysis of a silent verb generation PET activation protocol conducted in six right-handed subjects. HMSD detection performances on stereotactically intersubject averaged data were compared to that obtained with the 2D and 3D version of SPM and demonstrate that the combination of amplitude and size informations increases detection sensitivity. Applied to single-subject data, HMSD provides a first approximation of the activated areas extent, offers the opportunity to look at detailed correlation between brain anatomy and function, and reveals significant individual differences in the functional anatomy of silent verb generation.

I. INTRODUCTION

Due to the low sensitivity of 2D PET scanners and the limited radiation dose that may be delivered to a subject during a PET activation experiment, most of the functional imaging cognitive studies with PET so far have been conducted on groups of subjects. Such studies require intersubject brain scan averaging, for which various schemes have been proposed (Fox *et al.*, 1988; Friston *et al.*, 1991; Worsley *et al.*, 1992; Mazoyer *et al.*, 1993) that allow us to establish, for a given cognitive task, the average functional neuroanatomy in a population. Despite the numerous results it has provided, however, this approach remains somewhat limited by between subject variability in terms of both brain anatomy and brain function localizations (Galaburda *et al.*, 1990).

Detection algorithms used for the analysis of PET brain activation maps are usually based on the formation of a difference image, and changes in regional cerebral blood flow (rCBF) are evaluated by assessing the significance of signal amplitude in every voxel composing this image. Due to the intrinsically low signal-to-noise ratio of individual PET difference images, it is difficult to detect voxels where changes occurred in single-case analysis with this kind of approach. Detection procedures have been developed that combine low-pass filtering and averaging brain maps across subjects (Fox *et al.*, 1988; Friston *et al.*, 1991), spatial transformations being applied to individual brain maps to bring them into the so-called standard Talairach space (Talairach and Tournoux, 1988). However, all these methods are based on the extremal values of the image (or volume) and do not take into account any morphological information about the size or the shape of the signal to be detected.

Our group recently proposed a new two-dimensional individual-detection algorithm named *hierarchical*

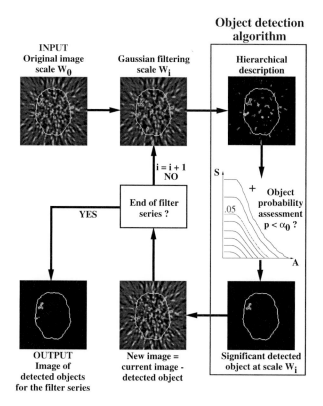

Object detection algorithm

INPUT
Original image
scale W$_0$

Gaussian filtering
scale W$_i$

Hierarchical
description

i = i + 1
NO

End of filter
series ?

YES

S

.05

+ Object
probability
assessment
p < α$_0$?

A

OUTPUT
Image of
detected objects
for the filter series

New image =
current image -
detected object

Significant detected
object at scale W$_i$

FIGURE 1   General overview of the hierarchical multiscale detection (HMSD) algorithm applied to the PET difference image of subject 4. The box contains the detection algorithm at a given scale including the 2D hierarchical description of the filtered image into connected objects and the object probability assessment by simultaneously testing their size and amplitude with respect to a Monte-Carlo derived bidimensional frequency distribution established under the null hypothesis. The cluster represents the parameters of the significant object located in the right inferior frontal gyrus.

multiscale detection, or HMSD (Poline and Mazoyer, 1994b), which is based on a hierarchical description of the PET difference image in terms of connected objects (clusters). Cluster sizes and magnitudes are simultaneously tested with respect to a Monte-Carlo derived bidimensional frequency distribution under the null hypothesis, an iterative procedure being used to control the overall Type I errors. In addition, because brain activation maps usually contain signals with different sizes, a multifiltering strategy is incorporated in HMSD to further improve the detection sensitivity (Poline and Mazoyer, 1994a); for a general overview see Figure 1. In a recent paper (Poline and Mazoyer, 1994b), Monte-Carlo simulations of signal and noise images were used to demonstrate that the HMSD method has better sensitivity than either SPM or change distribution analysis (CDA; Fox *et al.*, 1988). In the same study, we also showed that the combined use of size and amplitude

information can provide an estimate of the spatial limits of the activation signals.

In the present chapter, we evaluate the performances of the HMSD algorithm on experimental data and compare them to those of the standard statistical parametric mapping (SPM) averaging approach using both the 2D and the newer 3D version (SPM94) of this software.

II. Methods

A. PET Activation Experiment

Data were collected within the framework of an EU Concerted Action undertaken by nine PET centers from Europe running the same activation paradigm. Prior to the PET experiments, noun lists to be presented to the subjects were derived by testing a group of 20 volunteers. Starting from the 260 Snodgrass–Vanderwart pictures (Snodgrass and Vanderwart, 1980), a list of 100 unambiguous nouns was selected. One or two syllable nouns inducing the generation of at least three verbs within the 10 sec following noun presentation and having high associative strength for the first response were retained for the lists to be presented during the PET experiment.

Six right-handed young male French volunteers (aged from 21 to 25 years) participated in this study, their right-handedness being assessed with the Edinburgh inventory (Oldfield, 1971). The mean verb generation task performance across these six subjects was 4.0 ± 0.7 verbs/noun/10 sec. Using PET and 2.22 GBq bolus of oxygen-15-labeled water, normalized regional cerebral blood flow (NrCBF) was measured on an ECAT 953B (Mazoyer *et al.*, 1991) six times (15 min interscan) in each subject by replicating three times a series of two conditions: (1) silent rest control, eyes closed; (2) silent generation of verbs semantically associated to nouns presented at 0.1 Hz via earphones. All measurements were performed in total darkness, the condition serial order being defined using a Latin square and different noun lists being used for each verb generation task. In addition to the PET data, axial and sagittal series of 3 mm thick T$_1$-weighted high-resolution magnetic resonance images (MRI) covering the whole brain were acquired for each subject on an 0.5T GE-MRMAX imager.

B. Data Analysis

As a preprocessing step, the AIR package (Woods *et al.*, 1993) was used to perform PET-MRI registra-

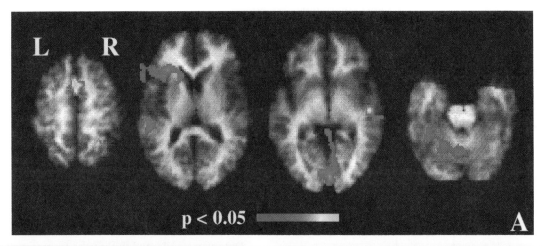

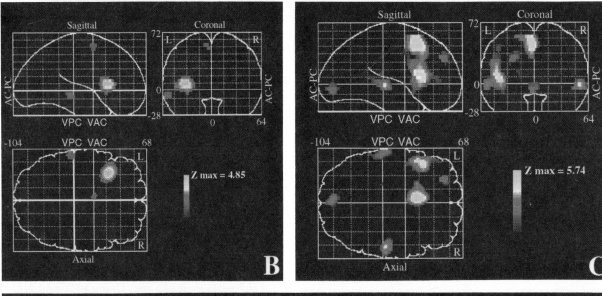

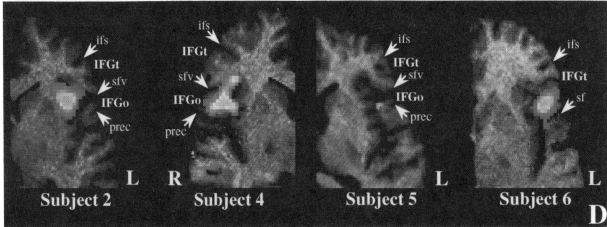

FIGURE 2   A: 2D HMSD analysis of the stereotactically intersubject averaged data. The significant activated areas detected while comparing silent verb generation and control task are superimposed on the standard SPM MRI normalized into the Talairach space at four different brain levels. From left to right, levels are AC–PC + 48 mm, + 8 mm, −4 mm, and −24 mm. Objects detected at a Bonferroni corrected significance level of $p < 0.05$ per plane are located in the SMA extending to the left anterior cingulate, the left inferior frontal gyrus, the right and left superior frontal gyrus, the left cerebellar cortex and the primary visual cortex.

B: 2D SPM analysis of the stereotactically intersubject averaged data obtained during verb generation versus control. Voxels that are significant at the given threshold of $p < 0.05$ corrected for the multiple comparisons per plane are displayed on single

tion. The PET data analysis was then conducted in two different ways.

1. Intersubject Stereotactically Averaged Data: Comparison between HMSD and SPM

For HMSD analysis, PET count images in each condition were normalized using the whole brain volume counts. Individual difference images were stereotactically averaged across replicates and across subjects, and the resulting mean difference image was processed with the HMSD algorithm with a Bonferroni corrected significance level set at 0.05 per plane. In this study, we successively applied Gaussian filters of width $w = 1.5, 2, 2.5, 3$ pixels, w being related to the Gaussian function full-width at half-maximum (FWHM) by $W = \text{FWHM}/\sqrt{8\log_e(2)}$ (Worsley et al., 1992).

The results obtained using HMSD on the intersubject averaged image were compared to those provided by SPM. Data were first analyzed with the 2D version of SPM (Friston et al., 1991) with the same significance level of 0.05 per plane and with the newer 3D version (Friston et al., 1995) with a level of significance set at 0.001 (uncorrected). For the SPM analysis, scans from each subject were realigned and stereotactically normalized in the Talairach's space and subsequent images were smoothed using a 12 mm FWHM isotropic Gaussian kernel. An ANCOVA model was fitted and a t-statistic image (SPM$\{t\}$) for contrast condition effect constructed.

2. Single-Case Analysis Using HMSD

In a second step, the HMSD detection algorithm was applied to the individual NrCBF difference images averaged across the three replicates. The significance level was set at 0.05 per plane after Bonferroni correction. The statistical threshold applied to each cluster defined by the hierarchical description was assessed by estimating the number of voxels composing the gray matter in each plane of the brain and then the number of independent comparisons made in the Bonferroni

correction. The filter series used for this analysis was set at $w = 1.5, 2, 2.5, 3$ pixels.

An accurate localization of the objects detected with the HMSD method was made based on a detailed anatomical analysis of each subject's brain anatomy. Using dedicated software (Voxtool), MRI axial slices were used to reconstruct a three-dimensional brain volume that was further segmented and allowed the display of both hemisphere's surfaces together with sections in three orthogonal directions (Mazoyer et al., 1993). The principal sulci, in particular those limiting the inferior frontal gyrus were identified in each subject's MRI.

III. RESULTS AND DISCUSSION

A. HMSD on Intersubject Averaged Data

Objects detected using HMSD in the intersubject averaged image are illustrated in Figure 2(A). A set of continuous leftward activations (+60 to 36 mm relative to AC–PC line) was detected from the supplementary motor area (SMA) down to the anterior cingulate gyrus. A second activated area was detected in the left inferior frontal gyrus extending inward to the left caudate nucleus. In the temporal lobes, bilateral activations were found in the left and right superior temporal gyrus. Furthermore, cerebellar activations were found in both the cerebellar vermis and in the cortex on the left side. Finally, a visual cortex activation was observed extending to the internal face of the temporal lobe.

B. 2D SPM on Intersubject Averaged Data

Figure 2(B) illustrates the regions showing significant increases in rCBF during the silent verbal generation task as compared to the control task with the 2D version of SPM on the same intersubject averaged data. The main activation found with SPM was located in the left inferior frontal gyrus; this activation remained

sagittal, coronal, and axial projections of the brain. Activations are located in left inferior frontal gyrus, the left SMA and in the left middle temporal gyrus.

C: 3D SPM analysis of the stereotactically intersubject averaged data obtained for the verb generation versus control comparison. Threshold is set to $p < 0.001$, uncorrected. Activations are located in the left SMA, the left inferior frontal gyrus, and the bilateral superior temporal gyri, as well as in the superior frontal gyrus and the visual cortex. Note the increase of sensitivity in the 3D SPM analysis as compared to the 2D one.

D: HMSD results for the single case analysis. After realignment of the MRI and PET volumes in the same coordinates space, the inferior frontal gyrus activations detected in four subjects are zoomed and superimposed on their corresponding axial MRI slice. A detailed anatomical analysis after sulcal identification allows precise localization of these activations in the left inferior frontal gyrus for subjects 2, 5, and 6 and in the right inferior frontal gyrus for subject 4. In subjects 2 and 6, the activation lies in the pars triangularis and in the pars opercularis for subject 5. Right inferior frontal gyrus activation of subject 4 covers both the pars opercularis and the pars triangularis.

significant when the significance level was lowered to 0.001. Small and low *Z*-score activations were found located in the left SMA and in the left middle temporal gyrus. No activations were found in the right temporal cortex, in the cerebellum, or in the visual cortex.

C. 3D SPM on Intersubject Averaged Data

Results obtained with SPM94 are illustrated in Figure 2(C). With the 3D version of SPM running at a 0.001 significance level, results are comparable to that of HMSD and a common set of activations was detected. The major activations were located in the left SMA, the left inferior frontal gyrus, and the right superior temporal gyrus. The verb generation task led to smaller rCBF increase in the left superior temporal gyrus and in the superior frontal gyrus as well as in the primary visual cortex. It is noteworthy that the unexpected primary visual cortex activation was detected using either SPM94 or HMSD.

D. Single-Case Analysis Using HMSD

The characteristics of the detected objects in terms of size and mean amplitude are given in Table 1. An SMA activation was found in five of the six subjects. This activation was leftward lateralized for all of them, but the location along the *z*-axis of these individual activations shows a large intersubject variability. In the same vein, a left precentral activation was observed in subject 2 and a right superior frontal activation in subject 4. Significant objects were detected in the left inferior frontal gyrus for subjects 2, 5, and 6 and in the right side in subject 4. The superior temporal gyrus was activated in the right side for subject 4 and bilaterally for subject 5. Single-subject cerebellum activations were found in the cerebellar vermis in subject 5, in the left cerebellar cortex in subject 4, and in the right one for subject 2. Figure 2(D) gives the detailed anatomical analysis for the four subjects who activated the inferior frontal gyrus. In subjects 2, 5, and 6 the activations lay in the left inferior frontal gyrus. Subject 4 is remarkable in that his activation was located in the right inferior frontal gyrus (see Fig. 2(D)). This, together with the presence of right-sided temporal and left-sided cerebellar cortex activations, suggests a rightward language dominance in a right-handed subject. A primary visual cortex activation was detected in one subject only (subject 5).

Taking the results obtained with the 3D version of SPM as a reference, it appears that the HMSD algorithm has a higher detection sensitivity than SPM for analyzing 2D images. Using the same significance level, the pattern of activations provided by HMSD was very

TABLE 1 Single Case Data Analysis

Detected Objects	Subjects					
	1	2	3	4	5	6
L SMA	112[a]	146	51		135	6
	1.86[b]	*2.77*	*2.73*		*2.64*	*3.43*
L Prec		115				
		2.71				
R SFG				43		
				2.63		
L IFG		81			3	62
		2.41			*3.67*	*2.56*
R IFG				113		
				2.70		
L STG					50	
					2.66	
R STG				22	229	
				2.05	*1.97*	
L CC				75		
				2.49		
R CC		384				
		2.44				
Vermis						39
						2.91
PVC					549	
					2.03	

Notes. Anatomical localization, size and mean amplitude of detected objects with the HMSD method while comparing silent verb generation and control task. Bonferroni corrected significance level was set at $p < 0.05$ per plane.

L is left, R is right; Prec is precentral; SFG is superior frontal gyrus; IFG is inferior frontal gyrus; STG is superior temporal gyrus; CC is cerebellar cortex; PVC is primary visual cortex.

[a]Size of the detected objects in voxels.

[b]Mean amplitude in image voxel standard deviation.

close to that given by 3D SPM, whereas the 2D version of SPM found only a restricted subset of regions. We believe this sensitivity improvement is due to the use of the two-parameter (size *x* amplitude) detection scheme in HMSD detection, which seems to compensate for the lack of sensitivity in the 2D analysis as compared to the 3D one. Looking at the limited difference in the activation pattern provided by the 2D implementation of HMSD and the 3D version of SPM, we can anticipate that a 3D implementation of HMSD would have further enhanced detection sensitivity for stereotactically averaged images.

Even though the data were acquired with septa extended, which results in reduced sensitivity as compared to full 3D acquisition, the HMSD algorithm was sensitive enough to reveal areas activated in single case analysis. The combination of size and amplitude allows us to discriminate objects with very small size and high amplitude, like the inferior frontal gyrus activation in subject 5, as well as objects characterized by a large extent and a low amplitude, such as the SMA activation in subject 1 (see Table 1 for detailed characteristics of size and magnitude). In this respect, it is important to recall that these two parameters play equivalent roles in the detection procedure: Increasing the weight of one of the parameters would be a way to introduce some *a priori* information on what should be considered a signal and would, thus, increase the detection sensitivity of such signals.

The averaged results partly reflect the regions that were found activated in a majority of subjects like SMA (five of the six subjects) and the left inferior frontal gyrus (three of the six). But intersubject averaged activations may also result from a strong activation present in one or two subjects only, as was observed for the superior temporal cortex or the visual cortex activation in subject 5. Such activations could be false positives but, we believe, in this present case, they are true activations. In fact, although the protocol was designed to limit the activation of the auditory areas, one can still expect the temporal cortex to be activated to some degree (Price *et al.*, 1992) at the word presentation rate of 0.1 Hz. As for the visual cortex activation present in subject 5, it most likely reflects the fact that the laser beams had unfortunately not been turned off during one of the verb generation tasks for this subject.

In addition, some areas were found activated in only one subject and had no corresponding activations detected in the intersubject averaged image. Again, these activations may be either true positives, thereby revealing significant individual differences in functional neuroanatomy, or false positives. For instance, the left precentral and right cerebellar cortex activations observed in subject 2 are consistent with the left inferior frontal gyrus and left SMA activations observed in this subject and reveals, we believe, an activation of the motor network for language. A similar argument can be used to interpret the right inferior frontal and left cerebellar activations observed in subject 4, leading to the conclusion of a right hemisphere dominance for language in this right-handed subject. Consistent with this conclusion is the right superior temporal and right superior frontal activation observed in this particular subject.

The multiscale description strategy used in the algorithm allows us to detect signals of different sizes and amplitudes, and the hierarchical description approach provides a first estimate of the activation morphology. This last feature, together with a detailed analysis of the subject's brain anatomy, can provide an accurate localization of the activated areas, as has been demonstrated in the present study regarding the precise localization of the inferior frontal activation during verb generation. This last result demonstrates that individual functional neuroanatomy is an important complement of intersubject averaging because it may help to solve questions about the exact location of an area detected on a group-averaged image. In the present case, for instance, we think we have demonstrated that Broca's area (Brodmann's areas 44 and 45) is the major site of activation during silent verb generation and not the left dorsolateral prefrontal cortex (Brodmann's areas 9, 10 and 46). Interestingly, the right equivalent of Broca's area was found activated in the subject presenting a right hemisphere dominance for language.

HMSD certainly appears to be a good tool both for the investigation of the intersubject variability of the functional neuroanatomy for various cognitive functions and for a better understanding of the interindividual averaged results. At this stage, however, the presence or absence of activated areas in a single case must still be interpreted with caution. In the present protocol, data were acquired on the ECAT 953B operated in the 2D mode. For the same total dose given to the subjects, 3D acquisition would have provided difference images with better statistics, in which more activated areas might have been detected. For instance, taking the individual 2D data set and setting the significance threshold of the HMSD detection to 0.2 instead of 0.05 results in additional objects detected in the right superior temporal gyrus of subjects 3 and 6. In this respect, it is clear that 3D acquisition and 3D implementation of HMSD would dramatically improve the degree of confidence one could have in single-case analysis.

The HMSD approach also presents some current limitations related to the shape of the bidimensional frequency distribution derived with Monte-Carlo simulations. Another limitation comes from the differences in the edge effects one can expect between the Monte-Carlo simulated images and the experimental ones. A 3D version of HMSD, which will be based on a more realistic noise model of the 3D simulated images accounting for the voxel anisotropy, the nonstationarity effects, and the effects of voxel variance on the edges of the image is under development. The HMSD principle is quite general and can be applied to brain activation maps obtained with other modalities such as functional MRI as long as the autocovariance function assessed in experimental noise images can be approximated by a Gaussian function. Whenever the autocovariance function is thought to be too different from the Gaussian kernel, a series of new simulations should provide some adequate distribution.

References

Fox, P. T., Mintun, M. A., Reiman, E. M., and Raichle, M. E. (1988). Enhanced detection of focal brain response using intersubject averaging and change-distribution analysis of substracted PET images. *J. Cereb. Blood Flow Metab.* **8**: 642–653.

Friston, K. J., Frith, C. D., Liddle, P. F., and Frackowiak, R. S. J. (1991). Comparing functional (PET) images: The assessment of significant changes. *J. Cereb. Blood Flow Metab.* **11**: 690–699.

Friston, K. J., Holmes, A. P., Worsley, K. J., Poline, J. B., Frith, C. D., and Frackowiak, R. S. J. (1995). Statistical parametric maps in functional imaging: A general approach. *Human Brain Mapping* **2**: 189–210.

Galaburda, A. M., Rosen, G. D., and Sherman, G. F. (1990). Individual variability in cortical organization: its relationship to brain laterality and implications to function. *Neuropsychologia* **28**: 529–546.

Mazoyer, B. M., Trebossen, R., Deutch, R., Casey, M., and Blohm, K. (1991). Physical characteristics of the ECAT 953B/31: A new high resolution brain positron tomograph. *IEEE Trans. Med. Imaging* **10**(4): 499–504.

Mazoyer B. M., Tzourio N., Poline J. B., Petit L., Levrier O., and Joliot M. (1993). Anatomical regions of interest versus stereotactic space: A comparison between two approaches for brain activation maps analysis. *In:* "Quantification of Brain Function. Tracer Kinetics and Image Analysis in Brain PET." Elsevier, Amsterdam.

Oldfield, R. C. (1971). The assessment and analysis of handedness: The Edinburgh inventory. *Neuropsychologia* **9**: 97–113.

Poline, J. B., and Mazoyer, B. M. (1994a). Enhanced detection in brain activation maps using a multifiltering approach. *J. Cereb. Blood Flow Metab.* **14**: 639–642.

Poline, J. B., and Mazoyer, B. M. (1994b). Analysis of individual brain activation maps using hierarchical description and multiscale detection. *IEEE Trans. Med. Imaging* **13**(4): 702–710.

Price, C., Wise, R., Ramsay, S., Friston, K. J., Howard, D., Patterson, K., and Frackowiak, R. S. J. (1992). Regional response differences within the human auditory cortex when listening to words. *Neurosci. Lett.* **146**: 179–182.

Snodgrass, J. G., and Vanderwart, M. (1980). A standardized set of 260 pictures: Norms for name agreement, image agreement, familiarity and visual complexity. *J. Exp. Psychol. Hum. Learning Memory* **2**: 174–215.

Talairach J., and Tournoux J. (1988). "Co-planar Stereotaxic Atlas of the Human Brain." Thieme, Stuttgart.

Woods, R. P., Mazziotta, J. C., and Cherry, S. R. (1993). MRI-PET registration with automated algorithm. *J. Comput. Assist. Tomogr.* **17**(4): 536–546.

Worsley, K. J., Evans, A. C., Marrett, S., and Neelin, P. (1992). A three-dimensional statistical analysis for CBF activation studies in human brain. *J. Cereb. Blood Flow Metab.* **12**: 900–918.

67

Transformations to Normality and Independence for Parametric Significance Testing of Data from Multiple Dependent Volumes of Interest

G. PAWLIK and A. THIEL

*Max Planck Institute for Neurological Research
and Neurology Clinic of the University of Cologne
D-50931 Cologne, Germany*

PET image data can hardly be analyzed reliably by conventional parametric test procedures because they typically do not conform with fundamental statistical assumptions of normality, homogeneity of variances, and independence among volumes of interest. Therefore, we developed a strategy of stepwise transformations to make multiple volume-of-interest data normally distributed (Box–Cox transformation) and mutually independent (Mahalanobis transformation), thus permitting efficient parametric analysis. This approach was tested in an activation PET study of 106 patients, whose cerebral glucose metabolism was measured in a resting state and during continuous visual recognition, in order to investigate the relationships both among the functional changes of selected regions and between regional and global responses, using a regression model, with whole brain change representing the independent variable. At the original data level, most variables exhibited significantly nonnormal distributions and correlations ranging from r = 0.46 for the thalamus or primary visual cortex to r = 0.69 for the cerebellum or parietal cortex. The Box–Cox algorithm including a χ² test indicated the significant need for transformation, mostly by square root transformation, of global and regional metabolic changes. Following Box–Cox transformation, the variables approximated a normal distribution. Their correlations were then completely removed and their variances standardized to unity by Mahalanobis transformation. Therefore, after corresponding transformations of the original null hypotheses, conventional parametric tests could be applied independently to each volume of interest.

The strategy proposed is highly efficient, produces unconditional statistical results, and holds great promise for future application to PET image analysis at the pixel level.

I. INTRODUCTION

PET image data sets typically neither satisfy the requirements of parametric procedures nor do they represent statistically independent measures so as to warrant the repeated application of univariate parametric significance tests without adjustment for the heterogeneous, mutual dependence of all tested picture elements (Pawlik, 1988; Ford *et al.*, 1991). Nonparametric randomization tests offer a possible solution to this problem, but they are very computer intensive and typically rather conservative when applied to nearly normally distributed data (Holmes *et al.*, Chapter 65 in this book). Most of all, however, they are conditional tests whose results cannot be generalized; that is, their significance statements hold only for the actual test sample and any change of, say, reconstruction parameters may change the statistical outcome. Most parametric tests, by contrast, are both efficient and unconditional, and their results are reliable, as long as their fundamental assumptions are not too heavily violated. With regard to the normality requirement this means that the variables under investigation must be (nearly) normally distributed either in the population from which the test sample was taken or in the test sample itself. Therefore, we developed a strategy of stepwise transformations to normality and independence among volumes of interest (VOIs), permitting the efficient application of multiple conventional parametric significance tests.

II. METHODS

A. Transformation to Normality

First, using an algorithm proposed by Box and Cox (1964), for the sample data within each registered VOI an exponent is estimated so that the data being raised to that power approximates a normal distribution. Depending on the kind of statistical analysis one wishes to perform, different Box–Cox transformations must be applied, all of which follow the same principle. If only j dependent variables are of interest, that is, one PET measure per subject i in each of j VOIs, the exponents λ_j of the power transformation

$$y_{ij}^O = [(y_{ij} + c)^{\lambda(j)} - 1]/\lambda_j \qquad \text{for } \lambda_j \neq 0 \qquad (1)$$

or

$$y_{ij}^O = \ln(y_{ij} + c) \qquad \text{for } \lambda_j = 0$$

are determined, after adding a constant $c = |\min(y_{ij})| + 1$ to all variable values y_{ij} to eliminate negative values, by iteratively maximizing the following log likelihood function:

$$L_{\max} = -[(n-1)/2] \ln(s^O)^2 \\ + (\lambda_j - 1)[(n-1)/n] \sum \ln(y_{ij} + c) \qquad (2)$$

where $(s^O)^2$ represents the variance of lambda transformed y_j. This transformation can be performed either individually for each variable or simultaneously for all j variables by replacing $(s^O)^2$, the variance of a single variable, by the error mean square (Sokahl and Rohlf, 1980).

If there are both dependent and independent variables, say, some measure of whole brain function, and bivariate normal distribution is required for parametric analysis, say, for regression, the power transformation must be applied to the independent variable as well:

$$x_{ij}^O = [(x_i + c)^{\kappa(j)} - 1]/\kappa_j \qquad \text{for } \kappa_j \neq 0 \qquad (3)$$

or

$$x_{ij}^O = \ln(x_i + c) \qquad \text{for } \kappa_j = 0$$

In this case, as illustrated in Figure 1, the log likelihood function is maximized by simultaneously iterating λ and κ:

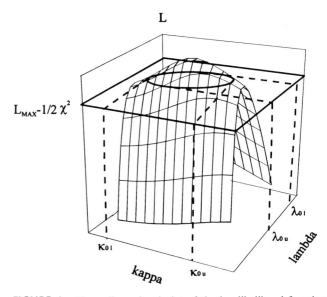

FIGURE 1 Three-dimensional plot of the log likelihood function [equation (4)] in the vicinity of its maximum, obtained by simultaneous iteration of λ and κ, also illustrating iterative root finding procedure to estimate lower (index $0l$) and upper (index $0u$) confidence limits around λ_j and κ_j, respectively.

$$L_{\max} = -[(n-2)/2] \ln(s_r^O)^2 \\ + (\lambda_j - 1)[(n-1)/n] \sum \ln(y_{ij} + c) \qquad (4)$$

where the sample variance of equation (2) is replaced by the residual variance of the linear regression of the transformed variables y_{ij}^O on x_{ij}^O (Box and Cox, 1964):

$$(s_r^O)^2 = SQ_{res}(\lambda_j, \kappa_j)/(n-2) \qquad (5)$$

with $SQ_{res}(\lambda_j, \kappa_j)$ = residual sum of squares of linear regression of transformed variables. Using equation (4), the lower and upper 95% confidence limits around κ_j and λ_j, respectively, are obtained (Fig. 1) by iterating κ and λ to solve for the roots of

$$L = L_{\max} - 1/2 \, \chi_{0.05}^2 \qquad (6)$$

A confidence interval comprising unity would indicate no significant departure from normality at the 0.05 level, and therefore no Box–Cox transformation of that particular variable would be necessary.

B. Transformation to Independence

To eliminate any correlations among the j dependent variables (and to make their variances equal unity, which may be important for certain parametric procedures; e.g., analysis of variance without adjustment of degrees of freedom), the Box–Cox transformations are followed by linear Mahalanobis transformation (Mardia *et al.*, 1979) according to

$$\mathbf{y}_i^{OO} = \mathbf{S}^{-1/2} \cdot \mathbf{y}_i^{O'} \qquad (7)$$

where $\mathbf{y}_i^O$ is the *i*th row vector of the matrix of Box–Cox transformed dependent variables and $\mathbf{S}$ is the Box–Cox sample covariance matrix across those variables. The term $\mathbf{S}^{-1/2}$ is obtained by inverse symmetric square root decomposition:

$$\mathbf{S}^{-1/2} = \mathbf{\Gamma} \mathbf{\Lambda}^{-1/2} \mathbf{\Gamma}', \qquad \text{with } \mathbf{\Lambda}^{-1/2} = \text{diag}(\mathbf{e}^{-1/2}) \quad (8)$$

where $\mathbf{\Gamma}$ is the orthogonal matrix of eigenvectors and $\mathbf{e}$ the vector of eigenvalues of $\mathbf{S}$.

C. Transformation of Test Hypotheses

The addition of constant c as well as the subsequent power and linear transformations cause a shift of origin that must be accounted for by adjustment of the null hypotheses in significance tests at the level of Mahalanobis transformation. Therefore, the origins are Box–Cox transformed according to

$$y_{0j}^O = 1/\lambda_j(c^{\lambda(j)} - 1) \qquad (9a)$$

$$x_{0j}^O = 1/\kappa_j(c^{\kappa(j)} - 1) \qquad (9b)$$

At the Mahalanobis level, this becomes

$$\mathbf{y}_0^{OO} = \mathbf{S}^{-1/2} \mathbf{y}_0^{O'} - \text{diag}(\mathbf{b}^{OO}) \mathbf{x}_0^O \qquad (10)$$

where $\mathbf{y}_0^O$ and $\mathbf{x}_0^O$ are the vectors across VOIs of Box–Cox transformed origins y_{0j}^O and x_{0j}^O, respectively, and $\mathbf{b}^{OO}$ is the slope vector of the linear regressions of $\mathbf{y}^{OO}$ on $\mathbf{x}^O$.

D. Exemplary Application

To demonstrate the effects of those transformations, selected PET data were analyzed from 106 patients (50 each with senile dementia or temporal lobe epilepsy, 6 with no cerebral pathology; $i = 1, \ldots, 106$) aged 12 to 86 years and representing a wide range of global brain function. Using the 2-[^{18}F]fluoro-2-deoxy-D-glucose method and a Scanditronix PC 384–7B PET scanner, their cerebral glucose consumption was investigated both in a standard resting condition and while performing a difficulty-adjusted continuous visual rec-

ognition task (Kessler *et al.*, 1991). Comprehensive VOI mapping (Herholz *et al.*, 1985) was performed to compute global metabolic rates and, averaged across sides, four exemplary VOIs ($j = 1, \ldots, 4$) that were very small (0.22–0.83%) compared to the total scanned brain volume were chosen for regional assessment: primary visual cortex, thalamus, cerebellum, and parietal cortex. Metabolic changes from rest to activation were obtained by subtraction of scans matched within and among patients (Pawlik *et al.*, 1986). Without adjustment for repeated testing, Shapiro–Wilk's test was performed before and after each transformation step to test the null hypothesis of no deviation from a normal distribution. Likewise, the correlations among VOIs were analyzed after each transformation. For transformation to normality, the model with one independent variable (global metabolic change) and several dependent variables (metabolic changes in the four selected VOIs) according to equation (4) was applied. We used a downhill simplex algorithm (Press *et al.*, 1989) for rapid maximization of the log likelihood function and the secant method (Press *et al.*, 1989) for root finding to iteratively estimate confidence limits. The program was written in Turbo-Pascal (Borland Inc.) and implemented on a 486DX/66 CPU. The Mahalanobis transformation was programmed in SAS-IML (interactive matrix language, SAS Institute, Cary, North Carolina). SAS was also used for all statistical testing.

III. RESULTS AND DISCUSSION

As summarized in Table 1, the Box–Cox algorithm produced distinct maxima of the log likelihood function in all tested brain regions. All λ values and the κ values in cerebellum and parietal cortex were significantly different from unity, thus emphasizing the need for transformation to normality. Likewise, Shapiro–Wilk's tests revealed numerous departures from a normal distribution at the original data level that were remedied by transformation (Table 2). At the original data level, the correlations between regions were quite heterogeneous, ranging from $r = 0.46$ (thalamus or primary visual cortex) to $r = 0.69$ (cerebellum or pari-

TABLE 1 Box–Cox Exponents and 95% Confidence Limits

Region	Kappa	Lambda
Primary visual cortex	0.316 [−0.523 ⇔ 1.181]	−0.454 [−0.953 ⇔ 0.024]
Thalamus	0.724 [−0.252 ⇔ 1.814]	0.657 [0.434 ⇔ 0.903]
Cerebellum	−0.627 [−1.184 ⇔ −0.057]	0.499 [0.043 ⇔ 0.993]
Parietal cortex	0.269 [−0.345 ⇔ 0.861]	0.602 [0.306 ⇔ 0.907]

TABLE 2   Distribution Parameters of Regional and Global Metabolic Changes

Region	Original data Skewness kurtosis significance			Box–Cox transformed Skewness kurtosis significance			Mahalanobis transformed Skewness kurtosis significance		
Primary visual cortex	1.13	0.93	**	0.09	−0.83	*	0.12	0.10	n.s.
Thalamus	1.34	5.24	**	0.43	2.13	n.s.	0.70	3.63	n.s.
Cerebellum	0.05	−0.28	n.s.	−0.32	0.02	n.s.	−0.35	0.18	n.s.
Parietal cortex	0.75	0.92	**	0.22	0.43	n.s.	0.03	0.23	n.s.
Whole brain	1.04	1.87	**						
Global$_{primary\ visual\ cortex}$				0.34	0.57	n.s.			
Global$_{thalamus}$				0.76	1.19	*			
Global$_{cerebellum}$				−0.61	0.93	n.s.			
Global$_{parietal\ cortex}$				0.03	0.53	n.s.			

Note. Shapiro–Wilk's test for normal distribution: $*P < 0.05$; $**P < 0.01$; n.s. $P > 0.10$.

etal cortex), and they became 0 after Mahalanobis transformation.

The proposed transformations provide the formal justification for analyzing typical PET data sets by multiple application of efficient parametric statistical methodology. Even though in the present study a data set comprising only a few VOIs was used for illustration, the described methodology can readily be extended to large image matrices. Should singular covariance matrices occur, which will always be the case when the number of VOIs exceeds the number of subjects, conventional statistical methodology would suggest generating a limited number of spatial hypotheses about the location of some regional effect in a small pilot sample, using any of the pixel-based exploratory algorithms in common use. Those hypotheses could then be tested reliably in a larger study as described above. However, matrix reduction might prove to be a more efficient alternative. In that strategy, for calculation of $S^{-1/2}$ only columns with nonzero eigenvalues are used—an approach well known from multiple correlation analysis (Tucker *et al.*, 1972; Raju, 1983).

References

Box, G. E. P., and Cox, D. R. (1964). An analysis of transformations. *J. R. Statist. Soc.* **268**, *Ser. B:* 211–243.

Ford, I., McColl, J. H., McCormack, A. G., and McCrory, S. J. (1991). Statistical issues in the analysis of neuroimages. *J. Cereb. Blood Flow Metab.* **11**: A89-A95.

Herholz, K., Pawlik, G., Wienhard, K., and Heiss, W.-D. (1985). Computer assisted mapping in quantitative analysis of cerebral positron emission tomograms. *J. Cereb. Blood Flow Metab.* **9:** 154–161.

Kessler, J., Herholz, K., Grond, M., and Heiss, W.D. (1991). Impaired metabolic activation in Alzheimer's disease: A PET study during continuous visual recognition. *Neuropsychologia* **29:** 229–243.

Mardia, K. V., Kent, J. T., and Bibby, J. M. (1979). "Multivariate Analysis." Academic Press, New York.

Pawlik, G. (1988). Positron emission tomography and multiregional statistical analysis of brain function: From exploratory methods for single cases to inferential tests for multiple group designs. *In:* "Progress in Computer-Assisted Function Analysis"(J. L. Willems, J. H. van Bemmel, and J. Michel, Eds.), pp. 401–408. Elsevier Science Publishers, Amsterdam.

Pawlik, G., Herholz, K., Wienhard, K., Beil, C., and Heiss, W.-D. (1986). Some maximum likelihood methods useful for the regional analysis of dynamic PET data on brain glucose metabolism. *In* "Information Processing in Medical Imaging" (S. L. Bacharach, Ed.), pp. 298–309. Nijhoff, Dordrecht.

Press, W. T., Flannery, P. B., Teukolsky, S. A., and Vetterling, W. T. (1989). Numerical Recipes in PASCAL: The Art of Scientfic Computing. Cambridge University Press, Cambridge.

Raju, N. S. (1983). Obtaining the squared multiple correlations from a singular correlation matrix. *Educ. Psychol. Meas.* **34:** 127–130.

Sokahl, R. R., and Rohlf, F. J. (1980). "Biometry," 2nd ed. Freeman, New York.

Tucker, L. R., Cooper, L. G., and Meredith, W. (1972). Obtaining squared multiple correlations from a matrix which may be singular. *Psychometrika* **37:** 143–148.

68

Improved Analysis of Functional Activation Studies Involving Within-Subject Replications Using a Three-Way ANOVA Model

R. P. WOODS,[1] M. IACOBONI,[1] S. T. GRAFTON,[4] and J. C. MAZZIOTTA[1,2,3]

[1]*Department of Neurology and Division of Brain Mapping*
[2]*Department of Pharmacology*
[3]*Department of Radiological Sciences*
UCLA School of Medicine
Los Angeles, California 90095
[4]*Departments of Neurology and Nuclear Medicine*
University of Southern California

Compared to a two-way AN(C)OVA model, a three-way model allows for explicit modeling of subject–task and subject–replication interactions present in functional imaging data. The major potential disadvantages of a three-way model are the requirement that tasks be replicated within all subjects and the possibility that the reduction in the number of degrees of freedom in the model might not be offset by improvements in the estimate of intrinsic variance in the data. In the data we have examined, the reduction in the number of degrees of freedom has not proven to be problematic, even with as few as 10 degrees of freedom in the full three-way model. Advantages of the three-way model include the ability to make more precise inferences by using a model that makes no assumptions that are unlikely to be correct, the ability to realistically predict the reproducibility of a study in a new group of subjects, and the ability to distinguish task, replication, and task–replication interaction effects in the absence of specific a priori contrast hypotheses by performing separate analyses of variance for each effect. In addition, false negative results that can result from the use of a two-way AN(C)OVA as a masking procedure prior to contrast analysis can be avoided. This latter problem can also be resolved by simply eliminating masking procedures, because they are not required for the validity of a priori contrast analyses.

I. INTRODUCTION

The analysis of functional imaging data commonly employs analysis of variance (ANOVA) or related (e.g., analysis of covariance or ANCOVA) techniques to identify areas of significant change in group analyses. The models still typically used to analyze such data were initially implemented at a time when it was relatively uncommon to replicate tasks within subjects. In the absence of within-subject replications, intersubject variability in the signal response to behavioral tasks cannot be assessed and must be assumed to be negligible to statistically quantify the responses themselves (Neter, 1990). Improved positron emission tomography (PET) imaging techniques and the use of functional magnetic resonance imaging (fMRI) have now led to fairly routine use of within-subject replications. Although it is possible to continue to use older analysis techniques by treating each replication as if it were a new task, replacement of the older two-way ANOVA or ANCOVA models with three-way models offer theoretical and practical advantages when analyzing group functional imaging data.

An essential component of both the two-way and the three-way models is the explicit recognition of considerable task-independent variability between subjects. This task-independent variability is potentially larger than the task-dependent effects of interest. Consequently, both models employ a block design in which task-independent differences can be ignored in computing the amount of intrinsic variability in the measurements. This intrinsic variability is then compared to the task-dependent changes to assess the statistical significance of these changes.

II. TWO-WAY ANOVA AND CONTRAST ANALYSIS

For the simplest possible experimental design involving multiple subjects, each subject performs each task only once. To estimate the magnitude of measurement errors (against which task-related changes are calibrated in performing an analysis of variance), it is assumed that each real measurement can be broken down into four components: (1) a global baseline, (2) a subject effect, (3) a task effect, and (4) an error term. This is generally represented in the form of a model:

$$Y_{ij} = \mu_{...} + \rho_i + \tau_j + \varepsilon_{ij}$$

where the subscript i refers to subjects, j refers to tasks, Y refers to measurements; μ is the global mean across all measurements; each subject has a subject effect, ρ; each task has a task effect, τ; and each measurement is associated with an error, ε. It should be noted that this model does not allow for the possibility that subjects and tasks might interact (i.e., that the magnitude of a task-related change in signal might truly differ from one subject to another) because such effects cannot be distinguished from measurement errors in this situation. An analysis of covariance can be used instead of an analysis of variance to remove the effects of a confounding factor, but this distinction is unimportant to the discussion here, with all arguments being similarly applicable to ANCOVA models. The assumption that subjects and tasks do not interact is unavoidable in the statistical analysis of data sets where tasks are not replicated within subjects; and to the extent that this assumption is incorrect, the results of such analyses will be biased. Unfortunately, this assumption is unlikely to be true in general, because it contradicts our everyday experience, in which individuals often display cognitive, sensory, and motor abilities or disabilities that are unexpected on the basis of that particular individual's typical performance of other tasks.

In analyzing data with no replications, two different tools are available to look for the presence of task-related signal changes. The first tool is the analysis of variance, which provides a general screening for task-related differences without any consideration to the specific hypotheses of the investigator. The second tool is a contrast analysis, which uses the estimated variances from the AN(C)OVA model to specifically test explicit hypotheses about linear combinations of various task effects. A statistically significant general AN(C)OVA assures the existence of at least one significant set of linear contrasts, but a negative AN(C)OVA does not preclude the existence of a significant result by linear contrasts. Nonetheless, the general AN(C)OVA has historically been used to screen or mask data, with linear contrasts computed only if the AN(C)OVA is positive.

In applying the two-way AN(C)OVA model to data with multiple replications per subject, each replication of the task within a subject is treated as if it were a different task, so the total number of "tasks" is equal to the product of the number of unique tasks and the number of replications. The AN(C)OVA is typically computed to look for a "task" effect; and if such an effect is identified, the investigator's specific hypotheses are tested. By assigning the same linear contrast to each replication of a given task, replications can be properly combined to look for specific task effects. Conversely, if replication effects are of interest, contrasts can be assigned on the basis of replication number, independent of task, to test hypotheses of interest. Finally, if specific hypotheses regarding task–replication interactions are of interest, these can be tested by the appropriate assignment of contrasts. Subject–task and subject–replication interactions cannot be tested because the model explicitly must assume that no such interactions are present.

In reviewing the assumptions underlying the two-way method of analysis, we have identified several distinct issues that persuade us that a two-way model is suboptimal for analyzing functional imaging data involving replications within multiple subjects and also persuade us that within-subject replications should be incorporated into study designs whenever possible. The first set of arguments relates to the less restrictive set of assumptions required by a full three-way model. The second set of arguments relates to the issue of intersubject variability and its impact on the reproducibility of findings across laboratories. The third set of arguments is based on the fact that a three-way model allows independent AN(C)OVA analysis of task effects, replication effects, and task–replication interactions. We have found empirically that the two-way AN(C)OVA model can fail to identify robust task effects due to the confounding treatment of replications as separate tasks. The use of the AN(C)OVA to mask areas for subsequent contrast analysis makes this an issue of particular concern.

III. THEORETICAL ARGUMENTS IN FAVOR OF A THREE-WAY MODEL

Using a three-way multivariate design, it is possible to simultaneously control for intersubject variability while explicitly identifying and accounting for subject–task interactions. Indeed, at the same time, it is also possible to allow for subject–replication interactions and task–replication interactions (Neter, 1990). Some examples of such interactions will be provided later. The full three-way ANOVA model can be represented by a series of factors including (1) a global baseline, (2) a subject effect, (3) a task effect, (4) a replication effect, (5) subject–task interactions, (6) subject–replication interactions, (7) time–task interactions, and (8) an error term:

$$Y_{ijk} = \mu_{...} + \rho_i + \alpha_j + \beta_k + (\rho\alpha)_{ij} + (\rho\beta)_{ik} + (\alpha\beta)_{jk} + \varepsilon_{ijk}$$

(Note that terms in parentheses denote interaction terms and should not be interpreted as numerical products.) Only three-way interactions between subject, task and replication cannot be modeled with this method.

To get a sense of the differences between this model and the two-way, it is useful to consider some concrete examples of circumstances that might result in certain types of interactions:

Subject–task interactions. This is the situation described already, in which a particular subject might be particularly good or particularly poor in performing one task when compared to some other task and when compared to other subjects.

Subject–replication interactions. These interactions would be expected to arise in relation to idiosyncratic responses during an imaging session. For example, one subject might become tired more easily than the others, another might be particularly anxious during acquisition of the initial images, and yet another might experience a full bladder toward the end of the imaging session. Likewise, slow random drift in calibration of imaging equipment would give rise to such effects.

Task–replication interactions. These interactions are likely to arise when one of the tasks is differentially subject to learning, memory, or treatment effects. In some cases, this may be a deliberate aspect of study design, but in other cases may simply be a confound of no primary interest. As noted earlier, linear contrasts can be used to test for specific task–replication interactions predicted *a priori*, but general screening for task–replication interactions isolated from task or replication effects using a two-way AN(C)OVA is not possible.

Subject–task–replication interactions. These interactions, which cannot be identified with the two-way or three-way AN(C)OVA model, would arise from learning or memory effects idiosyncratic to a particular subject.

Given that human brains and behavior are highly individual and highly sensitive to learning and memory and that instruments used for functional imaging are subject to drift over time, the most conservative approach is to always utilize a full three-way AN(C)OVA model. There are few, if any, circumstances under which a reduced model can be justified by a theoretical argument that certain effects or interactions cannot occur. It should be noted that this is quite different from other areas of science, such as physics or chemistry, where it can often be safely assumed that all replications of a given observation should be treated equivalently. In such cases, it is possible to use conventional analysis of variance (with multiple observations per cell instead of the single observation per cell required when subjects are used as blocking factors) because replication main effects and all interactions involving replications can be assumed to be zero.

All other things being equal, inclusion of the various interaction terms of the full three-way model should decrease the estimate of intrinsic variance of the data and thereby increase statistical significance. However, this will not necessarily be the case because the three-way model reduces the number of degrees of freedom involved in estimating the intrinsic variance. When the number of degrees of freedom is already small, this can offset or even reverse the improvement in statistical significance that should otherwise result from accounting for subject–task and subject–replication interactions. To the extent that certain interactions are negligible, consideration can be given to a reduced model that recovers degrees of freedom associated with such interaction terms. For example, it is possible to use a reduced three-way model that makes the same assumptions as the two-way model (i.e., no subject–task or subject–replication interactions). This model will have exactly the same number of degrees of freedom as the two-way model and, for contrast analyses of main task effects, can be shown to be mathematically identical (the reduced AN(C)OVA is not mathematically equivalent to the two-way model, as will be discussed later). However, it is also possible to continue to include subject–task interactions while excluding subject–replication interactions or vice versa. Likewise, it is possible to exclude task–replication interactions. This latter option might be more appropriate than excluding subject interactions for tasks that do not involve learning or memory effects (note that within-subject analyses often assume no task–replication interaction). In general, restricted models should be used only when the number of degrees of freedom is unavoidably small or when the assumptions of the reduced model can be supported by independent data confirming the absence of an interaction. As a final comment with regard to reduced models, it should be noted that computing significance with the full three-way model and various reduced models and then choosing the most significant answer is not good statistical practice. In general, the choice of model should be made in advance of the data analysis.

In performing analyses of task or replication effects, we have empirically found the full three-way ANOVA and full three-way contrast models to be similar to the reduced three-way models that exclude subject–task and subject–replication interactions (when using a fixed effects model for subjects). At worst, a mild reduction in the F score or t-statistic can be seen when the full model is compared to the reduced model and the opposite effect may be seen at other locations. This has been true for 2D PET data with only two replications and for 3D PET data with as many as six replications. The data sets that we have evaluated have involved six to eight subjects. This suggests that the decrease in the variance estimate will generally offset losses due to the smaller number of degrees of freedom. For studies with larger numbers of subjects, the results with the three-way model should be even more favorable because the effect of the number of degrees of freedom asymptotically approaches a constant value as the degrees of freedom become large.

In directly comparing the ANOVA results from the two-way model to those from the three-way model, we have consistently identified an additional effect that strongly favors the three-way model. This effect is restricted to the general ANOVA and is not seen in comparing contrast analyses from the two-way and three-way models unless the contrast analysis is preceded by ANOVA-based masking of the data. The basis for this effect will be detailed in Section V, discussing the separation of task, replication, and task–replication interactions in the three-way AN(C)OVA model.

IV. REPRODUCIBILITY—FIXED VS RANDOM EFFECTS MODELS

Numerical estimates of statistical significance are intended to give a quantitative sense of the reproducibility of a set of experimental observations. If we accept that there is intersubject variability in responses to various functional tasks (subject–task interactions),

then there are two different ways that the experiment could be reproduced. The first way would be to take exactly the same subjects and repeat the study; the second way would be to recruit a new set of subjects and repeat the study. Barring interference effects due to repeating the study in the same subjects, we would expect reuse of the same subjects to give the more consistent results with the original study because the same set of subject–task interactions will be present. In contrast, the use of a new set of subjects could reasonably be expected to give somewhat different results because a new random set of subject–task interactions will be introduced. The reproducibility when using the same set of subjects can be addressed by using a fixed subject effects model when performing AN(C)OVA or contrast analysis, whereas the reproducibility for a new, random set of subjects can be addressed using a random subject effects model (Neter, 1990). Probability values calculated with the fixed effects model will always be less than or equal to values calculated with the random effects model.

It should be noted that most functional imaging data published to date using AN(C)OVA methods has implicitly used a fixed effects model for subjects in computing significance. Because two-way AN(C)OVA analyses assume from the outset that no subject–task interactions occur, they necessarily predict identical reproducibility when reusing the old subjects as when recruiting new ones, since task related changes are assumed to be identical across all subjects in the population. Consequently, the equations for computing "random effects" in a two-way block design AN(C)OVA are identical to the fixed effects equations because the relevant factor (intersubject variability in the form of subject–task interactions) has been declared nonexistent in order to be able to perform a valid two-way analysis in the first place. Similarly, single-subject analyses based on fMRI or PET represent a fixed effects model because they provide no statistical analysis of the likelihood that others in the population will show similar effects. With a three-way model, the fixed and random effects models are mathematically different from one another because the model explicitly allows for the existence of the relevant subject–task interactions. (The fixed and random effects models for task effect will become identical if subject–task interactions are negligible, as will the models for replication effect if subject–replication interactions are negligible. Task–replication interactions are assumed constant across all subjects in three-way models because three-way task–replication=subject interactions cannot be differentiated from error and are assumed to be 0.)

Both the fixed and random effects results are potentially of interest in functional imaging. Although potentially not representative of the entire population, results obtained with the fixed effects model are valid for the individuals involved in the study. In some sense, results using the fixed effects model are analogous to those obtained in case studies of deficits after brain injury or in electrophysiologic recordings of primates. To the extent that other evidence suggests that functional organization of a particular system is highly stereotyped across subjects (even if there are subtle quantitative details), a significant result using the fixed effects model suggests that the observation will likely generalize to the population. Likewise, to the extent that fixed effect results of separate experiments are concordant, the likelihood that the findings are representative of the population increases. However, if the results cannot be replicated in a new group of subjects, this could indicate either a false positive outcome in the original study, a false negative outcome in the new study, or that intersubject differences are responsible for the different outcomes. In contrast, a positive random effects result confirms a much more robust effect that can be generalized to the entire population without the need for further evidence. Results obtained with the random effects model should be more consistently replicable than similarly significant results with the fixed effects model. Results from a fixed effects model can help to confirm an existing hypothesis about the general population or to generate a new hypothesis about the general population but do not provide sufficient evidence to independently support inferences about the general population.

Even though everyone would be pleased to find that their results were sufficiently robust to give a significant random effects result, current typical functional imaging strategies are suboptimal for obtaining such results with the random effects model. Except in areas where intersubject variability is extremely low, studies involving only six to eight subjects are unlikely to generate positive results with a random effects model because of the low number of degrees of freedom associated with the denominator in the AN(C)OVA F test or contrast t-statistic. Unlike the fixed effects model, where subjects, tasks, and replications all contribute to the denominator degrees of freedom for task effects, in the random effects model, only the subjects contribute. Consequently, a low number of subjects is likely to be problematic even if the effects within subject are extremely well defined by performing a large number of replications.

One context in which the use of a random effects model is particularly important is in the comparison of one population to another. If such comparisons are based on fixed effects, the detected difference between the populations may represent merely the effect of ran-

domly selecting individuals from the two populations who happened to be significantly different from one another (i.e., the subjects in the two groups might truly be different from one another but this fact might have no relationship to true differences between the groups). In fact, it is even possible (though unlikely) that the true population difference might be in the opposite direction from the direction indicated by the individual fixed effects result.

If random effects estimates are of interest, it is critical to utilize more than one observation of each task per subject and use more than one subject. If only one observation per task per subject is made, a three-way model cannot be utilized to analyze the data and proper random effects cannot be estimated.

V. SEPARATION OF TASK, REPLICATION, AND TASK-REPLICATION AN(C)OVA ANALYSES IN THE THREE-WAY MODEL

If each replication of a given task is treated as a new "task" in a two-way AN(C)OVA, the resulting AN(C)OVA analysis for "task" effects will reflect the pooled contributions of task, replication, and task–replication interactions. In contrast, in a three-way AN(C)OVA, each of these three effects can be tested independently. Although contrast analyses can be used to isolate the various effects of interest, such analyses require specific *a priori* hypotheses about the nature of the effects. Whereas the investigator is likely to have quantitatively precise hypotheses for identifying task related effects (e.g., contrasting stimulation states to appropriate controls), replication effects and especially task–replication interactions indicative of learning or memory will not generally have magnitudes that can be estimated *a priori*. This is the specific situation for which AN(C)OVA is more useful than linear contrasts, so the ability to test for the designated effects independently is a significant advantage of the three-way model.

It also turns out to be the case that lumping all three of these effects together increases the likelihood that the AN(C)OVA result will be negative despite the existence of significant results by linear contrast analysis. We have found that this problem is especially likely to arise when task effects and replication effects are localized in distinct regions in the images. For example, in an area dominated by task effects, the replication terms in the two-way AN(C)OVA model contribute very little to the ability of the "task–replication" terms to account for variance in the data thereby substantially decreasing the average amount of variance accounted for by the "task–replication" terms. We have found that the three-way task ANOVA consistently gives substantially more significant results than the two-way "task–replication" ANOVA based on combined tasks and replications. Likewise, we have found that the three-way replication ANOVA also give consistently more significant results than the two-way "task–replication" ANOVA. These findings suggest that the use of a two-way ANOVA to mask data for subsequent contrast analysis may be especially likely to inappropriately exclude areas of true task- or replication-related effects. In some of our data with a large number of replications (six), the magnitude of this effect has been sufficient to exclude areas that would have withstood correction for multiple comparisons. Because of this and because contrast analyses do not require a positive AN(C)OVA to be interpreted as valid, we have abandoned the use of AN(C)OVA in situations where we are interested in testing specific hypotheses with a contrast analysis.

VI. ADDITIONAL STATISTICAL REFINEMENTS

Two additional statistical issues need to be considered in assessing the statistical significance of changes in functional imaging studies. The first is the now familiar issue of correcting for the multiple number of hypotheses tested when a voxel-by-voxel analysis of images is performed. These issues have already been addressed in detail for the two-way model by Friston, *et al.* (1991) and Worsley *et al.* (1992). For contrast analyses, the issues for the three-way model are identical, and recent work by Worsley *et al.* (1995) allows for similar corrections of two-way and three-way AN(C)OVA analyses. The second issue has received little attention in the voxel-by-voxel analysis of functional images and relates to specific problems that can arise when repeated measurements are made on the same subjects. In this setting, the validity of the statistical inferences made by contrast or AN(C)OVA analyses is dependent on certain assumptions about the covariance structure of the data that may not necessarily be true. Ideally, the validity of these assumptions should be tested by evaluating the "sphericity" (also known as "circularity") of the data at each voxel. If the criteria for sphericity are not met, the number of degrees of freedom in the model should be reduced according to established criteria to allow for correct statistical inferences. This concern about sphericity is equally applicable to two-way and three-way AN(C)OVA and contrast analyses and is discussed in detail in most chapters and treatises on repeated measures analysis of variance (Girden, 1992). Sphericity corrections have been applied only rarely to the voxel-by-voxel analysis of functional images (Grafton *et al.*, 1994), but the need for such corrections is well established in the statistics literature and deserves closer attention in the future.

Acknowledgments

Our research has been supported by grants to RPW (1 K08 NS01646–02) and STG (1K08 NS01568–03) from the Institute of Neurological Disorders and Stroke, a contract (DE-FC03–87ER60615) with the Department of Energy, gifts from the Ahmanson Foundation and the Jennifer Jones Simon Foundation, and grants from the International Human Frontier Science Program and the Brain Mapping Medical Research Organization.

References

Friston, K. J., Frith, C. D., Liddle, P. F., and Frackowiak, R. S. J. (1991). Comparing Functional (PET) Images: The Assessment of Significant Change. *J. Cereb. Blood Flow Metab.* **11:** 690–699.

Girden, E. R. (1992). ANOVA: Repeated Measures. Sage University Paper Series on Quantitative Applications in the Social Sciences, 07–084. Sage, Newbury Park, CA.

Grafton, S. T., Woods, R. P., and Tyszka, M. (1994). Functional imaging of procedural motor learning: Relating cerebral blood flow with individual subject performance. *Hum. Brain Mapping* **1:** 1–14.

Neter, J., Wasserman, W., and Kutner, M. H. (1990). "Applied Linear Statistical Models," 3rd ed. Irwin, Burr Ridge, Illinois.

Worsley, K. J., Evans, A. C., Marrett, S., and Neelin, P. (1992). A Three-Dimensional Statistical Analysis for CBF Activation Studies in Human Brain. *J. Cereb. Blood Flow Metab.* **12:** 900–918.

Worsley, K. J., Marrett, S., Neelin, P., and Evans, A. C. (1995). A unified statistical approach for determining significant signals in location and scale space images of cerebral activation. *Neuro-Image* **2:** S71.

Smoothness Variance Estimate and Its Effects on Probability Values in Statistical Parametric Maps

J-B. POLINE,[1] **K. J. WORSLEY,**[2] **A. P. HOLMES,**[1] **R. S. J. FRACKOWIAK,**[1] **and K. J. FRISTON**[1]

[1]*Wellcome Department of Cognitive Neurology*
Institute of Neurology,
London WC1N 3BG, United Kingdom
[2]*Department of Mathematics and Statistics*
McGill University, Montreal H3A 2K6, Canada

Correcting for the number of pixels tested in statistical parametric maps requires a measure of the spatial dependency of pixel values. This measure is more often than not done through the measure of the smoothness parameter, which is estimated empirically from the data. This method implies that the parameter is random (and has a variance), therefore casting some uncertainty on the p-values computed in the statistical analysis of the data. We have derived a first-order approximation of the variance of the smoothness parameter estimator and have investigated the effect of this variability on the p-values computed for a cerebral activation using a PET activation experiment. This work is presented in full detail in (Poline et al., 1995).

I. INTRODUCTION

To compute a valid statistical threshold when testing for a significantly activated area of the brain in statistical parametric maps (SPM), it is essential to take into account the number of voxels tested in the volume analyzed (this is a solution to the well-known multiple comparison problem). To do so, the spatial dependency of the voxels is assessed from the data and the parameter that measures this dependency is called the *smoothness* (Friston *et al.*, 1991; Worsley *et al.*, 1992). It is a key parameter because usually it is the only one estimated from the data and it is needed for all statistical strategies, based either on the height of a region (Friston *et al.*, 1991; Worsley *et al.*, 1992), or on the spatial extent of clusters defined above a given thresh-

old (Poline and Mazoyer, 1993; Friston *et al.*, 1994), or indeed on a mixed strategy (Poline and Mazoyer, 1994a).

Because the true value of the smoothness is unknown, an estimate of its variance is essential and should provide some useful bounds for the *p*-values computed using this parameter. In this work, we have derived and validated a first-order approximation of the smoothness variance and have shown the effect on the assessment of significant changes in SPMs using (1) the spatial extent of the activated region and (2) its peak intensity value or height.

II. MATERIALS AND METHODS

In this section, we will provide the equations and describe the method to compute a first approximation of the variance of the smoothness estimate. The *smoothness parameter* is defined as the determinant of the variance covariance matrix of the gradient of the volume to be analyzed (Worsley *et al.*, 1992). When the main axis of the autocovariance function (ACF) of the process is parallel to the axis of the volume, the smoothness (W) is computed with

$$W = \prod_i [\Sigma_x \tau(\mathbf{x})^2 / \Sigma_x \tau_i(\mathbf{x})^2] \qquad (1)$$

where $\mathbf{x}$ is the position in the space, $\tau(\mathbf{x})$ is the value of the volume at position $\mathbf{x}$, $\tau_i(\mathbf{x})$ is the value of the gradient of the volume along the ith direction (i ranges from 1 to D, the dimension of the space), and Σ_x means the sum over all **x**. To simplify the notations, we denote u_0 the sum $\Sigma_x \tau(\mathbf{x})^2$ and u_i the sum $\Sigma_x \tau_i(\mathbf{x})^2$, such that we have $W = f(u_0, u_1, u_2, \ldots) = u_0^D/\Pi_i u_i$.

To compute a first approximation of the variance of W we proceed in three steps:

1. Assume a shape for the ACF of the process (or use an empirically assessed function).
2. Compute the mean and the variance covariance matrix of the vector $\mathbf{u} = (u_0, u_1, u_2, \ldots)$ using the ACF computed or assumed shape.
3. Compute an estimate of the variance of W using the results obtained in step 2 and a first-order Taylor expansion of the function f.

A. Mean and Variance–Covariance Matrix of u

To compute the mean and the variance covariance matrix of u, assuming $\rho(x)$ to be the autocorrelation function of the process (and $\rho_i(x)$ the autocorrelation function of the gradient of the process in the ith direction), we use a spectral representation where $g(\mathbf{w})$ is the spectral density function of the process and $g_i(\mathbf{w})$ is spectral density function of the gradient field.

Using this spectral representation, we have

$$E(u_0) = \Sigma\, g(\mathbf{w}) = N \text{ (N: number of points in}$$
$$\text{the volume, sum over } \mathbf{w})$$
$$E(u_i) = \Sigma\, g_i(\mathbf{w})$$
$$\mathrm{cov}(u_k, u_j) = 2\Sigma\, \mathbf{w}_k^2 \mathbf{w}_j^2\, g(\mathbf{w})^2 = 2\Sigma\, g_k(\mathbf{w}) \cdot g_j(\mathbf{w})$$

A full description of the derivation of these equations can be found in Poline *et al.* (1995).

We then use a first-order approximation of the Taylor expansion around the expectation of **u**:

$$\mathrm{var}(W) = \mathrm{var}[f(\mathbf{u})] \approx \Sigma_{kj}(\partial f/\partial u_k)(\partial f/\partial u_j)\,\mathrm{cov}\,(u_k, u_j)$$

The effect of the variability of the smoothness estimator on the *p*-values is computed through the equations

$$p_Z(W) \approx S\,(2\pi)^{-(D+1)/2}\,W^{-1/2}\,Z^{D-1}\,e^{-Z^2/2}$$

where S is the volume of the SPM (the number of voxels) and Z the SPM intensity. The expression for the *p*-value based on the size of the region k above a threshold Z is given by

$$p_k(W) \approx 1 - \exp[-p_Z(W) \cdot e^{-\beta k^{2/D}}]$$

where

$$\beta = [\Gamma(D/2 + 1) \cdot p_Z(W)/S \cdot \Phi(-Z)^{2/D}$$

See Friston *et al.* (1994), for a review of the development of these equations.

TABLE 1　Mean and Variance–Covariance of the Vector **u**

	u_0	u_1	u_2	u_3
Experimental mean ($\times 10^5$)	1.3112	0.0516	0.0689	0.1459
Theoretical mean ($\times 10^5$)	1.3107	0.0515	0.0688	0.1457
Experimental covariance ($\times 10^7$)				
u_0	9.118	0.186	0.241	0.559
u_1		0.010	0.005	0.011
u_2			0.018	0.015
u_3				0.095
Theoretical Covariance ($\times 10^7$)				
u_0	8.670	0.170	0.228	0.661
u_1		0.010	0.005	0.010
u_2			0.018	0.014
u_3				0.083

Note. Top: from simulations, below: computed with the first-order approximation.

III. RESULTS

We first validate the approximate expression for the variance of W by simulating 1000 3D SPMs (uncorrelated Gaussian noise convolved with a Gaussian kernel, volume size $64 \times 64 \times 32$ voxels), and compare the predicted values for the mean and variance covariance matrix of **u** to the results of the simulations. Table 1 demonstrates the good agreement between the variance–covariance matrices computed experimentally using simulations (C_{exp}) and those predicted theoretically (C_{theo}) in 3D. The first-order approximations of W's standard deviation ($W = 4369$, SD $= 579.8$) compared well to the empirically determined values (SD $= 607.4$).

In Figure 1, we look at the impact of varying W, within the range of two standard deviations, on the *p*-values, for 3D processes (50000 pixels, $W = 18432$, $\mathrm{SD}_W = 6766$) corresponding to standard values for the resolution of PET based SPMs. Values of z and cluster size (k) have been chosen so that the probabilities come out around 0.05. Figure 1 shows that an overestimation of W has an opposite effect on the *p*-values for the two methods: it decreases the estimated *p*-value for the intensity method but it increases the estimated *p*-value for the cluster size assessment. Also, overestimating W has a stronger effect that an underestimation. In both cases, these effects are far from being negligible.

We computed the variation of the *p*-values obtained in an experimental activation study data set when W lies in the range $W \pm 2\mathrm{SD}_W$. In this case, SD_W was

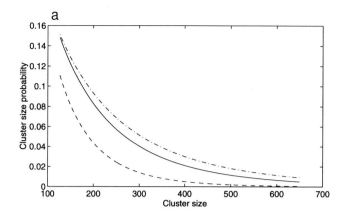

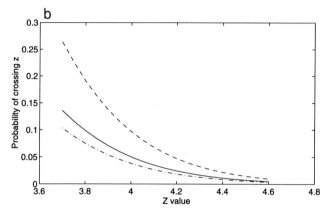

FIGURE 1   (a): Variation of cluster size probability for 3D data with the cluster size and with the variation of the smoothness estimate in ± 2 SD (SD_W), threshold $Z = 3$, size of the process; 50000 pixels, $W_0 = 18432$, $SD_W = 6766$; dashed line, min. p-value, dot–dashed line, maximum p-value.

(b): Variation of the z-value probability for 3D data with z and the variation of the smoothness estimate in $\pm 2SD_W$. In this example, $W_0 = 18432$, $SD_W = 6766$; dashed line; $W = W_0 + 2SD_W$; dot–dashed line, $W = W_0 - 2SD_W$.

1706 with $W = 7634$, the size of the process (number of voxels) was 60545. In Table 2 we give a few examples of local maxima or cluster probability with p-values around 0.05 and their variation with the smoothness estimate $\pm 2SD_W$.

TABLE 2   Range of Variation for P-Values Assessed from the Peak intensity (p_z) or Spatial extent (p_n) of an SPM Taken from an Activation Study

$(x, y, z) = (-38\ -68\ -8)$	$p_z = 0.049$	range: [0.041 0.066].
$(x, y, z) = (22\ -38\ 28)$	$p_z = 0.021$	range: [0.018 0.028].
$(x, y, z) = (-38\ -68\ -8)$	$p_n = 0.059$	range: [0.040 0.070].

IV. DISCUSSION AND CONCLUSION

Other important factors can affect the outcome of the statistical analysis performed on an SPM. The most important ones are the low-pass filter choice (with FWHM ranging usually from 6 to 20 mm) which must be made before starting the analysis (note that it is not a valid statistical method to adapt the filter to the data *a posteriori*; Poline and Mazoyer, 1994b), the spatial stereotactic normalization algorithm (and its implementation), and the normalization for the global activity in the brain. From our experience, the statistical outcome is very sensitive to these factors. However, none of these are random, and the smoothness variability is unique in that sense. Uncertainty on the smoothness estimation should have the same kind of effect on the analysis of functional MRI studies.

In this work, we have confirmed that estimating the smoothness on the data is a reasonable way to proceed and found that the p-values, "confidence intervals," due to the assessment of this parameter are of the order of 20%. This should be taken into account when reporting results and should moderate the role associated with a "knife-edged" 5% α-risk threshold.

Acknowledgments

JBP was funded by an EU grant, Human Capital and Mobility, No ERB4001GT932036. APH, KJF and RSJF were funded by the Wellcome Trust.

References

Friston, K. J., Frith, C. D., Liddle, P. F., and Frackowiak, R. S. J. (1991). Comparing functional (PET) images: The assessment of significant change. *J. Cereb. Blood Flow Metab.* **11:** 690–699.

Friston, K. J., Worsley, K. J., Frackowiak, R. S. J., Mazziotta, J. C., and Evans, A. C. (1994). Assessing the significance of focal activations using their spatial extent. *Hum. Brain Mapping* **1:** 214–220.

Poline, J. B. and Mazoyer, B. M. (1993). Analysis of individual positron emission tomography activation maps by high signal to noise ratio pixel cluster detection. *J. Cereb. Blood Flow Metab.* **13:** 425–437.

Poline, J. B., and Mazoyer, B. M. (1994a). Analysis of brain activation maps using multiscale detection and hierarchical description method. *IEEE Trans. Med. Imag.* **13**(4), 702–710.

Poline, J. B., and Mazoyer, B. M.· (1994b). Enhanced detection in brain activation maps using a multi filtering approach. *J. Cereb. Blood Flow Metab.* **14:** 639–641.

Poline J. B., Worsley K. J., Holmes A. P., Frackowiak R. S. J., and Friston, K. J. (1995). Estimating smoothness in statistical parametric maps: Variability of p values. *J. Comp. Assist. Tomogr.* **19:** 788–796.

Worsley, K. J., Evans, A. C., Marrett, S., and Neelin, P. (1992). A three-dimensional statistical analysis for rCBF activation studies in human brain. *J. Cereb. Blood Flow Metab.* **12:** 900–918.

Proportionality of Reaction CBF to Baseline CBF with Neural Activation and Deactivation

IWAO KANNO, JUN HATAZAWA, EKU SHIMOSEGAWA, KAZUNARI ISHII, and HIDEAKI FUJITA

Department of Radiology and Nuclear Medicine
Akita Research Institute of Brain and Blood Vessels
Akita 010, Japan

We will demonstrate the proportionality of activation CBF to baseline CBF and the symmetric feature of activation CBF in response to neural activation and deactivation. We used two data sets, which consisted of quantitative CBF measured during two neural activities and $PaCO_2$ perturbation. The first data set was obtained from 12 normal volunteers during 8 Hz flicker stimulation and periods of rest with subjects' eyes closed for various $PaCO_2$ levels to modify the baseline CBF. We found that the increment of CBF at the primary visual cortex was proportional to the baseline CBF. The second data set was retrospectively selected from clinical stroke studies in which $PaCO_2$ responsiveness was evaluated in patients with the crossed cerebellar hypoperfusion (CCH) and with the affected to nonaffected CBF ratio (ANR) at rest being < 0.9. We found that ANR of each patient was constant despite the change in $PaCO_2$. These results confirmed (1) reaction of CBF to the neural activation was proportional to the baseline CBF, and (2) this proportionality was preserved in deactivation for the CCH-affected cerebellum. These results further suggested a hemodynamic analogy between neural activity and $PaCO_2$; that is, physiological compatibility between these two factors. In addition, the proportionality of activation CBF to the baseline CBF will support the validity of the widely applied preprocessing of normalization in functional activation study; that is, division by global CBF within and between subjects.

I. INTRODUCTION

Since Lassen, Ingvar, and Skinhoj (1978) demonstrated regional CBF responses increased by psycho-physiological stimulation in humans using the Xe-133 clearance method, the reaction of CBF to neural activation has been used widely for mapping of functional anatomy. However, our knowledge based on this evidence is very limited, not only as a physiological mechanism for CBF reaction in linkage with local neural activity but also the quantitative features of the behavior of CBF change. Recently, our two independent papers concerning this issue were published, one relating neural activation that dealt with CBF during photic stimulation under various $PaCO_2$ levels (Shimosegawa et al., 1995) and the other with neural deactivation that dealt with CBF during steady deactivation under various $PaCO_2$ levels in stroke patients affected by crossed cerebellar hypoperfusion (CCH) (Ishii et al., 1994). The purpose of this chapter is to combine the two data sets to postulate a general concept concerning reaction CBF in a quantitative manner in relation to baseline CBF and to elucidate a physiological role of activation CBF.

II. METHOD AND MATERIALS

A. CBF Measurement

Both data sets consisted of quantitative CBF. The CBF was measured using an intravenous bolus $H_2^{15}O$, a continuous arterial blood sampling and a 90 sec accumulation image of $H_2^{15}O$ by PET (Kanno et al., 1987). The measurement was repeated with a 15 min interval. The PET scanner used was Headtome IV, 8.5 mm in effective in-plane FWHM and 10 mm in axial FWHM. All subjects underwent an MRI scan as the anatomical reference and to confirm the absence of cerebral infarction. The scan was done parallel to the AC–PC line using the MRI mid-sagittal plane and lateral X-ray view, and performed using an immobilizing head form to minimize head motion between scans. The $PaCO_2$ level was perturbed by voluntary hyperventilation for hypocapnia, resting for normocapnia, and 7% CO_2 inhalation for hypercapnia. $PaCO_2$ was measured by two arterial samplings before and after PET data acquisition.

B. Photic Stimulation Data Set

We measured 12 normal volunteers. The activation condition was photic stimulation 8 Hz flicker given by a goggle-mounted red LED. The control condition involved rest with subjects' eyes closed and covered by a black cloth. Ears were plugged with small earphones and fed binaurally with white-noise during measurement. Combining three breathing conditions (hyperventilation, rest, and CO_2 inhalation) and two functional conditions (flicker stimulation and eye closure), a total of six CBF measurements were carried out. The scan sequence was randomized. The regional CBF in the primary visual cortex was obtained from multiple ROI defined on corresponding MRI slices.

C. Crossed Cerebellar Hypoperfusion Data Set

We retrospectively selected data from clinical PET studies carried out to evaluate hemodynamic reserve in stroke patients. The criteria for selection of patients were as follows: (1) Deficit in the infratentorial areas was confirmed to be free angiographically as well as by T_2-weighted MRI. (2) Major infarction of the supratentorial area was in a single hemisphere. And, (3) the CBF ratio between CCH-affected and nonaffected cerebellum (ANR) was < 0.9. Seventeen patients fulfilled these criteria from 30 recent stroke patients who underwent three sets of CBF studies for hypo-, normo-, and hypercapnia. The CBF measurements were usually performed in the fixed order of breathing; that is, resting, CO_2 inhalation, and hyperventilation. Two ROIs of 2 × 3 cm were selected on the bilateral cerebellar cortices.

III. RESULTS AND DISCUSSION

A. Neural Activation

The absolute CBF in the primary visual cortex for flicker stimulation and eye closure with various levels

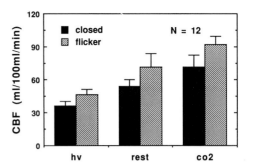

FIGURE 1   The absolute CBF in the primary visual cortex under two neural conditions, eye closure (solid) and flicker-on (hatched) each for hyperventilation (hv), rest, and CO_2 inhalation (co2). The error bar shows 1 SD. Data were obtained from 12 healthy volunteers.

of $PaCO_2$ is plotted in Figure 1. Slight differences in global CBF between flicker and eye closure for each $PaCO_2$ level were corrected by multiplying the ratio of global CBF; that is, normalization confined within a pair of CBF images of flicker and eye closure. An increase in CBF in the primary visual cortex area during flicker over that during eye closure became larger with elevating $PaCO_2$ levels from hypocapnia to hypercapnia (Fig. 1). The data suggested the increment of CBF caused by neural activation should be proportional to the baseline CBF.

B. Neural Deactivation

The absolute cerebellar blood flow (CeBF) of the cortex was taken from CBF images for hypocapnia, normocapnia, and hypercapnia and sorted into the CCH-affected side and the nonaffected side, depending on the supratentorial cerebrovascular lesion(s) (Fig. 2). The difference between the CeBF of the CCH-affected side and that of the nonaffected side was enlarged with elevating $PaCO_2$ levels. As the CCH-affected side was considered to be neural deactivation (Baron et al.,

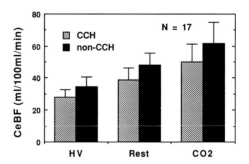

FIGURE 2   The cerebellar blood flow (CeBF) of bilateral cerebellar cortices after sorting into the crossed-cerebellar hypoperfusion (CCH) affected side (hatched) and the non-CCH side (solid), each for hyperventilation (HV), resting, and CO_2 inhalation (CO_2). The error bar represents 1 SD, and data were taken from 15 patients.

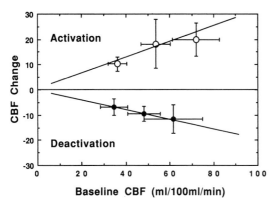

FIGURE 3 The results of the two data sets were replotted as blood flow difference between two neural conditions on the ordinate and the baseline blood flow on the abscissa. Photic stimulation caused positive CBF change and CCH caused negative CeBF change. Both blood flow changes were proportionate to the baseline blood flow and symmetrical to each other.

1980) and the nonaffected side to be the control, the difference between CeBF of the CCH-affected side and that of the nonaffected side was considered to correspond to a CeBF decrease due to neural deactivation. The data again suggested that this decrement of CeBF was proportional to the baseline CBF.

C. Proportionality

The two data sets were replotted on a common graph (Fig. 3). Figure 3 clearly demonstrated the proportionality between baseline CBF and reaction CBF in both directions, positive for neural activation and negative for deactivation. The proportionality will hold statistical rationality of normalization, which is a widely accepted preprocessing step in PET activation studies. The normalization, that is, division of whole images by each ratio of global CBF, is a procedure to equalize mean CBF within and between subjects. To date, this has been required by statistical procedure and the present study physiologically validates the rationality of this hypothesis (Friston *et al.*, 1990; Tempel *et al.*, 1991). In addition, because modern PET activation studies provide only relative CBF distribution or relative $H_2^{15}O$ distribution without arterial sampling, the proportionality is an essential property indispensable in CBF activation study.

D. Hemodynamic Considerations

We need to elucidate a few physiological analogies and discrepancies between the two data sets, before we take into account the observations to postulate the hemodynamic mechanism as triggered by neural activation and deactivation. Concerning cerebellar blood flow vs. cerebral blood flow, we confirmed elsewhere that both exhibited the same hemodynamic reactivity to $PaCO_2$ (Kanno *et al.*, 1985). Concerning the relationship between neural activity and $PaCO_2$, because both acting sites are known to exist on the resistance vessels, that is, the arterioles, the hemodynamic roles of the two components might be compatible.

IV. CONCLUSION

We can conclude that the reaction CBF induced by neural activation and deactivation is proportionate to the baseline CBF. This is also pertinent to statistical analysis using CBF data for functional mapping in PET activation studies.

Acknowledgment

The study was supported by grant 2A-10, 1995, the National Center of Neurology and Psychiatry of the Ministry of Health and Welfare, Japan.

References

Baron, J. C., Bousser, M. C., Comar, D., and Castaigne, P. (1980). "Crossed cerebellar diaschisis" in human supratentorial infarction. *Ann. Neurol.* **8**: 128.

Friston, K. J., Frith, C. D., Liddle P. E., Dolan, R. J., Lammertsma, A. A., and Frackowiak, R. S. J. (1990). The relationship between global and local changes in PET scans. *J. Cereb. Blood Flow Metab.* **10**: 458–466.

Ishii, K., Kanno, I., Uemura, K., Hatazawa, J., Okudera, T., Inugami, A., Ogawa, T., Fujita, H., and Shimosegawa, E. (1994). Comparison of carbon dioxide responsiveness of cerebral blood flow between affected and unaffected sides with crossed cerebellar diaschisis. *Stroke* **25**: 826–830.

Kanno, I., Iida, H., Miura, S., Murakami, M., Takahashi, K., Sasaki, H., Inugami, A., Shishido, F., and Uemura, K. (1987). A system for cerebral blood flow measurement using $H_2^{15}O$ autoradiographic method and positron emission tomography. *J. Cereb. Blood Flow Metab.* **7**: 143–153.

Kanno, I., Uemura, K., Murakami, M., Miura, S., Iida, H., Takahashi, K., Hagami, E., Sasaki, H., Shishido, F., and Inugami, A. (1985). Regional cerebrovascular reactivity to $PaCO_2$ change in man using $H_2^{15}O$ autoradiographic method and positron emission tomography. *J. Cereb. Blood Flow Metab.* **5**: S659–S660.

Lassen, N. A., Ingvar, D. H., and Skinhoj, E. (1978). Brain function and blood flow. *Sci. Amer.* **239**: 62–71.

Shimosegawa, E., Kanno, I., Hatazawa, J., Fujita, H., Iida, H., Miura, S., Murakami, M., Inugami, A., Ogawa, T., Itoh, H., Okudera, T., and Uemura, K. (1995). Photic stimulation study of changing the arterial partial pressure level of carbon dioxide. *J. Cereb. Blood Flow Metab.* **15**: 111–114.

Tempel, L. W., Snyder, A. Z., and Raichle, M. E. (1991). PET measurement of regional and global cerebral blood flow at rest and with physiological activation. *J. Cereb. Blood Flow Metab.* **11**: S367.

Counts vs. Flow

When Does It Matter?

RICHARD D. HICHWA,[1] DANIEL S. O'LEARY,[2] LAURA L. BOLES PONTO,[1] STEPHAN ARNDT,[2]
TED CIZADLO,[2] RICHARD R. HURTIG,[3] G. LEONARD WATKINS,[1] SCOTT D. WOLLENWEBER,[1]
and NANCY C. ANDREASEN[2]

[1]P.E.T. Imaging Center, Department of Radiology
[2]Department of Psychiatry
[3]Department of Speech, Pathology and Audiology
University of Iowa Hospitals and Clinics
Iowa City, Iowa 52242

Ten normal right-handed volunteers were studied with [15O]water and PET imaging during simultaneous presentation of auditory and visual stimulation paradigms. Arterial blood sampling was performed over the image acquisition period. PET count and absolute flow images were created. Region of interest (ROI) and function of interest (FOI) methods were evaluated to determine when and if quantitative flow values (arterial input function required) provided different or better information over normalized image data when similar strategies were employed for analyzing each of two data types (count and flow images). The FOI approach resulted in similar patterns of activation from either the normalized count, normalized flow, or absolute flow data. To achieve equivalent results from the ROI count or flow data, respective normalization by mean global count or flow is required. If only normalized FOI analyses will be applied, arterial blood data and absolute flow calculations are not needed. To measure changes in global flow, absolute flow data is necessary.

I. INTRODUCTION

Brain regions responding to stimuli (i.e., activation paradigms) exhibit increased neuronal activity and, therefore, increased metabolic demand. This elevated metabolic activity results in enhanced blood flow to these regions (Roland *et al.*, 1987).

[15O]water is a freely diffusible, positron-labeled tracer that permits absolute and relative blood flow to be globally or regionally monitored, noninvasively, under a multitude of activation conditions (Fox and Raichle, 1984; Fox *et al.*, 1987a; Fox *et al.*, 1987b). Even though widely used, [15O]water is not the perfect tracer to study brain activation (Herscovitch *et al.*, 1983) for the following reasons: (1) at high flows, it is not completely extracted and is considered to be flow limited (Raichle *et al.*, 1983); (2) a single-compartmental model is inadequate to fully describe the kinetic behavior of the tracer (Gambhir *et al.*, 1987); (3) the radiation burden to the subject limits the amount of [15O]water injected and, therefore, the statistical quality of the images (Herscovitch, *et al.*, 1993; Smith *et al.*, 1994; Brihaye *et al.*, 1995); and (4) quantitative assessment of absolute blood flow requires knowledge of the arterial input function (Herscovitch *et al.*, 1983). Errors in image acquisition (e.g., timing mismatch between initiation of activation stimulus and arrival of brain radioactivity) and in the characterization of the arterial input function (e.g., delay between arrival of radioactivity at the arterial sampling site and arrival of brain radioactivity; dispersion) can potentially result in significant errors in blood flow quantitation (Meyer, 1989; Iida *et al.*, 1988; Koeppe *et al.*, 1987; Iida *et al.*, 1986; Herscovitch *et al.*, 1983; Raichle *et al.*, 1983).

Despite these difficulties, the issue of quantitation is important and remains one of the particular strengths of the PET methodology. The need for arterial sampling to obtain absolute quantitative results for brain blood flow is often debated (Lammertsma, 1994). Further, numerous schemes for data analysis are employed to extract meaningful information from less than optimal [^{15}O]water images (Fox *et al.*, 1988; Worsley *et al.*, 1992; Friston *et al.*, 1991; Poline and Mazoyer, 1993; Cherry *et al.*, 1995).

In this study, region of interest (ROI) methods were evaluated along with function of interest (FOI) methods to determine when and if quantitative flow values (arterial input function required) provide different or better information over normalized image data when similar strategies were employed for analyzing each of the data types (counts vs. flow images).

II. MATERIALS AND METHODS

Ten normal right-handed volunteers, nine male and one female, gave informed consent to participate in this study. Subjects were positioned in the PET scanner with the assistance of laser light guides such that the orbital–meatal line was parallel to the plane of the tomograph detectors. PET images from eight 1850 MBq bolus injections of [^{15}O]water in 5–7 ml saline were acquired with a GE 4096 Plus 15 slice whole body tomograph (resolution = 6.5 mm FWHM in *x*, *y*, and *z*; *z*-axis FOV = 10 cm; sensitivity = 5,000 counts/sec/ μCi/ml). The tracer was injected via a venous catheter into the antecubital vein of the right arm. Injections were repeated at approximately 15 min intervals. Arterial blood was withdrawn from a catheter placed in the radial artery of the left wrist (nondominant hand) at a

rate of 12 ml/min (20 samples at 0.5–1.0 ml/sample/ 5 sec). Sampling was initiated with the onset of each injection and continued for 100 sec. The arterial input function was derived by decay correcting the discrete arterial blood samples from the time of measurement of blood radioactivity to the time each sample was collected. The bolus arrival time was individually determined by injecting 550 MBq of [^{15}O]water and measuring the time from injection to rapid rise of activity in brain. The arrival time was determined prior to performing the activation paradigms. Images were acquired in 20 5-sec frames. Based on time–activity curves derived from a ROI placed over major cerebral arteries, the eight sequential frames that reflect the first 40 sec after bolus transit through the brain were summed and PET count images formed by reconstructing sinograms into 2 mm pixels in a 128 × 128 matrix using a Butterworth filter (order = 6, cutoff frequency = 0.35 Nyquist). Cerebral blood flow images were calculated on a pixel-by-pixel basis by using the PET count images, the arterial input function, an assumed brain–blood partition coefficient of 0.9, and applying the autoradiographic method (Herscovitch *et al.*, 1983).

During PET scans, subjects were instructed to fixate on a central field while auditory stimulation was presented binaurally, monaurally, or dichotically (auditory duration of 500 msec followed by 300 msec of silence) and simultaneous visual information was presented in the right and left visual fields from a video monitor suspended over the PET couch (visual stimulation on for 200 msec followed by 600 msec of blank screen). An activation paradigm for a specific injection was initiated at 24 sec prior to bolus arrival in brain and

TABLE 1   Specific ROIs

Region	Normalized counts		Normalized flow		Absolute flow	
	t	*p*<	*t*	*p*<	*t*	*p*<
L HeG	7.49	0.0001*	7.59	0.0001*	4.43	0.0008*
L PT	7.32	0.0001*	6.97	0.0001*	3.92	0.0017*
L Str	2.49	0.0172*	2.46	0.0180*	1.43	0.0928
L aR	−0.40	0.3490	−0.35	0.3680	−0.33	0.3760
R HeG	3.49	0.0034*	3.46	0.0036*	2.06	0.0347*
R PT	6.58	0.0001*	6.09	0.0001*	2.96	0.0079*
R Str	1.38	0.0999	1.54	0.0785	0.51	0.3122
R aR	−0.02	0.4920	0.04	0.4860	−0.43	0.3384

*Significant at *p* < 0.05 level. L = left; R = right; HeG = Heschl's gyrus; PT = planum temporale; Str = striate; aR = ascending ramus

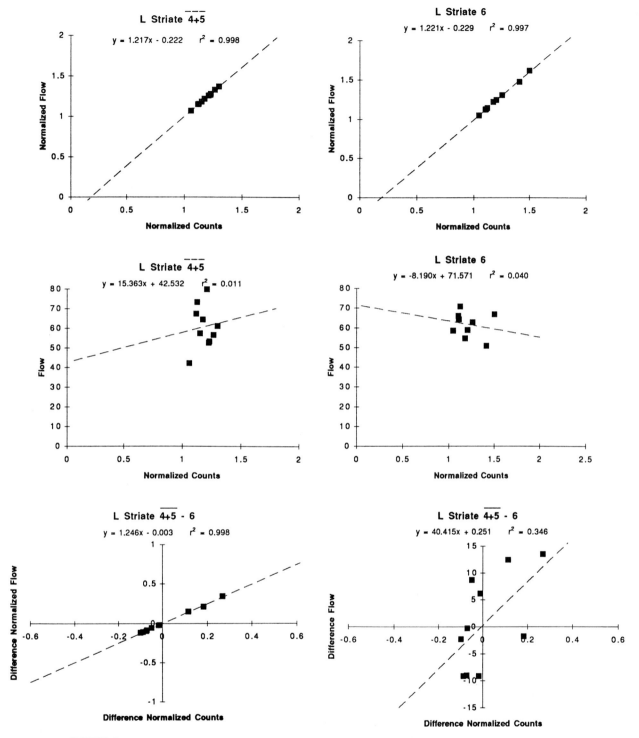

FIGURE 1   Plots of normalized flow or absolute flow values vs. normalized PET counts. Each data point represents a flow or count value for a particular subject and ROI. The ROI, injection (either the average of injections 4 and 5 or a baseline, which is injection 6), and regression information are specified in each panel. Normalized flow values are obtained by dividing absolute ROI flow values by the whole brain mean flow values. Normalized counts are obtained by dividing ROI count values by the mean whole brain count values. Difference data are obtained by subtracting the baseline (injection 6) from the average value obtained from injections 4 and 5.

TABLE 2   Flow vs. Counts

Region	Injection 4 and 5 (average)		Injection 6	
	Slope	r^2	Slope	r^2
Normalized Flow vs. Normalized Counts				
L HeG	1.207	0.994	1.174	0.989
L PT	1.334	0.946	1.111	0.976
L Str	1.217	0.998	1.221	0.997
L aR	1.393	0.900	1.330	0.995
R HeG	1.168	0.989	1.148	0.989
R PT	1.326	0.989	1.184	0.996
R Str	1.253	0.994	1.275	0.997
R aR	1.332	0.959	1.246	0.996
Absolute Flow vs. Normalized Counts				
L HeG	9.2	0.010	87.8	0.249
L PT	84.4	0.373	70.9	0.480
L Str	15.4	0.011	−8.2	0.040
L aR	142.6	0.416	126.2	0.736
R HeG	61.0	0.339	52.4	0.340
R PT	105.1	0.444	60.7	0.282
R Str	7.5	0.005	7.1	0.006
R aR	126.0	0.314	100.5	0.545

Normalized Flow vs. Normalized Counts
(Average of Injection 4 and 5 − Injection 6)

	Slope	r^2
L HeG	1.231	0.984
L PT	1.305	0.887
L Str	1.246	0.998
L aR	1.235	0.958
R HeG	1.282	0.992
R PT	1.386	0.987
R Str	1.230	0.993
R aR	1.154	0.974

Note. See Table 1 for region of interest definitions.

continued for 24 sec following bolus arrival in brain. An [^{15}O]water injection was associated with each of the following activation paradigms in the following order:

1. Binaural consonant–vowel–consonant (CVC) sound, ignore bilateral visual field;
2. Monaural CVC in right ear, ignore bilateral visual field;
3. Monaural CVC in left ear, ignore bilateral visual field;
4. Dichotic CVC, attend to left ear, ignore bilateral visual field;

5. Dichotic CVC, attend to right ear, ignore bilateral visual field;
6. Baseline, eyes closed, ears occluded, no auditory input;
7. Right visual field CVC, look for letter combination *FAW*, ignore dichotic CVC;
8. Left visual field CVC, look for letter combination *FAW*, ignore dichotic CVC.

MR scans were obtained for each subject using a standard T_1-weighted three-dimensional SPGR sequence on a 1.5 T GE Signa scanner (TE = 5, TR = 24, flip angle = 40, NEX = 2, FOV = 26, matrix = 256 × 192, slice thickness = 1.5 mm).

Flow and count images were coregistered with MR images using the BRAINS software package (Cizadlo *et al.*, 1994) by first outlining the brain on the MR images using a combination of edge detection and manual tracing techniques. Brains of all subjects were aligned to a standard position and orientation in Talairach coordinate space (Talairach and Tournoux, 1988). PET images were fitted to the MR images for each subject. Any head movement from scan to scan was accounted for by repositioning the PET data set and repeating the coregistration process.

FOI analyses of PET images were performed using an adaptation of the method developed by Worsley and co-workers (1992). An 18 mm Hanning filter was applied to PET flow and count images. These images were resampled into 128 × 128 × 80 voxels using the Talairach atlas bounding box with a calculated resolution element (resel) of 2.47 cc (after filtering). For this study, a within-subject subtraction of the baseline (injection 6) from the activation sequence (average of injections 4 and 5) was then performed, followed by across-subject averaging of the subtraction images and computation of voxel-by-voxel *t*-tests of the flow or count changes. Significant regions of activation were calculated on the *t*-map images. Because the activation paradigms for injections 4 and 5 were nearly identical, the average of the two injections was considered to constitute a representative data set for analysis. Injections 2 and 3 or 7 and 8 could also have been used as representative cases.

ROI analyses were accomplished by drawing ROIs (specific ROIs are defined in Table 1) on individual MR images and telegraphing the region location to the original coregistered PET images (unfiltered images) to obtain regional count or flow information. Mean ROI values were normalized by dividing the region-based values (total counts or flow values in region/region area) by the global mean count or flow value (whole brain mean count or flow), respectively.

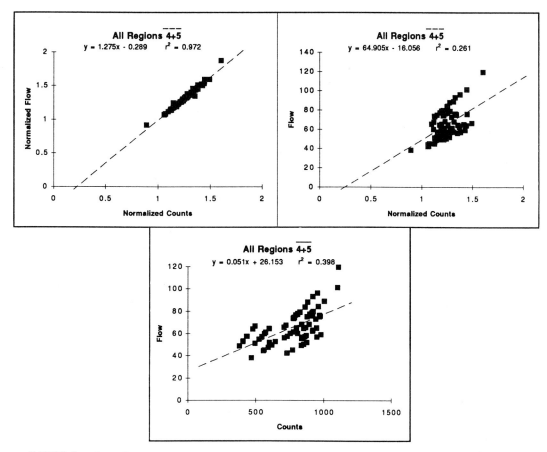

FIGURE 2 Plots of normalized flow or absolute flow vs normalized PET counts for all ROIs. Variables are defined in Figure 1. Plots depict 80 data points (8 ROIs × 10 subjects).

Significant peaks in the FOI analyses were defined by standard criteria (Worsley *et al.*, 1992) and compared with respect to the magnitude of the t-statistic and significance level. The regions identified in the FOI approach were used to sample the normalized counts, normalized flow, and absolute flow images for the activated (injections 4 and 5) and baseline (injection 6) states. Comparisons were made between ROI values obtained from normalized count and normalized flow images, as well as from normalized count and absolute flow images by regression analysis.

III. RESULTS AND DISCUSSION

For the FOI approach, analyses of normalized count data and normalized flow data depicted patterns of activation as shown in Table 1. However, small differences were apparent in the magnitude of the t-values and level of significance. Subtle differences between count and flow images due to the nonlinearity of the lookup table for conversion of counts to flows and round-off errors accounted for most of the observed effects. Analyzing nonnormalized flow images (absolute blood flow images) yields similar trends in significant areas of activation differing only in one region not reaching significance (left striate). The absolute flow images possess increased variance over the normalized flow or count images, which account for the left striate not being included.

Typical results obtained using ROI techniques from normalized flow, normalized counts, and normalized difference images are shown in the upper panels of Figure 1. Nearly identical results are obtained for all regions when normalized flow and normalized counts are compared to each other ($r^2 > 0.90$ in all eight regions that were compared), as shown in Table 2. This straightforward finding is consistent with the fact that flow images are derived from the count images. Most flow values fall within a moderate flow region and are not appreciably affected by the nonlinearity of $[^{15}O]$-water response at high flows. The ROI values cluster about an average value for each region. Differences in injection techniques, amount of activity injected, and individual response to a specific injection are taken into account by the arterial input function for determination of absolute flows and are eliminated by the normalization procedure. The slope and intercept of the regression line indicate the extent of the nonlinearity of the lookup table for the cluster of flow values. When normalized, count and flow images differ only by a multiplicative scalar. When flow values were not normalized to global mean flow and were compared to normalized count images, there existed little relationship between absolute flows and normalized counts ($0.005 < r^2 < 0.74$) as shown in the lower panels of Figure 1. The relationship was poorer when absolute flow and count images were compared, because normalization (activity in region/activity in brain) is not equivalent to an absolute representation of the measured value: This is clearly seen in Figure 2. The arterial input function accurately represents the time course of activity input to the region. Without accounting for specific arterial input differences, correlation between flow and counts or normalized counts is poor. To measure changes in global flow, analysis of absolute flow data is necessary, which requires knowledge of the arterial blood input function.

FOI approaches that normalize the data result in no significant differences between analyses based on flow or count data. FOI analyses of absolute flow data yield nearly equivalent regions, but increased variance tends to reduce the number of significant regions. To achieve equivalent results from ROI count or flow data, respective normalization by global count or flow is required, which in turn requires an arterial blood input function. Knowledge of the type of analyses that will be applied to the data is critical to the choice of data acquisition. If only normalized FOI analyses will be applied, arterial blood data and absolute flow calculations are not needed.

Acknowledgments

This research was supported in part by NIMH Grants MH40856 and MH43271.

References

Brihaye, C., Depresseux, J. C., and Comar, D. (1995). Radiation dosimetry for bolus administration of oxygen-15 water. *J. Nucl. Med.* **36**: 651–656.

Cherry, S. R., Woods, R. P., Doshi, N. K., Banerjee, P. K., and Mazziotta, J. C. (1995). Improved signal-to-noise in PET activation studies using switched paradigms. *J. Nucl. Med.* **36**: 307–314.

Cizadlo, T., Andreasen, N. C., Zeien, G., Rajarethinam, R., Harris, G., O'Leary, D., Swayze, V., Arndt, S., Hichwa, R., Ehrhardt, J., and Yuh, W. T. C. (1994). Image registration issues in the analysis of multiple-injection [^{15}O]H$_2$O PET studies: BRAINFIT. (1994). *SPIE—The Int. Soc. Opt. Eng.* **2168**: 423–430.

Fox, P. T. and Raichle, M. E. (1984). Stimulus rate dependence of regional cerebral blood flow in human striate cortex, demonstrated by positron emission tomography. *J. Neurophysiol.* **51**: 1109–1120.

Fox, P. T., Burton, H., and Raichle, M. E. (1987a). Mapping human somatosensory cortex with positron emission tomography. *J. Neurosurg.* **67**: 34–43.

Fox, P. T., Miezin, F. M., Allman, J. M., Van Essen, D. C., and Raichle, M. E. (1987b). Retinotopic organization of human visual cortex mapped with positron-emission tomography. *J. Neurosci.* **7**: 913–922.

Fox, P. T., Mintun, M. A., Reiman, E. M., and Raichle, M. E. (1988). Enhanced detection of focal brain responses using intrasubject averaging and change-distribution analysis of subtracted PET images. *J. Cereb. Blood Flow Metab.* **8**: 642–653.

Friston, K. J., Frith, C. D., Liddle, P. F., and Frackowiak, R. S. J. (1991). Comparing functional (PET) images: The assessment of significant change. *J. Cereb. Blood Flow Metab.* **11**: 690–699.

Gambhir, S. S., Huang, S. C., Hawkins, R. A., and Phelps, M. E. (1987). A study of the single compartment tracer kinetic model for the measurement of local cerebral blood flow using [^{15}O]water and positron emission tomography. *J. Cereb. Blood Flow Metab.* **7**: 13–20.

Herscovitch, P., Markham, J., and Raichle, M. E. (1983). Brain blood flow measured with intravenous H$_2$^{15}O. I. Theory and error analysis. *J. Nucl. Med.* **24**: 782–789.

Herscovitch, P., Carson, R. E., Stabin, M., and Stubbs, J. B. (1993). A new kinetic approach to estimate the radiation dosimetry of flow based radiotracers. *J. Nucl. Med.* **34**: 155P.

Iida, H., Kanno, I., Miura, S., Murakami, M., Takahashi, K., and Uemura, K. (1986). Error analysis of a quantitative cerebral blood flow measurement using H$_2$^{15}O autoradiography and positron emission tomography, with respect to the dispersion of the input function. *J. Cereb. Blood Flow Metab.* **6**: 536–545.

Iida, H., Higano, S., Tomura, N., Shishido, F., Kanno, I., Miura, S., Murakami, M., Takahashi, K., Sasaki, H., and Uemura, K. (1988). Evaluation of regional differences of tracer appearance time in cerebral tissues using [^{15}O]water and dynamic positron emission tomography. *J. Cereb. Blood Flow Metab.* **8**: 285–288.

Koeppe, R. A., Hutchins, G. D., Rothley, J. M., and Hichwa, R. D. (1987). Examination of assumptions for local cerebral blood flow studies in PET. *J. Nucl. Med.* **28**: 1695–1703.

Lammertsma, A. A. (1994). Noninvasive estimation of cerebral blood flow. *J. Nucl. Med.* **35**: 1878–1879.

Meyer, E. (1989). Simultaneous correction for tracer arrival delay and dispersion in CBF measurements by the H$_2$^{15}O autoradiographic method and dynamic PET. *J. Nucl. Med.* **30**: 1069–1078.

Poline, J. B. and Mazoyer, B. M. (1993). Analysis of individual positron emission tomography activation maps by detection of high signal-to-noise-ratio pixel clusters. *J. Cereb. Blood Flow Metab.* **13**: 425–437.

Raichle, M. E., Martin, W. R. W., Herscovitch, P., Mintun, M. A., and Markham, J. (1983). Brain blood flow measured with intravenous H$_2$^{15}O. II. Implementation and validation. *J. Nucl. Med.* **24**: 790–798.

Roland, P. E., Eriksson, L., Stone-Elander, S., and Widen, L. (1987). Does mental activity change the oxidative metabolism of the brain? *J. Neurosci.* **7**: 2373–2389.

Smith, T., Tong, C., Lammertsma, A. A., Butler, K. R., Schnorr,

L., Watson, J. D. G., Ramsay, S., Clark, J. C., and Jones, T. (1994). Dosimetry of intravenously administered oxygen-15 labelled water in man: A model based on experimental human data from 21 subjects. *Eur. J. Nucl. Med.* **21:** 1126–1134.

Talairach, J. and Tournoux, P. (1988). "Co-planar Stereotaxic Atlas of the Human Brain." Thieme-Medical Publishers Inc., New York.

Worsley, K., Evans, A., Marrett, S., and Neelin, P. (1992). A three-dimensional statistical analysis for CBF activation studies in human brain. *J. Cereb. Blood Flow Metab.* **12:** 900–918.

Analyzing a European PET Activation Study

Lessons from a Multicenter Experiment

EUROPEAN CONCERTED ACTION ON FUNCTIONAL IMAGING
COLOGNE, COPENHAGEN, DÜSSELDORF, ESSEN, GROENINGEN, LEUVEN, LIEGE,
LONDON, LYON, MILAN, ORSAY, STOCKHOLM
(RAPPORTEUR: J.-B. POLINE)

J-B. Poline is at the Wellcome Department of Cognitive Neurology,
WC1N 3BG, United Kingdom and part of the work was done at the
MRC Cyclotron Unit, Hammersmith Hospital, London W12ONN United Kingdom

PET activation studies are widely performed to study human cognitive functions. The question of reproducibility or reliability of the results of such experiments has rarely been addressed on a large scale. Recently, 12 PET centers agreed to perform the same cognitive activation experiment. We have analyzed each center's data set and the pooled data set using statistical parametric mapping. We present some first results showing how consistent the output of these analyses is and the increased sensitivity due to the increased number of subjects. We used a MANOVA to test for center, condition, and center by condition effects and found a predominant center effect.

I. INTRODUCTION

During 1994, a European Union (EU) concerted action was undertaken by 12 PET centers scattered in eight European countries. These centers agreed to perform the same silent verbal fluency activation experiment. The aims were manifold and included methodological issues such as reproducibility, confounding factors, and differential sensitivity and neurolinguistic issues relating to differences between languages. Data produced by the PET scanners from different centers had very different characteristics, such as field of view (ranging from 5.4 to 15.0 cm), number of planes

(from 7 to 47), or number of scans per subject (from 4 to 12). In this chapter, we will concentrate on three questions:

- How reproducible are the results from one center to another, despite all the center differences?
- What increase in sensitivity do we get when pooling all the data?
- How is the variance of this data set decomposed?

The large number of centers involved in this experiment (77 subjects, more than 450 scans) is unique and has allowed us to draw some conclusions on the reproducibility of this PET activation study.

II. MATERIALS AND METHODS

Table 1 presents some characteristics of the centers. Data were analyzed with the latest version of statistical parametric mapping (SPM94) (Friston *et al.*, 1995). Scans were stereotactically normalized into Talairach space in preparation for pixel-by-pixel analyses. First, each center's data set was analyzed using a completely randomized block design. ANCOVA was fitted and a *t*-statistic for the contrast condition effect constructed. Equivalent *z*-statistic volumes were assessed for significant regions by voxel intensity and suprathreshold cluster size separately (Worsley *et al.*, 1992; Friston

TABLE 1 Characteristics of the PET Centers

Center	Subjects × scans	Language	Camera	Axial FOV (cm)	2D/3D
Cologne	7 × 6	Ger	Exact HR	15.0	3D
Copenhagen	10 × 6	Dan	GE-ADVANCED	15.2	3D
Düsseldorf	6 × 6	Ger	Scandi.PC4096-15	9.2	2D
Essen	6 × 12	Ger	CTI-953	5.4	2D
Gronigen	6 × 4	Dut	CTI-951	10.8	2D
Hammersmith	6 × 8	Eng	CTI-953B	10.8	3D
Karolinska	6 × 6	Swe	Exact HR	15.0	2D
Leuven	6 × 6	Dut	CTI-931	10.8	2D
Liege	6 × 6	Fre	CTI-951	10.8	2D
Lyon	6 × 6	Fre	TTV03	8.1	2D
Milan	6 × 6	Ita	CTI-93	5.4	2D
Orsay	6 × 6	Fre	CTI-953B	10.8	2D

et al., 1994). A direct comparison of each center's results was performed using the set of regions found at the 5% significance level. Second, a group of nine centers with similar PET FOVs were analyzed together (57 subjects, 347 scans) using a split plot design implemented in SPM94 with a regression coefficient specific to each center for global effects. Within this model, inferences regarding overall activation, activation by center interaction, and comparisons between languages can be performed using appropriate contrasts. Third, a singular-value decomposition (SVD) was performed on the whole series of scans (after correction for the global activity and the block effect), and the variance was decomposed into orthogonal axes. We also performed a multivariate analysis of variance on the first eight scores obtained with the SVD analysis (explaining more than 75% of the variance) and some ANOVAs on the first four scores (explaining respectively 24.6, 23.1, 12, and 8.6% of the variance).

III. RESULTS

Figure 1 shows the SPM projections in the sagittal and coronal orientations. The high consistency between these patterns is clearly seen on the maps, especially among the centers with 3D acquisition scanners. Note that the last row is made of the centers with small fields of view: This explains the absence of signal in the higher or lower parts of the brain. For results from these individual centers, highest z scores ranged from 3.9 to 9.2 (average, 5.4), the resolution of the z-map was between 15 and 25 mm (FWHM) for an initial Gaussian filter of 12 mm FWHM.

Figure 2 presents the results of the pooled analysis: In this figure, the threshold was set such that each voxel above this threshold survived the correction for multiple comparisons. In particular, an important number of structures in the right hemisphere were found highly significant. The highest z score was about three times the average z score in an individual analysis.

A. Singular Value Decomposition

The singular value decomposition (SVD) of the data from seven centers with similar fields of view and number of scans per subject is summarized in Figure 3, showing the scores for the first four axes explaining 68% of the total variance. In this figure, each gray level corresponds to one center, and for each of them the first three observations relate to the activation state and the last three correspond to the resting state. We observe that the condition (activation) effect is concentrated on the first two axes (especially in the second axis), but is mixed with a center effect.

B. Multivariate Analysis of Variance (MANOVA)

The results of the MANOVA performed on the data set were all highly significant (center, condition, and center by condition interaction), but the center ex-

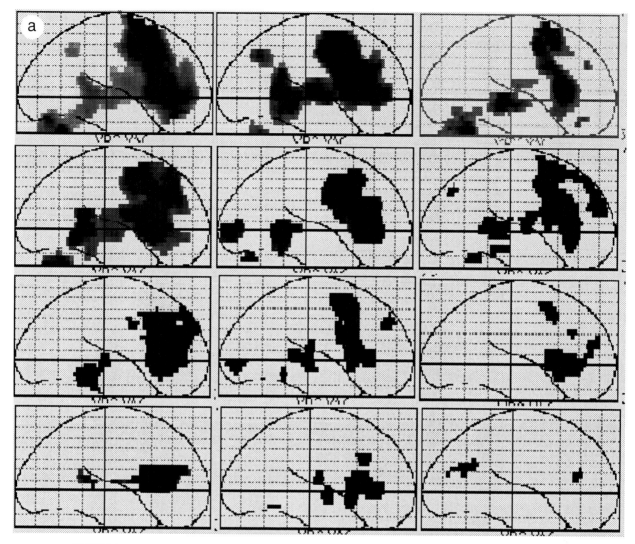

FIGURE 1   (a): Sagittal sections of the statistical parametric maps (maximum intensity projection) for each of the 12 center analyses. The z-maps were thresholded at $z = 3.09$. Row by row, from top to bottom and left to right: Copenhagen, Hammersmith, Cologne, Liege, Leuven, Karolinska, Groningen, Orsay, Düsseldorf, Essen, Lyon, Milan. (*Continues.*)

plained most of the variance. Although the interaction effect was significant in the MANOVA results, this effect was not found in the first two axes resulting from the SVD. This means that the interaction term (in other words, the differences of the subjects' responses between centers) does not contribute to the variance of the data along the two main axes.

IV. DISCUSSION AND CONCLUSION

The high consistency found in the pattern of the SPM maps was also reflected by a consistent set of regions, which reached the significance level of 5% in most of the center-by-center analyses. In particular, the left middle temporal gyrus, the left inferior and medial frontal gyri, the cingulate, the supplementary motor area, and the cerebellum on the right were found respectively in 8, 11, 6, 7, and 7 centers (note that some centers have not scanned the SMA or the cerebellum, the corresponding figure would have probably been greater).

Some of the variability observed in the set of regions found is due to the difference in sensitivity among the centers. When we lower the risk of error from 5 to 20 or 40%, the set of regions found is even more consistent, decreasing the number of false negatives.

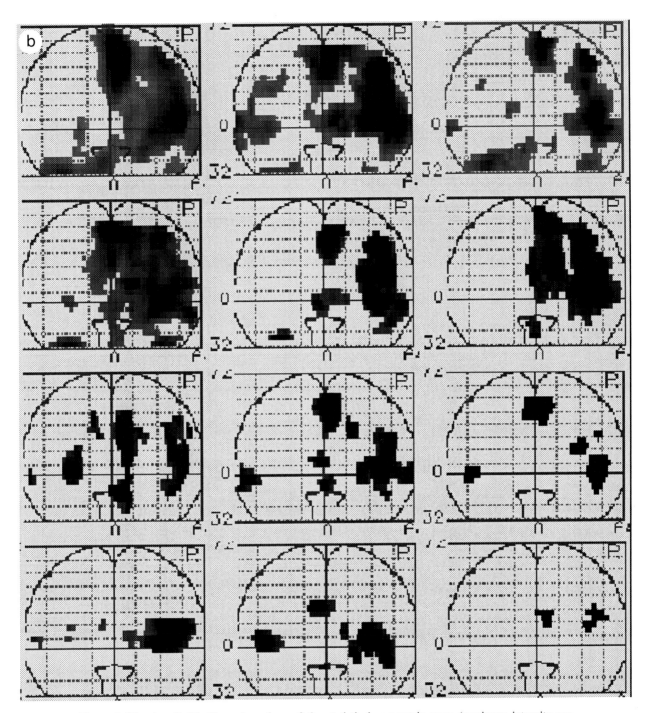

Figure 1 (*Continued*) (b): Coronal sections of the statistical parametric maps (maximum intensity projection) for each of the 12 center analyses. The z-maps were thresholded at $z = 3.09$. Row by row, from top to bottom and left to right: Copenhagen, Hammersmith, Cologne, Liege, Leuven, Karolinska, Groningen, Orsay, Düsseldorf, Essen, Lyon, Milan. The left side of the brain is on the right of each image.

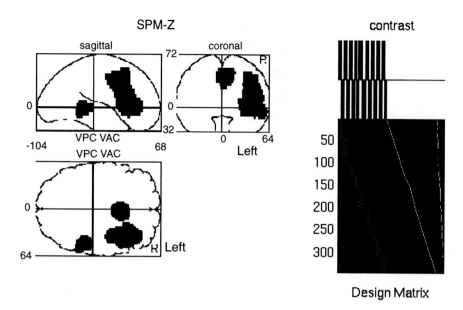

Regional Effects

region	size {k}	P(n max > k)	Z	P(Z max > u)	(Uncorrected)	{x,y,z mm}		
1	9665	0.000	17.27	0.000	(0.000)	2	6	48
			17.06	0.000	(0.000)	44	16	8
			13.38	0.000	(0.000)	38	-2	44
2	155	0.082	6.77	0.000	(0.000)	-60	-22	0
			6.67	0.000	(0.000)	-52	-28	0
			5.79	0.000	(0.000)	-60	-34	4
3	615	0.014	6.55	0.000	(0.000)	-34	12	4
			5.74	0.000	(0.000)	-48	12	-8
			4.80	0.001	(0.000)	-14	-6	4
4	7	0.216	4.17	0.010	(0.000)	-42	-38	4
5	9	0.211	4.02	0.017	(0.000)	32	-68	32

Threshold = 3.09; Volume [S] = 44316 voxels; df = 231
FWHM = [29.4 27.8 28.8] mm (i.e. 30 RESELS)

FIGURE 2 Pooled SPM analysis of the nine centers with large fields of view. The design matrix implemented a study (center) specific ANCOVA for the correction of the global activity in the brain. Notice the very high z score reached by this analysis. The z-map has been thresholded so that every voxel seen on this figure survived the multiple comparison correction.

The main source of variability in the data set being the center effect, this raises the question of the source of variability: Can it be attributed to an instrumental factor or to some characteristics of the group of subjects selected for the experiment? We performed some preliminary analyses that showed no simple relation between a set of instrumental factors or subject charac-teristics and the center effect (having removed the condition and the interaction effect).

This study, the largest one of its kind, showed that highly consistent results can be found when analyzing a cognitive protocol, despite all the differences between the center scanners, group of subjects, and scanning procedure. These results also suggest that an im-

Axis : 1 - % of variance : 24.6

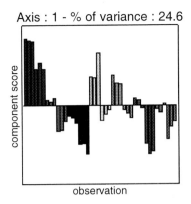

Axis : 2 - % of variance : 23.1

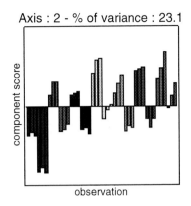

Axis : 3 - % of variance : 12.9

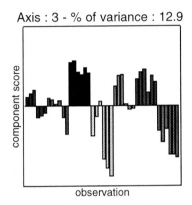

Axis : 4 - % of variance : 8.6

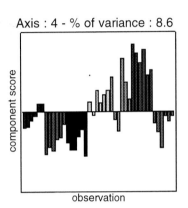

FIGURE 3 Singular value decomposition. The first four axes accounted for 68% of the variance. Each gray level corresponds to one center, and the first three observations of each correspond to the activation state and the last three observations correspond to the resting state. The condition (activation) effect is clearly seen on the first and second axes, but these axes are not free from a center effect, which is also observed in the axes 3 and 4.

portant part of the variability found in cognitive PET activation studies between different centers is due to the variation in sensitivity (due to the scanners' sensitivity, the scanning session, the subjects' selection, etc.).

Acknowledgments

The EU concerted action on Functional Imaging was funded by the European Union and coordinated by B. Mazoyer and R. Frackowiak (EU Biomed 1 Concerted Action on Positron Emission Tomography of Cellular Degeneration and Regeneration). JBP was funded by an EU grant, Human Capital and Mobility, No ERB4001GT932036. The author is very much in debt to A. Holmes, K. Friston and R. Frackowiak for their great help and support as well as to all the participants of this EU concerted action.

References

Friston, K. J., Worsley, K. J., Frackowiak, R. S. J., Mazziotta, J. C., and Evans, A. C. (1994a). Assessing the significance of focal activations using their spatial extent. *Hum. Brain Mapping* **1:** 214–220.

Friston, K. J., Holmes, A. P., Worsley, K. J., Poline, J. B., Frith, C. D., and Frackowiak, R. S. J. (1995). Statistical parametric maps in functional imaging: A general linear approach. *Hum. Brain Mapping.* **2:** 189–210.

Worsley, K. J., Evans, A. C., Marrett, S., and Neelin, P. (1992). A three-dimensional statistical analysis for rCBF activation studies in human brain. *J. Cereb. Blood Flow Metab.* **12:** 900–918.

[^{15}O]Water PET

More "Noise" Than Signal?

S. C. STROTHER,[1,3] **J. J. SIDTIS,**[2] **J. R. ANDERSON,**[1] **L. K. HANSEN,**[4] **K. SCHAPER,**[1] **and D. A. ROTTENBERG**[1,2,3]

[1]*PET Imaging Section*
VA Medical Center
Minneapolis, Minnesota 55417
[2]*Neurology and* [3]*Radiology Departments*
University of Minnesota
Minneapolis, Minnesota 55455
[4]*Electronics Institute*
Danish Technical University
Lyngby, DK-2800, Denmark

For the analysis of functional activation [^{15}O]water PET studies we demonstrate that, by not using hypothesis-testing techniques based on the mathematically tractable assumptions of parametric noise models, such as statistical parametric mapping (SPM), it is possible to gain important insights into the underlying signal structure of [^{15}O]water PET images of a sequential finger opposition task. Using a nonparametric exploratory analysis based on singular value decomposition (SVD) within the scaled subprofile model (SSM) framework we show that (1) most of the nonrandom signal structure and random PET reconstruction noise seem to play only a minor role in determining spatial patterns of functional activation; (2) the differences between current hypothesis-testing approaches, which produce extensive negative regions, and SSM, which does not, predominantly reflect different normalization procedures; and (3) the spatial activation patterns associated with current hypothesis-testing approaches may be accurately predicted within the SSM framework.

I. INTRODUCTION

Most analyses of functional activation data sets from [^{15}O]water PET studies are based on mathematically tractable parametric models for the noise, such as Gaussian random fields (Friston *et al.*, 1994), and calculate detection thresholds for the null hypothesis that only noise is present. These approaches do not define a specific alternate signal hypothesis. As a result, difficulties in choosing the "true" spatial activation pattern may be encountered if several different patterns can be derived from a single data set. We demonstrate that inconsistent activation patterns may be derived from the same data set as a result of choosing different normalization procedures; for example, global mean (the mean of all brain voxels) normalization compared to that of the scaled subprofile model (SSM; Strother *et al.*, 1995a, 1995b, 1995c). In Strother *et al.* (1995b) both global mean and analysis of covariance (ANCOVA, Friston *et al.*, 1990) normalization procedures are shown to introduce large negative biases into calculated spatial activation patterns relative to the results obtained from SSM.

We shall refer to normalization by the global mean followed by subtraction of averaged activation and averaged baseline images as intersubject averages of paired image subtractions (IAPS); this approach, which is still widely used, was first proposed in the context of change–distribution analysis (CDA; Fox *et al.*, 1988). In this paper we will focus on the relationship between IAPS and SSM, but similar results apply in comparing other normalization procedures, i.e.,

ANCOVA and factor analysis of variance (FANOVA; Strother et al., 1995b,c).

II. MATERIALS AND METHODS

[¹⁵O]water baseline–activation PET scans were acquired from 21 young normal right-handed volunteer subjects using a Siemens-ECAT 953B PET scanner operated in its 3D acquisition mode. For baseline studies, subjects had their eyes patched and ears plugged with insert earphones and were instructed to lie still and remain awake. For activation studies, the subjects performed a simple motor task consisting of sequential finger–thumb opposition between the thumb and successive digits of the left hand at a rate of one opposition per second. Ten-milliliter boluses of 370–925 MBq [¹⁵O]water were infused intravenously at 1 ml/sec; scanning began when the radioactivity reached the brain and continued for 90 sec. Each subject's scanning session consisted of eight 90 sec PET scans separated by 10 min "rest" periods to allow for ¹⁵O decay. The first, third, fifth, and seventh scans were acquired in the "baseline state," the second, fourth, sixth, and eighth scans in the "activated state." For a more detailed account of scanning and stimulus methods, see Strother et al. (1995b).

The eight scans from each subject were aligned to the first baseline-state scan using the intramodality image ratio technique described by Woods, Cherry, and Mazziotta (1992). For each of the 21 subjects, the eight "intrasession aligned image volumes" were summed and 21 intersubject transformations were calculated. Intersubject registration to a single simulated reference PET image volume was accomplished using our own implementation of the general 12-parameter linear transformation described by Woods, Mazziotta, and Cherry (1993). The simulated PET image volume was obtained by applying the sampling, resolution parameters, and reconstruction algorithm from our PET scanner to projections derived from a higher resolution, segmented, reference MRI scan (Bonar et al., 1993). The simulated PET volume was transformed to Talairach space using transformation parameters derived from the reference MRI scan (Strother et al., 1994). Aligned intrasession image volumes were normalized by the injected dose/kilogram and smoothed. These images were then transformed to Talairach-aligned volumes using the 21 intersubject transformations, and voxels below 45% of each slice's maximum voxel value were discarded; only Talairach voxel locations that were nonzero in all image volumes were considered in subsequent analyses.

Our analysis is based on the SSM framework described in Moeller and Strother (1991) and Strother et al. (1995b, 1995c). The relevant equations are briefly outlined:

$$v_{iq} = g_q(r_i + z_{iq} + e_{iq})$$

$$i_{iq} = z_{iq} + e_{iq} = \sum_{k=1}^{Q-1} h_{ik} \sqrt{c_k} s_{kq} \qquad (1)$$

$$i_{iq} = \sum_{k=1}^{Q-1} h_{ik} \mathrm{ssf}_{kq}$$

where

$$\mathrm{ssf}_{kq} = \sqrt{c_k} s_{kq} \qquad (2)$$

v_{iq} = voxel value for region i and scan q (1 to Q), g_q = global scaling factor, r_i = group mean pattern, z_{iq} = true interaction term, e_{iq} = error, i_{iq} = interaction term with error, h_{ik} = value of kth orthonormal eigenimage for region i, c_k = eigenvalue, s_{kq} = qth scan weight for kth orthonormal eigenvector, ssf_{kq} = qth scan scaling factor for kth eigenvector with length $\sqrt{c_k}$. Procedures for estimating the model parameters in equations (1) and (2) are described in Moeller and Strother (1991) and Strother et al. (1995b). The eigenimages, eigenvectors, and eigenvalues also could be obtained using principal component analysis (Strother et al., 1995c). We shall use the phrase principal component (PC) to refer to the eigenimage and eigenvector pair associated with each of the eigenvalues.

From equations (1) and (2), normalization by the global voxel mean ($v._q$) may be written as

$$\frac{v_{iq}}{v._q} \approx \left(\frac{1}{r.}\right)\left[r_i + \sum_{k=1}^{Q-1}\left(h_{ik} - \frac{h._k r_i}{r.}\right)\mathrm{ssf}_{kq}\right] \qquad (3)$$

using $(1 + x)^n \approx (1 + nx)$ for $x \ll 1$ and retaining only first-order interaction terms (i_{iq}). The result of normalization by $v._q$ is the addition of a negative offset to all eigenimages (h_{ik}). This result was first derived and its consequences discussed in Moeller and Strother (1991). From equation (3), the widely used IAPS spatial activation pattern (e.g., Worsely et al., 1992) is given by

$$\overline{(v_{iq}/v._q)}_{q=\text{activation}} - \overline{(v_{iq}/v._q)}_{q=\text{baseline}} = \left(\frac{1}{r.}\right)\sum_{k=1}^{Q-1}$$
$$\left(h_{ik} - \frac{h._k r_i}{r.}\right)\left((\overline{\mathrm{ssf}_{kq}})_{q=\text{activation}} - (\overline{\mathrm{ssf}_{kq}})_{q=\text{baseline}}\right) \qquad (4)$$

III. RESULTS AND DISCUSSION

Multiple SSM analyses were performed to study the signal variation and subspace structure of the interac-

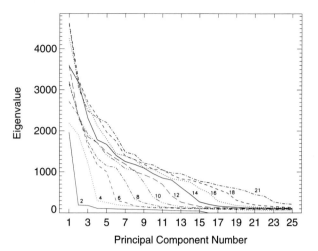

FIGURE 1   The eigenspectra of 10 scaled subprofile model (SSM) analyses of the true interaction term plus error [i_{iq}, equation (2)] performed for groups of 2 to 21 subjects; eigenvalues are plotted against principal component numbers. The labels represent the number of subjects analyzed to produce each curve and are located at the point on the curve where the component number equals the number of subjects analyzed. From Strother *et al.* (1995c); reprinted with permission of Kluwer Academic Publishers.

tion term (i_{iq}; equation (2)) as a function of number of subjects analyzed. For every SSM analysis performed, the eigenvalues (i.e., an eigenspectrum) and intersubject variation [$\Sigma_{\text{subjects}} ((\overline{\text{ssf}}_{kq})_{q=\text{intrasubject}})^2$] were plotted as a function of PC number. Figure 1 presents the eigenspectra from the 10 SSM analyses performed for groups of 2, 4, 6, 8, 10, 12, 14, 16, 18, and 21 subjects. All spectra appear to approach a plateau of eigenvalues with values from 100 to 200 that represent random error effects in the interaction term. Fifty simulated PET images (Strother *et al.*, 1994) with different samples from the same noise distribution produced approximately flat eigenspectra with values in the 150–250 range (unpublished data), suggesting that the plateau in Figure 1 is due to reconstruction noise. A break or elbow is seen in these eigenspectra plots, especially in the spectra of the smaller groups, just before or at the point where the component number equals the number of subjects being analyzed.

Figure 2 demonstrates the structure underlying the breaks in the eigenspectra in Figure 1. These breaks represent the transition from an intersubject to an intrasubject subspace with the former having a dimension of 1 less than the number of subjects being analyzed. As the group size increases the transition between the spaces becomes less distinct and spreads over several PCs.

Two independent groups of eight subjects were analyzed separately. The first group corresponds to the

eigenspectrum and subspace partition shown for eight subjects in Figures 1 and 2. For the first group of eight subjects, Figure 3 shows the abrupt transition in the underlying ssf distributions (cf. Figure 2) that occurs between the values of PC_k for $k = (\# \text{ subjects} - 1)$ and $k = (\# \text{ subjects})$. Figure 4 displays the distribution of differences between successive baseline and activation scans derived from the ssf values plotted in Figure 3. For equal numbers of paired baseline and activation scans per subject, the distributions in Figure 4 determine the weight, $[(\overline{\text{ssf}}_{kq})_{q=\text{activation}} - (\overline{\text{ssf}}_{kq})_{q=\text{baseline}}]$ from equation 4, with which each offset eigenimage contributes to the IAPS spatial activation pattern.

The mean activation–baseline ssf differences in Figure 4 demonstrate that the IAPS spatial pattern is predominantly influenced by PC 8, the first component of the intrasubject subspace. It is tempting to conclude that the distributions of ssf differences for the other components are not significantly different from 0 as suggested by the *t*-test results in Strother *et al.* (1995c). However, the calculated *p*-values are inaccurate, because the values of ssf for a given eigenvector are likely to be correlated (Jackson, 1991). Therefore, while verifying the prediction of negative offsets from equations (3) and (4) we shall also address the question of the relative importance of components other than PC 8 by demonstrating that they contribute only minor changes to the IAPS spatial pattern.

Equation (4) together with Figure 4 indicate that the IAPS spatial pattern should be quite closely approximated by the offset eighth eigenimage derived from an SSM analysis (i.e., $(h_{i8} - h_{.8} r_i/r_.)$).

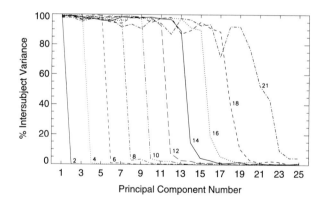

FIGURE 2   From SSM analyses of groups of 2 to 21 subjects with labels representing the number of subjects analyzed to produce each curve, the percent of intersubject variation ($[\Sigma_{\text{subjects}} ((\overline{\text{ssf}}_{kq})_{q=\text{intrasubject}})^2]/c_k$) of each principal component (PC_k) is plotted against k. Labels are located at the point on the curve where the component number equals the number of subjects analyzed. From Strother *et al.* (1995c); reprinted with permission of Kluwer Academic Publishers.

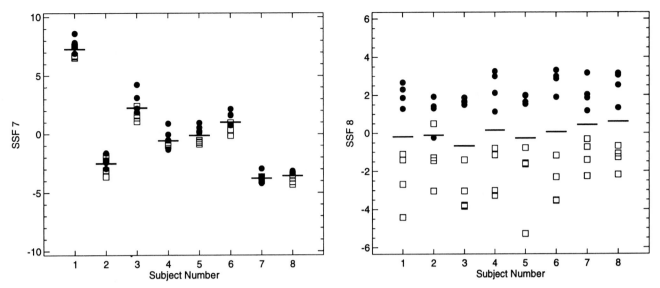

FIGURE 3 Scan scaling factor (ssf_k) distributions for the last ($k = 7$) and first ($k = 8$) principal components of the inter- and intrasubject subspaces, respectively, plotted for each subject from an SSM analysis of eight subjects (64 scans). The filled circles represent scans performed with motor activation; the open squares are baseline scans without motor activation. Each subject's mean ssf value is displayed as a short black horizontal bar.

In Figures 5 and 6, the offset introduced by normalization with the global mean ($v._q$) is seen to introduce large negative biases in the lingual gyrus (lG) and other

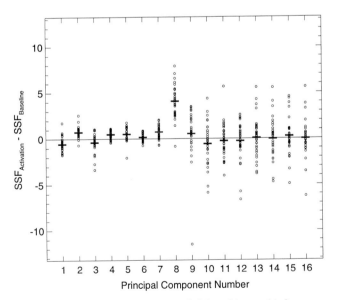

FIGURE 4 From an SSM analysis of eight subjects with four successive baseline–activation scan pairs per subject, the change in scan scaling factor (ssf) for each pair is plotted for principal components from 1 to 16. The mean change across all pairs for each PC, or $[(ssf_{kq})_{q=\text{activation}} - (ssf_{kq})_{q=\text{baseline}}]$ from Equation (4), is represented by the bold horizontal bar.

areas seen in Figure 2 of Strother *et al.* (1995b). In addition, relative to the eighth eigenimage from an SSM analysis, many voxels below the maximum in the spatial pattern have had their relative significance either reduced by moving them toward zero or increased by moving them from zero to negative values.

Figures 5 and 6 also demonstrate that equation (4) predicts the form of the IAPS spatial activation pattern and that the single offset eighth eigenimage can provide a good approximation to this pattern. Figure 5(B) further demonstrates that, in the summation of equation (4), almost all of the IAPS activation pattern is contributed by the intrasubject subspace components 8–11 (thin line) with little added by the intersubject subspace components 1–7 ([1–7] + [8–11] ≡ dot–dashed line). These results provide preliminary evidence that the intersubject subspace contributes only random effects to calculated activation patterns. This conclusion is reinforced by Figure 6, which demonstrates that in the second group of eight subjects the offset eighth eigenimage is almost identical to the IAPS activation pattern; other eigenimage components contribute even less than for the first group's data (Figures 4 and 5).

It has commonly been assumed that global means are negligibly effected by small regional activation changes, and therefore their use as normalization factors will have little effect on derived spatial activation patterns. We have shown that this assumption is not true. Activation data sets are mostly "noise" in the

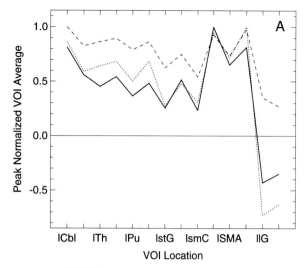
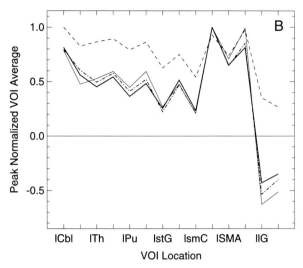

FIGURE 5 Relative volume of interest (VOI) values placed on activated foci identified for the motor task in Strother *et al.* (1995b) are plotted from the first group of eight subjects: IAPS calculated directly (left side of equation (4); heavy line), eighth eigenimage (h_{i8}) from SSM analysis (dashed line), and for (A) offset eighth eigenimage ($h_{i8} - h_{.8} \, r_i/r_.$; dotted line), and (B) sum of offset eigenimages 8–11 (equation (4); thin line), and sum of offset eigenimages 1–11 (equation (4); dot–dashed line). VOIs are normalized by the peak value for each profile and represent the average of all voxel values greater than 50% of the maximum value within a 1 cm³ ellipsoid centered on the Talairach coordinates listed in Table 1 of Strother *et al.* (1995b). Region identifiers: Cbl, cerebellum; Th, thalamus; Pu, putamen; stG, superior temporal gyrus; smC, sensorimotor cortex; SMA, supplementary motor area; IG, lingual gyrus; *l* refers to left and the right VOI is adjacent and unlabeled.

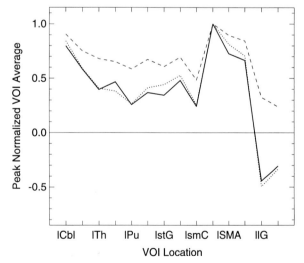

FIGURE 6 For the second independent group of eight subjects, the relative volume of interest (VOI) values (normalized by peak VOI values) from the activated foci identified for the motor task in Strother *et al.* (1995b): IAPS calculated directly (left side of equation (4); heavy line), eighth eigenimage (h_{i8}) from SSM analysis (dashed line), and the offset eighth eigenimage ($h_{i8} - h_{.8} \, r_i/r_.$; right side of equation (4), dotted line). For VOI identifiers see Figure 5.

form of unwanted nonrandom signal structure—the activation signal constitutes only a few percent of the total variation in the interaction term and may, therefore, be significantly changed by "small regional effects" in global means.

Acknowledgments

We wish to acknowledge helpful discussions with Claus Svarer, Niels Moerch, Nicholas Lange, and Fred Bookstein. This work was supported by NIH grant DA09246.

References

Bonar, D. C., Schaper, K. A., Anderson, J. R., Rottenberg, D. A., and Strother, S. C. (1993). Graphical analysis of MR feature space for the measurement of CSF, gray-matter and white-matter volumes. *J. Comput. Assist. Tomogr.* **17:** 461–470.

Fox, P. T., Mintun, M. A., Reiman, E. M., and Raichle, M. E. (1988). Enhanced detection of focal brain responses using intersubject averaging and change-distribution analysis of subtracted PET images. *J. Cereb. Blood Flow Metab.* **8:** 642–653.

Friston, K. J., Frith, C. D., Liddle, P. F., Dolan, R. J., Lammertsma, A. A., and Frackowiak, R. S. J. (1990). The relationship between global and local changes in PET scans. *J. Cereb. Blood Flow Metab.* **10:** 458–466.

Friston, K. J., Worsley, K. J., Frackowiak, R. S. J., Mazziotta, J. C., and Evans, A. C. (1994). Assessing the significance of focal activation using their spatial extent. *Hum. Brain Mapping.* **1**: 210–220.

Jackson, J. E. (1991). "A Users Guide to Principal Components." Wiley, New York.

Moeller, J. R., and Strother, S. C. (1991). A regional covariance approach to the analysis of functional patterns in positron emission tomographic data. *J. Cereb. Blood Flow Metab.* **11**: A121–A135.

Strother, S. C., Anderson, J., Xu, X-L., Bonar D. C., and Rottenberg, D. A. (1994). Quantitative comparisons of image registration techniques based on high-resolution MRI of the brain. *J. Comput. Assist. Tomogr.* **18**: 954–962.

Strother, S. C., Kanno, I., and Rottenberg, D. A. (1995a). Principal component analysis, variance partitioning and "functional connectivity." *J. Cereb. Blood Flow Metab.* **15**: 353–360.

Strother, S. C., Anderson, J. R., Schaper, K. A., Sidtis, J. J., Liow, J-S., Woods, R. P., and Rottenberg, D. A. (1995b). Principal component analysis and the scaled subprofile model compared to intersubject averaging and statistical parameteric mapping: I.

"Functional connectivity" of the human motor system studied with [^{15}O] PET. *J. Cereb. Blood Flow Metab.* **15**: 738–753.

Strother, S. C., Anderson, J. R., Schaper, K. A., Sidtis, J. S., and Rottenberg, D. A. (1995c). Linear models of orthogonal subspaces and networks from functional activation PET studies of the human brain. *In:* "Information Processing in Medical Imaging. 14th Int. Conf." (Y. Bizais, C. Barillot, and R. Di Paola, Eds.), pp. 299–310. Kluwer Academic, Dordrecht, The Netherlands.

Woods, R. P., Cherry, S. R., and Mazziotta, J. C. (1992). A rapid automated algorithm for accurately aligning and reslicing positron emission tomography images. *J. Comput. Assist. Tomogr.* **16**: 620–633.

Woods, R. P., Mazziotta, J. C., and Cherry, S. R. (1993). Automated image registration. *In:* "Proceedings of Brain PET '93 AKITA: Quantification of Brain Function" (K. Uemura, N. A. Lassen, T. Jones, and I. Kanno, Eds.), pp. 391–400. Excerpta Medica. Elsevier Science Pub. B. V., Amsterdam.

Worsley, K. J., Evans, A. C., Marrett, S., and Neelin, P. (1992). A three-dimensional statistical analysis for CBF activation studies in human brain. *J. Cereb. Blood Flow Metab.* **12**: 900–918.

74

A Comparison of Four Pixel-Based Analyses for PET

T. J. GRABOWSKI,[1] R. J. FRANK,[2] C. K. BROWN,[2] H. DAMASIO,[1] L. L. BOLES PONTO,[3] G. L. WATKINS,[3] and R. D. HICHWA[3]

[1]*Department of Neurology, Division of Behavioral Neurology and Cognitive Neuroscience*
[2]*Department of Preventive Medicine and Environmental Health*
[3]*Positron Emission Tomography Imaging Center*
University of Iowa, Iowa City, Iowa 52242

Four pixel-based methods for estimating regional activation in positron emission tomography images were compared using a verb generation paradigm. Quantitative $[^{15}O]H_2O$ imaging was performed on a GE4096 tomograph. Eighteen normal subjects performed "generate verb" and "read noun" tasks, four times each. The sample was analyzed as a whole and also as independent samples of 9 subjects with one, two, or four task pairs per subject (9×1, 9×2, 9×4). Parallel analyses were carried out with same-task (noise) pairs. Four methods and their published variants were implemented, including change distribution analysis (CDA), Worsley's method (WOR), a pixelwise general linear model (GLM), and Holmes's rerandomization method (RER). The following factors were held constant: coregistration algorithm, smoothing, stereotactic transform, search volume, and volumetric alpha level. Methods were highly concordant for the detection of activation in sample sizes 9×2 and larger. Type II errors were common at the lower sample sizes, especially using GLM and RER, methods dependent on local variance estimates. Repeating tasks led to marked improvement in the power to detect activation and in the stability of its location. These pixel-based methods are concordant and specific in localizing activation, but their power is modest in samples of conventional size.

I. INTRODUCTION

The analysis of brain activation images generated by positron emission tomography (PET) frequently re-lies on pixel-based methods of statistical analysis. In general, reports have been compatible with observations previously made in subjects with acquired brain lesions, and in some cases, PET results have been cross-replicated. However, result discrepancies have also emerged (e.g., see Petersen *et al.*, 1988 vs. Raichle *et al.*, 1992; Pardo *et al.*, 1990 vs. Bench *et al.*, 1993; and Petersen *et al.*, 1990 vs. Howard *et al.*, 1992 and Price *et al.*, 1994), and as more activation studies with similar paradigms are undertaken in different centers, such discrepancies require an explanation. Are PET activation results sensitive to small differences in the paradigm, or are technical factors of image analysis responsible for these discrepancies? Understanding the effect of technical factors would be useful in evaluating the existing literature on functional brain activation, in informing the design of new studies, and in improving the performance of existing techniques. The objective of this study was to compare the performance of four pixel-based statistical methods for analyzing PET activation images, using identically prepared data sets.

II. METHODS

We studied 18 normal subjects with PET using a GE 4096 tomograph. Each received eight injections of 1850–2775 MBq $[^{15}O]$water. Arterial sampling was performed and images of rCBF were calculated by the autoradiographic method (Herscovitch *et al.*, 1983; Hichwa *et al.*, 1995). Magnetic resonance (MR) images were obtained for each subject, reconstructed in three

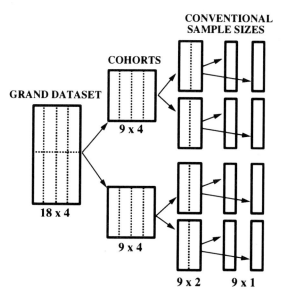

CONVENTIONAL SAMPLE SIZES

COHORTS

GRAND DATASET

18 x 4

9 x 4

9 x 4

9 x 2   9 x 1

FIGURE 1 The grand data set was partitioned into samples of conventional size. The grand dataset had sample size 18 × 4 (subjects × "generate–read" pairs). Two cohorts of nine subjects were formed by random assignment. Within a cohort, data were partitioned, at random, to data sets of size 9 × 1 and 9 × 2. Same-task pairs were also studied with an identical design (not illustrated).

dimensions with Brainvox (Damasio and Frank, 1992), and used for PET slice orientation, Talairach transformation, anatomical interpretation of clusters, and search volume definition (Damasio *et al.*, 1993; Grabowski *et al.*, 1995a).

Subjects performed "generate verb" and "read noun" tasks of a verb generation paradigm (Petersen *et al.*, 1988). Concrete nouns were presented visually at one per 2 sec. Four replicates of each task were performed. Stimuli were not repeated.

The grand data set comprised 144 rCBF images; that is, 18 subjects × 4 "generate–read" pairs. The data were partitioned into two independent cohorts of nine subjects (sample size 9 × 4). Within cohort, data were further randomly partitioned into independent samples of sizes 9 × 2 and 9 × 1. Because most published PET activation studies have used samples of this magnitude, we refer to 9 × 1 and 9 × 2 as *conventional sample sizes* (Fig. 1). In addition, same-task pairs (i.e., noise images) were studied with a completely parallel design.

The following methods were implemented according to their published descriptions: Change distribution analysis (CDA; Fox *et al.*, 1988); Worsley's method (WOR; Worsley *et al.*, 1992), a pixelwise general linear model (GLM; Friston *et al.*, 1991; Friston, 1994), and Holmes's rerandomization method (RER; Holmes *et al.*, 1995). GLM implements the same statistical model as SPM94 but not its other features, notably the nonlin-

ear spatial standardization algorithms. We also investigated the following modifications of the primary methods. We explored the effect of the SPM anatomical preprocessing routines by passing our data through the SPM94 transforms and then performing statistical analysis with our implementations of GLM, WOR, and RER [GLM(S), WOR(S), RER(S)]. We also studied GLM and WOR using spatial extent thresholds rather than magnitude thresholds [GLM(E), WOR(E); Friston *et al.*, 1994]; Worsley's method with local variance [WOR(L)]; and CDA with one-tailed omnibus tests [CDA(1)]. (For more detail, see Grabowski *et al.*, 1996.)

To compare methods in terms of their inferential statistics, we held the following technical factors constant: (1) MR–PET coregistration was accomplished with a local *a priori* alignment algorithm (Grabowski *et al.*, 1995a), corrected with Automated Image Registration (AIR) (Woods *et al.*, 1993); (2) images were smoothed to 20 mm FWHM in-plane, no axial smoothing was done; (3) a piecewise linear Talairach transformation (Talairach and Tournoux, 1988), based on MR landmarks, was used; (4) the search volume comprised all shared intracerebral stereotactic voxels, defined with reference to coregistered 3D MR; (5) finally, we imposed a volumetric alpha level of 0.05 (two-tailed), we considered that activation might be manifested as either blood flow increases or decreases.

The operation of these methods yielded sets of activation clusters; that is, sets of contiguous suprathreshold voxels. Each cluster was mapped onto coregistered MR images and given an anatomical interpretation. In this way, 27 distinct activation regions were identified. Activation regions were classified according to whether they were internally replicated. A *replicated region* was one found in data sets not sharing any injections of labeled water. We also distinguished *consensus regions*, those detected by all four primary methods in the grand data set; and *marginal regions*, those that were not replicated but were nevertheless found in the grand data set.

We compared the methods with the following indices. (1) *Type I errors* were indexed by counting clusters in same-task analyses. (2) Between-method *concordance of activation region detection* was assessed by the κ statistic for interrater reliability. Each method was considered to be an independent rater and was polled as to the presence or absence of activation in each dataset in each of the 27 unique activation regions. Within-method concordance was assessed with within-method replication rates, which express the overall probability (percent) that activations were replicated in independent datasets of the same sample size. (3) *The extent of detected activation* was indexed by the

TABLE 1   Classification of Activation Clusters

Classification	Regions (N)	Clusters N	Clusters %
Replicated and consensus	12	411	87
Other replicated regions	3	37	8
Not replicated but marginal	6	19	4
Other nonreplicated regions	6	7	1
Total	27	474	100

number and cumulative volume of activation regions. (4) *Type II errors* were evaluated with respect to the roster of consensus regions. The relative power of these methods in data sets of conventional size was indexed by the proportion of consensus regions that were detected in them. (5) In looking for *spatial stability*, our best estimate of the "true" location of activation was the within-cohort average location of the region's center of mass. The radius around this locus that would envelope 95% of exemplars (the "radius of 95% confidence") was calculated as the mean plus 1.65 standard deviations of the vector distance between detected centers of mass and cohort-specific mean centers of mass.

III. RESULTS AND DISCUSSION

A total of 474 activation clusters were identified in 27 distinct anatomical regions. Seven regions, corre-

TABLE 3   Concordance of Primary Methods in Detecting Activation

Regions	Sample size	κ	Z
All	9 × 1	0.33	4.80
	9 × 2	0.61	11.05
	9 × 4	0.65	11.38
	18 × 4	0.61	6.78
Increases	9 × 1	0.37	4.62
	9 × 2	0.70	10.52
	9 × 4	0.67	8.74
	18 × 4	0.63	5.34
Decreases	9 × 1	0.23	1.87
	9 × 2	0.48	4.79
	9 × 4	0.67	7.26
	18 × 4	0.59	4.19

sponding to only 1.5% of all clusters, were probably false positives because they were neither replicated nor marginal. But the great majority (87%) of activation clusters were in 12 replicated, consensus regions. These were a superset of the foci reported by Petersen *et al.* (1988). There were both consensus increases and consensus decreases in rCBF (Tables 1 and 2). In contrast, the action of the four primary methods on all 15 noise data sets yielded only three suprathreshold clusters, a false positive rate equal to the nominal α (0.05).

The κ statistics were consistently 0.6–0.7 in samples 9 × 2 and higher. These values were highly significant (Table 3). The values of κ fell to about 0.3 at 9 × 1

TABLE 2   Consensus Regions

	Abbreviation	Talairach 1988 coordinates X	Y	Z
Blood flow increases				
Left inferior frontal	LIFG	−39	+21	+5
Right cerebellum	RCBLM	+27	−65	−33
Left dorsolateral prefrontal	LDPF	−44	+15	+25
Anterior cingulate	ACING	−1	+21	+31
Cerebellar vermis	CVERM	−1	−57	−21
Ventral thalamus or midbrain	VTHAL	−1	−14	−1
Blood flow decreases				
Right mesial posterior sylvian	RMPSYL	+45	−13	+11
Right lateral parietal	RLPAR	+49	−55	+26
Right lateral temporal	RLTEMP	+55	−25	−10
Right mesial orbital	RMORB	+2	+37	−11
Mesial parietal	MPAR	+2	−56	+30
Left mesial posterior sylvian	LMPSYL	−45	−16	+12

TABLE 4 Within-Cohort Method Replication Rates of Activation Regions

Regions	Sample size	Within cohort	Between cohorts
Increases	9 × 1	57%	47%
Increases	9 × 2	78%	80%
Increases	9 × 4	—	93%
Decreases	9 × 1	39%	23%
Decreases	9 × 2	54%	52%
Decreases	9 × 4	—	80%

and were relatively low for decisions about blood flow decreases. The overall within-method, within-cohort replication rate for increases in rCBF was approximately 60% for 9 × 1 data sets and 80% for 9 × 2 data sets. For blood flow decreases, the corresponding rates were about 40 and 50%, respectively (Table 4). Between-cohort replication rates were lower than within-cohort rates only at the 9 × 1 level.

The number of detected activations increased with increasing sample size, but not uniformly for the four methods (Fig. 2(A); Color plate). Gains were least for CDA and most rapid for the methods dependent on local variance estimates; that is, RER and GLM. WOR had the best overall performance, especially in conventional sample sizes. Derived methods did not detect larger numbers of foci but did increase their volume (Figure 2(B); Colorplate).

The power of these analyses to detect consensus activations was modest (about 40%) for a 9 × 1 sample, especially for GLM and RER (Fig. 2(C); Color plate). Dramatic improvement in power resulted from repeating tasks (even once). Blood flow increases were detected more powerfully than decreases. Using spatial extent thresholding improved the sensitivity of GLM from 15 to 40% for the 9 × 1 data sets. The SPM transforms increased its sensitivity for the consensus increases from 15 to 60%. Worsley's method made modest gains with these modifications. However, even with these improvements, power $(1-\beta)$ was only about 0.6 with any of the methods.

A final index of comparison is the spatial stability of activation regions. The 95% radius of confidence for rCBF increases was 10–15 mm and ranged from 5 to 19 mm. This distance was larger for sample size 9 × 1. It also tended to be larger for methods depending on local variance estimates. This observation is consistent with those of Taylor, Minoshima, and Koeppe (1993). The same confidence radius for blood flow decreases

was greater (13–18 mm, range 11–28 mm). Effects of sample size and method were less apparent for blood flow decreases (Table 5).

Significant, spatially discrete regional decreases in rCBF were detected. Although these were not normalization artifacts (Grabowski *et al.*, 1996), they had less stable locations and were detected less powerfully than blood flow increases.

The performances of these methods were distinguishable on the basis of Type II error rates in conventional sample sizes and the spatial stability of activation regions. The methods dependent on local variance estimates (GLM, RER) had lower power and less stability. The use of spatial extent thresholding and nonlinear anatomical standardization increased the power of all methods but especially GLM and RER. In practice, the success of these methods in studies with conventional sample sizes is strongly influenced by variance reduction techniques, notably nonlinear spatial normalization.

Contrary to the assumption of stationary variance underlying Worsley's method, variance was higher in gray matter than in white matter. Gray matter variance was itself heterogeneous, being higher in the visual cortex and activated regions (Fig. 3; Color plate). Although this assumption was not correct, it did not lead to spurious activations in this study. As long as a pooled variance estimate was used, WOR performed well in all sample sizes. WOR(L) was the least powerful method of all (Fig. 2), for reasons that have been well discussed by Worsley *et al.* (1993).

TABLE 5 Spatial Stability of Activation Regions

	Method	Sample size	95% Confidence radius (mm)
Increases	CDA	9 × 1	9.9
	WOR	9 × 1	14.2
	GLM	9 × 1	13.5
	RER	9 × 1	19.0
	CDA	9 × 2	5.2
	WOR	9 × 2	9.5
	GLM	9 × 2	10.1
	RER	9 × 2	16.4
Decreases	CDA	9 × 1	12.0
	WOR	9 × 1	13.4
	GLM	9 × 1	*
	RER	9 × 1	28.0
	CDA	9 × 2	11.2
	WOR	9 × 2	14.9
	GLM	9 × 2	16.6
	RER	9 × 2	17.5

*Insufficient observations.

In small samples, CDA performed well, despite the lack of formal control over Type I error. However, its performance improved relatively little when sample size increased. CDA(1) gave results very similar to CDA, except for reduced sensitivity for blood flow decreases (Fig. 2).

Our data suggest that these pixel-based methods are highly specific in localizing activation and are highly concordant with one another, but their power is modest in samples of conventional size.

Acknowledgments

We thank Andrew Holmes for providing information on the rerandomization method and for helpful correspondence, Julie Fiez for many helpful discussions about the paradigm, Jon Spradling and Kathy Jones for dedicated technical assistance, and Ann Reedy for preparing the manuscript.

References

Bench, C. J., Frith, C. D., Grasby, P. M., Friston, K. J., Paulesu, E., Frackowiak, R. S. J., and Dolan, R. J. (1993). Investigations of the functional anatomy of attention using the Stroop test. *Neuropsychologia* **31:** 907–922.

Damasio, H., and Frank, R. (1992). Three-dimensional in vivo mapping of brain lesions in humans. *Arch Neurol.* **49:** 137–143.

Damasio, H., Grabowski, T. J., Frank, R., Knosp, B., Hichwa, R. D., Watkins, G. L., and Boles Ponto, L. L. (1993). PET-Brainvox, a technique for neuroanatomical analysis of positron emission tomography images. *In:* "Quantification of Brain Function. Tracer Kinetics and Image Analysis in Brain PET." (K. Uemura *et al.*, Eds.). Elsevier Science Publishers, Amsterdam.

Fox, P. T., Mintun, M. A., Reiman, E. M., and Raichle, M. E. (1988). Enhanced detection of focal brain responses using intersubject averaging and change-distribution analysis of subtracted PET images. *J. Cereb. Blood Flow Metab.* **8:** 642–653.

Friston, K. J., Frith, C. D., Liddle, P. F., and Frackowiak, R. S. J. (1991). Comparing functional (PET) images: The assessment of significant change. *J. Cereb. Blood Flow Metab.* **11:** 690–699.

Friston, K. J. (1994). Statistical parametric mapping. *In:* "Functional Neuroimaging" (R. W. Thatcher, M. Hallett, T. Zeffiro, E. R. John, and M. Huerta, Eds.), pp. 79–93. Academic Press, San Diego.

Friston, K. J., Worsley, K. J., Frackowiak, R. S. J., Mazziotta, J. C., and Evans, A. C. (1994). Assessing the significance of focal activations using their spatial extent. *Hum. Brain Mapping* **1:** 210–220.

Grabowski, T. J., Damasio, H., Frank, R., Hichwa, R. D., Boles Ponto, L. L., and Watkins, G. L. (1995a). A new technique for PET slice orientation and MRI-PET coregistration. *Hum. Brain Mapping* **2:** 123–133.

Grabowski, T. J., Frank, R. J., Brown, C. K., Damasio, H., Boles Ponto, L. L., Watkins, G. L., and Hichwa, R. D. (1996). Reliability of PET activation across statistical methods, subject groups, and sample sizes. *Hum. Brain Mapping,* in press.

Herscovitch, P., Markham, J., and Raichle, M. E. (1983). Brain blood flow measured with intravenous H$_2$^{15}O. I. Theory and error analysis. *J. Nucl. Med.* **24:** 782–789.

Hichwa, R. D., Boles Ponto, L. L., and Watkins, G. L. (1995). Clinical blood flow measurement with [^{15}O] water and positron emission tomography (PET). *In:* "Chemists' Views of Imaging Centers" (A. M. Emran, Ed.). Plenum, New York/London.

Holmes, A. P., Blair, R. C., Watson, J. D. G., and Ford, I. (1995). Non-parametric analysis of statistic images from functional mapping experiments. *J. Cereb. Blood Flow Metab.* **16:** 7–22.

Howard, D., Patterson, K., Wise, R., Brown, W. D., Friston, K., Weiller, C., *et al.* (1992). The cortical localization of lexicons: Positron emission tomography evidence. *Brain* **115:** 1769–1782.

Pardo, J. V., Pardo, P. J., Janer, K. W., and Raichle, M. E. (1990). The anterior cingulate cortex mediates processing selection in the Stroop attentional conflict paradigm. *Proc. Natl. Acad. Sci.* **87:** 256–259.

Petersen, S. E., Fox, P. T., Posner, M. I., Mintun, M., and Raichle, M. E. (1988). Positron emission tomographic studies of the cortical anatomy of single-word processing. *Nature (London)* **331:** 585–589.

Petersen, S. E., Fox, P. T., Snyder, A. Z., and Raichle, M. E. (1990). Activation of extrastriate and frontal cortical areas by visual words and word-like stimuli. *Science* **249:** 1041–1044.

Price, C. J., Wise, R. S. J., Watson, J. D. G., Patterson, K., Howard, D., and Frackowiak, R. S. J. (1994). Brain activity during reading; The effects of exposure duration and task. *Brain* **117:** 1255–1269.

Raichle, M. E., Fiez, J. A., Videen, T. O., and Petersen, S. E. (1992). Activation of left posterior temporal cortex in a verbal response selection task is rate dependent. *Soc. Neurosci. Abstr.* **18:** 933.

Talairach, J., and Tournoux, P. (1988). 3-Dimensional proportional system: An approach to cerebral imaging. *In:* "Co-Planar Stereotaxic Atlas of the Human Brain." Thieme Medical Publishers, New York.

Taylor, S. F., Minoshima, S., and Koeppe, R. A. (1993). Instability of localization of cerebral blood flow activation foci with parametric maps. *J. Cereb. Blood Flow Metab.* **13:** 1040–1042.

Woods, R. P., Mazziotta, J. C., and Cherry, S. R. (1993). MRI-PET registration with automated algorithm. *J. Comput. Assist. Tomogr.* **17:** 536–546.

Worsley, K. J., Evans, A. C., Marrett, S., and Neelin, P. (1992). A three-dimensional statistical analysis for CBF activation studies in human brain. *J. Cereb. Blood Flow Metab.* **12:** 900–918.

Worsley, K. J., Evans, A. C., Marrett, S., and Neelin, P. (1993). Detecting and estimating the regions of activation in CBF activation studies in human brain. *In:* "Quantification of Brain Function. Tracer Kinetics and Image Analysis in Brain PET" (K. Uemura *et al.*, Eds.). Elsevier Science Publishers, Amsterdam.

A. Number of Activation Regions

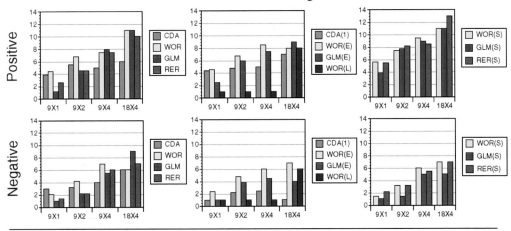

B. Cumulative Volume of Activation (mL)

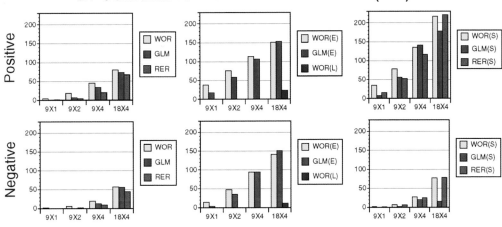

C. Percent of Consensus Regions Detected

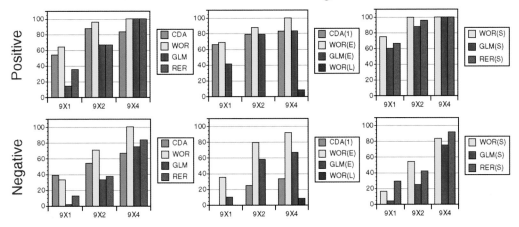

FIGURE 2   The figure summarizes the extent of activation detected by primary methods and their variants (A, B) and the relative power of the methods to detect consensus activation regions (C). Significant blood flow increases are shown in the upper tier of each panel, and blood flow decreases in the lower tier. Each primary method and its variants are depicted using the same color.

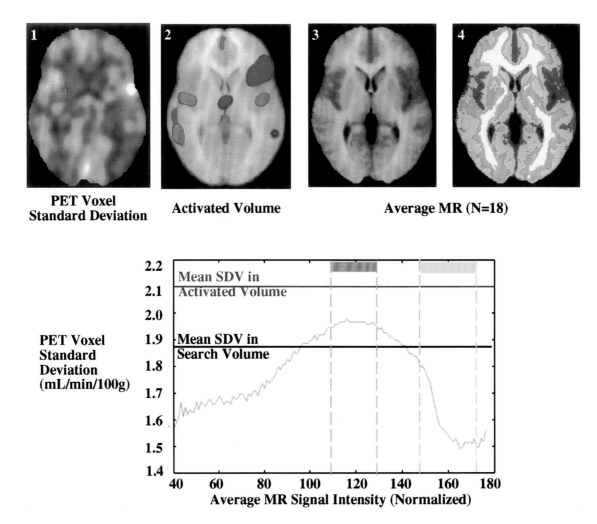

FIGURE 3 The figure demonstrates that variance was not stationary. The upper tier shows four images at $Z = +6$: (1) PET voxel standard deviation, as used by WOR, for the grand data set; (2) the activated volume(significant increases in red, decreases in blue/violet); (3) the average MR of our 18 subjects; (4) the average MR with two signal intensity intervals, corresponding to gray matter and white matter compartments, marked in pink and yellow, respectively. In the lower panel, PET voxel standard deviation is displayed as a function of coregistered MR signal intensity. The standard deviation is higher in the gray matter interval than in the white matter interval. Note also that the mean standard deviation in the activated volume (blue line) is higher than the mean standard deviation over the entire search volume (black line).

75

A Comparison of Approaches to the Statistical Analysis of Cognitive Activation Studies Using [^{15}O]H$_2$O with Positron Emission Tomography

STEPHAN ARNDT,[1,2] TED CIZADLO,[1] NANCY C. ANDREASEN,[1] GENE ZEIEN,[1] GREG HARRIS,[1] DANIEL S. O'LEARY,[1] G. LEONARD WATKINS,[3] LAURA L. BOLES PONTO,[3] and RICHARD D. HICHWA[3]

[1]*The Mental Health Clinical Research Center, Department of Psychiatry*
[2]*Department of Preventive Medicine and Environmental Health*
[3]*PET Imaging Center, Department of Radiology*
The University of Iowa Hospitals and Clinics
Iowa City, Iowa 52242

The use of [^{15}O]H$_2$O to study human cognition and emotion has given neuropsychiatrists a powerful tool for measuring and understanding brain function. As the "water method" has matured, sophisticated techniques for conducting statistical analysis of data have been developed. This study compares two of the most widely used, the Friston method (SPM94) and the Worsley method (Montreal). Both methods were applied to a single data set of 33 subjects, who have been studied in a paradigm designed to evaluate memory for word lists in order to determine the comparability of the two methods in the world of "real data." One subtraction from this study was compared: long-term memory for words minus reading words. The computer program SPM94 implemented the method developed by Friston et al. (1991). We used a locally developed version of the Montreal technique based on formulae provided in Worsley et al. (1992). Aspects of the analysis (e.g., filtering, spatial normalization) were held constant so that differences in statistical methods (e.g., intensity normalization, missing values) could be cleanly contrasted. The methods' location of peaks, volume of peaks, and size of t or z statistic characterizing the peak were compared. Neither method emerged as strikingly different or strikingly preferable. Both were found to produce generally similar results identifying brain regions active during long-term memory: frontal parietal, cingulate, and cerebellar. We discuss some of their underlying assumptions, as well as their strengths and weaknesses.

I. INTRODUCTION

The application of PET using [^{15}O]H$_2$O to studies of human cognition has already achieved a high degree of maturity. There is also a growing consistency of findings across studies. In spite of these advances, some inconsistencies across studies are evident, and it is difficult to determine if they are due to differences in design or methodology.

Two recent strategies are widely used for statistical analysis of PET imaging data. Statistical parametric mapping (SPM), developed by Friston *et al.* (1991) is perhaps the most popular method. A second approach (the Montreal method) is also used by a number of investigators and was developed by Worsley *et al.* (1992). This chapter is based on an earlier and more in-depth comparison of these two methods (Arndt *et al.*, 1995).

Both analysis strategies share a common general

TABLE 1   Montreal and SPM Methods Compared

	Montreal	SPM94
General		
Uses FOI approach	Yes	Yes
Omnibus test for image differences	Yes	Yes
Based on *t*-test	Yes	Yes
Correct for large number of tests	Yes	Yes
3D solutions	Yes	Yes
Use Talairach atlas for reporting	Yes	Yes
Sample based MR coregistration	Yes	No
Average PET coregistration	No	Yes
Preprocessing		
Controls for global CBF (gCBF)	Yes	Yes
Analysis of covariance	No	Yes
Normalizes images—ratio to CBF	Yes	Optional
Uses voxels with missing data	No	Yes
Statistical Assumptions		
Normally distributed data	Yes	Yes
Errors are independently and identically distributed	Yes	Yes
Uses Gaussian random field theory	Yes	Yes
Assume "stationarity"	Yes	Yes
Constant relation of rCBF with gCBF	Yes	Yes
Linear relation of rCBF with gCBF	No	Yes
Proportional relation of rCBF with gCBF	Yes	No
t-statistics based on small df	No	Yes
Voxel SDs are all equal	Yes	No

background. Both use the more exploratory function of interest (FOI) approach rather than the *a priori* region of interest (ROI) approach. The FOI strategy anticipates that PET studies are likely to identify unforeseen areas of activation possibly distributed throughout the brain.

Both SPM and the Montreal methods rely on the notion of image subtraction and tests of group averages. Because they rely on averages, they also require coregistration techniques. Both also use Talairach atlas coordinates for reporting. Table 1 shows a large number of similarities between the methods. There are, however, some important differences.

Statistical calculations are shown schematically in Figure 1 (Color plate). The Montreal method appears in the top row and SPM appears as the bottom row. Both begin with an average difference image, $\overline{\Delta}$. The first column shows the $\overline{\Delta}$ images. These differ because SPM omits voxel locations with missing data making the image smaller than the Montreal $\overline{\Delta}$ image. Also, different intensity normalization methods are used. SPM uses an ANCOVA to remove the effects of global CBF (gCBF) variance, and the Montreal image uses a ratio of rCBF to gCBF. The second column shows another important difference. Worsley *et al.*, suggest a constant pooled SD in the calculation of $S_{\overline{\Delta}}$ but SPM uses local SDs that vary across the image. The final *t*-image is a ratio of the $\overline{\Delta}$ and $S_{\overline{\Delta}}$ images. Therefore, the three major differences are (1) different normalization procedures; (2) the Montreal *t*-image considers more data than the SPM *t*-image because it includes voxels with some missing data; and (3) the Montreal *t*-image is less variable because voxels are divided by a constant. The present investigation was conducted to examine these two widely used methods for the statistical analysis of $[^{15}O]H_2O$ data collected using PET. A recent version of SPM developed by Friston and his colleagues, SPM94, and the Worsley (Montreal) method are applied to a single data set of 33 subjects studied in a memory paradigm designed to evaluate memory for word lists.

A. Subjects

Subjects were 33 healthy normal volunteers recruited from the community by newspaper advertising.

B. Memory Tasks

The complete study in which these subjects participated was designed to explore aspects of short-term and long-term memory (Andreasen *et al.*, 1995). For our comparison of methods, we focus on positive activations from one subtraction in this study: long-term memory for words minus reading words. In the "long-term memory" condition subjects were trained until they had perfect recognition memory of a list of 18 words during the week before the PET study; the list was reviewed on the day before the PET experiment to ensure that it was still well learned. The experimental comparison was reading common English words. All words were one- or two-syllable concrete nouns presented on a video monitor.

C. Implementation

We tried to make the comparison as commensurate as possible. For instance, thresholding voxels at some value separates the brain from background radiation and voxels below the threshold are dropped from consideration. Thus, changes in threshold vary the scene of the analysis and sometimes dramatically. The Montreal method uses a threshold of 1.5 times the image average, while SPM94 uses 80% of an analyst supplied value. We modified the SPM94 program's hardwired 80% cutoff to make the final output images analogous to the Montreal

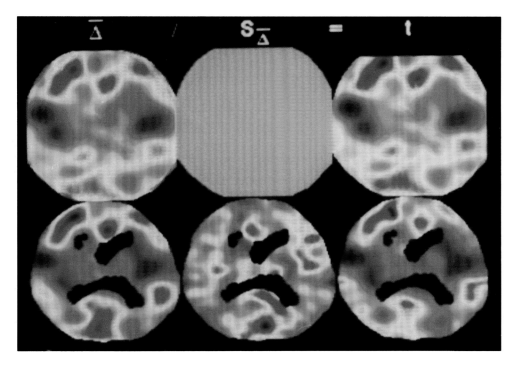

FIGURE 1 Schematic representation of the Montreal (top row) and SPM (bottom row) statistical calculations.

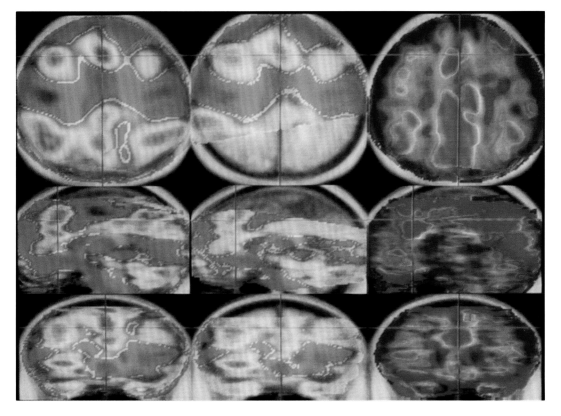

FIGURE 2 Three orthogonal views of the statistical images show the Montreal method's t=statistic (left column), SPM94 (middle column) z=statistic, and the variance map (right column). The images, based on 33 subjects' subtraction images, are superimposed on the subjects' average MR brain. The two methods show similar activation areas in the frontal, parietal, and cingulate regions. The left parietal activation noticeable in the Montreal image is truncated in the SPM's image because of missing data. Note that the variance image tends to be light (low) at the edges. The variance image also tends to resemble, somewhat, the activation image. This will make the locally based t-tests tend to be lower in high-variance regions and higher in low variance areas (the edges) than the Montreal t-test which is based on a constant pooled SD.

TABLE 2 Comparison of Long-Term Memory Activations Using the Montreal Method vs. SPM94

Region	Montreal					SPM 94				
	x	y	z	T_{max}	Vol (N pixels)	x	y	z	Z_{max}	Vol (N pixels)
R. Fr Med/10	26	47	−15	6.68	1595	22	46	−13	3.78	22
R. Fr Med/9	37	12	39	5.35	1572	35	24	32	5.53	2095
R. Fr Med/46	30	43	10	5.31	1329	29	49	8	5.46	3831[a]
R. Inf Fr/47	35	19	−5	5.84	670	31	22	−6	5.20	[a]
L. Inf Fr	−25	53	−13	5.83	740	−37	54	−19	4.28	73
L. Inf Fr	−34	50	1	4.44	390	−36	50	−0	5.20	1111
L. Sup Fr	—	—	—	—	—	−41	32	26	4.83	602
R. Parietal	42	−47	42	8.99	4284	53	−40	35	4.64	1017
L. Parietal	−42	−55	42	8.57	3411	—	—	—	—	—
L. Cerebellum	−10	−82	−25	6.80	6066	−13	−85	−24	6.07	6115
Ant Cingulate	−1	23	35	5.14	1771	−1	26	35	4.38	556
Postcingulate/Cuneus	−1	−72	41	6.25	1741	—	—	—	—	—

[a]SPM94 saw these two areas as contiguous; however, they were separated in the Montreal method.

image. The threshold for significance for both SPM94 and the Montreal method was chosen as 3.61.

II. RESULTS

The study's original purpose was to explore mechanisms of human memory, and the results of one image subtraction are shown in Table 2. This table shows all peaks identified by either method that exceed a t_{max} (Montreal) or z_{max} (SPM94) of 3.61 and that are larger than 500 pixels (approximately 1 cc). If a smaller peak in the same location was identified by either method, it is also shown in the table for purposes of comparison. Figure 2 (Color plate) shows the same information.

The major role of the right frontal regions in long-term memory would be evident from the use of either method, and investigators would be able to identify the role that the right frontal region plays in retrieval. The Montreal method finds a total of four right frontal peaks that are distributed on the lateral superior and inferior surface (Brodmann areas 9, 10, 46, and 47). The SPM method finds similar but larger and fewer sites of activity. The SPM method finds a single large (3831 pixels) peak at 29/49/8 that is divided into two smaller peaks using the Montreal method at 30/43/10 and 35/19/−5. Visual inspection of the SPM peak indicated that it has a dumbbell shape with two peaks linked by a line of pixels. The highest value in the other peak is at 31/22/

−6. A comparable situation also occurs for the large peak identified by the SPM method at 35/24/32.

Both methods also identify areas of activity in left frontal regions. Using the prespecified size and significance criteria, the Montreal method finds one relatively small left frontal region at −25/53/−13, and SPM finds two at somewhat different coordinates (−36/50/0 and −41/32/26). These differences in location appear to reflect their different approaches to handling $S_{\overline{\Delta}}$.

In addition to the frontal activations, both methods locate areas of activity in parietal association cortex. The Montreal method identifies activity bilaterally, whereas the SPM method identifies activity only on the right. This difference is particularly enlightening (see the transaxial section of Fig. 2). The results could lead to important differences in interpretation, because preferential involvement of the right parietal lobe for a verbal task is counterintuitive. This difference between the two methods is a direct consequence of the SPM approach to missing data. Figure 2 indicates that the brain area considered by the SPM method is considerably smaller because pixels with missing values were dropped. Yet an inspection of overall sample size for the missing pixels indicated that an adequate number was present to conduct statistical tests; data are present in 26 out of the 33 subjects. When we repeated the SPM analysis using these 26 subjects, the left parietal peak appeared at −37/−57/42. The SPM analysis omits valuable data and could lead to the inference that verbal memory does not involve biparietal association cortex but is instead selectively right sided, an inference that is likely to be wrong.

Both methods produce relatively similar results for the other major area that appears to be involved in long-term memory: the cerebellum. Both find large areas of activity (6066 and 6615 pixels), and both identify nearly identical coordinates. They also find a prominent active area in the anterior cingulate, although a larger area is identified by the Montreal method (see Fig. 2, coronal section). However, the Montreal method finds an area in the posterior cingulate at $-1/-72/41$, which is not found by the SPM analysis.

The previous discussion relied on finding "significant" peaks, which requires a somewhat arbitrary threshold. Modifying this threshold can considerably change the number of peaks and the volume of the activated area. Assuming a similar threshold, the two methods can potentially produce different results in three ways: location of peaks, size of peaks, and significance level assigned to them. A total of 14 clearly corresponding regions were identified by both methods and were used for numeric comparisons of location, size, and significance level. For an area found as a single peak in the Montreal method but split into four areas by SPM, we used a composite center of the four SPM peaks.

In general, the location of the peaks identified by both methods were in relatively close agreement. Using a straight-line distance between the two method's peaks, most (11/14) were within 10 mm of each other. The largest distance (15 mm) was caused by SPM94 truncating the image due to missing data.

Both methods yielded comparable estimates of the probability levels of the peaks identified (mean difference $< .00001$). However, the relative ranking of a peak's importance varied considerably from method to method. For instance, a peak's *p*-value might be considered a gross index of its relative importance in the set of activation areas. The Spearman correlation between SPM94 and Worsley assigned *p*-values was nearly 0 ($r = 0.04$). Similarly, region size did not show a strong correlation (Spearman $r = 0.29$).

III. CONCLUSIONS

Our results suggest that these two methods do not produce seriously discrepant results, although they dif-

fer in some ways. They found relatively similar answers as to which areas of the brain are involved in a long-term memory task. Both found similar locations that included predominantly frontal, parietal, and cerebellar regions. Neither identified activity in medial temporal regions, as might be predicted by lesion studies implicating a hippocampal role in long-term memory (Squire and Zola-Morgan, 1991). Both are consistent with a model suggesting that retrieval engages predominantly right frontal regions. Their major area of difference was in parietal regions, with SPM finding only right parietal activity, whereas the Montreal method localized activity biparietally. They also differed in their localization of the small area of activity observed in the left frontal region. Numeric comparisons of the two methods also suggest that they can produce relatively similar results. However, low correlations between methods suggest that assigning the relative importance to areas based on the region size in pixels or on the size of the test statistic (t_{max} or z_{max}) may not generalize from one method to the next.

Two differences between the methods, handling missing data and the local versus pooled variance estimates, did produce some consequences in the results. The choice by the SPM method to drop all pixels containing missing data leads to a loss of data and a smaller image set. The resulting image truncation can cut off areas of activation. In a large sample such as was used in the current study, this choice is a handicap.

References

Andreasen, N. C., O'Leary, D. S., Arndt, S., Cizadlo, T., Hurtig, R., Rezai, K., Watkins, G. L., Boles-Ponto, L. L., and Hichwa, R. D. (1995). Short-term and long-term verbal memory: A positron emission tomography study. *Proc. Nat. Acad. Sci.* **92**: 5111–5115.

Arndt, S., Cizadlo, T., Andreasen, N. C., Zeien, G., Harris, G., O'Leary, D. S., Watkins, G. L., Boles-Ponto, L. L., and Hichwa, R. D. (1995). A comparison of approaches to the statistical analysis of [^{15}O]H$_2$O PET cognitive activation studies. *J. Neuropsychiat. Clin. Neurosci.* **7**: 155–168.

Friston, K. J., Frith, C. D., Liddle, P. F., and Frackowiak, R. S. J. (1991). Comparing functional (PET) images: The assessment of significant change. *J. Cereb. Blood Flow Metab.* **11**: 690–699.

Squire, L. R., and Zola-Morgan, S. (1991). The medial temporal lobe memory system. *Science* **253**: 1380–1386.

Worsley, K. J., Evans, A. C., Marrett, S., and Neelin, P. (1992). A three dimensional statistical analysis for CBF activation studies in human brain. *J. Cereb. Blood Flow Metab.* **12**: 900–918.

76

Comparative Analysis of rCBF Increases in Voluntary Index Flexion Movements

J. MISSIMER,[1] U. KNORR,[2] R. J. SEITZ,[2] R. P. MAGUIRE,[1] G. SCHLAUG,[2] K. L. LEENDERS,[1] H. HERZOG,[3] and L. TELLMAN[3]

[1]PET Program, Paul Scherrer Institute, Villigen, Switzerland
[2]Department of Neurology, University of Düsseldorf, Düsseldorf, Germany
[3]Institute of Medicine Research Center, Jülich, Germany

Ten volunteers performed self-paced index flexions with their right hands. Regional cerebral blood flow (rCBF) was measured at rest and during finger movements by positron emission tomography (PET) using the tracer [^{15}O]butanol. The images of quantified rCBF were analyzed using the computerized brain atlas (CBA) (Seitz et al., 1990) and statistical parametric mapping (SPM) (Friston et al., 1991b). The comparison was divided into two stages: standardization and statistical analysis. In addition the effect of filtering was evaluated.

After spatial standardization using each method, the images were smoothed in-plane. Both sets of standardized images were analyzed by use of descriptive t-maps combined with cluster analysis (Roland et al., 1993) and with the analysis of covariance and smoothing techniques of SPM (Friston et al., 1991b). All four procedures detected activation in the left motor cortex and the right anterior lobe of the cerebellum. Using CBA procedures in both stages located additional functional regions (FRs) in the left supplementary motor area and in the left anterior cingulate gyrus; SPM procedures detected additional FRs only in the basal ganglia, in the temporal and occipital lobes, and in the frontal cortex.

Using a filter with a FWHM of 10 mm, the procedures yield similar estimates of the rCBF at rest and the percentage change. The difference in the number of FRs found by the procedures appears to be due largely to the method of standardization. The stereotactic normalization of SPM yields an order of magnitude more FRs and volumes of FRs that are typically a factor of 10 bigger than the CBA standardization.

The effects of filtering were more pronounced with the CBA standardization than with SPM. For the same spatial standardization, the CBA statistical analysis yields many more FRs than the ANCOVA analysis of SPM.

I. INTRODUCTION

The determination of regions of significant change in activation studies involving several individuals requires (1) mapping the images into a standard reference volume and (2) statistical evaluation. The computerized brain atlas (CBA) (Seitz et al., 1990) and statistical parametric mapping (SPM) (Friston et al., 1991b) were both designed to accomplish these tasks. Because mapping into a standard volume requires nonlinear as well as linear transformations of individual images, it is not obvious that these two conceptually different methods will yield comparable locations and sizes of regions of significant change nor that the amount of increase expressed as percent or differences of absolute quantities, that is, regional cerebral blood flow, will agree. An additional question is the effect of filtering on statistical comparisons (Poline and Mazoyer, 1994). Users of CBA employ no filtering of images (Seitz et al., 1990; Roland et al., 1993); a filter of 20 mm FWHM in-plane was suggested for SPM (Friston et al., 1991b) to accommodate the resolution of the scanner as well as the known scale of individual variations in human brain anatomy (Steinmetz et al., 1989). We report here a comparison of the two methods of evaluating activation studies. The comparison was divided into two stages, standardization and statistical analysis, and we analyzed the results of each method of standardization with both methods of statistical analysis. In addition, we investigated the effect of filtering.

II. METHODS

Ten healthy, right-handed volunteers performed self-paced index flexions with their right hands at 2 Hz. Patients were blindfolded; the ambient noise of the scanner was the only aural stimulation. The movements were analyzed by comparing the rCBF during activation with that at rest. The rCBF was measured using PET with the tracer [^{15}O]butanol. Arterial blood sampling permitted an absolute quantification of the rCBF (Herzog *et al.*, 1993).

The tomograph used was the Scanditronix PC-4096/15WB PET camera providing an optimal spatial resolution of 5.50 mm FWHM in the center of the field of view. The PET data sets had the following format: 15 slices, 6.50 mm slice width, 128 × 128 image matrix with pixels of 2 mm on a side and a 16-bit gray scale. The images were reconstructed by filtered back projection using a 6 mm FWHM Hanning filter, providing an in-plane resolution of 9 mm FWHM and an axial resolution of 8 mm FWHM (Rota Kops *et al.*, 1990).

The rCBF images were analyzed with CBA and SPM. Standardization using the CBA program has been described in the literature (Bohm *et al.*, 1986; Greitz *et al.*, 1991). This process created for each scan 14 transaxial standard shaped images with a voxel side length of 1.27 mm and a distance between the slices of 6.75 mm. The images were then smoothed in plane using a Gaussian filter with full-width at half-maximum (FWHM) of 0, 10, 15, 20, and 25 mm. Statistical evaluation was performed using the CBA and SPM methods that will be described. The complete analyses will be denoted CBA–CBA and CBA–SPM, respectively.

Stereotactic normalization, the designation for standardization in SPM, transformed the 15 planes into the 26 planes defined by the Talairach atlas (Talairach and Tournoux, 1988) by aligning the image volume with reference to a template image (Friston *et al.*, 1991a). The pixels of the standardized images are 2 mm on a side and the distance between planes is 4 mm. The images were then smoothed as described and analyzed using the CBA and SPM statistical methods.

From the spatially standardized PET images, the statistical analysis of CBA begins with the computation of images of mean rCBF in the rest and activation states, images of mean rCBF changes, and images of

the standard error of the mean. Then, a descriptive *t*-map is calculated as an omnibus test voxel-by-voxel according to

$$t = \Delta V_{(Act-Rest)}/SEM_{(Act-Rest)}$$

where ΔV denotes the mean rCBF change in a voxel and SEM the corresponding standard error. Regions of significant change were determined by selecting voxels for which the *t*-statistic exceeded 2.82, corresponding to $p = .01$, and requiring that the number of contiguous voxels fulfilling the threshold criteria exceed 12. The probability that pixel clusters of this size occur by chance in 14 image slices has been estimated by a simulation study not to exceed one in a thousand ($P < .001$) (Roland *et al.*, 1993).

In contrast to the usual SPM procedure, the quantification of the original rCBF images was preserved in the standardization and statistical analysis stages; the global mean of all studies was not fixed. The analysis of covariance, described in detail in the literature (Friston *et al.*, 1990), yields a voxel-by-voxel *t*-statistic. This is adjusted for the correlation of neighboring pixels due to the resolution of the scanner and the image reconstruction process (Friston *et al.*, 1991b; Worsley *et al.*, 1992), yielding a *z*-score. Regions of significant change satisfy the criteria that *z*-scores for each pixel in the region exceed a threshold, $z = 2.33$, corresponding to the given level of significance, $p = .01$. To facilitate the comparison with the CBA method of statistical analysis, only areas exceeding 5 pixels (corresponding in area to 12 CBA pixels) were included in the comparison.

III. RESULTS AND DISCUSSION

The number of spatially separated FRs for a filter with a FWHM of 10 mm were CBA–SPM 2 ($p < 0.05$), CBA–CBA 5 ($p < 0.01$), SPM–SPM 36 ($p < 0.01$), and SPM–CBA 45 ($p < 0.01$). Every method detected activation in the left motor cortex and the right parasagittal part of the cerebellum. The CBA–CBA method located additional FRs in the left supplementary motor area and in the left anterior cingulate gyrus; the SPM–SPM and SPM–CBA methods detected FRs in the basal ganglia, in the temporal and occipital lobes, and in the frontal cortex as well. The FR detected in the left anterior cingulate gyrus by the latter two methods was not the same FR detected by CBA–CBA.

A comparison of the volumes, rest rCBF and percentage change of the FRs evaluated by the three more sensitive procedures is presented in Table 1. The FR cereb I includes regions in three planes for both meth-

TABLE 1   Comparison of FR Volumes, Rest rCBF (ml/100g/min), and
Percentage Increase for Three Analysis Procedures at FWHM = 10 mm

Region	cereb I	cereb II	sma	motor
Volume (ml)				
CBA–CBA	.89	.25	.19	2.8
SPM–SPM	13	4.3	8.0	30
SPM–CBA	15.6	5.5	8.6	48
Rest rCBF				
CBA–CBA	51.3	54.6	62.0	52.2
SPM–SPM	49.4	51.4	66.9	54.1
SPM–CBA	47.6	51.2	58.2	38.6
Increase (%)				
CBA–CBA	23.0	22.0	20.1	30.2
SPM–SPM	22.0	22.9	16.1	28.0
SPM–CBA	24.9	24.4	23.2	35.2

ods of standardization; cereb II includes regions in one plane for CBA and two planes for SPM; the supplementary motor area (sma) includes regions in one plane for CBA and four planes for SPM; and the supplementary motor cortex (motor) includes regions in two planes for CBA and four for SPM. The table indicates that the three procedures yield reasonably good agreement on the rest rCBF and percentage increase of the four FR that could be compared; the deviation in the motor area of rest rCBF found by SPM–CBA can be attributed to voxels outside the brain. In contrast, the FR volumes are remarkably different with SPM–SPM, being typically 10 times those estimated by CBA–CBA. The SPM–CBA estimates of the FR volumes lie 10–40% higher than those of SPM–SPM.

We infer that the difference in the number of FRs found by the procedures is due largely to the method of standardization: the stereotactic normalization of

SPM yields an order of magnitude more FRs and volumes of the FRs that are as much as a factor of 10 bigger than the CBA standardization. Possibly, the SPM standardization is more effective at projecting the activation regions onto FRs but sacrifices realistic estimates of the volumes. It is also associated with a slight optimum in the maximum of the z-score, irregularity in the change in volumes of the FR, and in more pronounced decreases in the percentage change as a function of FWHM.

To access the influence of varying the FWHM, we determined the volumes of the FRs (Fig. 1), the maximum (Fig. 2), and the average of the statistical parameter, and the average rCBF and percentage change of the rCBF in the FR at FWHM between 0 and 30 in steps of 5 mm. As shown in Figure 1(a), the CBA–CBA procedure shows a smooth behavior of the volumes with increasing FWHM: they increase with increasing

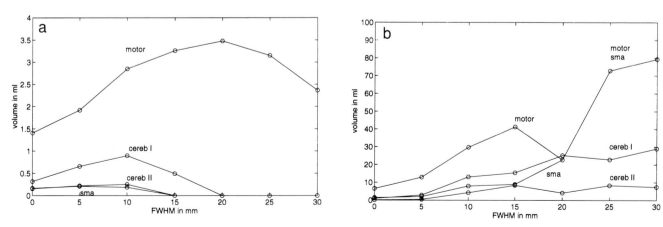

FIGURE 1   Areas of FRs vs. FWHM: (a) for CBA–CBA; (b) for SPM–SPM.

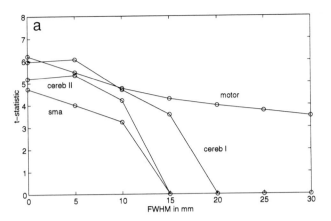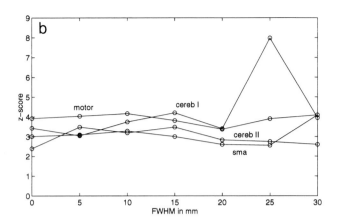

FIGURE 2   (a) *t*-statistic vs. FWHM for CBA–CBA; (b) *z*-score vs. FWHM for SPM–SPM.

FWHM until a maximum is reached whose position depends on the size of the FR, after which they decrease notably. The sizes of the smaller FR vanish at 15 or 20 mm. The SPM–SPM procedure exhibits irregular increases with no evidence of decrease at the largest FWHM (Fig. 1(b)). Although not evident in the figure, cereb I and cereb II merge partially beginning at FWHM = 15 mm; the sma begins to merge with the motor at FWHM = 10 mm and merges completely by FWHM = 20 mm. The SPM–CBA procedure, not shown, exhibited the smooth behavior of the CBA–CBA procedure.

Concerning the maximum statistical parameter, the CBA–CBA procedure yielded a monotonic decrease until the FR becomes insignificant (Fig. 2(a)). In contrast, the SPM–SPM procedure showed slight local maxima between 5 and 15 mm, after which the parameter remained almost constant (Fig. 2(b)) except for a large fluctuation in the FR cereb I. The SPM–CBA procedure showed a monotonic decrease similar to CBA–CBA.

The average statistical parameter, the average rest rCBF and percentage change for an FR showed similar behavior as a function of the FWHM in all three analysis procedures. The average statistical parameter and rest rCBF decreased regularly about 10% over the entire range; the percentage change exhibited decreases of as much as 50% for the CBA–CBA and CBA–SPM procedures and decreases of as much as 75% for SPM–SPM.

The effects of filtering were more pronounced with the CBA standardization than with SPM, which is consistent with the volumes being markedly smaller for CBA. With the CBA standardization, observing smaller volumes demands that the filter be less than 15 mm at FWHM. However, the SPM standardization does not appear to benefit from larger filters either:

maximum sensitivity either decreases slightly or occurs for filters between 5 and 15 mm for all the FRs observed in this study.

For the same spatial standardization, the CBA statistical analysis yields many more FRs than the ANCOVA analysis of SPM. A few FRs evaluated as quite significant by the CBA analysis do not appear using the ANCOVA of SPM at all. This suggests the surprising result that the CBA statistical analysis, which does not adjust for global differences, is more sensitive than the ANCOVA, which was invoked for this adjustment, or it may indicate that ANCOVA is more rigorous.

References

Bohm, C., Greitz, T., Blomqvist, G., Farde, L., Forsgren, P. O., and Kingsley, D. (1986). Applications of a computerized adjustable brain atlas in positron emission tomography. *Acta Radiol. Suppl.* **369:** 449–452.

Friston, K. J., Frith, C. D., Liddle, P. F., Dolan, R. J., Lammertsma, A. A., and Frackowiak R. S. J. (1990). The relationship between global and local changes in PET scans. *J. Cereb. Blood Flow Metab.* **10:** 458–466.

Friston, K. J., Frith, C. D., Liddle, P. F., and Frackowiak, R. S. J. (1991a). Plastic transformation of PET images. *J. Comput. Assist. Tomogr.* **15:** 634–639.

Friston, K. J., Frith, C. D., Liddle, P. F., and Frackowiak, R. S. J. (1991b). Comparing functional (PET) images: Assessment of significant change. *J. Cereb. Blood Flow Metab.* **11:** 690–699.

Greitz, T., Bohm, C., Holte, S., and Eriksson, L. (1991). A computerized brain atlas: Construction, anatomical content, and some applications. *J. Comput. Assist. Tomogr.* **15:** 26–38.

Herzog, H., Seitz, R. J., Tellmann, L., Rota Kops, E., Schlaug, G., Jülicher F., Jostes, C., Nebeling, B., and Feinendegen, L. E. (1993). Measurement of cerebral blood flow with PET and ^{15}O-butanol using a combined dynamic-single-scan approach. *In:* "Quantitation in PET" (K. Uemura, N. A. Lassen, T. Jones, and I. Kanno, Eds.), pp. 161–170. Elsevier, Amsterdam.

Poline, J. B., and Mazoyer B. (1994). Enhanced detection in brain activation maps using a multifiltering approach. *J. Cereb. Blood Flow Metab.* **14:** 639–642.

Roland, P. E., Levin, B., Kawashima, R., and Åkerman, S. (1993). Three-dimensional analysis of clustered voxels in ^{15}O-butanol brain activation images. *Hum. Brain Mapping* **1:** 3–19.

Rota Kops, E., Herzog, H., Schmid, A., Holte, S., and Feinendegen, L. E. (1990). Performance characteristics of an eight-ring whole body PET scanner. *J. Comput. Assist. Tomogr.* **14:** 437–445.

Seitz, R. J., Bohm, C., Greitz, T., Roland, P. E., Eriksson, L., Blomqvist, G., Rosenqvist, G., and Nordell, B. (1990). Accuracy and precision of the computerized brain atlas programme for localization and quantification in positron emission tomography. *J. Cereb. Blood Flow Metab.* **10:** 443–457.

Steinmetz, H., Fürst, G., and Freund, H. J. (1989). Cerebral cortical localization: Application and validation of the proportional grid system in MR imaging. *J. Comput. Assist. Tomogr.* **13:** 10–19.

Talairach, T., and Tournoux, P. (1988). "Co-Planar Stereotactic Atlas of the Human Brain." Thieme, Stuttgart.

Worsley, K. J., Evans, A. C., Marrett, S., and Neelin, P. (1992). A three-dimensional statistical analysis for CBF activation studies in human brain. *J. Cereb. Blood Flow Metab.* **12:** 900–918.

A High-Resolution Anatomic Reference
for PET Activation Studies

ARTHUR W. TOGA, JOHN C. MAZZIOTTA, and ROGER P. WOODS

Department of Neurology, Division of Brain Mapping
UCLA School of Medicine, Los Angeles, California 90024

Presently available anatomic atlases provide useful coordinate systems such as the ubiquitous Talairach system but are sorely lacking in both spatial resolution and completeness. An appropriately sampled anatomic specimen can provide the additional detail necessary to accurately localize activation sites as well as provide other structural perspectives such as chemoarchitecture. As part of the International Consortium for Brain Mapping (ICBM), whose goal it is to develop a probabilistic reference system for the human brain, we collected serial section postmortem anatomic data from several whole human head and brain specimens using a cryosectioning technique. Tissue was imaged so that voxel resolution was 200 microns or better at full color (24 bits/pixel). The collected data sets were used in one of several ways as an anatomic reference for functional studies: first, on an individual basis as a traditional, n = 1 structural atlas with unprecedented spatial resolution and complete coverage of the forebrain, midbrain, and hindbrain (the data set can be registered to a functional data set using either anatomic landmarks or an automatic approach); second, several of these high resolution data sets were placed within the Talairach system and used to produce a probabilistic representation (this approach represents anatomy within a coordinate system as a probability). Coordinate locations are assigned a confidence limit to describe the likelihood that a given location belongs to an anatomic structure based on the population of specimens. These data produce an anatomic reference that is digital, high in spatial and densitometric resolution, 3D, comprehensive, and in combination, probabilistic. The superior resolution makes it possible to delineate structures impossible to visualize in other structural modalities. These data are an important and necessary part of the comprehensive structural and functional analyses that focus on the mapping of the human brain.

I. INTRODUCTION

Accurate localization of brain structure and function in any modality is improved by correlation with higher resolution anatomic data placed within an appropriate spatial coordinate system. Recent brain mapping efforts have begun to explore this approach yet remain disadvantaged by the lack of readily available, spatially detailed 3D morphology of the normal human brain (Damasio *et al.*, 1991). In response to this need, several computerized atlases have been developed for neurosurgical applications or for analysis of metabolic studies such as PET and SPECT (Tiede *et al.*, 1993; Evans *et al.*, 1991; Lehmann *et al.*, 1991; Roland and Zilles, 1994). These atlases, based on data acquired using magnetic resonance imaging (MRI), have the advantage of intrinsic three-axis registration and spatial coordinates but have relatively low resolution and lack anatomic contrast in important subregions. High-resolution MR atlases, using up to 100–150 slices, a section thickness of 2 mm, and 256^2 pixel imaging planes (Evans *et al.*, 1991; Lehmann *et al.*, 1991) still result in resolutions lower than the complexity of many neuroanatomic structures.

Several digital atlases have been developed using photographic images of cryoplaned frozen specimens (Bohm *et al.*, 1989; Greitz *et al.*, 1991). The use of photographed material, although providing superior anatomic detail, has limitations. For accurate correlations, data must be placed in the equivalent plane as the image of interest. Digital imaging can overcome some of the limitations of conventional film photography methods. Using 1024^2, 24-bits/pixel digital color cameras, spatial resolution can be as high as 100 microns/pixel for whole human head cadaver preparations or higher for isolated brain regions (Toga *et al.*, 1994). Cryosectioning in micron increments permits collection of data with high spatial resolution in the axis orthogonal to the sectioning plane. Acquisition of images in series directly from the consistently positioned cryoplaned block face avoids the need for serial image registration prior to reconstruction. Serial images can be reconstructed to a 3D anatomic volume that is amenable to various resampling and positioning schemes.

The combination of cryosectioning and specimen surface photography provides both the means for acquiring anatomic image data and the potential to collect specimen tissue for histological analysis (Pech, 1987; Rauschning, 1986). Application of histochemical stains removes any remaining ambiguity in the identification of boundaries thus increasing the detail of segmentations.

We conducted experiments demonstrating the creation of spatially accurate, high-resolution anatomic reference volumes from postmortem cryosectioned whole human brain. They were conducted to examine the advantages of this approach and determine the value of the data as an anatomic reference for MR, PET, and other modalities. First, we examined anatomic image data (1024^2 24-bits/pixel) to see if it contained sufficient resolution to improve the ability to delineate neuroanatomic structures. Second, we tested whether 3D reconstruction, repositioning, scaling, and resampling could be performed while preserving accurate spatial relationships. Statistical morphometrics were calculated to determine the degree of precision in anatomic segmentation and placement within the Talairach coordinate system (Talairach and Tournoux, 1988). Finally, we evaluated tissue collected from the cryosectioned specimens for compatability with specific histochemical staining and analysis for cytoarchitectonic delineation. The goal was to produce a series of high resolution 3D anatomic volumes with potential to serve as an anatomic reference for comprehensive human brain mapping in a variety of imaging modalities.

II. METHODS

We collected high-resolution image data from frozen human cadaver preparations that included fixed and unfixed whole head, fixed whole brain, and fixed isolated regions of interest. Histologic sections were collected from fixed whole brain and brain regions. Image data were used for 2D anatomic segmentation, digital 3D reconstruction, and visual comparison to *in vivo* MRI. Five whole head and brain data sets were reconstructed into the Talairach and Tournoux stereotactic atlas space for comparison to 3D reconstructed *in vivo* MRI from 10 normal male subjects. We calculated morphometric statistics for a small sample of neuroanatomic structures from the cryosectioned anatomy, *in vivo* MRI, and a 3D reconstruction of the Talairach atlas plates.

A. Specimen Preparation and Cryosectioning

Cadavers were obtained through the Willed Body Program at the UCLA School of Medicine, optimally within 5–10 hr postmortem. All were adult or aged (54–90 years) with approximately equal representation of gender. Specimens were sectioned on a large sledge cryomacrotome (PMV, Stockholm, Sweden) equipped with a high-resolution color camera (DAGE MTI, Michigan City, Indiana), professional flat-field macro lenses, and a voltage regulated fiber optic illumination system. Whole human head specimens were sectioned in 50 micron increments with digital images acquired either every 100 microns or every 500 microns throughout the dorsal–ventral axis.

We collected histology from one fixed, decalcified head, one whole brain, cerebellum, and brain stem. Tissue sections were mounted on large glass slides and stained using modified cresyl violet or von Braunmuhl silver stain protocols. We photographed the histology through the microscope and digitized sections using the same camera and illumination system used for blockface imaging.

B. MRI Acquisition

MRI were obtained from 10 adult normal male subjects using a 1.5 T scanner (Signa, General Electric) with TR = 1500 msec, TE = 20 msec, and TI = 600 msec. Data for each subject (140 slices) were acquired in the horizontal plane in 1 mm thickness and 256^2 resolution.

C. Three-Dimensional Reconstruction

Image data from cryosectioned specimens were reconstructed to 3D anatomic volumes. Picture width (x) and height (y) in the imaging plane were determined by the camera field of view. The depth axis value (z)

corresponding to the position of each serial image in the volume was determined by the distance in microns between each image. We placed anatomic data from 5 of the whole head and brain data sets and reconstructed MRI from all 10 subjects into the spatial coordinate system described by Talairach and Tournoux (1988).

D. Anatomic Segmentation

Anatomic structures were identified in cryosectioned anatomy using visual cues provided by color, texture, and contrast differences to surrounding tissue. Cerebral cortex, cerebellum, brain stem, ventricular system, and selected subcortical structures including the anterior commissure, head and tail of the caudate, putamen, thalamus, hippocampus, and globus pallidus were outlined for segmentation. For *in vivo* MRI, structure boundaries were based on the line of highest intensity gradient visible. These boundaries were manually segmented and retained for surface model reconstruction, visualization, and morphometrics.

Surface models were generated using wireframe mesh triangulation methods based in UNIX software. Shading, texture, and pseudocolor were applied to enhance model visualization. Segmented structures were displayed individually or nested to emphasize spatial relationships. Texture mapping of cut planes was used to localize structures that had been demonstrated in histochemically stained data within the greater context of the 3D surface model.

E. Morphometric Analysis

We included data from 5 anatomic volumes of cryosectioned whole human heads, 10 MRI, and the 3D reconstructed Talairach atlas model in our calculations. Morphometric statistics were computed for the left and right globus pallidus, head and tail of the caudate, putamen, thalamus, anterior commissure, and ventricles. We compared values for surface area, volume, and center of mass within (interhemispheric) and between individual anatomic data sets, the Talairach atlas and *in vivo* MRI.

III. RESULTS AND DISCUSSION

A. Postmortem Cryosectioned Anatomy

Digital images of the whole head and brain possessed average spatial resolutions of 200 and 170 microns/pixel, respectively, in the imaging plane. This method produced anatomically detailed data sets for the brain stem, pons, cerebellum, cingulate cortex, and optic

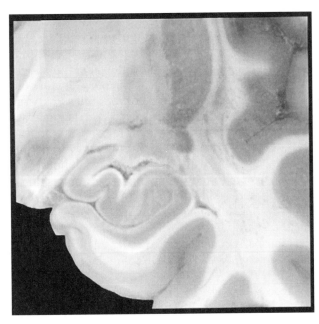

FIGURE 1 An optically magnified region of the hippocampus was captured with a small field of view (40 mm) to yield a spatial resolution approximately 40 microns/pixel. The optical nature of this technique permits collection of anatomic detail suitable for delineation of complex structures. At this resolution, it is possible to clearly observe structures not visible in tomographic images, such as the dentate granular layer. The white matter bundle of the alveus is sharply demarcated against white subcortical matter. Also note the tail of the caudate, claustrum, and putamen. Combined with histologically processed sections, these data can be used to study any region of interest.

tract and hippocampus (Fig. 1). Spatial resolution in the orthogonal axis was determined by frequency of image acquisition. For whole head imaging at a frequency of 500 microns, resolution in the reconstructed axis was 200 microns/pixel.

High-resolution cryosectioned anatomy demonstrated gyral and sulcal anatomy as well as laminar structures and nuclear regions. We were easily able to identify subcortical structures in high-resolution digital images based on color pigment differentiation and texture contrast to adjacent tissues. The densitometric gradations afforded by 24 bits provided subtle textural detail important in the segmentation of regional anatomy. This was especially apparent in deep subcortical structures such as the corpus striatum. It was possible to distinguish the internal capsule dividing the caudate and lentiform nuclei. In the thalamic region, we could observe the anterior, medial, lateral, and ventral nuclei as well as the lateral geniculate bodies and pulvinar. These visual distinctions allowed us to more precisely determine the boundaries of neuroanatomic structures in cryosectioned anatomy than *in vivo* MRI (Fig. 2).

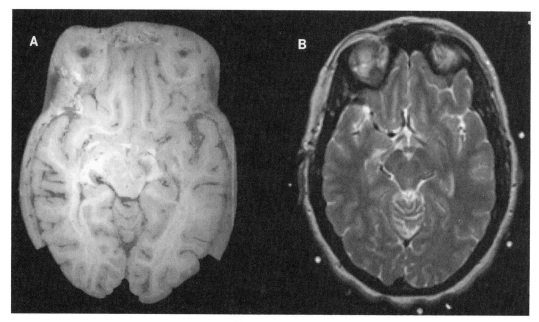

FIGURE 2   Nuclear and laminar boundaries of structures normally not visible in tomographic modalities can be seen in high-resolution color images of cryosectioned anatomy. Whole brain *in vivo* MRI (right), at a resolution of 256^2, does not provide the anatomic detail provided by high-resolution digital imaging. In addition the visual cues provided by texture and color are not available in 8-bit tomographic images. This horizontal slice through a whole human head (left) at the level of the superior colliculus shows the central tegmental tract, third nerve nucleus, and medial longitudinal fasciculus. The superior occipital region of bone was removed from this unfixed specimen to improve sectioning characteristics; however, the frozen brain has retained its *in situ* configuration and relevant bony landmarks such as the internal auditory meatus and infraorbital ridge are still intact.

B. Correlated Histology

To acquire whole brain sections from fixed tissue it was necessary to section in larger increments, producing sections up to 100 microns thick and difficult to maintain proper anatomic configuration. We were unable to obtain sections of the whole human head because the chemical decalcification process proved to be incompatible with section collection. Thinner sections (20–40 microns) were easily collected from the isolated brain region specimens such as brain stem and pons. The use of Nissl and modified silver stains enabled us to examine cell morphology under the light microscope (Fig. 3). For thicker whole brain sections, cytologic detail was suboptimal but we were able to appreciate the enhanced gray matter and white matter differentiation. By correlating each slide mounted section with the block face image acquired during cryosectioning, we were able to record the correct spatial localization of histologic data in the gross anatomic specimen.

C. Morphometry

Morphometric statistics describing anterior commissure, caudate, putamen, globus pallidus, and thalamus in image data from postmortem cryosectioned anatomy were relatively consistent across subjects and in general agreement with the Talairach atlas data. Mean surface area, volume, and center of mass demonstrated significantly less variability between hemispheres in comparison to intersubject variability. Volume was less susceptible than surface statistics to variance due to complicated geometries; for example, statistics calculated on the ventricular system were highly influenced by slight differences in the lateral extent of this structure and therefore unreliable.

The goals of the present experiments were to determine if postmortem cryosectioned anatomy could be used as a spatially detailed digital anatomic reference of the normal human brain. We were able to demonstrate a spatial resolution greater than 200 microns using large fields of view capable of imaging the whole horizontal plane of human brain. Equivalent resolutions in MR have been produced only for isolated postmortem specimens using a prototype 7.0 T superconducting magnet (Boyko *et al.*, 1994). In addition, by using a 24-bit color digital camera we were able to capture additional visual cues of texture and depth not available in tomographic imaging modalities.

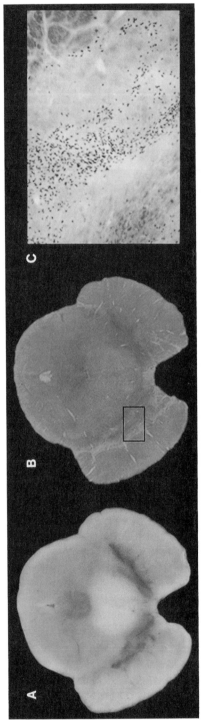

FIGURE 3   High-resolution images from the cryoplaned block face can be correlated with histology for three dimensional mapping of cytoarchitectonic fields. (A) This axial section through the human brain stem was captured in high resolution directly from the block face. Cryosections were stained with a modified von Braunmuhl silver stain, imaged, and digitally correlated with block face complements. Structures possessing simple geometry, such as the brain stem, are mapped using landmark based affine transformations and require no local deformations. (B) The block face and corresponding histochemically stained section each contribute 50% of this composite image. The box indicates the light microscope view shown in C. (C) Histochemically stained sections can be viewed through the light microscope to resolve ambiguities in delineation of specific nuclear regions. Here the substantia nigra is clearly seen in this 40 micron section photographed at 32×. Spatial relationships are retained for specific regions of two-dimensional histologic sections within the three-dimensional anatomic structure.

The ability to resolve neuroanatomic boundaries is critical for accurate structure delineation. The spatial and densitometric detail provided in high-resolution images of cryosectioned anatomy significantly improved our ability to differentiate structure boundaries. When compared to MRI, we found it easier to delineate structures in the cryosectioned anatomy, for example, laminar partitions of the basal ganglia and hippocampus. Subsequent histological processing of collected tissue sections proved even more valuable for localization of additional anatomic structure. By correlating digitized histology with block face images of it was possible to retain their respective spatial context. Histologic sections have previously been used as an anatomic reference to improve interpretation of MR and CT images (Rauschning, 1986); however, such correlations have been primarily visual. By using digital reconstruction and resampling techniques we were able to display high-resolution anatomy in specified planes to precisely match image data from other modalities.

Appropriate spatial coordinate systems facilitate localization of neuroanatomic structures and serve as a prerequisite for intersubject and between modality comparisons. We were able to accomplish accurate placement of the volumes by utilizing the same transformation that MR and PET methods employ. The spatial positioning scheme described by Talairach and Tournoux bases its registry and scaling on the bicommissural line (Talairach and Tournoux, 1988). Because this approach is so dependent on the selection of the superior and inferior margins of the AC and PC midsagittal points, the higher resolution afforded in cryomacrotomed data was advantageous.

The differences between tomographic images of *in vivo* human brain and surface imaging of cryoplaned postmortem specimens must be recognized. First, frozen preparation can induce changes in the configuration of anatomic specimens. Previous studies have suggested that alterations in size, shape, and attenuation values of specimens may not be significant (Ho *et al.*, 1988; Pech, 1987; Rauschning *et al.*, 1983). Our own morphometric measurements support this. However, many changes occur post mortem, such as loss of mean arterial pressure and uneven distribution of intracranial fluids, which contribute to differences between *in vivo* and *ex vivo* derived data.

These experiments demonstrated the use of postmortem anatomical volumes created from serial cryoplaned heads and brains. These data, in combination with histologically processed tissue from the specimen, provide a detailed high-resolution reference for tomographically acquired images. This approach, in combination with multimodality mapping techniques, will add to the growing data base being applied to the goal of mapping the human brain.

Acknowledgments

The Laboratory of Neuro Imaging thanks Annie Lee for her many hours with aromatic histological methods and specimen preparation and Edward Lee for keeping us organized. This work was supported in part by the Human Brain Project funded jointly by the National Institute of Mental Health, the National Institute on Drug Abuse (P20 MH52176), the National Library of Medicine (R01 LM05639), the National Science Foundation (BIR 9322434), and the Biomedical Research Technology Program of NCRR (R01 RR05956). Thanks also go to the Brain Mapping Medical Research Organization, the Pierson–Lovelace Fund and the Ahmanson Foundation.

References

Bohm, C., Greitz, T., and Eriksson, L. (1989). A computerized adjustable brain atlas. *Eur. J Med.* **15:** 687–689.

Boyko, O., Alston, S. R., Fuller, G., Hulette, C., Johnson, A., and Burger, P. (1994). Utility of postmortem magnetic resonance imaging in clinical neuropathology. *Arch. Pathol. Lab. Med.* **118:** 219–225.

Damasio, H., Kuljis, R. O., Yuh, W., and Ehrhardt, J. (1991). Magnetic resonance imaging of human intracortical structure *in vivo*. *Cereb. Cortex* **1**(5): 374–379.

Evans, A., Marret, S., Torrescorzo, J., Ku, S., and Collins, L. (1991). MRI-PET correlation in three dimensions using a volume of interest (VOI) atlas. *J. Cereb. Blood Flow Metab.* **11:** 169–178.

Greitz, T., Bohm, C., Holte, S., and Eriksson, L. (1991). A computerized brain atlas: construction, anatomical content, and some applications. *J. Comput. Assist. Tomogr.* **15**(1): 26–38.

Ho, P., Yu, S., Czervionke, L., Sether, L., Wagner, M., Pech, P., and Haughton, V. (1988). MR and cryomicrotomy of C1 and C2 roots. *Amer. J. Neur. Radiol.* **9:** 829–831.

Lehmann, E. D., Hawkes, D., Hil, D., Bird, C., Robinson, G., Colchester, A., and Maisley, M. (1991). Computer aided interpretation of SPECT images of the brain using an MRI derived neuroanatomic atlas. *Med. Informatics* **16:** 151–166.

Pech, P. (1987). Correlative investigations of craniospinal anatomy and pathology with computed tomography, magnetic resonance imaging, and cryomicrotomy. Uppsala University, Sweden.

Rauschning, W. (1986). Surface cryoplaning. A technique for clinical anatomical correlations. *Uppsala J. Med. Sci.* **91:** 251–255.

Rauschning, W., Bergstrom, K., and Pech, P. (1983). Correlative craniospinal anatomy studies by computed tomography and cryomicrotomy. *J. Comput. Assist. Tomogr.* **7**(1): 9–13.

Roland, P. E., and Zilles, K. (1994). Brain atlases—A new research tool. *TINS* **17**(11): 458–467.

Talairach, J., and Tournoux, P. (1988). "Co-Planar Stereotaxic Atlas of the Human Brain." Thieme Medical Publishers, New York.

Tiede, U., Bomans, M., Hohne, K. H., Pommert, A., Riemer, M., Schiemann, T., Schubert, R., and Lierse, W. (1993). A computerized three-dimensional atlas of the human skull and brain. *Amer. J. Neur. Radiol.* **14**(3): 551–559.

Toga, A. W., Ambach, K., Quinn, B., Hutchin, M., and Burton, J. S. (1994). Postmortem anatomy from cryosectioned whole human brain. *J. Neurosci. Methods* **54**(2): 239–252.

An Elastic Image Transformation Method for 3D Intersubject Brain Image Mapping

KANG-PING LIN,[1] HIDEHIRO IIDA,[2] IWAO KANNO,[2] and SUNG-CHENG HUANG[3]

[1]*Department of Electrical Engineering*
Chung-Yuan University, Taiwan
[2]*Research Institute for Brain and Blood Vessels, Akita, Japan*
[3]*Department of Molecular and Medical Pharmacology*
UCLA School of Medicine
Los Angeles, California 90024

Intersubject tomographic image registration can be applied to match corresponding tissue volumes in different subjects for specific structures. This study presents a two-step self-organizing method that can elastically map one subject's MR image, called the input image, to another subject's MR image. Linear transformation is first introduced to grossly match the input image to the reference image. Then the input image is divided into several smaller cubes of equal volume. A local correspondence is used to estimate the best matching position by moving individual cubes of the input image around a search neighborhood of the reference image. Based on local correspondence, coarse displacement vectors for each cube are determined by the position difference between the original and the new cube centers. The estimated vectors of all pixels are obtained by interpolation and thus provide a complete transformation that matches the entire input image to the reference image. As the process is repeated, a better transformation is obtained, which improves the matching. The registration accuracy of the method was examined by measuring the location of 16 anatomical structures in 10 sets of MR images that had all been registered by the present registration method to a common reference image set. The registered anatomical location has a standard deviation of ~2 mm in the x, y, and z directions. The accuracy of the elastic mapping method is ~30% better than that of a linear stretching method currently used at the Akita Research Institute of Brain and Blood Vessels. In summary, the present method is found to be effective in registering 3D MR image of different subjects.

I. INTRODUCTION

Many methods have been used to align PET to PET and PET to MR images. However, to examine the anatomical variation in sensory–motor stimulation or to obtain cross-subject signal averaging to enhance the detectability of focal brain activation, it is necessary to accumulate the image signal from different subjects (either for functional MR images or for the O-15 PET images). Because of the large shape variations from subject to subject, mapping brain images of different subjects to a standard brain image is nontrivial. Various techniques for image deformation and matching have been presented (Burr, 1983; Kosugi et al., 1993; Bajscy et al., 1983; Gee et al., 1993; Evans et al., 1992; Evans, 1993; Collins et al., 1994). They involved various degrees of sophistication and various amounts of user interactions and limitations.

In this study, we have developed a general automated elastic mapping method that can adjust local and global shape differences to allow accurate registration

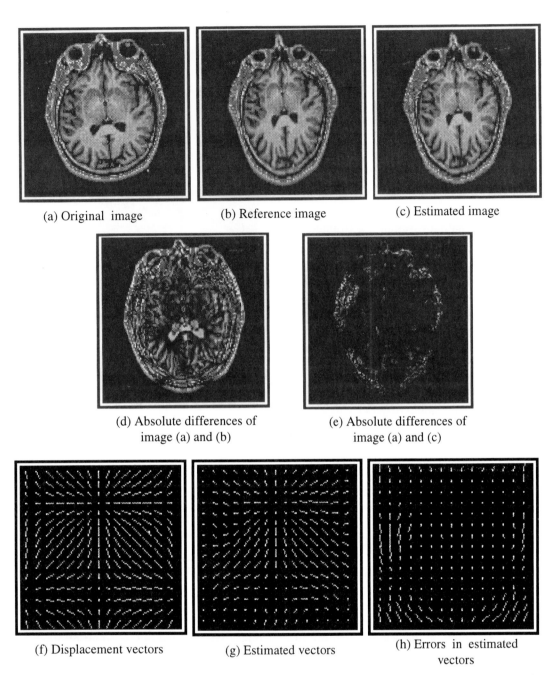

(a) Original image   (b) Reference image   (c) Estimated image

(d) Absolute differences of
image (a) and (b)

(e) Absolute differences of
image (a) and (c)

(f) Displacement vectors   (g) Estimated vectors   (h) Errors in estimated
vectors

FIGURE 1   Results of images and displacement vectors from the study of 2D computer simulation (see text for detailed description).

of 3D medical images of different subjects. The elastic image registration method (1) does not require internal and external fiducial markers, (2) does not use a head holder, (3) has few requirements of image preprocessing, such as edge detection or feature extraction, and (4) requires little user interaction. The method has been applied to register MR images of 10 different individuals to those of an 11th subject, considered the common reference image. The performance is evalu-

TABLE 1   Vector Errors (pixels) between the Estimated and Original Displacement Vectors in a 2D Registration Experiment

	Mean	Maximum
Within brain	0.02	2.11
Entire image	0.81	6.54

TABLE 2   Vector Errors (pixels) between the Estimated
and Original Displacement Vectors
in a 3D Registration Experiment

	Mean			Maximum		
	x	y	z	x	y	z
Within brain	0.01	0.02	0.09	0.72	0.94	1.54
Entire image	0.91	1.12	1.26	2.30	2.93	3.32

ated by examining the location variations of 16 anatomical structures of the elastically mapped images relative
to those of the reference images.

II. METHODS

The MR images used in this study were obtained
with a 1.5 T GE scanner. The MR T_1-weighted images
were acquired using a standard technique. The parameters for the scanning protocol were 500 msec pulse
repetition time (TR), 21 msec echo time (TE). The field
of view was 24 × 24 cm and the reconstruction matrix
was 256 × 256 pixels, resulting in a pixel size of 0.94
mm. The number of original slices was 19, and the slice
thickness was 6 mm. MR images were resampled using
linear interpolation to 128 × 128 × 64 pixels before the
registration process.

A. Linear Image Transformation

Before starting the elastic matching process, the images were coarsely scaled relative to each other. The
global image scaling factors in the x, y, and z directions
were roughly determined using three orthogonal 2D
images through the center of the subject's brain. A
linear stretch along each direction was used to adjust
the input image to similar size as that of the reference
image. The linear scaling procedure yielded a gross
alignment of the input images to the reference images.
With the scaled input image made similar in size to the
reference images, the next step of the elastic image
registration was easier than for the case without the
linear transformation step.

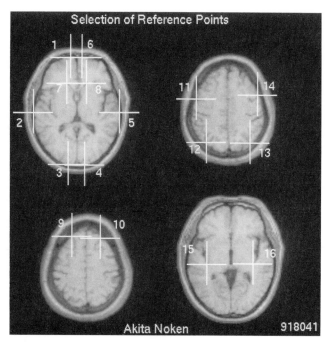

FIGURE 3   Anatomical structures on the most frontal, left most,
right most, and most posterior points in each hemisphere (1–6), most
frontal ventricle (7–8), most superior frontal sulcus, central sulcus,
and transverse occipital sulcus (9–14), and most posterior part of
the Sylvian fissure (15–16). The locations of these structural points
were examined among 10 sets of registered MR images to evaluate
the performance of the 3D elastic mapping program.

B. Elastic Image Mapping

The elastic image registration method searched optimal correspondence between two sets of 3D images.
The method first divided one 3D image into subimages
of equal volume. The size of each subimage (8 × 8 ×
4 for a 128 × 128 × 64 volumetric image) was fixed
during the entire elastic mapping procedure. Each subimage was moved independent of other subimages, to
the best matched location within a prespecified neighborhood of the reference image. The "best local
match" satisfied the criterion of having the minimal
sum of squared differences between the subimage and
the reference image values in the neighborhood of the
subimage. After the best match has been obtained for
each subimage, the procedure can be repeated until a
stable global match is achieved. Using this procedure,

FIGURE 4   Image results after elastic registration of the MR images of 10 different subjects to a reference image set. Only the images from
one image plane are shown for each registered image. A contour obtained from the reference image is superimposed on each registered image
to show the performance of the intersubject image registration method.

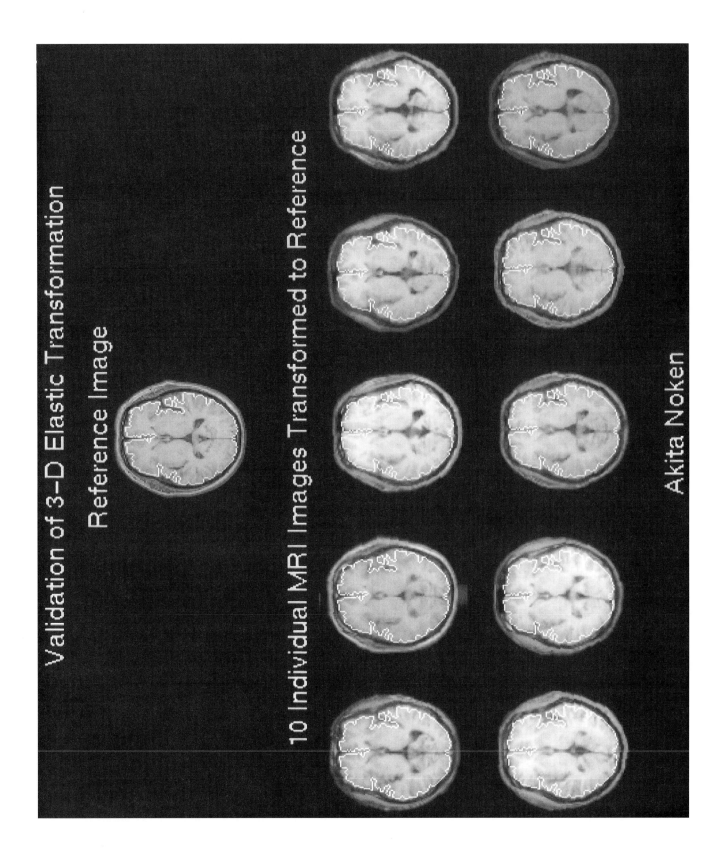

the method can elastically register two sets of 3D images of different subjects.

III. VALIDATION RESULTS

The registration accuracy of the present elastic transformation method was validated first by simulated images. The test not only examined the voxel correspondence in the entire image distribution but also measured the errors of the estimated transformation map. The mean square differences between the estimated image and the resampled image was used to measure the performance.

The simulated images were obtained by resampling an original MR image based on a set of predetermined displacement vectors (see later). The original images were then registered to the simulated reference image. An estimation of the transformation was obtained by the image registration procedure. The differences between the estimated displacement vectors and the actual displacement vectors were then used to measure the accuracy of the method.

The displacement vectors for transforming the original image to the reference image were defined by

$$\begin{aligned} x_1 &= x + A\sin(\pi x/32) \\ y_1 &= y + B\cos(\pi y/32) \\ z_1 &= z + C\sin(\pi z/64) \end{aligned} \qquad (1)$$

where x, y, and z were coordinates of a point in the original image and x_1, y_1, and z_1 were coordinates of the corresponding point in the transformed image. A, B, and C were the limits of the maximum displacement distances along the x, y, and z directions, respectively.

The method was first tested using one 2D MR image as depicted in Figure 1. The results show the original MR image (Fig. 1a) and the reference image (Fig. 1b), which was transformed from the original image according to a predetermined transformation matrix specified by equation (1) ($A = 8$ sample points, $B = 6$ sample points, and $C = 0$) and shown in Figure 1f. The final image (Fig. 1c) elastically transformed from the original image is shown to be close to the reference image (Fig. 1b). The difference images, both before and after transformation are shown in Figures 1d and 1e, respectively. Figure 1h shows the difference between the original transformation and the estimated transformation. Within the brain region, the errors are relatively small (i.e., larger vector errors are all outside of the brain region). The averaged errors within the brain and within the entire image are shown in Figure 1h. The vector error results are shown in Table 1.

The second simulation study was similar to the first one, except that it is for 3D images and the transformation matrices were obtained by assigning A and B as 6 pixel distances, and C as 2 plane separations in equation (1). The three-dimensional image registration was then applied. Table 2 summarizes the errors in the estimated transformation within an entire brain region.

The registration accuracy of the method was also validated using MR images in 11 subjects. One of the registration results obtained by the three-dimensional elastic mapping method is shown in Figure 2 (Color plate), which shows the registration of the MR images of two normal subjects. Subject 1 images were used as the reference images. The subject 2 images before and after elastic registration to the reference images are also shown.

The registration accuracy was examined by measuring the location of 16 anatomical structures in 10 sets of MR images, which had all been registered to a common reference image set. Figure 3 shows the anatomical landmarks of the most frontal, left most, right most, and most posterior in each hemisphere (1–6), most frontal ventricle (7–8), superior frontal sulcus, central sulcus, and transverse occipital sulcus (9–14), and most posterior part of the Sylvian fissure (15–16). The standard deviations of the locations of the 16 landmarks in 10 registered images were 1.29/3.43 mm (mean/max), 1.48/4.03 mm, and 1.14/2.94 mm, respectively, in the x, y, and z directions. The standard deviations (among the 10 registered image sets) of the location of one structure (9) were 1.93, 2.19, and 1.74 mm, respectively, in the x, y, and z directions as compared to 2.52, 2.48, and 3.90 mm, resulting from a linear stretching method developed by Kanno *et al.* (1993). Figure 4 shows a common image slice from each subject that has been elastically registered to the reference image. The outside brain contour obtained from the reference image was superimposed on each subject image to show the registration performance.

IV. DISCUSSION

An elastic transformation algorithm for tomographic image mapping is presented. The advantages of the algorithm described are its simplicity, flexibility, and ease of implementation. To assess the accuracy of the automated method, several simulations and direct assessments of intersubject image registrations were performed. The results of the present study indicate that the local image voxel matching algorithm is effective

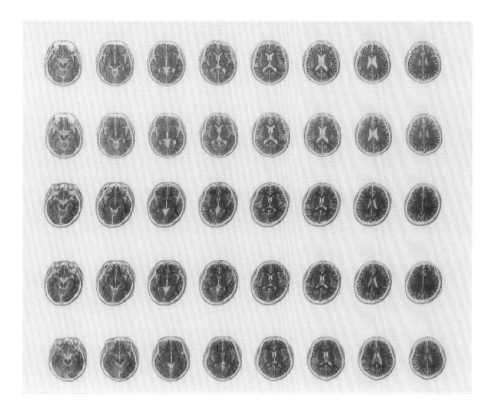

FIGURE 2 Intersubject image registration results obtained by the three-dimensional elastic mapping method. MR images of eight consecutive slices from one of two different normal subjects are shown in each row. The first and second rows are the images of subject 1 (reference images), with and without brain contour, respectively. The third and fourth rows show, respectively, the images of subject 2 (original images), without and with superposition of contours of the reference images. The bottom row shows the elastically registered subject 2 images that match the reference images and contours (of subject 1).

for elastically registering MR images of multiple subjects to a standard brain image. The algorithm can accurately and consistently estimate the transformation matrices for both global and local tissue localization in truly three-dimensional images. Minimal human interaction and no feature extraction are required. The computation time is approximately 2 min for linear scaling and 15–18 min for image elastic registration on a SUN Sparc-10 workstation. The short computation time allows a large number of intersubject images to be processed for signal integration.

Acknowledgment

This work was partially supported by DOE contract DE-FC03-87ER60615 and NIH grant CA56655.

References

Bajscy, R., Lieberson, R., and Reivich, M. (1983). A computerized system for the elastic matching of deformed radiographic images to idealized atlas images. *J. Comput. Assist. Tomogr.* **7:** 618–625.

Burr, D. J. (1983). Matching elastic templates. *In:* "Physical and Biological Processing of Images." pp. 260–271. Springer-Verlag, New York/Berlin.

Collins, D. L., Neelin, P., Peters, T. M., and Evans, A. C. (1994). Automatic 3D intersubject registration of MR volumetric data in standardized Talairach space. *J. Comput. Assist. Tomogr.* **18:** 192–205.

Evans, A. C., Marrett, S., Neelin, P., Collins, K. W., Weiqian, D., Milot, S., Meyer, E., and Bub, D. (1992). Anatomical mapping of functional activation in stereotactic coordinates space. *Neuroimage.* **1:** 43–53.

Evans, A. C. (1993). 3D multimodality human brain mapping: Past, present and future. *In:* "Proceedings of Brain PET '93 AKITA." pp. 373–386. Excerpta Medica, Amsterdam.

Gee, J. C., Reivich, M., and Bajcsy, R. (1993). Elastically deforming 3D Atlas to match anatomical brain images. *J. Comput. Assist. Tomogr.* **17:** 225–236.

Kosugi, Y., Sase, M., Kuwatani, H., Kinoshita, N., Momose, M., Nishikawa, J., and Watanabe, T. (1993). Neural network mapping for nonlinear stereotactic normalization of brain MR images. *J. Comput. Assist. Tomogr.* **17:** 634–640.

Kanno, I., Yoshiharu, Y., Hideaki, F., Kenji, I., Hugh, L., Shuichi, M., Keiichi, O., Norihiro, S., and Hinako, T. (1993). Comparison of three anatomical standardization methods regarding foci localization and its between subject variation in the sensorimotor activation. *In:* Proceedings of Brain PET '93 AKITA. pp. 439–447. Excerpta Medica, Amsterdam.

Individual Hemodynamic vs. Metabolic Functional Anatomy of Repeating Words
A Study Using MRI-Guided Positron Emission Tomography

G. R. FINK,[1,2] K. HERHOLZ,[1,2] K. WIENHARD,[1] J. KESSLER,[1] M. HALBER,[1] T. BRUCKBAUER,[1]
U. PIETRZYK,[1] and W.-D. HEISS[1,2]

[1]Max Planck Institute for Neurological Research
50931 Germany
[2]Neurology Clinic of the University of Cologne
Cologne, Germany

Transient increases in functional cerebral activity cause an increase in energy metabolism that is followed by an increase in blood flow. In humans, however, little is known about the interrelationship between metabolic and hemodynamic functional changes, both in spatial localization and magnitude. Using MRI-guided positron emission tomography (PET) measuring relative regional cerebral blood flow (rCBF), the anatomical localization of brain areas involved in repeating words was examined in seven nonaphasic subjects. Data on relative rCBF were compared with the results of a previous study measuring relative regional glucose metabolism (rCMR$_{glu}$) in a similar group of subjects using the same activation paradigm. In each individual, significant increases in relative rCBF were seen in the superior temporal gyrus bilaterally, the vocalization area in the sensorimotor cortex bilaterally, and the supplementary motor area. On average, the location and magnitude of functional relative rCBF and relative rCMR$_{glu}$ changes did not show any significant differences. This study demonstrates a consistent individual pattern of relative rCBF increases in each individual with a simple word repetition task. It further shows that glucose metabolism and regional cerebral blood flow increase in response to transient neuronal activation in a matched way.

I. INTRODUCTION

In humans, it has been demonstrated, that under normal conditions at rest, blood flow, oxygen metabo-lism, and glucose metabolism are tightly correlated (Lassen *et al.*, 1978) and that all three can be used for measuring regional cerebral activity. Although a physiological uncoupling of cerebral blood flow and oxidative metabolism has been demonstrated (Fox and Raichle, 1986) during states of functional activation, such an uncoupling of glucose metabolism and blood flow has never been demonstrated and measurements of glucose metabolism and blood flow are widely considered exchangeable. Very few studies, however, have looked into changes of glucose metabolism and blood flow during contrasting behavioral states, and therefore little is known about the interrelationship between metabolic and hemodynamic changes following transient neuronal activation. Attention to these questions has been refocused by functional MRI; questions of particular concern are the exact location, the spatial extent, and the magnitude of such stimulus-related functional changes.

In 1988, Ginsberg *et al.* investigated the local metabolic and hemodynamic changes following a unilateral discriminative somatosensory–motor task. They asked their subjects to sort mah-jongg tiles by the engraved design. In a regions-of-interest based analysis of the group they found a 17% increase in normalized regional glucose metabolism (rCMR$_{glu}$) and a 27% increase in normalized regional blood flow (rCBF) in the contralateral sensorimotor cortex. They concluded that the increments in rCMR$_{glu}$ and rCBF correlated poorly with one another and that the mean rCBF increment was significantly higher.

Autoradiographic and optical imaging studies in animals, however, suggest a tightly coupled match of metabolic and hemodynamic changes both in a normal state and following transient increases in functional cerebral activity in response to external or internal stimuli (e.g., Reivich, 1974; Grinvald *et al.*, 1988).

Using MRI-guided [18]FDG-PET measuring regional glucose metabolism, Herholz *et al.* (1994) investigated the metabolic anatomy of repeating words. In six individuals, they demonstrated consistent bilateral increases in glucose metabolism in the superior temporal gyrus, the vocalization area of the sensorimotor cortex, and the supplementary motor area (SMA).

The present study aimed at investigating the hemodynamic anatomy of repeating words using the same activation paradigm as Herholz *et al.* (1994), the same equipment, and the same data analysis, but measuring relative regional cerebral blood flow. This was done to compare the magnitude and location of metabolic and hemodynamic changes associated with a simple word repetition task.

II. SUBJECTS AND METHODS

While lying in the PET scanner, seven nonaphasic subjects (five men, two women; aged between 39 and 64 years) were asked to repeat aloud words, single German nouns, that they heard at an average rate of one word per 1.5 sec. Four subjects were neurologically normal. The remaining three subjects had suffered from ischemic stroke leading to lacunar lesions in the right thalamus ($n = 1$), left putamen ($n = 1$), and left parietal operculum ($n = 1$); none of these patients suffered or had suffered aphasia at any time of the disease (as assessed both clinically and by neuropsychological testing). The subjects were selected to match those chosen by Herholz *et al.* (1994). All subjects gave written informed consent after being instructed about the purpose of the study.

Eight $H_2^{15}O$-PET relative regional cerebral blood flow measurements were performed on a high-resolution scanner (ECAT EXACT HR, Siemens-CTI, Knoxville, Tennessee; 47 planes, field of view 15 cm; Wienhard *et al.*, 1994) following the intravenous injection of 370 MBq radioactive labeled water. PET scans were performed in a random order during four runs each of the word repetition task and a resting state (for control). Data were acquired in 3D-mode for 90 sec starting with the iv injection of the radioactive tracer. Data were scatter and attenuation corrected.

For morphological localization of PET measured changes in relative rCBF, magnetic resonance imaging (MRI) was performed in a superconducting 1 T instru-

ment (Magnetom, Siemens, Germany) using a FLASH sequence (flip angle 40°, TR 40 msec, TE 15 msec) producing 64 transaxial T_1-weighted tomograms.

Following image processing, maps of relative regional cerebral blood flow were derived for each run. After an initial image realignment of all PET images ($128 \times 128 \times 47$ voxels of $2.17 \times 2.17 \times 3.125$ mm voxel size), a mean PET image was calculated and brought into the standard position, as defined by the AC–PC line, using the MPI tool (multipurpose imaging tool; Pietrzyk *et al.*, 1994). All individual runs were then resliced to this PET mean image and normalized to global blood flow (scaling of each study to the average of all brain voxels). A percent increase image was calculated (division of activation through resting tasks) and smoothed in x, y, and z directions using a spherical 8 mm median filter. Following MRI to PET image coregistration, the resliced MRI, the PET mean image, and the percent increase image were simultaneously displayed. All activated brain areas were inspected on this simultaneous display in all three orthogonal plane directions using the VOI tool (Herholz *et al.*, 1996; Chapter 34). The following regions were selected as target volumes: superior temporal gyrus, vocalization area of the sensorimotor cortex, and the supplementary motor area (SMA). Within these areas local maxima of relative rCBF increase were searched and their anatomical location was checked on the MRI. The resulting coordinates of local maxima within regions of significant activation ($p < 0.05$, corrected for multiple comparisons) were determined both as individual coordinates and in standard stereotaxic space (Talairach and Tournoux, 1988), thus allowing comparability with other subjects and groups.

Noise images were created for each individual by dividing the average of two activated and two resting scans through the average of the remaining scans, using the same normalization and filtering procedures as for the activation images. The average standard deviation across voxels in these noise images was 3.24 ± 0.77 (mean $\pm$ standard deviation).

III. RESULTS

Consistent increases in relative rCBF with repeating words were seen in each individual bilaterally in the superior temporal gyrus (Fig. 1), the lower knee of the pre- and postcentral gyrus corresponding to the vocalization area of the sensorimotor cortex, and the supplementary motor area (SMA). The respective coordinates and percent increases in normalized rCBF are given in Table 1, together with the corresponding

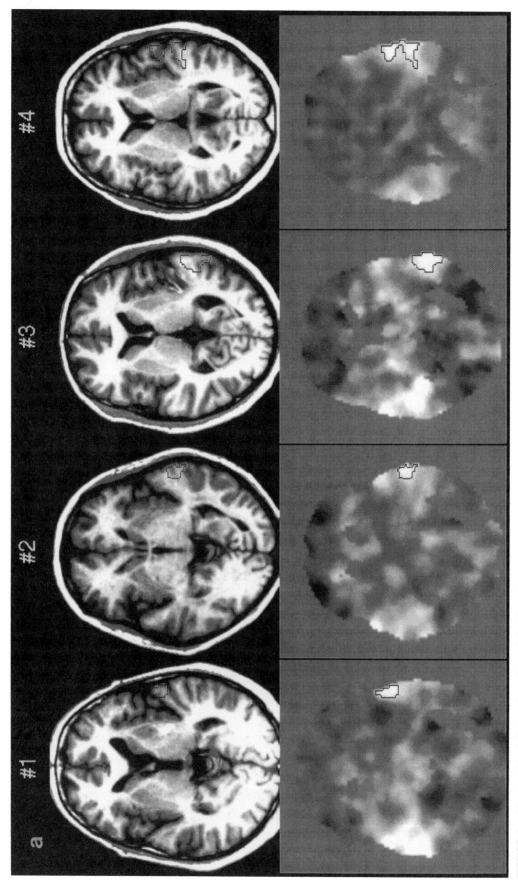

FIGURE 1 (a): 1–4; (b): 5–7. Local maxima of significant increase in normalized relative rCBF within the left superior temporal gyrus of all seven subjects. Upper row, individual MRIs; lower row, individual percent increase images. No stereotaxic procedures have yet taken place at this stage of data analysis. Left is right and right is left. Within the superior temporal gyrus a consistent pattern of relative rCBF increases with repeating words is seen in each subject with an anterior and a posterior local maximum within this area. Contours include all voxels with normalized relative rCBF increase >10%.

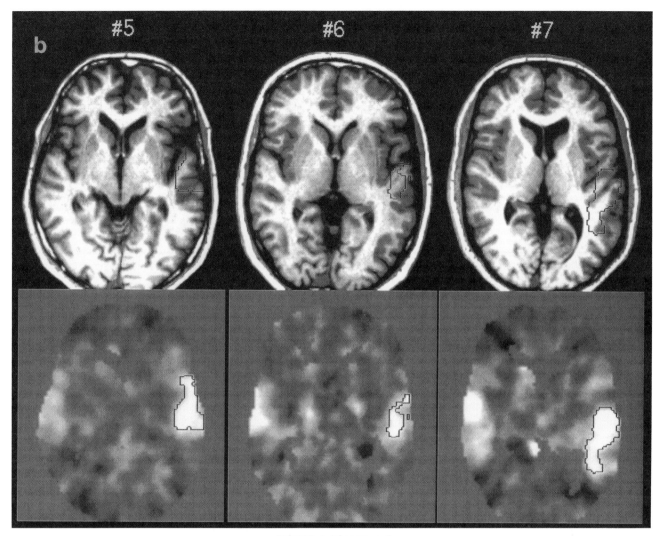

FIGURE 1 (*Continued*)

coordinates and percent increases in normalized rCMR$_{glu}$ obtained by Herholz *et al*. (1994) using the same paradigm but [18]FDG-PET. The location of the local maxima within the superior temporal gyrus, the vocalization area, and the SMA did not differ significantly from one another. The percent increases of normalized rCMR$_{glu}$ and normalized rCBF were comparable with each other although there was a trend for higher increases of rCMR$_{glu}$ in the vocalization area. Average percent normalized rCBF increases in activation maxima ranged from 15.2 to 19.1%, which is the 4.7- to 5.9-fold of noise standard deviation.

IV. DISCUSSION

The results of the present study are in good accordance with previous findings by Petersen and Fiez (1993), who in a group analysis showed that a simple word repetition task leads to increases in rCBF in the superior temporal gyrus, the vocalization area of the perirolandic cortex, and the SMA. These activations have now been demonstrated for a group of seven non-aphasic subjects and for each individual. Reproducible increases in rCBF in individuals are detected by four runs per condition using as little as 370 MBq of radioactive labeled water per run. The anatomical locations of the local maxima of regional rCBF increases are identified precisely in the cortices of the respective regions as proven by MRI-to-PET coregistration.

The results obtained in the present study using rCBF to identify neuronal activations associated with repeating words are similar to those obtained by Herholz *et al*. (1994) using the same paradigm but rCMR$_{glu}$. On average, both rCBF and rCMR$_{glu}$ increase in response to the activation task in a tightly matched way. The

TABLE 1   Location and Magnitude of Local Activation Maxima of Relative rCBF (mean ± SD) in a Word Repetition Task

Region	Side	Talairach coordinates (mm)			% Increase of normalized rCBF
		x	*y*	*z*	
Superior temporal gyrus	Left	−59 ± 5	−12 ± 19	4 ± 4	17.4 ± 1.7
		[−64 ± 5]	[−20 ± 11]	[5 ± 3]	[19.0 ± 4.3]
	Right	62 ± 7	−19 ± 12	4 ± 6	19.1 ± 3.9
		[52 ± 7]	[−25 ± 5]	[3 ± 6]	[18.7 ± 2.2]
Vocalization area	Left	−49 ± 6	−6 ± 7	40 ± 8	14.3 ± 3.7
		[−55 ± 5]	[−7 ± 6]	[34 ± 10]	[17.5 ± 2.8]
	Right	52 ± 10	−5 ± 7	36 ± 11	15.5 ± 4.5
		[50 ± 8]	[−8 ± 9]	[39 ± 12]	[20.4 ± 3.2]
SMA	Medial	−1 ± 8	0 ± 7	67 ± 6	15.2 ± 5.2
		[−1 ± 5]	[−4 ± 9]	[68 ± 8]	[14.7 ± 3.9]

Note. Values in brackets [. . .] indicate corresponding values of location and magnitude of local activation maxima of relative rCMR$_{glu}$ using the same activation paradigm (data taken from Herholz *et al.*, 1994).

location of the maxima and the magnitude of relative rCBF and rCMR$_{glu}$ increases did not show any significant differences. Furthermore, no difference in data variance were observed between ^{18}FDG and ^{15}O-PET.

The techniques applied in these two studies can easily be used for group and individual studies of language functions both in normals and in patients with aphasia.

References

Fox, P. T., and Raichle, M. E. (1986). Focal physiological uncoupling of cerebral blood flow and oxidative metabolism during somatosensory stimulation in human subjects. *Proc. Natl. Acad. Sci.* **83:** 1140–1144.

Ginsberg, M. D., Chang, J. Y., Kelley, R. E., Yoshii, F., Barker, W. W., Ingenito, G., and Boothe, T. E. (1988). Increases in both cerebral glucose utilization and blood flow during execution of a somatosensory task. *Ann. Neurol.* **23:** 152–160.

Grinvald, A., Frostig, R. D., Lieke, E., and Hildesheim, R. (1988). Optical imaging of neuronal activity. *Physiol. Rev.* **68:** 1285–1366.

Herholz, K., Pietrzyk, U., Karbe, H., Würker, M., Wienhard, K., and Heiss, W.-D. (1994). Individual metabolic anatomy of repeat-ing words demonstrated by MRI-guided positron emission tomography. *Neurosci. Lett.* **182:** 47–50.

Herholz, K., Dickhoven, S., Karbe, H., Halber, M., Pietrzyk, U., and Heiss, W.-D. (1996). Integrated quantitative analysis of functional and morphological 3D data by volumes of interest. *In:* "Quantification of Brain Function Using PET." (T. Jones Quantification of brain function, etc., Ed.), pp. 175–180. Academic Press, San Diego.

Lassen, N., Ingvar, D. H., and Skinhoj, E. (1978). Brain function and blood flow. *Sci. Am.* **239:** 62–71.

Petersen, S. E., and Fiez, J. A. (1993). The processing of single words studied with positron emission tomography. *Annu. Rev. Neurosci.* **16:** 509–530.

Pietrzyk, U., Herholz, K., Fink, G.R., Jacobs, A., Mielke, R., Slansky, I., Würker, M., and Heiss, W.-D. (1994). An interactive technique for three-dimensional image registration: Validation for PET, SPECT, MRI and CT brain studies. *J. Nucl. Med.* **35:** 2011–2018.

Reivich, M. (1974). Blood flow metabolism couple in brain. *In:* "Brain Dysfunction in Metabolic Disorders." (F. Plum, Ed.), pp. 125–140. Raven Press, New York.

Talairach, J., and Tournoux, P. (1988). "Co-Planar Stereotaxic Atlas of the Human Brain." Thieme, Stuttgart.

Wienhard, K., Dahlbom, M., Eriksson, L., Michel, C., Bruckbauer, T., Pietrzyk, U., and Heiss, W.-D. (1994). The ECAT EXACT HR: Performance of a new high resolution positron scanner. *J. Comput. Assist. Tomogr.* **181:** 110–118.

80

Dynamic Imaging of a PET Activation Experiment

Do rCBF Changes Persist after an Activation Paradigm?

G. F. EGAN,[1] G. J. O'KEEFE,[1] D. G. BARNES,[1] J. D. G. WATSON,[2,3] B. T. O'SULLIVAN,[4]
H. J. TOCHON-DANGUY,[1] and S. R. MEIKLE[5]

[1]Center for Positron Emission Tomography
Austin Repatriation Medical Center
Melbourne 3084, Australia
[2]Department of Medicine, University of Sydney, Sydney, Australia
Departments of [3]Neurology, [4]Psychiatry, and [5]Nuclear Medicine
Royal Prince Alfred Hospital, Sydney 2050, Australia

Improved sensitivity to changes in human brain function using PET activation studies may be achieved by continuing the PET scan for a short period immediately after the activation paradigm ends. An investigation of the statistical significance of rCBF changes occurring during, after, and both during and after an activation paradigm has been made. PET scans using repeated [H$_2$^{15}O] slow infusions and a lexical decision activation paradigm were undertaken in five normal male subjects. The 40 sec [H$_2$^{15}O] infusion produced a monotonically increasing brain count rate for 70 ± 5 sec. The 90 sec uptake acquisition commenced synchronously with the increasing brain count rate, whereas the 100 sec cognitive paradigm commenced 10 sec earlier. A further 20 sec tracer washout acquisition followed immediately. For the combined data acquisitions three large regions of highly significant rCBF change were identified. These three regions were also observed in the uptake data set, but only two smaller associated regions were observed in the washout data. One of the large regions was not identifiable using the washout data only, suggesting that rCBF changes in this region were more highly synchronised with the cognitive paradigm. Therefore, although continued PET scanning after the activation paradigm did not change the significance of the findings, it enabled identification of regions having greater or lesser synchronisation with the paradigm.

I. INTRODUCTION

Human brain function research using PET activation studies is limited due to the lack of temporal resolution of PET activation studies and by the limited sensitivity of PET scanners. Apart from constructing PET scanners of higher intrinsic sensitivity, improved sensitivity to subtle changes in brain function can be achieved by undertaking more scans per subject with lower infused radioactivity per scan. Higher noise equivalent counts are then obtained because the proportion of random coincidences in the total counts is then reduced.

Alternatively, more subjects can be scanned and included in the group analysis. Although this is always possible, the ability to obtain statistically significant results for a minimum number of research volunteers is both ethically motivated and logistically preferable. Finally, by continuing to scan for a short period after each completion of the activation paradigm, the statistical quality of the PET data may be improved. An investigation of the statistical significance of regional cerebral blood flow (rCBF) changes occurring during, after, and both during and after an activation paradigm has been undertaken. Determination of the optimal timing for PET data acquisition during and after the paradigm presentation is the primary focus of this study.

Studies of human brain function using PET require an infusion of radioactive water, subject stimulation using an appropriate paradigm, and acquisition of the γ ray coincidence data. The maximal sensitivity for detecting rCBF changes associated with the activation paradigm is dependent on the degree of synchronisation between the tracer infusion, paradigm presentation, and PET data acquisition. PET data are typically acquired for 60 to 90 sec after arrival of the radiotracer in the subject's brain, but the optimal duration and synchronisation of the paradigm has been less well established.

Measurement of activation regions in the brain using PET is based on detection of regions having increased rCBF (Roland, 1994). At the cellular level these regions must have higher $[H_2{}^{15}O]$ specific activity produced by increased perfusion from the vasculature into brain tissue. Therefore, because water is a freely diffusing agent, the back perfusion from the tissue must also be increased during the activation. Thus, the maximal specific activity in an activated brain region is produced by commencing the paradigm simultaneously with the arrival of radiotracer in the brain and stopping the paradigm when the tracer has cleared from the blood. Continued stimulation after tracer clearance from the blood may then decrease the specific activity in the activated region. Finally, if a relative higher specific activity persists in the activated region after the cessation of the paradigm, the statistical significance of the activation in that region may be improved by continued scanning.

Earlier studies (Volkow *et al.*, 1991; Silbersweig *et al.*, 1993; Cherry *et al.*, 1993; Hurtig, *et al.*, 1994) have confirmed that best results are obtained by limiting the activation paradigm to the duration of the radioactive tracer uptake in the brain. However, only one study (Silbersweig *et al.*, 1993) investigated the effects of continued imaging after cessation of the paradigm, and it concluded that results of greater significance were obtained with an additional 30 sec of PET data acquisition. The present study extends this earlier work by investigating the statistical significance of rCBF changes occurring during, after, and both during and after an activation paradigm. Comparison of the statistical parametric maps (SPM) (Friston *et al.*, 1990; Friston *et al.*, 1991) from data acquired during and data acquired after the paradigm may reveal activated regions that either (1) persist in the postparadigm data and thus maintain relatively higher specific activity in accordance with the simple perfusion model described earlier, (2) vanish in the postparadigm data and thus

may continue to be activated in accordance with the model, (3) appear for the first time in the postparadigm data, or (4) be statistically insignificant in either data sample but be statistically significant in the combined data sample. In the last case, the activated region will actually become detectable due to the increased scanning duration. Thus activation regions that persist may be considered more specific to the paradigm and activation regions that vanish in the postparadigm data may be less specific. Therefore, an analysis of the temporal evolution of an activated region may reveal new information about specificity of activation regions to the activation paradigm. This is of particular interest for subtle cognitive activations where multiple activation regions may be detected.

II. METHOD

PET activation scans using repeated $[H_2{}^{15}O]$ slow infusions and a lexical decision activation paradigm (Coltheart *et al.*, 1977) have been undertaken in five normal subjects (male; mean age, 29 ± 8 years). All subjects gave informed consent in accordance with the Austin Repatriation Medical Center human ethics in research guidelines. The lexical decision paradigm consisted of visual presentation of a random sequence of words and nonwords (each four or five letters in length) at a presentation rate of one every 3 sec. For each letter string the orthographic neighborhood value (N) can be determined by counting the number of real words that can be formed by the replacement of one letter only. For example, although "lune" is a nonword, six words ($N = 6$) can be formed by replacing one letter; tune, lone, lane, lure, line, and lung. The activation task consisted of words and nonwords having high N values, but the control task consisted of words and nonwords having low N values. For example, jazz ($N = 0$) and ilge ($N = 1$). The subject was required to press one of two predesignated keys on a computer keyboard to identify the stimulus as either a word or nonword, and the subject's reaction times and error rates were recorded.

For each subject an initial scan of a small $[H_2{}^{15}O]$ infusion (180 MBq) enabled determination of the time delay from commencement of infusion to detection of radioactivity in the brain, which was typically 40–60 sec. Six dynamic scans (three activation and three baseline scans) were then acquired in 3D mode and reconstructed using a standard image reconstruction algorithm (Kinahan and Rogers, 1989) and a Hanning filter with a cutoff frequency of 0.45 cycles/cm. Each scan consisted of three frames having durations of 30,

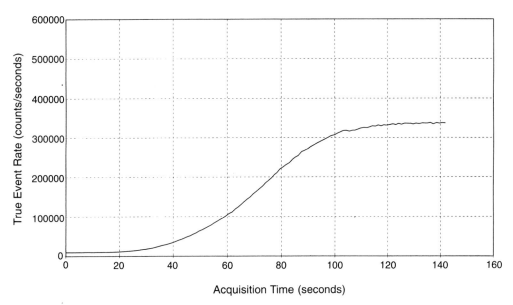

FIGURE 1 The temporal evolution of the brain true coincidences count rate calculated from the true counts, random counts, and the dead time correction factor each measured at 1 sec intervals, commencing immediately prior to the $[H_2^{15}O]$ infusion. The second acquisition frame extended from 30 to 120 sec, and the third acquisition frame extended from 120 to 140 sec.

100, and 20 sec, respectively. Data from the initial 30 sec acquisition frame was used to correct frame 2 and 3 data for background activity. Also the dead time correction factor measured in frame one was used to dead time correct data in frames 2 and 3.

The 40 sec $[H_2^{15}O]$ infusion (mean activity per infusion = 790 ± 60 MBq) using a highly reproducible automated water generator (Clarke and Tochon-Danguy, 1992) produced a monotonically increasing brain count rate for 70 ± 5 sec. The temporal evolution of the brain count rate was calculated from the true counts, random counts, and the dead time correction factor, which were each measured at 1 sec intervals commenc-

ing immediately prior to the $[H_2^{15}O]$ infusion. Thereafter, the dead time and decay corrected brain count rate was observed to be constant (Fig. 1). The acquisition was commenced to synchronise frame 2 with the increasing brain count rate. The 100 sec cognitive paradigm was visually presented 10 sec prior to the commencement of acquisition frame 2. The average radiation dose per subject was 4.6 ± 0.8 mSv (Smith *et al.*, 1994).

In this experiment the cognitive paradigm and the $[H_2^{15}O]$ infusion were highly synchronised with the second data acquisition frame, and the second and third data acquisition frames taken together were slightly

TABLE 1 Activation Regions Greater than 20 Voxels in Size (voxel threshold $Z > 2.33$, $p < 0.01$) for Different Synchronisation between the Cognitive Paradigm, $[H_2^{15}O]$ Infusion, and Data Acquisition

Frame	Acquisition (sec)	NEC[a] (Mc)	Region	Size (pixels)	Z_{max}	(x, y, z) (mm)
2	100	4.5	1	388	3.9	34, 30, 12
			2a[b]	30	2.8	−12, 10, 44
2 and 3	120	5.7	1	434	3.8	40, 32, 12
3	20	1.2	2b[b]	21	3.4	−20, 14, 24
			1[c]	25	2.8	50, 14, 0

[a]Noise equivalent counts.
[b]The superior medial frontal regions may be related due to their proximity.
[c]The small lateral insula region identified is wholly contained within a larger region identified in the longer acquisition.

TABLE 2 "Inhibition" Regions Greater than 20 Voxels in Size (Voxel Threshold $Z > 2.33$, $p < 0.01$) for Different Synchronisation between the Cognitive Paradigm, $[H_2{}^{15}O]$ Infusion, and Data Acquisition

Frame	Acquisition (sec)	NEC (Mc)	Region	Size (pixels)	Z_{max}	(x, y, z) (mm)
2	100	4.5	3a	49	3.0	−12, −70, 28
			4	100	3.0	−52, −12, 16
2 and 3	120	5.7	3	316	3.6	−14, −64, 24
			4	135	3.1	−58, −8, 12
3	20	1.2	3b	36	3.0	−22, −52, 28

less synchronised with the paradigm and the infusion. The significance of changes between the activation and control rCBF images were determined for three cases: (1) during $[H_2{}^{15}O]$ uptake (frame 2), (2) during $[H_2{}^{15}O]$ uptake and 20 sec of washout (frames 2 and 3 summed), and (3) for the 20 sec of $[H_2{}^{15}O]$ washout only (frame 3).

The reconstructed data volume was analyzed as a contiguous set of 31 images, each containing 128×128 voxels. An automated registration algorithm (Woods *et al.*, 1992) was used to align the second and subsequent scans to the first scan for each subject. Masking was then applied to each image to remove spurious signal outside the cortical surface by collapsing a 2D contour around the sum of all the images of the subject. The masking threshold was chosen seperately for each image slice as 35% or the maximum voxel value present in that slice. Centering and reslicing to 43 image planes was performed, and the volume data set was then transformed in stereotaxic space (Talairach and Tournoux, 1988) resulting in a voxel dimension of 2.0 mm $\times$ 2.0 mm $\times$ 4.0 mm. The images were then smoothed using an 18 mm Gaussian blurring function. Finally, statistical parametric maps (SPMs) (Friston *et al.*, 1990; Friston *et al.*, 1991; Friston *et al.*, 1995) of complimentary experimental designs (ABABAB and BABABA) were determined to enable identification of both activation and "inhibition" SPMs. An analysis of rCBF decreases ("inhibition") was included because the objective of this study is to determine the temporal evolution of significant rCBF changes (activations and "inhibitions") rather than only significant rCBF activations, although the original cognitive hypotheses related only to activations. SPMs were determined separately for both frames 2 and 3 and for the summed data set.

III. RESULTS AND DISCUSSION

Three large regions (regions 1, 3, and 4; see Tables 1 and 2) of highly significant rCBF change were identi-

fied for the uptake and summed data sets, although smaller associated regions were observed in the washout data. In the analysis of activation regions (experimental design ABABAB), the right frontal insula (region 1) was identified in all three SPMs and was most significant for the highest degree of tracer uptake/data acquisition synchronisation (frame 2). The inclusion of radiotracer washout data slightly increased the size of region 1 (434 voxels compared to 388), shifted the centroid of the region by 6 mm, but did not alter the maximum pixel Z-score for rCBF change ($Z_{max,2} = 3.8$, $Z_{max,2,3} = 3.8$). The spatial location of activation region 2 varied from frame 2 to frame 3, possibly due to rCBF changes occurring immediately post paradigm. This result suggests that an acquisition protocol in which additional shorter acquisition frames are acquired may

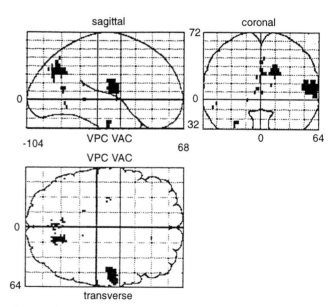

FIGURE 2 Statistical parametric map of the "inhibition" regions detected using the uptake data set only (voxel threshold $Z > 2.33$, $p < 0.01$).

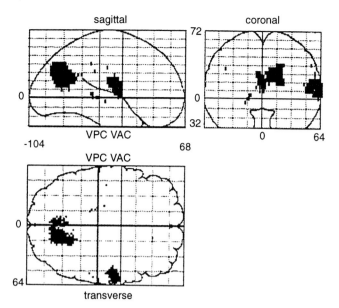

sagittal   coronal

VPC VAC

VPC VAC

transverse

FIGURE 3 Statistical parametric map of the "inhibition" regions detected using the summed uptake and washout data sets (voxel threshold $Z > 2.33$, $p < 0.01$).

determine if a temporal or a spatial evolution of the activated region occurs.

Regions of relative decrease in rCBF between the activation and control scans can be interpreted as either inhibitions occurring during the activation scans or as "spurious" activations occurring in the baseline scans but not present in the actual activation scans. Without absolute rCBF quantification we could not resolve this ambiguity of the identified "inhibitions" (Table 2). Even with absolute quantification it is difficult to measure changes from the complete resting state due to the difficulty of establishing such a state for each subject. Two significant "inhibition" regions were identified in the left lateral inferior parietal region (region 3) and in the left superior occipito–parietal junction (region 4) in an analysis of data from frame two (Fig. 2) and also in an analysis of the summed data set (Fig. 3). The size of region 3 significantly increased with the inclusion of washout data (316 voxels compared to 49) and subsequent analysis of only the washout data identified a proximate region (region 3b) 20 mm anterio-laterally, as determined from the Z_{max} voxel locations for each region. The analysis of the summed data set could not independently resolve ($p < 0.01$), the subregions observed in frames 2 and 3.

Conversely, for region 4, the inclusion of washout data did not significantly alter the size (135 voxels compared to 100), the maximum Z-value ($Z_{max,2} = 3.0$, $Z_{max,2,3} = 3.1$), or the location of the voxel of most significant rCBF (8 mm displacement). Not surpris-

ingly, region 4 was subsequently not identifiable using the washout data only, suggesting that rCBF changes in region 4 were more highly synchronised with the cognitive paradigm than the changes occurring in region 3. Continued PET scanning after an activation paradigm may enable identification of regions of significant rCBF change that are more specific or less specific to the paradigm. Furthermore, a degree of temporal resolution in PET activation studies may be possible by either acquiring data in list mode, or by acquiring multiframe scans, where the duration of each frame is adjusted to provide approximately equal average noise equivalent counts (NEC) per subject.

IV. CONCLUSION

The results of this study suggest that, to improve the sensitivity of detecting rCBF changes in PET activation studies, (1) the end of the cognitive paradigm should be approximately synchronised with the maximum brain count rate corrected for dead time and decay, (2) incorporating radiotracer washout data (postparadigm data) did not necessarily improve the detection of activation regions for the lexical decision paradigm but did improve the detection of inhibition regions (although we had no *a priori* hypothesis concerning this finding), (3) summation of paradigm and postparadigm data may conceal spatial and temporal variation of a region of significant rCBF change, and (4) additional acquisition frames (of approximately equal average NECs) acquired during and after the activation paradigm may provide additional important temporal information about each observed region of significant rCBF change.

References

Cherry, S. R., Woods, R. P., and Mazziotta, J. C. (1993). Improved signal to noise in activation studies by exploiting the kinetics of oxygen-15-labeled water. *J. Cereb. Blood Flow Metab.* **13**: S714.

Clarke, J., and Tochon-Danguy, H. J. (1992). "R2D2", A bedside [oxygen-15] water infuser. Proc. 6th Inter. Work. on Targetry and target chemistry. 91, ed. Weinreich, R. PSI, Switzerland.

Coltheart, M., Daveleer, E., Jonasson, J. T., *et al.* (1977). In "Attention and Peformance, VI." (S. Dornic, Ed.). Academic Press, New York.

Friston, K. J., Frith, C. D., Liddle, P. F., Dolan, R. J., Lammertsma, A. A., and Frackowiak, R. S. J. (1990). The relationship between global and local changes in PET scans. *J. Cereb. Blood Flow Metab.* **10**: 458–466.

Friston, K. J., Frith, C. D., Liddle, P. F., and Frackowiak, R. S. J. (1991). Comparing functional (PET) images: The assessment of significant change. *J. Cereb. Blood Flow Metab.* **11**: 690–699.

Friston, K. J., Holmes, A. P., Worsley, K. J., Poline J.-P., Frith, C. D., and Frackowiak, S. J. (1995). Statistical parametric maps in functional imaging: A general linear approach. *Hum. Brain Mapping* **2:** 189–210.

Hurtig, R. R., Hichwa, R. D., O'Leary, D. S., Boles Ponto, L. L., Narayana, S., Watkins, G. L., and Andreasen, N. C. (1994). Effects of timing and duration of cognitive activation in [^{15}O] water PET studies. *J. Cereb. Blood Flow Metab.* **14:** 423–430.

Kinahan, P. E., and Rogers, J. G. (1989). Analytic 3D image reconstruction using all detected events. *IEEE Trans. Nucl. Sci.* **36**(1): 964–968.

Roland, P. (1994). "Brain Activation." Wiley-Liss, New York.

Silbersweig, D. A., Stern, E., Frith, C. D., Cahill, C., Schorr, L., Grootoonk, S., Spinks, T., Clark, J., Frackowiak, R. S. J., and Jones, T. (1993). Detection of thirty-second cognitive activations in single subjects with positron emission tomography: A new low-dose [H_2^{15}O] regional cerebral blood flow three-dimensional imaging technique. *J. Cereb. Blood Flow Metab.* **13:** 617–629.

Smith, T., Tong, C., Lammertsma, A. A., Butler, K. R., Schnorr, L., Watson, J. D. G., Ramsay, S., Clark, J. C., and Jones, T. (1994). Dosimetry of intraveneously adminstered oxygen-15 labelled water in man: A model based on experimental human data from 21 subjects. *Eur. J. Nucl. Med.* **21:** 1126–1134.

Talairach, J., and Tourneaux, P. (1988). 3-Dimensional proportional system: An approach to cerebral imaging. "Co-planar Stereotaxic Atlas of the Human Brain." (M. Rayport, trans.), Thieme Medical, New York.

Volkow, N. D., Mullani, N., Gould, L. K., Adler, S. S., and Gatley, S. J. (1991). Sensitivity of measurements of regional brain activation with oxygen-15-water and PET to time of stimulation and period of image reconstruction. *J. Nucl. Med.* **32:** 58–61.

Woods, R. P., Cherry, S. R., and Mazziotta, J. C. (1992). A rapid automated algorithm for accurately aligning and reslicing positron emission tomography images. *J. Comput. Assist. Tomogr.* **16:** 620–634.

81

Mapping of Change in Cerebral Glucose Utilization Using [¹⁸F]FDG Double Injection and New Graphical Analysis

K. MURASE, H. KUWABARA, E. MEYER, A. C. EVANS, and A. GJEDDE

Positron Imaging Laboratories
McConnell Brain Imaging Centre
Montreal Neurological Institute
McGill University
Montreal, Quebec, H3A 2B4, Canada

We proposed a method for mapping the change in cerebral glucose utilization at two different physiological states using double injection of [¹⁸F]fluorodeoxyglucose and graphical analysis. The proposed method allows simple and reliable mapping of change in cerebral glucose utilization during physiological stimulation of the brain.

I. INTRODUCTION

An activation study using positron emission tomography (PET) requires comparison of two different physiological states measured in the control (baseline) and activated (stimulation) sessions. In general, this study requires repeated PET procedures in a subject, thereby increasing the burden on both subjects and investigators as well as the complexity of the procedure. However, a method using double injection of the tracer has several advantages over repeating PET studies in the same subject at different times, because this method allows two PET studies with different physiological states to be performed sequentially and conveniently without moving the subject out of the scanner (Chang *et al.*, 1987).

The purpose of the present study was to develop a simple and reliable method for mapping the change in cerebral glucose utilization at two different physiological states within one scanning sequence using double injection of [¹⁸F]fluorodeoxyglucose (FDG) and graphical analysis.

II. MATERIALS AND METHODS

A. Kinetic Model

The rates of change of FDG content in the precursor ($M_e^*(t)$) and metabolic compartments ($M_m^*(t)$) are given by the following differential equations, with the dephosphorylation of FDG-6-phosphate to FDG being neglected:

$$\frac{dM_e^*(t)}{dt} = K_1^* \, C_a^*(t) - (k_2^* + k_3^*)M_e^*(t) \tag{1}$$

$$\frac{dM_m^*(t)}{dt} = k_3^* \, M_e^*(t) \tag{2}$$

where $C_a^*(t)$ is the FDG concentration in arterial plasma at time t; K_1^*, the unidirectional clearance of FDG from the blood to the brain; k_2^*, the fractional clearance from the brain to the blood; and k_3^*, the phosphorylation coefficient. The FDG content per unit volume of brain measured by PET ($A^*(t)$) is given by $A^*(t) = M_e^*(t) + M_m^*(t) + V_0 C_a^*(t)$, where V_0 is the brain vascular volume.

B. Parameter Estimation

When $t \gg 0$, the brain FDG activity at time t ($A^I(t)$) in the first session divided by $C_a^*(t)$ can be approximated as (Gjedde, 1982; Patlak *et al.*, 1983)

$$\frac{A^I(t)}{C_a^*(t)} = K^I \Theta^I(t) + \left(\frac{K_1^I - K^I}{\beta^I} + V_0^I \right) \tag{3}$$

where $\Theta^I(t) = \int_0^t C_a^*(u)\,du/C_a^*(t)$, $K^I (= K_1^I k_3^I/(k_2^I + k_3^I))$ is the net clearance of FDG to the brain in the first session and $\beta^I = k_2^I + k_3^I$. The superscript I in these equations denotes the first session. Therefore, K^I can be estimated from the slope of the straight part in the plot of $A^I(t)/C_a^*(t)$ vs. $\Theta^I(t)$.

Analysis of the second session requires correction for the FDG content remaining from the first session, which is given by $K^I \int_0^{t_z} C_a^*(u)\,du$ for $t \gg t_z$ (t_z is the end time of the first session). Therefore, when $t \gg t_z$, the brain FDG activity at time t ($A^{II}(t)$) in the second session divided by $C_a^*(t)$ can be approximated as

$$\frac{A^{II}(t) - K^I \int_0^{t_z} C_a^*(u)\,du}{C_a^*(t)} = K^{II}\Theta^{II}(t) + \left(\frac{K_1^{II} - K^{II}}{\beta^{II}} + V_0^{II}\right) \tag{4}$$

where $\Theta^{II}(t) = \int_{t_z}^t C_a^*(u)\,du/C_a^*(t)$ and the superscript II denotes the second session. Therefore, K^{II} can be estimated from the slope of the straight part in the plot of $(A^{II}(t) - K^I \int_0^{t_z} C_a^*(u)\,du)/C_a^*(t)$ versus $\Theta^{II}(t)$.

With the constrained FDG method (Kuwabara *et al.*, 1990), the *y*-intercept of the straight part in the preceding plots can be theoretically obtained by (Yasuhara *et al.*, 1994)

$$\frac{V_d(\alpha - 1)^2}{\alpha(\alpha + \mu)} + V_0 \tag{5}$$

where $\alpha = (\tau - \varphi)/(\Lambda - \varphi)$; and V_d, μ, τ, and φ are the constraint constants (Kuwabara *et al.*, 1990). To stabilize the K^* values against statistical noise, we employed the *y*-intercept determined by equation (5) in addition to the straight part of these plots. In the present study, we assumed that the constraint constants had little regional or intersubject variation (Kuwabara *et al.*, 1990) and the lumped constant did not change during the second session. Furthermore, Λ and V_0 were fixed to 0.52 (Reivich *et al.*, 1985) and 0.036 ml/g (Yasuhara *et al.*, 1994), respectively.

C. PET Studies

First, PET studies were performed without vibrotactile stimulation (baseline–baseline group) to investigate the reliability of the present method. We studied five, right-handed, young normal subjects (age 22.4 ± 1.4 years old). Permission to conduct the study was granted by the Ethics and Research Review Committee of Montreal Neurological Institute and Hospital, and signed consent forms were obtained from the subjects before the study. The tracer was prepared with a Japanese Steel Works Medical Cyclotron (BC-107), and the PET studies were performed with a Scanditronix PC-

2048 15B eight-ring, 15-slice BGO head tomograph with a spatial resolution of about 6 mm FWHM in all three dimensions (Evans *et al.*, 1991a). After correction for tissue attenuation, dead time, scatter, and coincident counts, each PET image was reconstructed in a 128 × 128 matrix of 2 × 2 mm pixels (25.6 mm^3 in volume) using the filtered back projection method with a 20 mm FWHM Hanning filter. The subjects were positioned in the tomograph with their heads immobilized by a customized self-inflating foam headrest. A short indwelling catheter was placed into the left radial artery for blood sampling. FDG uptake was measured during two consecutive 30 min periods of a combined 60 min session. A 185 MBq bolus of FDG was partitioned into two, with the first portion containing approximately 50% of the total dose administered slowly at 0 min and the second portion containing the remainder administered slowly at 29.5 min. The scan schedule was six 30 sec, seven 1 min, five 2 min, and two 5 min scans (first session) immediately followed by six 30 sec, seven 1 min, five 2 min, and two 5 min scans (second session). Plasma samples were taken every 10 sec for the first 3 min after injection of FDG, then with increasingly prolonged intervals of time.

Second, PET studies were performed with vibrotactile stimulation (baseline–stimulation group). We studied five, right-handed, young normal subjects (age 24.5 ± 0.5 years old) as previously described. Vibrotactile stimulation was performed during the second session with a mechanical vibrator (Model 91, Daito, Osaka, Japan) fixed to the five fingertips of the right hand and held in place with tape to maintain a uniform pressure throughout the stimulation period. A vibration frequency of 110 Hz was chosen, and the vibrator was intermittently turned on and off at 1 sec intervals (1 sec on, 1 sec off) to avoid adaptation. The nominal vibration amplitude was 2 mm. The subjects were asked to focus their attention on the vibrotactile stimulus to generate a maximum change in cerebral activity (Meyer *et al.*, 1991).

D. Generation of *t*-Statistic Images

Each PET image data set was first coregistered with its corresponding MRI image volume using a three-dimensional landmark-matching algorithm (Evans *et al.*, 1988, 1991b). The K^* images, calculated from the raw PET data using the present method, were projected into Talairach's stereotaxic coordinates (Talairach and Tournoux, 1988) using the MRI volume for identification of the bicommissural plane (Evans *et al.*, 1991b). For each subject, subtraction images of each K^* map were obtained by subtracting the first-session (baseline) images from the second-session (activation) images. Those subtraction images were then averaged across all subjects and analyzed according to the method of Worsley *et al.* (1992). This analysis yielded a mean percentage change image of K^*. From this result, a *t*-statistic image was calculated by dividing the average change image by the average standard deviation across voxels. For a directed search in the cortex of the postcentral gyrus, which, in Talairach space, occupies approximately 24 cm³, the difference of the K^* value between baseline and activation was statistically significant at $p < 0.05$ for $t > 3.3$ (Worsley *et al.*, 1992).

III. RESULTS AND DISCUSSION

We previously reported a coupling between blood flow and glucose metabolism during vibrotactile stimulation (Kuwabara *et al.*, 1991). In this study, we extended the double injection FDG study to visually compare glucose utilization maps of two different physiological conditions using graphical analysis.

The FDG double-injection method was first introduced by Chang *et al.* (1987). Their method, however, is based on population average rate constants. Therefore, the accuracy of their method is dependent on the discrepancies between the subject and population average rate constants. Additionally, their method requires over a 30 min period in each session to minimize error that arises from the use of population average rate constants, thereby increasing the burden on the subject and investigators.

To investigate the reliability of the present method, we compared the estimates of K^* obtained in the first and second sessions in the baseline–baseline group. To do this, we selected 340 regions of interest (ROIs) on the parametric image of K^* from the five studies in the baseline–baseline group. The average size of the ROIs was 3.5 cm² (thickness 6.4 cm). Regional K^* values in the first and second sessions were strongly correlated ($r = 0.976, n = 340$), indicating the reliability of this method.

In the baseline–stimulation group, the K^* values in the left primary somatosensory cortex (SI) significantly ($p < 0.05$) increased during stimulation from 3.28 ± 0.50 to 3.94 ± 0.77 ml/100 g/min, but those in the right SI did not change significantly (from 3.41 ± 0.52 to 3.39 ± 0.34 ml/100 g/min). These changes corresponded to percent changes of 19.66 ± 6.23 and $-0.07 \pm 6.91\%$, respectively. In this case, a circular ROI with an area of 3.3 cm² was drawn in the left and right postcentral gyrii by aid of MRI–PET registration for anatomical identification of the cerebral structures (Evans *et al.*, 1991b). Ginsberg *et al.* (1988) reported

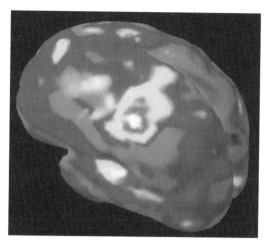

FIGURE 1   Three-dimensional display of the *t*-statistic map of K^*.

that the somatosensory stimulus elevated cerebral glucose utilization by $16.9 \pm 3.5\%$ in the contralateral sensorimotor cortical focus in humans. Our results strongly support the findings of Ginsberg *et al.* (1988).

Fox, Perlmutter, and Raichle (1985) introduced the stereotactic method for PET images and optimized the method of [¹⁵O]water studies of neuronal activation. They further developed an intersubject averaging technique for such studies to increase the signal-to-noise ratio (Fox *et al.*, 1988). In the present study, we used almost the same technique to generate the *t*-statistic map of K^*. Figure 1 shows the three-dimensional display of the *t*-statistic map of K^*. A significant increase in the left SI was clearly demonstrated ($t > 3.3$).

In conclusion, we demonstrated a method for mapping of change in cerebral glucose utilization using FDG double injection and graphical analysis, and the proposed method allows simple and reliable mapping of change in cerebral glucose utilization during physiological stimulation of the brain.

References

Chang, J. Y., Duara, R., Barker, W., Apicella, A., and Finn, R. (1987). Two behavioral states studied in a single PET/FDG procedure: Theory, method, and preliminary results. *J. Nucl. Med.* **28:** 852–860.

Evans, A. C., Beil, C., Marrett, S., Thompson, C. J., and Hakim, A. (1988). Anatomical functional correlation using an adjustable MRI-based region of interest atlas with positron emission tomography. *J. Cereb. Blood Flow Metab.* **8:** 513–530.

Evans, A. C., Thompson, C. J., Marrett, S., Meyer, E., and Mazza, M. (1991a). Performance evaluation of the PC-2048: A new 15-slice encoded-crystal PET scanner for neurological studies. *IEEE Trans. Med. Imag.* **10:** 89–98.

Evans, A. C., Marrett, S., Torrescorzo, J., Ku, S., and Collins, L. (1991b). MRI-PET correlation in three dimensions using volume-of-interest (VOI) atlas. *J. Cereb. Blood Flow Metab.* **11:** 69–78.

Fox, P. T., Perlmutter, J. S., and Raichle, M. E. (1985). A stereotactic method of anatomical localization for positron emission tomography. *J. Comput. Assist. Tomogr.* **9:** 141–153.

Fox, P. T., Mintun, M. A., Reiman, E. M., and Raichle, M. E. (1988). Enhanced detection of focal brain responses using intersubject averaging and change-distribution analysis of subtracted PET images. *J. Cereb. Blood Flow Metab.* **8:** 642–653.

Ginsberg, M. D., Chang, J. Y., Kelley, R. E., Yoshii, F., Barker, W. W., Ingenito, G., and Boothe, T. E. (1988). Increase in both cerebral glucose utilization and blood flow during execution of a somatosensory task. *Ann. Neurol.* **23:** 152–160.

Gjedde, A. (1982). Calculation of glucose phosphorylation from brain uptake of glucose analogs in vivo: A re-examination. *Brain Res. Rev.* **4:** 237–274.

Kuwabara, H., Ohta, S., Meyer, E., and Gjedde, A. (1991). Attenuation of flow-glucose metabolism coupling studied by PET. *J. Nucl. Med.* **32:** 910P.

Kuwabara, H., Evans, A. C., and Gjedde, A. (1990). Michaelis-Menten constraints improved cerebral glucose metabolism and regional lumped constant measurements with [^{18}F] fluorodeoxyglucose. *J. Cereb. Blood Flow Metab.* **10:** 180–189.

Meyer, E., Ferguson, S. S., Zatorre, R. J., Alivisatos, B., Marrett, S., Evans, A. C., and Hakim, A. M. (1991). Attention modulates somatosensory cerebral blood flow response to vibrotactile stimulation as measured by positron emission tomography. *Ann. Neurol.* **29:** 440–443.

Patlak, C. S., Blasberg, R. G., and Fenstermacher, J. D. (1983). Graphical evaluation of blood-to-brain transfer constants from multiple-time uptake data. *J. Cereb. Blood Flow Metab.* **3:** 1–7.

Reivich, M., Alavi, A., Wolf, A., Fowler, J., Russell, J., Arnett, C., MacGregor, R., Shiue, C., Atkins, H., and Anand, A. (1985). Glucose metabolic rate kinetic model parameter determination in humans: The lumped constants and rate constants for [^{18}F]fluorodeoxyglucose and [^{11}C]deoxyglucose. *J. Cereb. Blood Flow Metab.* **5:** 179–192.

Talairach, J., and Tournoux, P. (1988). "Co-Planar Atlas of the Human Brain." Thieme, Stuttgart.

Worsley, K. J., Evans, A. C., Marrett, S., and Neelin, P. (1992). A three-dimensional statistical analysis for CBF activation studies in human brain. *J. Cereb. Blood Flow Metab.* **12:** 900–918.

Yasuhara, Y., Kuwabara, H., Reutens, D., Murase, K., and Gjedde, A. (1994). Constructing glucose metabolism images with single PET scan and single arterial sample. *J. Nucl. Med.* **35:** 185P–186P.

82

PET Imaging of Neuromodulation
Designing Experiments to Detect Endogenous Transmitter Release

EVAN D. MORRIS,[1] RONALD E. FISHER,[1] SCOTT L. RAUCH,[2] ALAN J. FISCHMAN,[1] and NATHANIEL M. ALPERT[1]

[1]*Radiology and* [2]*Psychiatry Departments, Massachusetts General Hospital and Harvard Medical School, Boston, Massachusetts 02114*

This simulation study examines the possibility of using PET and bolus injections of a receptor ligand to detect changes in release of an endogenous neurotransmitter caused by the performance of a cognitive or motor task. Simulations were generated using a compartmental model for receptor binding that had been expanded to include competition between exogenous ligand and endogenous transmitter. Cognitive activation was modeled as causing a step-change in transmitter concentration. The dopamine system was simulated because the kinetics of the D_2 receptor ligand, $[^{11}C]$-raclopride, are well characterized. Estimates were made regarding the concentration and kinetics of intrasynaptic dopamine based on existing neurophysiological and biochemical literature. The χ^2 parameter was used to measure the differences between simulated time–activity curves of the resting and activated states. Larger differences indicate better detectability of transmitter release. We first examined the detectability of dopamine release due to a 7 min activation task beginning at the time of $[^{11}C]$raclopride injection. Next, we investigated the relationship between the binding characteristics of radioligands and detectability. Interestingly, detectability did not correlate with the equilibrium affinity constant, K_D. Rather, simulations indicated that detectability could be maximized by the use of an irreversible ligand, that is, a ligand with a very small dissociation rate constant. The timing of the activation task was examined for various ligands. To optimize detectability, a task must be started when the bolus of radioligand is injected. Simulations showed that the effect of transmitter release could be masked by the likely simultaneous increase in rCBF, thus, changes in blood flow during activation must be accounted for by the model. Finally, we demonstrated

that the prospects for detecting transmitter release are not affected by raclopride binding sites (i.e., the D_2 receptor) being distributed both intra- and extrasynaptically. We feel that these simulations should encourage further theoretical investigations into the use of PET for detection of transmitter release with cognitive activation as well as provide some guidelines on how to proceed experimentally.

I. INTRODUCTION

Until recently, receptor-specific ligands have been used qualitatively in PET to localize binding sites and quantitatively to assay for the density of (available) receptor sites *in vivo*. Recent work, however, has shown PET measurements with dopamine ligands to be sensitive to changes in basal release of endogenous dopamine (Ross and Jackson, 1989; Seeman *et al.*, 1989; Dewey *et al.*, 1993). Dewey *et al.* (1992) have taken advantage of this phenomenon to indirectly explore the interaction of various neurotransmitter systems *in vivo*. Following on this body of work, we investigated the possibility of using PET to detect increased release of endogenous neurotransmitter that we presume will accompany cognitive activation.

The main neuromodulatory transmitters such as norepinephrine, acetylcholine, dopamine, and serotonin have been implicated in numerous brain functions such as attention, arousal, learning, and memory. Currently, PET can investigate how various cognitive tasks activate which brain regions by measuring changes in regional cerebral blood flow. From these studies the links between particular neurotransmitters and cognitive

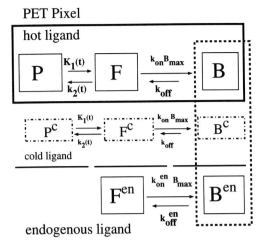

FIGURE 1 Schematic diagram of compartmental model. Model includes compartments to account for the effect of endogenous neurotransmitter (e.g., dopamine) on radioligand binding.

functions can be only inferred from the predominance of certain types of neuromodulatory synapses in those brain regions shown to have increased rCBF.

This simulation study was designed first to determine whether PET could be used to assess the role of neuromodulatory neurons in human brain function by identifying changes in transmitter release associated with a cognitive or motor task. To do so, we modified existing receptor binding models that have hitherto assumed that endogenous neurotransmitter levels remained in steady state during the PET experiment. Second, we sought to optimize the likelihood of detecting the phenomenon. We examined the effect of changing the radioligand's kinetics on the PET output and the importance of the length and timing of the task. Finally, we used simulations to consider the possible impact of changes in blood flow or distribution of (intra- versus extrasynaptic) receptors on the PET signals from experiments that we propose here to compare resting and activated states.

II. METHODS

A. Theory

The model used for the simulations presented here is diagrammed in Figure 1. This model is adapted from the one published by Delforge *et al.* (1990) for describing kinetics of labeled and unlabeled ligand in PET studies designed to measure the density of available receptor sites. To the existing model, we have two added compartments (below the long dashed line) to

account for the presence of endogenous transmitter in either the free state (i.e., in the synapse) or bound to the receptor in question. As indicated in Figure 1, the three species are modeled as competing for the same limited number of binding sites and it is through the term for receptor availability ($B_{max} - B - B^c - B^{en}$) that the three segments of the model are coupled, mathematically. The model equations follow. For labeled ligand compartments,

$$\frac{dF}{dt} = K_1 C_p(t) - k_2 F - k_{on} F [B_{max} - B - B^c - B^{en}] + k_{off} B - k_5 F + k_6 NS - \lambda F \quad (1)$$

$$\frac{dB}{dt} = k_{on} F [B_{max} - B - B^c - B^{en}] - k_{off} B - k_5 F + k_6 NS - \lambda B \quad (2)$$

For unlabeled ligand compartments,

$$\frac{dF^c}{dt} = K_1 C_p^c(t) - k_2 F^c - k_{on} F^c [B_{max} - B - B^c - B^{en}] + k_{off} B^c - k_5 F^c + k_6 NS^c \quad (3)$$

$$\frac{dB^c}{dt} = k_{on} F^c [B_{max} - B - B^c - B^{en}] - k_{off} B^c - k_5 F^c + k_6 NS^c \quad (4)$$

For endogenous transmitter compartments,

$$\frac{dB^{en}}{dt} = k_{on}^{en} F^{en} [B_{max} - B - B^c - B^{en}] - k_{off}^{en} B^{en} \quad (5)$$

$$F^{en} = F^{en}(0) + A * U(t - t_{up}) - A * U(t - t_{down}) \quad (6)$$

The superscripts *c* and *en* refer to cold ligand and endogenous chemical, respectively; λ is the decay constant for the isotope and it appears only in the equations pertaining to hot ligand. Equation (6) describes the step change in free endogenous transmitter that we attribute to a change in activation state.

B. Parameter Values

To perform simulations of the proposed experiments, model parameters were needed to describe the kinetics of both the radioligand, [^{11}C]raclopride, and the endogenous transmitter, dopamine. For the raclopride parameters, we used the rate constants published by Farde *et al.* (1989) for binding in the putamen of human subjects. Our model differs from the standard three-compartment model for receptor binding in its inclusion of terms for free and bound endogenous neurotransmitter. We define B_{max} differently from the way it is defined in Farde *et al.* (1989). In this chapter, B_{max}

refers to all the receptors, either free, bound to the exogenous ligand, or bound to the endogenous transmitter. In our simulations, we took B_{max} to be double the number published by Farde on the assumption that 50% of receptors are bound to endogenous dopamine at any one time and therefore were not measured by the classical PET receptor assay.

The K_D for binding of dopamine to the D_2 receptor has been measured in various *in vitro* and other preparations. We have chosen an average value of 100 nM (for a review of the pertinent literature, see Fisher *et al.*, 1995), this is the value measured *in vitro* by Ross and Jackson (1989) in mouse striatal preparations. The resting concentration of dopamine in the free space, $F^{en}(0)$ (i.e., in the synaptic cleft), and the increase in concentration due to activation needed to be estimated before the simulations could be run. Of course, the synaptic dopamine concentration is not a constant but fluctuates with every firing of a presynaptic neuron. For slow neuromodulatory synapses, the firing rate is roughly 5 Hz at rest and approximately 10 Hz in activation. Nevertheless, on the time scale of a PET scan we can talk about average dopamine concentrations. For the current simulations, we have taken the resting concentration to be 100 nM rising to 200 nM during activation. In addition to being derived from many studies in the literature (see Fisher *et al.*, 1995), these numbers have the added appeal of dictating that at rest exactly half of all receptors exist in the bound state.

The simulations of the proposed experiments that follow correspond to a single high specific activity injection of [^{11}C]raclopride (or other theoretical ligand). Dynamic PET scanning was simulated as consisting of 60 contiguous 1 minute acquisitions. Activation was modeled as causing a step change in endogenous neurotransmitter, which, unless otherwise noted, begins at the moment of injection of the radioligand. The simulations are compared on the basis of the predicted detectability of the activation phenomenon. Detectability is measured via the χ^2, $\chi^2 = \Sigma_i [(a_i - r_i)/\sigma_i]^2$, which is a measure of the difference between the resting (r_i) and activated (a_i) curves, inversely weighted by their respective variances σ_i^2. The χ^2 parameter is unitless.

III. RESULTS AND DISCUSSION

A. Simulated Experiments with [^{11}C]Raclopride

In Figure 2 we show the simulated PET data that we would expect from a pair of neurotransmitter release experiments (resting and activated) using a bolus injec-

tion of [^{11}C]raclopride. In this simulation, activation lasts for the first 7 min of imaging. Cessation of activation, which would be accomplished experimentally by termination of a dopaminergic cognitive task, leads to nearly immediate drop in endogenous dopamine. This, in turn, leads to increased receptor availability—shown in dashed line in Figure 2(a). Note that even at rest (after minute 7), the number of available receptors does not reach the total number of receptors, B_{max} (solid line), because a considerable number of receptors are assumed to be occupied at any moment by dopamine. Figure 2(b) shows the resting PET concentration of [^{11}C]raclopride in filled circles and the PET output expected for the 7 min activation task (solid curve). As expected, the presence of increased dopamine during activation leads to greater competition with the labeled ligand, lower binding to the receptor than in the resting case and therefore lower tissue activity. Figure 2(c) displays the normalized residuals for the data in Figure 27(b). The residuals (defined as resting - activated) are negative everywhere because transmitter release lowers labeled ligand binding.

B. Effect of Ligand Kinetics on Activation Detectability

Although Figure 2 suggests that the degree of increase in dopamine we have hypothesized will cause significant changes in the measured PET signal, we sought to optimize these changes to guarantee detectability of the activation phenomenon and understand the role of the ligand characteristics in this process. We examined the effects of kinetics by simulating the resting and activated curves (as in Fig. 2) for theoretical ligands whose association and dissociation rates we varied. Figure 3 shows the results of a theoretical ligand whose kinetics are the same as raclopride except that its dissociation rate from the D_2 receptor is 10 times slower. Careful examination of the receptor availability plot in Figure 3(a) reveals that the receptor sites are recovered more slowly following the termination of activation than in the comparable plot in Figure 2(a). However, the striking finding is evident in Figures 2(b) and 2(c). These figures show that the effect of competition by dopamine with a PET ligand that is fairly irreversible persists throughout a 40 min study as compared to the resting scan with the same ligand. The magnitude of the fractional residuals in Figure 3(c) reflect this persistent difference between curves, which could be used to identify activation.

Our investigations into the effect of various modifications to the D_2 receptor ligand kinetics are catalogued by the bar graph in Figure 4. The top horizontal bar, labeled *Raclopride*, indicates the χ^2 value ($\chi^2 \sim 5,300$)

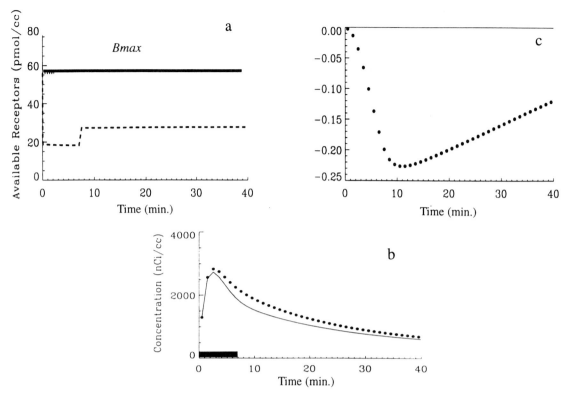

FIGURE 2   Simulations of model in Figure 1 based on kinetic parameters for [¹¹C]raclopride: (a) predicted
receptor availability (dashed line) plot, sharp increase in available receptors corresponds to termination of
activation; (b) simulated PET activity curves for resting (filled circles) and activated (solid curve). Length
and timing of activation task (0–7 min) indicated by heavy solid bar along *x*-axis. (c) Normalized residuals:
(activated value - resting value)/resting value.

associated with the difference between the resting and
activated curves shown in Figure 2(b). The bar labeled
90% lower k_{off} corresponds to the measure of the difference between the curves in Figure 3(b). The largest χ^2
value resulted from a simulation using a ligand with
completely irreversible binding to the receptor ($\chi^2 \sim$
18000). The second group of two bars correspond to
simulations where the K_D is fixed at the raclopride
value (9.9 n*M*) but the on and off rates are either decreased or increased 10-fold, in unison. Neither of
these simulations gives a larger χ^2 value than the raclopride simulation. The third tier of bars is for ligands
whose off rates are slower than raclopride. The result
is that the slower is the dissociation of the radioligand,
the larger is the difference between rest and activation.
Of course, by changing either the association or dissociation rate constants in our simulations, we change
the equilibrium constant, K_D. The K_D associated with
each simulation is annotated to the right of the corresponding bar. The bottom tier grouping of bars is for
ligands whose K_D is the same as the previous group,

but in this case the on rates have been increased. Only
the simulation with a k_{on} value twice that of the control
is even marginally better than raclopride. The others
yield lower χ^2 values. Comparison of equilibrium constant values with their χ^2 values reveals no apparent
correlation between K_D and detectability of transmitter
release. These simulations lead us to realize that what
is critical in our experiment are transient and not equilibrium phenomena. Recall that these stimulations reflect the behavior of tracer pursuant to bolus injections—not infusions—and the impact of activation
tasks that alter the endogenous transmitter briefly. No
steady state is achieved for either tracer or transmitter
during these simulated studies. In the case of irreversible tracers, we believe that the "success" of these
simulations lies in the coalescence of two kinetic properties: (1) increased competition at the beginning of the
study when lots of the radioligand is still in the free state
and (2) predominance of (irreversibly) bound tracer in
the overall PET signal at later time in the study (see
Morris *et al.*, 1995, for more explanation).

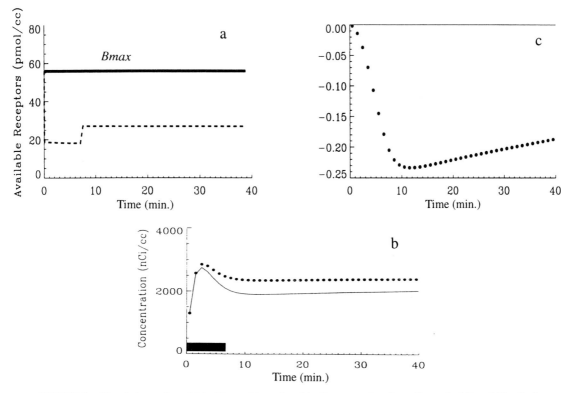

FIGURE 3   Simulations of model in Figure 1 based on kinetic parameters for a theoretical ligand identical to raclopride in all respects except that its dissociation rate constant, k_{off}, is one-tenth that of raclopride. (a) Receptor availability; (b) simulated PET activity curves; (c) normalized residuals.

C. Effects of Activation Timing

The apparent importance of system dynamics in the first minutes of the study led us to investigate the effects of task timing on detectability. For raclopride, the χ^2 value increases almost linearly with the task length. For more irreversible ligands, the effect of extending the task diminishes with tasks longer than 7–10 min (data not shown here). We investigated the effect of delaying the task following injection of radioligand. For these simulations, the task length was fixed at 7 min. Figure 5 shows the relationship between χ^2 value and task delay time for theoretical ligands of different dissociation rate constants. In all cases examined, the consequence of delaying the "turning on" competition (i.e., beginning the task) is catastrophic. In our bolus injection scheme, delay of the task by 10 or more min would be sufficient to obliterate all effects of activation.

D. Effects of Blood Flow Changes with Activation

To this point, we have ignored any possible change in regional cerebral blood flow during our simulated PET studies, although such changes seem likely. Figure 6 displays the simulation output for the case where change in blood flow in the region of interest is modeled as directly paralleling the change in transmitter concentration. That is, during the 7 min period of activation, the blood flow parameters, K_1 and k_2, are modeled as increasing by 100%. The kinetic parameters used for this simulation are otherwise those of raclopride. Figure 6(a) shows that receptor availability for this simulation is identical to that in Figure 2(a). Figure 6(b) shows the comparison between a resting PET scan and an activated scan that includes both increased competition and increased flow for 0–7 min. The PET curves are nearly indistinguishable; the χ^2 measure of difference in the curves is only about 200. The minimal differences between these resting and activated PET curves should serve as a warning to experimenters that effects of rCBF changes must be removed from the activated curve—or added to the control curve—before the changes due to transmitter release can be assessed. How do we know whether blood flow has changed during activation? The characteristic pattern of residuals for this simulation (see Figure 6(c)), which includes positive values at early times followed by negative val-

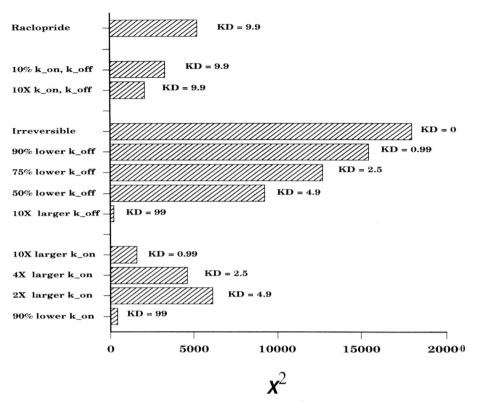

FIGURE 4 Optimal ligand kinetics. Comparison of χ^2 values for simulated experiments with various theoretical ligands. The χ^2 parameter measures the difference between the resting and activated curves and therefore is a measure of detectability of activation.

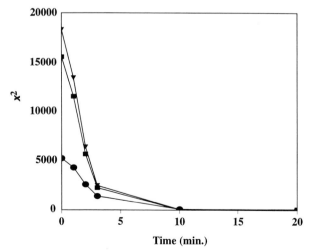

FIGURE 5 Optimal task delay. Comparison of detectability vs. time delay (min) of task from time of injection. Ligands with three different dissociation rate constants are examined: native raclopride, $k_{off} = 0.099$ (●), $k_{off} = 0.0099$ (■), and irreversible $k_{off} = 0$ (▼).

ues, reflects the competing forces of increased delivery of radioligand by high flow and decreased retention of radioligand due to competition with endogenous dopamine. We suggest that this recognizable pattern of residuals in an actual experiment can serve as an indicator of increased blood flow. To properly analyze these studies, however, it is advisable to perform complementary blood flow measurements (e.g., with [^{15}O] before and during activation task) so that the changes in rCBF due to activation can be taken into account. Once such measurements have been made, we propose that a proper "resting" curve can be simulated by using time-varying values for K_1 and k_2 that increase during activation. It is this corrected curve that should be compared to the activated curve shown (solid curve) in Figure 6(b).

E. Intra- vs. Extrasynaptic Receptors

This simulation study is a preliminary attempt to anticipate the likelihood of detecting neurotransmitter release with PET. To keep the model tractable, we have necessarily simplified our portrayal of the receptor ligand binding system. One of the simplifications

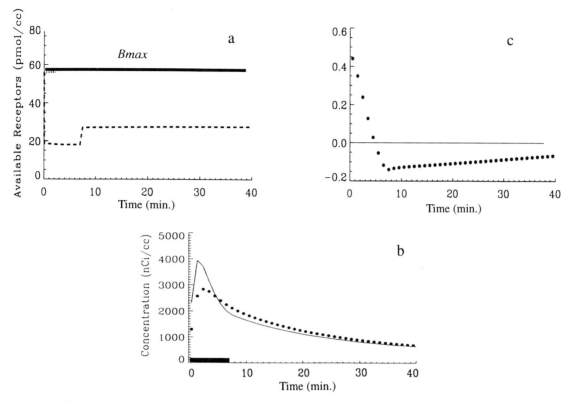

FIGURE 6   Simulations of model in Figure 1 for variable flow parameters K_1, k_2. The same parameters are used as in Figure 3, except that K_1 and k_2 are increased 100% during activation (0–7 min) to reflect increased rCBF during that time. (a) Receptor availability, (b) simulated PET activity curves, (c) normalized residuals.

made to this point was to assume that all D_2 receptors are located within the synapse so that the pertinent concentrations of dopamine to estimate were the intrasynaptic ones. In fact, it has been demonstrated that the D_1 receptor may exist primarily extrasynaptically (Smiley *et al.*, 1994). We attempted to determine whether the presence of extrasynaptic D_2 receptors would significantly alter our findings. If D_2 receptors were distributed both intra- and extrasynaptically, then a comprehensive model of the system would need to include two free and two binding compartments. The resulting model would be quite complicated. A simpler approach is displayed in Figure 7. Here we assume that all D_2 receptors are extrasynaptic. Although the kinetic parameters for this simulation are the same as those used for Figure 2, the concentrations of dopamine during rest and activation were chosen to reflect estimates of extrasynaptic dopamine levels. Studies suggest that the appropriate levels are 30 and 90 nM, respectively (Gonon and Buda, 1985). The receptor availability plot in Figure 7(a) is higher than in previous figures, reflecting the lower average dopamine levels extrasynaptically. Figure 7 shows that the difference between rest and activated PET curves is actually

slightly larger ($\chi^2 = 7400$) than for the simulation of Figure 2. We suggest that the simulations in Figures 2 and 7 can be taken together to bracket the possible distributions of D_2 receptors between the intra- and extrasynaptic space. This possibility seems not be be a cause for concern.

F. Other Neurotransmitters

Finally, we conclude with some speculation as to the importance of the proposed experiments to the investigation of other neurotransmitter systems. Recent articles by Jacobs and Fornal (1993, 1994) have elucidated the importance of the serotonin system in cats in maintaining muscle tone and facilitating repetitive movements. During REM sleep, when cats are devoid of muscle tone, their serotonin neurons are silent. Based on these findings and the success of selective serotonin reuptake inhibitors in alleviating symptoms of some people with obsessive–compulsive disorder, Jacobs (1994) hypothesizes that there is a connection between the two. He questions whether certain individuals might be engaging in repetitive actions such as hand washing in an attempt to up-regulate

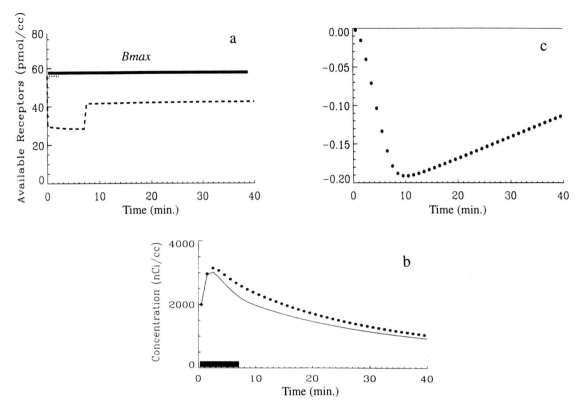

FIGURE 7 Simulations of model in Figure 1 for extrasynaptic concentrations of dopamine. The same parameters are used as in Figure 3, but the resting dopamine level $F^{en}(0) = 30$ nM and the change in dopamine due to activation (from 0–7 min) $A = 60$ nM. (a) Receptor availability, (b) simulated PET activity curves, (c) normalized residuals.

their serotonin systems; that is, to self-medicate. The close association of obsessive and compulsive symptomatology leads him to speculate similarly about the cause of repetitive obsessional thoughts. With the appropriate PET ligand for serotonin, one might be able to test this hypothesis in humans. The ligand [18F]-setoperone has been used to image 5-HT$_2$ receptors in humans (Fischman *et al.*, 1995). Conveniently, it has been found to be fairly irreversible in preliminary modeling attempts (personal communication, A. Bonab).

We believe that the simulation study presented here provides some good basis for further investigation into the possibility of detecting endogenous neurotransmitter release with PET. As we have suggested, even if initial attempts at these experiments are unsuccessful, there may be various ways to optimize the likelihood of detecting this phenomena that should be considered.

Acknowledgments

Dr. Morris wishes to acknowledge support of PHS training grant T32 CA 09362.

Dr. Rauch wishes to acknowledge NIMH grant MH01215 and the Pfizer-sponsored Harvard-MIT Clinical Investigator training Program.

References

Delforge, J., Syrota, A., and Mazoyer, B. M. (1990). Identifiability analysis and parameter identification of an in vivo ligand-receptor model from PET data. *IEEE Trans. Biomed. Eng.* **37**(7): 653–661.

Dewey, S. L., Smith, G. S., Logan, J., Brodie, J. D., Fowler, J. S., and Wolf, A. P. (1993). Striatal binding of the PET ligand 11C-raclopride is altered by drugs that modify synaptic dopamine levels. *Synapse* **13**: 350–356.

Dewey, S. L., Smith, G. S., Logan, J., Brodie, J. D., Yu, D.-W., Ferrier, R. A., King, P. T., MacGregor, R. R., Martin, T. P., Wolf, A. P., Volkow, N. D., Fowler, J. S., and Meller, E. (1992). GABAergic inhibition of endogenous dopamine release measured in vivo with 11C-raclopride and positron emission tomography. *J. Neurosci.* **12**:(10): 3773–3780.

Farde, L., Eriksson, L., Blomqvist, G., and Halldin, C. (1989). Kinetic analysis of [11C]raclopride binding to D2-dopamine receptors studied by PET—A comparison to the equilibrium analysis. *J. Cereb. Blood Flow Metab.* **9**: 696–708.

Fischman, A. J., Bonab, A. A., Babich, J. W., Callahan, R. J., and Alpert, N. M. (1995). PET imaging of human pituitary 5-HT2 receptors with F-18 setoperone. *J. Nucl. Med.* **36**: 15 (abstr.).

Fisher, R. E., Morris, E. D., Alpert, N. M., and Fischman, A. J. (1995). In-vivo imaging of neuromodulatory synaptic transmission using PET: A review of relevant neurophysiology. *Hum. Brain Mapping* **3:** 24–34.

Gonon, F. G., and Buda, M. J. (1985). Regulation of dopamine release by impulse flow and by autoreceptors as studied by in vivo voltammetry in the rat striatum. *Neurosci.* **14**(3): 765–774.

Jacobs, B. L. (1994). Serotonin, motor activity and depression-related disorders. *Am. Scientist* **82:** 457–463.

Jacobs, B. L., and Fornal, C. A. (1993). 5-HT and motor control: A hypothesis. *TINS* **16:** 346–352.

Morris, E. D., Fisher, R. E., Alpert, N. M., Rauch, S. L., and Fischman, A. J. (1995). In vivo imaging of neuromodulation using positron emission tomography: Optimal ligand characteristics and task length for detection of activation. *Hum. Brain Mapping* **3:** 35–55.

Ross, S. B., and Jackson, D. M. (1989). Kinetic properties of the in vivo accumulation of 3H-(—)-N-n-propylnorapomorphine in mouse brain. *Naunyn-Schmiedeberg's Arch. Pharmcol.* **340:** 13–20.

Seeman, P., Guan, H.-C., and Niznik, H. B. (1989). Endogenous dopamine lowers the dopamine D2 receptor density as measured by [3H]raclopride: Implications for positron emission tomography of the Human brain. *Synapse* **3:** 96–97.

Smiley, J. F., Levey, A. I., Ciliax, B. J., and Goldman-Rakic, P. S. (1994). D1 dopamine receptor immunoreactivity in human and monkey cerebral cortex: Predominant and extrasynaptic localization in dendritic spines. *PNAS (USA)* **91:** 5720–5724.

83

Statistical Analysis Summary

A. C. EVANS

Montreal Neurological Institute
McGill University
McConnell Brain Imaging Centre
Montreal, Quebec, H3A 2B4, Canada

I. INTRODUCTION

The final part of the meeting was a mixture of papers on statistics and biology with occasional overlap, where the physiological basis of statistical models were considered. In the statistical domain, there were noticeable trends and occasionally surprising omissions in the presentations. The session is summarized under the three headings of statistics, physiology, and anatomy.

II. COMPARISONS OF STATISTICAL METHODS

The choice of statistical methods (in general) usually proceeds as follows:

- Design of the experiment; that is, how we assign treatments to the subjects.
- Exploratory analysis of data to suggest features to look for, such as principal components.
- Choice of test statistic to detect features, such as peak height, region size, but also including such issues as voxel vs. pooled standard deviation.
- Setting the false positive rate, either by theory (validated by Monte-Carlo simulations) or by simulations themselves.
- Estimating the parameters of interest, once detected, such as location of activation, including errors for these estimates if possible.

In this session we saw contributions to all these aspects of statistical methods. The simplest methods

to apply are those that reduce the data to ROI averages. This allows us to open the full toolbox of "traditional" statistical methods to apply to the problem. Pawlik and Thiel (Chapter 67) emphasized the need to ensure proper normality and independence before applying those tools, using a Box–Cox transformation to impose normality and a Mahalanobis transformation on ROI values to eliminate regional correlations. Strother *et al.* (Chapter 73) approached the problem with a nonparametric approach using the SSM method based on principal components. They reported data indicating that these task-independent differences (subject effects) are considerably larger than the common task-specific response being sought, throwing doubt on the simple noise models employed in current parametric approaches.

Although the ROI techniques are much more manageable, both in computing time and variety of available methods, they do require a subjective decision on region boundaries. Most of the other contributions looked at voxel data analysis, where such decisions are avoided, usually at the expense of a greater number of independent tests. Experimental design was studied by Woods *et al.* (Chapter 68), who advocated replication of conditions within subjects and a corresponding extra dimension in three-way ANOVA or ANCOVA (subject × task × replication) to reduce error variance. This should be encouraged, if for no other reason than to allow the practitioner to check the statistician by making sure that no activation is detected when replicates of the same condition are compared.

Once the design has been chosen, the data are collected and then handed to the statistician to find inter-

434

esting features. Worsley *et al.* (Chapter 64) derived a precise general formula for the *p*-value or false positive rate of peak activation in the commonly used random fields (Gaussian, χ^2, *t*, and *F*) over search regions of any shape or size in four dimensions and over a range of scales. Notwithstanding the intimidating array of equations, Worsley reassured the audience that the method is straightforward to use within the limits dictated by its parametric assumptions. It generalizes earlier special cases for assessing single peak significance derived by Worsley and by Friston but does not directly address issues related to correlated activation of a number of regions (i.e., networks) or to peak extent.

Region extent and peak height have been combined in the methods suggested by Crivello *et al.* (Chapter 66), who report the interesting fact that signal location is more variable than signal height across subjects. If this is due to intersubject differences in neuroanatomy, then it suggests that much is to be gained by nonlinear warping methods that can better align the images before analysis is performed.

All methods of analyzing smooth images, using either region size or peak height, need to estimate the smoothness so that proper allowance can be made for searching over voxels. In most methods, the smoothness enters the calculation through the resels, or resolution elements, equal to the volume searched divided by the effective FWHM of the point spread function. The latter is estimated from the derivatives of the images, and Poline *et al.* (Chapter 69) have reminded us that this, too, is random and hence contributes to the overall variability of the test. Fortunately, its effect seems to be a slight reduction in sensitivity but not in specificity, with a range of $\pm 20\%$ in *p*-value.

Validating the false positive rate on null data is only one side of the coin; the other is examining the true positive rate or sensitivity at detecting features of interest. Antoine *et al.* (not submitted for publication) have taken up this arduous task and used some massive simulations to show us how the detection probability depends on the signal height and width and on the filter width.

The studies of statistical detection power and the use of scale space as an extra search dimension generally addressed the problem of detecting a single peak. Given a peak of a particular size, there will be a smoothing filter that is optimal for detecting that peak. However, in general one does not know the number, size, or separation of individual foci *a priori*. Hence, there will always be a trade-off between detectability and peak discrimination.

All the elegant theory discussed so far does not come without a price; namely, the assumption of some fairly strong conditions. The practitioner should always be aware that departures from these conditions may weaken the methods, but not totally invalidate them; the main question is how sensitive they are to these departures. This sort of question perhaps can be resolved only by validation on real data, which is why replicated conditions are so valuable. Fortunately Holmes *et al.* (Chapter 65) have provided us with a guaranteed assumption-free procedure that pays only a small price in sensitivity. The main cost is computational effort, which always seems to detract from these methods; as soon as computer power increases to make the necessary randomizations feasible, the theoreticians come up with a yet more complex method for which the feasibility of randomization is just out of reach.

This wealth of different techniques for registration, standardization, filtering, test statistic, and interpretation have been grouped into several "approaches" or even coded into "packages" such as SPM. Often the methods are very similar, but there are enough small differences in the details to make the practitioner wonder about which one to choose. Three presentations have compared these "approaches." Missimer *et al.* (Chapter 76) compared the SPM and computerized brain atlas (CBA) methods and the effect of varying the filter width with a voluntary index flexion task. Both packages use roughly similar methods of *t*-maps followed by test of region extent (or cluster size), using all permutations of spatial standardization or statistical analysis from SPM or CBA. The results suggested a greater number of peaks (≥ 21) when using the SPM spatial standardization as opposed to the CBA method (≤ 4). Conversely, the CBA statistical analysis resulted in about twice as many peaks as the SPM approach for the same standardization procedure. As always, lacking knowledge of the right answer, the interpretation of these results is difficult. Arndt *et al.* (Chapter 75) compared the Montreal method (Worsley *et al.*; Chapter 64) and SPM and reported that "neither method emerged as strikingly different or strikingly preferable." Grabowski *et al.* (Chapter 74) made a more extensive comparison of four methods: CDA Montreal, SPM, and RER (i.e., rerandomization, Holmes *et al.*; Chapter 65) and concluded that they were "remarkably concordant."

What about the more fundamental question of how the same analysis method performs in the hands of different investigators at different centers using different subjects and different languages? The EU Concerted Action on Functional Imaging group (Poline Chapter 72) reported the results of a very large study where 12 PET centers performed the same verbal fluency task. They concluded that "intercenter scanner sensitivity seems to be the most crucial factor." The author reported that, despite these confounding methodological factors, the results obtained at different centers were "strikingly similar." This was somewhat at odds with a table, showing from 1 to 16 peaks from individual sites, which caused some discussion. This apparent discrepancy was presumably a consequence of the effect of variations in scanner sensitivity on noise levels and the binary decision for inclusion or rejection of a suprathreshold peak as significant. This emphasizes the inherent dangers of traditional threshold analysis, which can exaggerate small differences in peak height and cause misleading conclusions.

III. PHYSIOLOGY

Egan *et al.* (Chapter 80) reminded us that magnitude and persistence of a focal activation observed in an image is dependent upon many factors. They suggested that comparing scans acquired during and after stimulation may discriminate task-specific from more generalized responses. Because the observed signal is a complex function of duration and timing for injection and stimulus, input function shape, and the temporal profile of the physiological response, it is not clear how to predefine an optimal schedule for frame acquisition. Of course, list mode acquisition is always possible at the expense of disk space.

A much-discussed issue in recent years in the statistics of PET activation studies has been the relationship between the magnitude of focal CBF change (ΔCBF) and the resting CBF value. Kanno *et al.* (Chapter 70) measured ΔCBF in a region as a function of its baseline CBF and demonstrated proportionality under both activation and deactivation conditions over a baseline CBF range of 30–60 ml/100 g/min. A lively discussion followed on the implications of this finding for statistics based on ANOVA (proportional, one-parameter) or ANCOVA (additive two-parameter) models. The study did not compare the validity of the two models for fitting the results. Also, Friston noted that the work did not regress local flow on global flow, implying that baseline CBF in a region may not be proportional to global CBF over the same range and, by extension, that the ANCOVA model may still be correct. The work of Ramsay *et al.* (*J. Physiol,* **471:**521–534, 1993) was raised as support for the ANCOVA method. Evans responded that the conclusion of this paper acknowledged an inability to reject either hypothesis. Holmes noted that the models perform comparably over the typical range of flows observed in activation studies.

A number of groups investigated the possibility of

activating changes in physiological measures other than blood flow. Murase *et al.* (Chapter 81) demonstrated focal changes in SI and SII glucose utilization during vibrotactile stimulation using an FDG double-injection paradigm. In a word-repetition task, Fink *et al.* (Chapter 79) demonstrated that the CBF and CMR$_{glu}$ responses had similar magnitude, although the latter changes showed greater spatial extent. Perhaps the most exciting new area concerns the possibility of altering receptor ligand binding by inducing changes in endogenous transmitter concentration during stimulation. Morris *et al.* (Chapter 82) performed simulation studies with compartmental models of ligand kinetics to design experiments that optimize the detectability of such transient signals. They concluded that stimulation tasks should last at least 7 min, commencing at injection time, although these results were specific to their model, which requires an irreversible ligand. It was not clear how displacement studies with reversible ligands should be performed. Questions were raised regarding the omission of noise in the simulations, the assumption of 50% occupancy, and the extent to which concomitant changes in CBF might mask any changes in ligand binding caused by changes in endogenous transmitter concentration. Other chapters in the Kinetic Analysis part discussed this topic with real data. For instance, Malizia *et al.* (Chapter 52) explored the capability of SPM, combined with a single compartmental model adjusted for time-dependent changes, to detect focal changes in model parameters for [^{11}C]flumazenil, elicited by preloading or displacement challenge. Weeks *et al.* (not submitted for publication) used a related approach to study differences in binding of [^{11}C]diprenorphine between normal and disease states. Here, however, the authors derived model parameters using a spectral analysis approach before voxel-statistic analysis of the parametric maps with SPM. The results were consistent with the known pathophysiology of Huntington's disease and suggested the involvement of previously unsuspected cortical regions in Tourette's syndrome.

IV. ANATOMY

Toga, Mazziotta, and Woods (Chapter 77) presented current progress in the use of cryosectioned cadaver heads to generate digital volumes of 50–100 micron resolution. Such data sets may play an important role in bridging the gap between macroscopic human imaging *in vivo* and traditional microanatomical techniques. For instance, using histochemical staining techniques, 3D chemoarchitectural maps can be constructed and analyzed in stereotaxic space in a manner analogous to that used for studying MRI and PET data. The labor-intensive and artifact-prone aspects of data acquisition still limit the technique at present but integration of this data type with other modalities is proceeding within the framework of the International Consortium for Brain Mapping (ICBM) as described by Evans, Collins, and Holmes (Chapter 25 in the Data Processing session). The latter paper discussed the application of an automated nonlinear 3D warping (ANIMAL) algorithm to MRI data, a topic also covered in this session by Lin *et al.* (Chapter 78). The two 3D warping chapters adopt quite similar strategies, dividing one volume into subcubes arranged on a 3D grid and then finding a local shift that optimally maps each subcube to a neighboring region in the other volume. The Lin algorithm represents each subcube by three orthogonal 2D planes intersecting the subcube center whereas the ANIMAL algorithm operates on the whole volume. Also, the Lin algorithm further divides each 2D image into subimages, presumably to obtain finer local deformations, whereas ANIMAL operates in a multiscale heirarchy, choosing progressively smaller 3D volumes to achieve this goal. These chapters, and other work, say, by Minoshima and Friston, indicate the considerable current interest in automated nonlinear image matching algorithms, both for the methodological goal of removing anatomical differences among subjects in functional mapping studies and for direct studies of the nature of these morphological differences.

V. CONCLUSION

In summary, the session demonstrated a degree of convergence on statistical analysis of activation data. Issues that have caused some consternation in the past (e.g., ANOVA vs. ANCOVA; pooled vs. voxel-based variance estimates) appear to be less important. New initiatives related to spatial extent or smoothing provide complementary perspectives to the traditional magnitude-base criteria. In this context, it might be useful to review previous and ongoing research in computer vision on the nature of object structure over scale space. New nonparametric approaches will provide a solid foundation with which to assess the validity of assumptions made by the faster, analytic techniques. Progress is also being made in applying the statistical methodology developed for CBF activation in other physiological domains, notably task-specific changes in ligand binding. These techniques will test the limits of PET signal detectability, and it is likely that the new techniques for optimizing signal/noise by improved 3D acquisition, spatial standardization, and statistical analysis all will be much in demand in the near future.

Index